B&T
50.95
3-26-90

# DICTIONARY OF AMERICAN TEMPERANCE BIOGRAPHY

# DICTIONARY OF AMERICAN TEMPERANCE BIOGRAPHY

From Temperance Reform
to Alcohol Research,
the 1600s to the 1980s

MARK EDWARD LENDER

GREENWOOD PRESS
Westport, Connecticut • London, England

NI

**Library of Congress Cataloging in Publication Data**

Lender, Mark E., 1947-
   Dictionary of American temperance biography.

   Bibliography: p.
   Includes index.
   1. Temperance—Biography. 2. United States—
Biography. 3. Temperance—Bibliography. I. Title.
HV5293.A2L46   1984        363.4'1'0922 [B]        83-12589
ISBN 0-313-22335-1 (lib. bdg.)

Library of Congress Catalog Card Number: 83-12589
ISBN: 0-313-22335-1

First published in 1984

Greenwood Press
A division of Congressional Information Service, Inc.
88 Post Road West, Westport, Connecticut 06881

Printed in the United States of America

10  9  8  7  6  5  4  3  2  1

For Penny,
with gratitude and love

Were it possible for me to speak with a
voice so loud as to be heard from the river
St. Croix to the remotest shores of the
Mississippi, which bound the territory of
the United States, I would say, "Friends
and fellow citizens! avoid the habitual
use of those seducing liquors."

> Benjamin Rush, *An Inquiry into the*
> *Effect of Ardent Spirits upon the*
> *Human Body and Mind...* (1785)


The devil of drink has seized me, and
I cannot get free from the grip of
his terrible hand!

> T. S. Arthur, *Strong Drink: The*
> *Curse and the Cure* (1877)

# Contents

# Preface

Drinking has always been part of America. From the first European colonists to the present era, beverage alcohol has found its place in national culture, and sometimes a prominent place. It has been a dietary staple, a standard "social lubricant," an important part of the national economy, and for many Americans the basis of a series of social, religious, and ethical questions. Indeed, no chapter of the American past has escaped at least some discussion of the proper roles of drinking and alcohol in society, and there were occasions when the "liquor question" was of paramount concern. From roughly the 1820s to the 1930s, the Temperance Movement emerged cyclically as one of the strongest and most broadly-based forces in American social and political life. Millions followed its banner over the years, lifting it to the peak of its influence during the era of National Prohibition (1920–33). Yet even after Repeal the movement never disappeared. Greatly diminished in strength, it has survived late into the twentieth century and shows few signs of dying out completely. Apart from the remnants of the antiliquor crusade, however, many more Americans also remained acutely aware of the problems of drinking and alcoholism in a complex society and anxious over their potential for personal tragedy and social disruption. The concerns were justified: After the collapse of Prohibition, alcohol consumption in American slowly increased over time, and by the early 1980s some estimates placed the number of alcoholics in the United States at as many as nine million (or more); and while some critics have challenged these figures, there has been no disputing the presence of a national drinking problem of serious magnitude. In response, an active (though loosely organized) alcoholism research and treatment movement has grown in the decades following the demise of the "noble experiment" and has become the vehicle for the expression of a variety of modern drinking-related questions. Thus, in one form or another, temperance (or at least some concern over alcohol problems) has left its mark on generations of Americans. Quite clearly, the matter has been one of the most enduring social issues in the history of the United States.

As the nation grappled with its "liquor question" over the years, a considerable number of individuals rose to public prominence through their involvement with the issue. This volume contains brief biographies of 373 of them, men and women active in the cause of temperance and efforts against alcoholism from the 1670s to the 1980s. Until this publication, there has been no compilation of historical data on American temperance figures in a single edition. In each biography, my goal was to present a concise overview of the life and chief contributions of each individual, offering both accurate factual information and historically sound interpretive judgements on their careers. As a group, however, those treated in the *Dictionary* do not constitute a random sample of temperance leaders; that was never my intention. Rather, the selections represent a conscious effort to introduce the many intellectual, ethnic, religious, and political variations that characterized the antiliquor struggle. The only preconceived notion inherent in the work is that, with due regard for certain important commonly held ideas among its followers, the Temperance Movement successfully attracted a re-markably varied and dynamic mass popular base. And if much of its intellectual outlook was antipluralist, movement rank and file nevertheless reflected some of the pluralist society from which they came.

Each entry is fairly short, and none is definitive. Lengthy, in-depth accounts would have forced a major reduction in the number of individuals included and consequently lessened the scope and usefulness of the volume. Yet most readers, I think, will find enough information. I modeled the biographies on the format developed by historian Henry Bowden in his *Dictionary of American Religious Biography* (1977)—and like an old army duffle bag, that format holds quite a bit if you pack it carefully. The sketches begin with an outline paragraph which provides dates and places of birth and death, as well as basic data on education and careers. Narrative paragraphs follow, going deeper into the individual's life and explaining his or her most important connections with the dry reform. For the advanced researcher, or for anyone interested in further detail, a third section (also *à la* Bowden) provides bibliographical references. Part A offers books and article-length publications by the particular temperance worker, generally up to a total of six titles. Many dry figures wrote considerably more than this admittedly arbitrary limit, but space considerations forced a cut-off point; and at any rate, the selected references do present the most important and representative works by a given author, at least in regard to temperance activities. Part B, again usually with a six-citation limit, lists secondary materials. Standard references are abbreviated (a key to all abbreviations follows the Preface), and with the exceptions of master's theses, doctoral dissertations, and a few manuscript col-lections, all Part B entries are published sources. While brief, then, each bi-ography conveys a good deal of information itself and (for those desiring it) offers a firm point of departure for additional inquiry. An asterisk next to a name in the text denotes an individual accorded a full biographical entry elsewhere in the *Dictionary*.

It was impossible, however, to include all Americans active on behalf of the dry crusade in this *Dictionary*. They numbered in the millions, with thousands acquiring, to a greater or lesser extent, credentials as leaders in the cause. In selecting names for inclusion, I have no doubt overlooked some who might well have belonged, while accepting others whose claims on the reader's attention seem less than compelling. Yet the criteria for selection assured that, from the almost two thousand names initially considered, a good representation of movement activists finally emerged. In general, all of the historical figures had died by 1980. The only exceptions were some of the more recent officers of the Woman's Christian Temperance Union and several members of the modern alcoholism treatment or research community. All either compiled impressive leadership records, made contributions of an intellectual nature, or had careers illustrative of significant trends in the course of the dry reform effort. In several instances, biographies appear with incomplete or questionable data—usually date of death. It was ironic that after compiling distinguished careers on the national scene, a number of temperance figures later faded into obscurity and their deaths went unrecorded by any major source. In such cases, the missing information is denoted with a question mark, as is material that I could not verify. For example: "worked in liquor business, 1890–93(?.)."

This volume, then, offers a biographical overview of one of the most controversial social issues in American history. And to say the least, it lists some of the most ardent and dedicated reform champions the nation has ever seen: political organizers, agitators, intellectuals, authors, clergymen, feminists, and, in some cases, even cranks. Still others saw temperance as a means of rebuilding American life and society, and as a keystone in bringing about a multitude of other reforms. Morevover, few of them stood second to anyone in their attachments to the antiliquor cause. No matter what popular views of the Temperance Movement may be today (and in America's wet society, the old temperance ideas generate little public support), the dry reformers were honestly convinced of the righteousness and necessity of the battle against "the demon rum"—and that victory would bring a better life for all. Recalling their careers is thus to remind ourselves that vision coupled with dedication can indeed prove a powerful force for social change.

Many friends offered invaluable assistance and advice during the preparation of this volume. Professor Henry Bowden of Rutgers University encouraged me to launch the *Dictionary* project, and scholars familiar with his *Dictionary of American Religious Biography* will quickly recognize the extent of my debt to him. Other colleagues who offered help with factual or interpretive questions were Leonard Blumberg (Temple University), Tim Coffey (Rutgers), Jed Dannenbaum (Georgia Institute of Technology), Harry Levine (Queens College), Jim Martin (University of Houston), Gail Milgram, Penny Page, and Jill Schumann (all of Rutgers). For research assistance, I had the benefit of help from Jill Schumann, Philip Hughes, Richard Grubb, and John Dennington, all of whom also wrote initial drafts of many of the biographies. Ernie Paolino, a fine historian, wrote drafts as well, and I always found his judgments sound. Mark Keller, editor emeritus of the *Journal of Studies on Alcohol*, kindly read drafts of a number of entries and made helpful comments. Lucille Hynda and Tim Coffey were consistently helpful in finding the means to support my research, and they have my deepest thanks. When I began the project, Jane Armstrong was librarian at the Center of Alcohol Studies, and Penny Page took over at midpoint. Both offered me their fullest assistance in tracking down an uncounted number of details. Penny Page saw the toughest duty, providing reference service over the telephone and digging continuously for me through the superb collections of the Rutgers Center of Alcohol Studies Library. This book is dedicated to her, and a dedication was never better earned. In preparing the manuscript, Rose Ullrich patiently endured my constant revisions (and frequently abominable handwriting) while helping with typing. At Kean College of New Jersey, Frances Siburn did all of the typing and proofreading with care and interest beyond the call of duty. I owe all of these individuals quite a bit; their contributions made a long project go faster and helped make it much more enjoyable.

# Abbreviations for Standard Reference Sources

BDAC     *Biographical Directory of the American Congress, 1774–1971* (Washington, Dc, 1971).

DAB     *Dictionary of American Biography*, ed., Allen Johnson and Dumas Malone, 20 vols. (New York, 1928–37; 4 supplements, 1944–74).

DARB     *Dictionary of American Religious Biography*, Henry Bowden (Westport, CT, 1977).

NAW     *Notable American Women, 1607–1950: A Biographical Dictionary*, ed. Edward T. James, 3 vols. (Cambridge, 1971).

NCAB     *National Cyclopedia of Americna Biography*, 55 vols. (New York, 1982–1974; current series, vols. A–L, 1930–72).

NYT     *New York Times*, 1851 to present.

SEAP     *Standard Encyclopedia of the Alcohol Problem,* ed. Ernest Hurst Cherrington, William Eugene Johnson and Frances Cora Stoddard, 6 vols. (Westerville, OH, 1925–30).

WW     *Who Was Who in America*, historical vol. and 6 vols. (Chicago,

# BIOGRAPHIES

# A

**ACHESON, Ernest Francis**  (19 September 1855, Washington, PA—16 May 1917, Washington, PA). *Education*: B.A., Washington and Jefferson Coll., 1875; A.M. (honorary), Washington and Jefferson Coll., 1889. *Career*: law practice, 1877–79; publisher and editor, *Washington* (PA) *Daily Observer*, 1879–1917; publisher and editor, *Daily Reporter*, 1902–12; member, U.S. House of Representatives, 1895–1909.

After finishing his education, Acheson rose quickly to prominence in his native Washington, Pennsylvania. A brief legal career soon gave way to a business opportunity as co-owner of the *Washington Daily Observer*, which he edited for years thereafter; he later became sole owner of the local *Daily Reporter* as well. Acheson's reputation as a journalist grew steadily, and in the early 1890s he served jointly as president of the Pennsylvania Editorial Association and as recording secretary of the parent National Editorial Association. Civically active, he served as a trustee of his alma mater, Washington and Jefferson College, as well as on the board of a local seminary. He devoted the bulk of his community involvement, however, to antiliquor efforts. A man of stern prohibitionist sympathies, he used his newspapers, particuarly the *Reporter*, to champion the dry cause and became a leading scourge of the Pennsylvania liquor traffic. His uncompromising editorial position on the liquor question established Acheson as one of the most prominent dry journalists of the period. He was also a major voice in a number of local temperance organizations, including the Pennsylvania chapter of the Anti-Saloon League. Acheson's views on the liquor issue propelled him to a national political career as well. A life-long Republican, he remained loyal to his party rather than transfer his allegiance to the Prohibition Party: Like other Anti-Saloon League members, he thought that more results would flow from work in the major parties than from efforts with the zealous but politically weak third party. Between 1895 and 1909 he represented his local district in Congress, where, in addition to taking an active (if not particularly prominent) role in party affairs, he gained a reputation as a staunch enemy of the drink trade. He was one of the first congressmen to introduce—albeit unsuccessfully—a national prohibitionary bill.

**Bibliography:**

A. *Trips of a Congressional Party to Panama...* (Washington, PA, 1907); *Pioneers and Patriotism* (Washington, PA, 1909).

B. SEAP 1, 46; WW 1, 4.

**AGNEW, Daniel**    (5 January 1809, Trenton, NJ—9 March 1902, Beaver, PA). *Education*: B.A., Western Univ. of Pennsylvania (now Univ. of Pittsburgh); LLD., Dickinson Coll.; LLD., Washington and Jefferson Coll. *Career*: legal practice, 1829–1851; jurist, 1851–79, including period as chief justice, Supreme Court of Pennsylvania, 1873–79.

The career of Daniel Agnew illustrates the caliber of professional individuals attracted to the temperance cause and how at key times members of the bar allied decisively with those opposed to the liquor traffic. Born to a family of Welsh and Irish descent, Agnew became one of the most respected Pennsylvania jurists of his generation. Admitted to the bar in 1829, he established a successful legal practice first in Pittsburgh and then in Beaver, where he lived the rest of his life. His professional stature was such that he served as a member of the state constitutional convention in 1837–38 and then received appointment to the bench as a district court judge from 1851 to 1863. He then moved on to the State Supreme Court in late 1863 and served as chief justice from 1874 to 1879. There is no direct evidence of how he came to sympathize with the Temperance Movement, but during his years on the bench he staunchly supported it. Not widely identified with other reform activities, Agnew focused his efforts solely on the prohibition question. He lectured and wrote extensively on the subject, advocating strict legislation against the liquor traffic. In court, he made an even greater impact, most notably in his decision on a local option law in 1872. In 1847, the Pennsylvania Supreme Court had found such legislation unconstitutional; Agnew, however, reversed the finding, which earned him the plaudits of state dry forces. Retiring from the bench in 1879, the old judge never wavered in his advocacy of the reform position. Even in his advanced years, he continued with other state temperance workers to fight for a prohibition amendment to the federal Constitution.

**Bibliography:**

B. SEAP 1, 75; WW 1, 10.

**ANDERSON, Elizabeth Preston**    (27 April 1861, Decatur, IN—?). *Education*: studied at Fort Wayne Coll., De Pauw Univ., Univ. of Minnesota. *Career*: temperance worker and organizer, 1889–1926.

Elizabeth Anderson's dedication to organized Temperance was almost total, an example of the depth of commitment that gave the movement its professional full-time cadre. She was evidently not directly involved with temperance work in her early youth; but she was a staunch Methodist, and like so many others of her denomination, she became a determined foe of "the demon rum" later in life. After moving from Indiana to North Dakota, she joined the WCTU in 1889. It was only the first step in a long WCTU career. Once a member, she launched herself into most of the group's activities and within four years (1873) rose to the presidency of the state chapter. She was consistently reelected to the post until the mid-1920s. In that capacity, she was a vigorous organizer and a formidable advocate for prohibition. Anderson's zeal was well illustrated by her almost constant lobbying in the North Dakota legislature. She attended almost all of its sessions from the time the state was admitted to the Union down to the 1920s. (Such was her presence in the state capital that the WCTU presented the legislature with a life-sized oil portrait of her.) Her marriage in 1901 to the Reverend James Anderson, a Methodist minister, did nothing to deter her dry career. Indeed, shortly thereafter it reached new heights. In 1903 the National WCTU recognized her ample talents and elected her assistant recording secretary, and between 1906 and 1926 she served as recording secretary (while continuing in her capacity as North Dakota chapter president). Her labors brought some impressive results, not all of which were confined to temperance legislation. In fact, Anderson's most singular achievement came on behalf of suffrage reform which she, like many other WCTU members, considered essential to the dry cause. In 1917, she was instrumental in the passage of a state presidential and municipal voting law, allowing women the ballot in those elections for the first time. Her energy and ability to produce results earned her a deserved reputation as one of the foremost dry proponents in her region and a respected voice in national temperance councils.

**Bibliography:**

B. SEAP 1, 163; WW 4, 28.

**ANDERSON, William Hamilton**    (8 August 1874, Carlinville, IL—4 September 1959, Yonkers, NY). *Education*: B.S., Blackburn Coll., Carlinville, IL, 1892; LLB., Univ. of Michigan, 1896; LLD. (honorary), Illinois Wesleyan Univ., 1919. *Career*: taught school, 1892–94; law practice, 1896–1900; legal and supervisory positions with Anti-Saloon Leagues of Illinois, New York, and Maryland, 1902–26; general secretary and founder, American Christian Alliance, 1926–59.

The achievements of William Hamilton Anderson are testimony to the political power the temperance crusade could generate when its sense of moral right was joined with a practical sense of the legal system and an appreciation of the impact of public relations. In the steady movement toward prohibition from the turn of the twentieth century, Anderson played leading roles in the public-policy and legislative functions of the Anti-Saloon League in Illinois, Maryland, and New York and at the national level. His sense of commitment stemmed from his membership in the Methodist Church, and over his long years of service he devoted considerable time to its temperance activities (in the 1920s, for example, he was a member of the Church Board of Temperance, Prohibition and Public Morals). His practical contributions to the cause, however, grew from his knowledge of the law. Trained as a lawyer, he made his mark first as the attorney for the Anti-Saloon League of Illinois in 1900, and shortly after rose to state superintendent. He drafted the Illinois local option statute and then played a central role in marshalling the regional churches behind a lobbying effort on behalf of the law. It passed, and league officials correctly marked Anderson as a man with a future. They were right. He next helped league organizing drives in New York and Maryland and served briefly (1909) as acting legislative superintendent of the National League office in Washington, D.C. He then settled back in New York in 1914 as state superintendent, preparing for the fight that would come with the drive for National Prohibition.

The struggle over the Eighteenth Amendment brought Anderson his greatest notoriety. He quickly mastered state politics, using his well-established skills as a lobbyist and organizer of religious opinion to push through a New York City local option law which wet forces had managed to stave off for twenty years. He greatly strengthened support for Prohibition among New York congressmen and in his most stunning coup secured state legislative ratification of the Eighteenth Amendment in 1919. It was a humiliating defeat for wets, as it seemingly dispelled their longstanding argument that small rural states were forcing Prohibition on the more populous urban areas. In defense of the dry experiment, he effectively organized public opinion in support of the antiliquor statutes and held violators (as well as less than enthusiastic civil and enforcement officials) up to the glare of scathing publicity and ridicule. His so-called Yonkers Plan made full use of this technique, exposing evidence of corrupt or indifferent enforcement efforts not to legal authorities but to the press and public opinion. Anderson's energetic approach carried great appeal with New York voters, and his endorsement of dry gubernatorial candidate Nathan L. Miller was instrumental in his 1920 victory over wet Democrat Alfred E. Smith. Anderson was, as the 1920s advanced, apparently the consummate dry leader, a prohibitionist success story.

As well as friends, however, Anderson's triumph made him enemies. Especially bitter were the Democrats of the Tammany organization, who had long held Prohibition in contempt. They succeeded in having him indicted in 1923 for the "alteration" of league books, charging that he diverted organization funds for personal use. The league supported him strongly, denouncing the charges as "a monstrous perversion of justice." Nevertheless, he was convicted in 1924 and served nine months in state prison. The sentence gave Tammany more than revenge, for it put their erstwhile effective opponent out of action during the 1924 Democratic Convention (held in New York City) and the presidential election of that year. Indeed, although they could not have known it at the time, they had destroyed Anderson politically. The stint in jail seemed to have cooled his enthusiasm for public life, and he never again took an active leadership role with the league. Yet he remained interested in church-related work and in 1926 founded the American Christian Alliance, a group with nativist, anti-immigrant leanings. This final attempt at launching a crusade, however, made little progress, and Anderson, once a genuine power in New York, passed his final years in relative obscurity.

**Bibliography:**

A. *The Church in Action Against the Saloon* (Westerville, OH, 1906; 2nd ed., 1910); *The "Yonkers Plan" for Prohibition Enforcement* (Westerville, OH, 1921).
B. SEAP 1, 165; WW 3, 27.

**ANTHONY, Susan Brownell**   (15 February 1820, Adams, MA—13 March 1906, Rochester, NY). *Education*: local private school, Battenville, NY, 1837–38; Friends' Boarding School, West Philadelphia, PA, 1830s. *Career*: taught school, 1835–1850; temperance, women's rights, and antislavery reform work, 1852–69; co-founder, National Woman Suffrage Association, 1869; suffrage reform activities, 1869–1906.

The life of Susan B. Anthony offers a striking example of temperance work serving as a catalyst in the generation of other reform activities. For it was in the Temperance Movement that the great women's suffrage leader first launched her reform career and pioneered many of the ideas that carried her to international fame. She had her first temperance lesson at home: Her father was a total abstainer and he insisted that his household conform. Susan did and subsequently became involved in organized temperance activities. In the 1840s she joined a local (Canajoharie, New York) Daughters' Union, a woman's auxiliary to the Sons of Temperance fraternal organization, and assumed her first leadership role. With her fellow women, she worked to support and finance the activities of the men's group, although the efforts of the Daughters' Union rarely came out of the shadow cast by the larger male society. When, in 1849, Anthony actually addressed a temperance gathering, the event created a minor sensation; previously, women had not played vocal roles in the cause, and many drys considered her action too forward. But Anthony continued to press for female leadership in the movement. In 1852, when a Sons of Temperance Convention (in Albany, New York) refused to let her speak because of her sex, she and other women bolted and organized the nation's first state-wide woman's temperance society. The new group quickly proved effective, revealing the potential power of women in the movement. Under Anthony's leadership, it soon collected some 28,000 names on a pro–Maine Law petition, which also called for the right of females to vote.

After the Civil War, women temperance workers were generally in the van of other reform movements as well; but in the 1840s and 1850s many women were hesitant, either out of conviction or fear of giving offense, to assume leadership positions alongside male reformers. It was on this issue that Anthony eventually broke with the Temperance Movement. During her antiliquor work she had also become sympathetic to the antislavery and women's suffrage crusades, and her own experience had shown that women could contribute as much toward these reforms as men. Her arguments, however, met continual male intransigence and determined opposition from some conservative women. Frustrated, she became convinced that women could realize their potential, and reform movements benefit accordingly, only when they had the right to vote. Finally, when the group she had founded, the New York Woman's State Temperance Society, failed to endorse strong women's rights positions at its 1853 convention, she left the dry standard. Fellow suffrage reformer Elizabeth Cady Stanton, also present at the convention, left with her. Thereafter, Anthony devoted her life to the women's rights cause, and it was in this battle that she emerged as a truly national (and later international) figure. Yet she had also left her mark on the dry crusade: Many temperance workers ultimately affirmed her faith in equal suffrage, making it part of their own struggle (especially with the subsequent rise of the WCTU); and during the later nineteenth century, the importance of female leadership to the antiliquor cause could hardly be denied.

**Bibliography:**

A. with Elizabeth Cady Stanton and Matilda Joslyn Gage, eds., *The History of Woman Suffrage*, 6 vols. (Rochester, NY, 1881–1922), vol. 4 with Ida Husted Harper.

B. SEAP 1, 172–74; WW 1, 28; Katherine Susan Anthony, *Susan B. Anthony: Her Personal History and Her Era* (Garden City, NY, 1954); Rheta Louise Childe Dorr, *Susan B. Anthony: The Woman Who Changed the Mind of a Nation* (New York, 1928); Ida Husted Harper, *The Life and Work of Susan B. Anthony*, 3 vols. (Indianapolis, 1898–1908); Alma Lutz, *Susan B. Anthony: Rebel, Crusader, Humanitarian* (Boston, 1959).

**APPLETON, James**    (14 February 1785, Ipswich, MA—25 August 1862, Ipswich, MA). *Career*: jewelry business, circa 1800–1812; army officer (promoted to brigadier general), 1812–14; landowner and farmer.

Appleton combined a high sense of moral rectitude, patriotism, and zeal in his reform career. He grew up on the family farm in Ipswich, Massachusetts, a descendant of English settlers who landed in 1635. As a substantial landholder and businessman, he rose to local prominence, and although a Federalist in politics, used his influence to organize the defenses of his native region during the War of 1812. He fought in several engagements during that conflict and ended the war as a brigadier general. The coming of peace, however, hardly diminished his taste for leadership. Indeed, like many other Federalists in these years, Appleton grew alarmed over the state of public affairs (especially with the decline of the Federalists as a national party) and committed himself to the establishment of moral and social norms in accord with his own view of the good life. This, in his eyes, meant a society purged of imperfections and social evils of all kinds, which in turn called for civic-minded citizens to lead their countrymen in a massive reform effort. Appleton was only too glad to take the van. Over the years, he repeatedly ran for public office, and sat in the legislatures of both Massachusetts (1813–14) and Maine (1836–39), where he moved in 1833. He became known as a staunch, unyielding enthusiast for temperance, trying hard to legislate for prohibition (he was one of the more radical members of the Maine Temperance Union), antislavery (he ran for governor of Maine three times on the Liberty Party ticket between 1841 and 1843), public education, and relief legislation for the poor. His zeal was such that other reformers listed him among the most energetic of their number: Neal Dow* recalled that Appleton was always "found in the thickest of the Fray, always leading toward closer and more effective fighting."

Temperance, however, was his chief interest. Destroy the liquor traffic, he reasoned, and most other evils would also wither away. While still living in Massachusetts in the 1830s, he urged a "Thirty Gallon Law" on the state legislature, a measure hoping to make liquor sales too expensive for most people by limiting purchases of distilled spirits to minimums of thirty gallons. At the time (1832), the proposal was considered too radical even to gain the support of the Massachusetts Society for the Suppression of Intemperance. But Appleton, while rebuffed in this initial effort, returned to the legislative wars after moving to Maine. Upon election to the Assembly, he became one of the nation's first politicians to introduce a state prohibition law (1837), a measure for which he fought long and hard during his tenure in office. Dow credited his effort with being the first to suggest the "true method of dealing with the liquor traffic." And while Appleton never saw his law enacted, his was the foundation upon which Neal Dow subsequently built a successful prohibition movement in the following decade. Later in life he returned to his farm in Ipswich, but he never stopped crusading. He died in the midst of active support for the Lincoln administration's war effort in 1861.

**Bibliography:**

B. DAB 1, 327; SEAP 1, 187–89; John A. Krout, *The Origins of Prohibition* (New York, 1925); *Origin of the Maine Law and of Prohibitionary Legislation* (New York, 1886); John G. Woolley and William E. Johnson, *Temperance Progress of the Century* (1903).

**ARMOR, Mary Harris**   (9 March 1863, Penfield, GA—?). *Education*: educated privately, and in public schools of Greensboro, GA; LLD. (honorary), Wesleyan Coll., 1918. *Career*: school teacher, 1880?–83; president, Georgia WCTU, 1905–9; organizer and lecturer, National WCTU, beginning 1909.

Coming from a family that was strongly church oriented (it included several ministers of the Gospel), Mary Armor gravitated almost naturally toward proselytizing. Her chosen field, however, was not religion but temperance, in which she worked indefatigably for most of her adult life. She began her climb to prominence in her native Georgia, where she proved an effective WCTU organizer. From 1905 to 1909 Armor was president of the Georgia state chapter, but she left the post to assume wider responsibilities. She became an organizer and lecturer for the National WCTU, where she was able to give her talents as a powerful orator full reign. She was a tireless speaker and campaigner with genuine eloquence on the public rostrum. Over her years of labor, Armor served the dry cause with addresses to audiences in no fewer than forty-two states in addition to the District of Columbia. With true missionary zeal, Armor also lent her skills to the international work of the WCTU. Foreign nations were no strangers to her message against alcohol, as she spoke in Canada, Mexico, and Western Europe. Often when speaking she had recourse to interpreters, but this did not seem to dilute the gospel of sobriety and abstinence that she carried to the men in the shops and factories of other cultures. She represented the Georgia and National WCTUs at three world conventions and at the Fourteenth International Congress Against Alcoholism in Milan, Italy (1913), where she was one of two American women representatives. In 1922, at age sixty, Mrs. Armor capped a lifetime of temperance work with a speaking tour of New Zealand.

**Bibliography:**

B. SEAP 1, 203.

**ARTHUR, Timothy Shay**    (6 June 1809, Newburgh, NY—6 March 1885, Philadelphia, PA). *Career*: bank agent, 1833; edited *Baltimore Athenaeum* and *Baltimore Sunday Visitor*, mid-1830s; edited *Baltimore Book* and *Baltimore Literary Magazine*, 1838–39; headed *Baltimore Merchant*, a Harrison campaign daily, 1840; wrote for *Godey's*, *Graham's Magazine*, *Saturday Courier*, 1841–45; began *Arthur's Ladies' Magazine*, 1845; began *Arthur's Home Gazette*, 1850; established *Arthur's Home Magazine*, 1853; began *Children's Hour*, 1867; founded *Once a Month*, 1867; published a farmer's and mechanic's journal, *The Workingman*, 1870; published extensively on behalf of the temperance cause.

As a child in school, Timothy Shay Arthur's academic performance led his parents and teachers to conclude that he was dull. His apprenticeship to a watchmaker proved equally futile: He could not master the trade. The close benchwork hurt his eyes and young Arthur's future looked bleak (to say the least). Yet he loved to read, a habit which provided his real education, and while in his apprenticeship he discovered a love of writing. He continued in his avocation after taking a position with a Baltimore, Maryland, bank (1833), which he hoped would improve his income. He travelled West as the bank's agent for several years, returning after the bank failed. In need of another job, he turned to editing a succession of local publications, beginning with the short-lived *Baltimore Athenaeum*. The work suited him, and still writing, Arthur became a recognized if minor figure in the city's younger literary circle. The experience was a tonic for the aspiring author and brought him into contact with the likes of Rufus Dawes, W. H. Carpenter, and Edgar Allan Poe. His career gathered momentum steadily as he also began contributing articles and short stories to a series of popular magazines of the period, notably *Godey's Lady's Book* and the *Saturday*

*Courier*. In 1841, with a modest literary reputation established, he moved to Philadelphia and began the writing effort that made him one of the most prolific and popular authors of the late nineteenth century.

Over his long career, Arthur wrote on any number of questions. His repertoire included women's rights, religion, finance, smoking, and gambling, to list only a few topics. In general, his stories were moralizing in tone and supportive of middle-class values. In addition, he was editor of a number of successful publications catering to popular literary tastes, such as *Arthur's Ladies' Magazine* (begun in 1845), *Arthur's Home Gazette* (1850), and several others. Yet his chief claim to fame was as a writer of Temperance Movement fiction. He was not originally a total abstainer, but he was repulsed at the social conditions surrounding the saloon. Arthur consequently joined the Baltimore Temperance Society, the first dry organization in Maryland, during his days as a bank agent. And as his literary talents grew, he increasingly used his pen in favor of the cause. His first notable success in this regard was *Six Nights with the Washingtonians, and Other Temperance Tales* (1842), a volume portraying, in fiction, the work of the Washingtonian temperance revival of the 1840s. He eventually wrote scores of other short stories and novels on the antiliquor reform, some of which became best-selling titles in their day. His "masterpiece" (if we can use that term in this context), was *Ten Nights in a Bar-Room, and What I Saw There* (1854), written to stimulate public sympathy for Maine Law legislation. *Ten Nights*, which traced the impact of liquor sales on a rural town over the course of ten years, captivated tens of thousands of readers with the story of drinking-related mayhem, tragedy, and, after local prohibition, redemption. It was a huge success as a novel and over the next few years did equally well as a stage production (one version of which had a musical score). While other antiliquor authors were quite successful as well, Arthur was arguably without peer. Upon his death, he had over seventy-five books to his name, and no one was better known as a temperance writer.

Arthur's writings epitomized a distinct genre of reform literature of the period loosely known as the Temperance Tales. The Tales (a term drawn from the titles of some of the most popular works of dry fiction) sought to convince popular audiences of the Temperance Movement's views of the impact of alcohol on man and society. None, including Arthur's, is today classed as significant literature: Plots were standard, characters stereotyped, and the lessons and moralizing constant. But they were extremely popular in their day, and they incorporated and publicized the temperance belief that alcoholism was a disease and an addiction. Drinkers, they explained in hundreds of melodramatic stories, risked progressive addiction, leading to consequent physical, moral, and social deterioration and death. The only prevention was total abstinence. The Tales drew their medical ideas generally from the early works of Benjamin Rush* but also relied heavily on the later (although similar) arguments of other antiliquor medical authorities. The *Quarterly Journal of Inebriety*, for example, the official organ of the American Association for the Study of Inebriety, actually endorsed

Arthur's novel, *Strong Drink: The Curse and the Cure*, because it so accurately portrayed current scientific views of alcohol addiction. There seems little doubt that Arthur, in league with most other dry writers, largely believed in the lessons of the Temperance Tales.

**Bibliography:**

A. *Six Nights with the Washingtonians; and Other Temperance Tales* (Philadelphia, 1842, and many subsequent editions); *Married and Single: Or Marriage and Celibacy Contrasted* (Philadelphia, 1845); *The Maiden* (Philadelphia, 1848); *Ten Nights in a Bar-Room, and What I Saw There* (Philadelphia, 1854, and many subsequent editions); *Woman to the Rescue* (Philadelphia, 1874); *Strong Drink: The Curse and the Cure* (Philadelphia, 1877).

B. D. A. Koch, ed. (editor's introductory essay), Timothy Shay Arthur, *Ten Nights in a Bar-Room, and What I Saw There* (Cambridge, MA, 1964); Mark Edward Lender and Karen R. Karnchanapee, " 'Temperance Tales,' Antiliquor Fiction and American Attitudes Toward Alcoholics in the Late 19th and Early 20th Centuries," *Journal of Studies on Alcohol* 38 (1977): 1347–70.

**ASBURY, Francis**    (20 August 1745, Handsworth, Staffordshire, England— 31 March 1816, Spotsylvania, VA). *Career*: itinerant Methodist preacher as a young man; Methodist missionary in America, beginning 1771; general assistant, Methodist Church in America, 1772–84; appointed joint superintendent (with Thomas Coke), with self-assumed title of bishop, 1784–1816.

An intensely devout and dedicated founder of Methodism in America, Francis Asbury was in no small way responsible for the cultivation of some of the earliest temperance sentiments in the country. Asbury grew up in England under the sheltered care of his deeply religious mother, who encouraged him toward an ardent faith in Methodism. By his late teens, he was already a local preacher and, after being admitted to the Wesleyan Conference at twenty-one, spent four years as an itinerant minister. His rise to prominence, however, began when John Wesley appointed him as general assistant to the small and struggling Methodist community in the American colonies. While other leaders had arrived earlier to labor on behalf of the new denomination, Asbury proved the most energetic and strong-willed and gradually, against occasional opposition, emerged as the de facto leader of the church in America. In 1784, Wesley named him, along with Thomas Coke, joint superintendent of American Methodists. Asbury, however, referred to himself thereafter as bishop, and while Wesley had not sanctioned it, the Americans allowed him the title. Never noted as an innovative theologian, or even as a dynamic preacher, he was a master organizer and a tireless proselytizer. During his long tenure of leadership, he travelled some 300,000 miles as a missionary and administrator and played an instrumental role in developing his denomination (which had numbered only 316 souls upon his arrival in 1771) into a fellowship of over 214,000 members. Upon his death, Methodism was among the fastest growing church groups in the United States.

Part and parcel of Asbury's Methodist zeal was a hatred of drunkenness and of distilled liquors. Wesley had cautioned against them in England, and his disciple carried the same message to his American flock. In his sermons and private journals, Asbury repeatedly denounced intemperance and the retailing of hard liquor as "productive of so many evils, that we judge it our indispensable duty to form a regulation against them." At the same time, he insisted that all Methodist ministers get out of the distilling business (there were, apparently, some whiskey-making parsons). In their day, his views on the question were quite radical, as most Americans were used to fairly heavy drinking as the social norm. The bishop's words thus were not always taken kindly and even produced an occasional brawl in his audiences. We should note, however, that he was no prohibitionist; Asbury held no brief against the moderate use of wines, beers, and beverages with lighter alcoholic contents. Yet his pronouncements established the Methodists, along with the Quakers, as one of the earliest religious groups to speak out on the liquor question in any respect. He by no means sparked a reform movement against alcohol abuse—there is evidence to suggest that even some of his fellow Methodists were less than enthusiastic about his ideas on the liquor question—but he had some impact. In his many travels he did meet Dr. Benjamin Rush,* and it is possible that the church leader provided some inspiration in forming Rush's views on alcohol. It is certain that Rush admired the Methodist position on distilled beverages. And at the very least, Asbury could take credit for helping lay the foundations for a temperance sentiment which, in later generations, would make his denomination one of the staunchest foes of "the demon."

## Bibliography:

A. *The Doctrines and Discipline of the Methodist Episcopal Church in America: With Explanatory Notes by Thomas Coke and Francis Asbury* (Philadelphia, 1789); *The Journals and Letters of Francis Asbury*, ed. Elmer T. Clark, J. Manning Potts, and Jacob Payton, 3 vols. (Nashville, TN, 1958).

B. DAB 1, 379–83; DARB, 18–20; Herbert Asbury, *A Methodist Saint* (New York, 1927); William L. Duren, *Francis Asbury: Founder of American Methodism* (New York, 1928); L. C. Rudolph, *Francis Asbury* (Nashville, TN, 1966); George G. Smith, *Life and Labors of Francis Asbury* (Nashville, TN, 1898); Ezra S. Tipple, *Francis Asbury: The Prophet of the Long Road* (New York, 1916).

**AUSTIN, Henry Warren**    (1 August 1828, Skaneateles, NY—24 December 1889, Oak Park, IL). *Career*: hardware business, real estate interests, 1840s–1889.

Austin entered the Temperance Movement by way of a business career, a not unknown avenue for many in the nineteenth century. After attempting various enterprises in Connecticut, Canada, and New York State, he finally launched a thriving hardware business in Chicago. He did quite well and branched out into real estate with equal success, even creating a Chicago suburb which he named after himself. There is no direct evidence on why he became interested in temperance, although it is a reasonable surmise that, like many other businessmen of the age, he saw the results of alcohol abuse as socially disruptive and economically wasteful. At any rate, his first efforts on behalf of the dry reform fully mirrored his commercial background: In his own residence of Oak Park, Illinois, (outside of Chicago), he cleansed the area of saloons by the simple expedient of buying them out or leasing them and installing other forms of business. While a member of the Illinois legislature, Austin also pioneered statutes known today as "dram shop" laws. Such legislation put the burden of legal responsibility for the damages or injury caused by the intoxicated upon the saloonkeeper or landlord of a tavern who supplied alcoholic beverages. This law was a forerunner of modern efforts to hold bartenders or liquor establishments liable (under certain conditions) for the actions of their inebriated patrons. In Austin's day, Illinois courts indeed awarded damages under the law, usually on behalf of the wives and children of alcoholics. Austin felt so strongly on the liquor question that, when the Republicans equivocated on the issue, he severed his longtime affiliation with the GOP and joined the Prohibition Party in 1884. Until his death in 1889 he devoted himself to the Prohibitionists' fund-raising and publicity efforts.

**Bibliography:**

B. SEAP 1, 225.

# B

**BACKUS, James Emory Norton** (13 September 1835, Minden, NY—16 February 1899, Linchlaen Center, NY). *Career*: founder (1851), organizer, and lecturer, Independent Order of Good Templars, 1851–99.

From boyhood on, James Backus was involved in one way or another with temperance work. While still very young he became a member of the Cadets of Temperance and shortly thereafter was a charter member of a new temperance group, the Knights of Jericho, formed in Utica, New York. These organizations were typical of the many dry national lodges that arose in the aftermath of the Washingtonian temperance revival of the 1840s. But where the Washingtonians had failed to institutionalize, the temperance brotherhoods tried to provide members with a stable social network, enabling them to better resist drink. Some even had youth organizations (thus Backus could join a group such as the Cadets) or women's auxiliaries if females were not allowed in the men's lodge. Just as fraternal lodges do in modern America, these dry groups often became important in the social life of local communities and frequently adopted secret oaths, signs, and elaborate uniforms for members. Over the late 1840s and 1850s, a major part of the nation's antiliquor strength was embodied in these organizations, a fact for which Backus could claim a great deal of credit. While only sixteen years old, in a meeting at Oriskany Falls, New York, Backus was one of a handful of the Knights of Jericho that laid the foundations for yet another group, the Independent Order of Good Templars. It was destined to emerge as the leading nonsectarian temperance organization in the world. The Good Templars became Backus's first love, and he devoted most of his life to speaking and organizing chapters. In addition to his organizing activities, which sometimes took him to Europe, Backus also served in major lodge offices on both the national and international levels and as the editor of the first publication of the IOGT, *The Crystal Fount*. Backus died in 1899, and the order honored the man who was probably most responsible for its phenomenal growth by erecting a monument to his memory at his resting place in De Ruyter, New York.

**Bibliography:**

B. SEAP 1, 252.

**BACON, Leonard**    (19 February 1802, Detroit, MI—24 December 1881, New Haven, CT). *Education*: B.A., Yale Coll., 1820; B.D., Andover Sem., 1823; postgraduate study, Andover Sem., 1823–24. *Career*: minister, First Congregational Church, New Haven, CT, 1824–81; editor, *Independent*, 1848–61; taught theology and church history, Yale Divinity Sch., 1866–81.

Although born in the Old Northwest, Leonard Bacon found his home and career in the New England of his ancestors. After an education at Yale and Andover, he took the pulpit of the First Congregational Church in New Haven and held the post (emeritus after 1866) for the rest of his life. Over his long tenure at First Church, his name became synonymous with New England Congregationalism, and justifiably so: No one worked harder to direct the affairs of the denomination and to reconcile its differences with other Protestant groups. Within his generally tolerant theological outlook, however, Bacon always insisted that local churches retain control over their own policies. He also became noted for the breadth of his ministry; the duties of the church, the New Haven pastor believed, stretched far beyond the pulpit. He was a leading proponent of evangelical reform, seeking a rebirth in Christian precepts in national morality, and he lent his talents to that end, not only as a speaker but as an editor in the Congregationalist press. In the public eye, he was probably most closely identified with antislavery reform activities. Bacon reviled slaveholding as an abomination and considered it every Christian's duty to renounce the practice. Yet he was never really a true radical on the question. Rather, he advocated gradual emancipation followed by the colonization of freed blacks in Africa. Moderate or not, however, Bacon was committed to the cause until the Civil War swept away the "peculiar institution." He was equally committed to the early Temperance Movement and very likely felt his initial enthusiasm after hearing a Lyman Beecher* sermon on the issue. He decried the spread of drunkenness and its attendant evils in New Haven, and his writings on the subject garnered a significant measure of public recognition. Without ever condemning the liquor traffic generally, he leveled a withering fire at illegal beverage sales, denouncing them as sources of immorality, poverty, and crime. The battle against intemperance, he insisted, was nothing less than a fight to "preserve from corruption the rising youth of our New England city." To enlist in the cause was a Christian citizen's duty.

Throughout his ministry, Bacon insisted that the church hold the rudder of America's reform movements. Only the firm guide of the pulpit, he believed, would keep reformers on their proper course and thus guarantee maximum benefits to the nation. Were the churches ever to lose control, he feared a further spread of national disorder as ill-trained or (worse) even unchurched individuals rose to leadership positions in the various social crusades. Linked with this was another concern: Bacon considered legal coersion an impractical reform technique. It was more indicative of Christian morality at work, he argued, when reform came voluntarily through citizens altering their views and behavior in order to enhance the public good. Bacon's involvement with the antiliquor cause fully reflected his views in this regard. In the early days of the antebellum movement, he approved not only of the church's involvement but also of its influence with the temperance societies. The societies, the New Haven minister felt, worked wonders in changing American drinking patterns by inducing a spontaneous movement among the citizenry. People voluntarily adopted total abstinence and advanced the reform (and thus struck a blow at alcohol-related social problems) through personal example. Yet as temperance organization increased and the movement became an "institution" with "corporate interests and a corporate spirit," Bacon saw trouble. The rise of "professional reformers," he warned in the 1860s, and of "stipendiary agitators," with their legal solutions to social problems, would lead to change by the involuntary imposition of an organization's views on all—a substantial difference from Bacon's preference for reform based on changes in personal conduct and belief. He also deplored the activities of the Washingtonian and fraternal temperance groups, which he claimed lessened the direct control of the movement by the established societies and the churches. Finally, he became outraged at the movement's emphasis on the liquor traffic and moderate drinking—and its sympathy for the drunkard. Such a view, Bacon claimed, merely excused immoral personal conduct and falsely established legal coercion as the only approach to the liquor question. He ended up holding that society would actually see less drunkenness by supporting properly regulated liquor businesses rather than enacting prohibitory "Maine Laws." Still, if he was disappointed in the eventual course adopted by organized temperance, the old crusader always spoke out against drunkenness and retained his faith in reforming the nation through reforming the morals of its citizens.

## Bibliography:

A. *A Plea for Africa* (New Haven, CT, 1825); *A Discourse on the Traffic in Spiritous Liquors...* (New Haven, CT, 1838); *Thirteen Historical Discourses* (New Haven, CT, 1839); *Slavery Discussed in Occasional Essays* (New York, 1846); *Mistakes and Failures of the Temperance Reformation* (New York, 1864); *The Genesis of the New England Churches* (New York, 1874; 1972).

B. DAB 1, 479–81; DARB, 22–23; NCAB 1, 176; NYT, Dec. 25, 1881; Theodore D. Bacon, *Leonard Bacon: A Statesman in the Church* (New Haven, CT, 1931); Daniel Dorchester, *The Liquor Problem in All Ages* (New York, 1888).

**BACON, Selden Daskam**    (10 September 1909, Pleasantville, NY— ). *Education*: B.A., Yale Univ., 1931; M.A., Yale Univ., 1935; Ph.D., Yale Univ., 1939. *Career*: field fellow, Social Science Research Council, 1936–37; instructor, Dept. of Sociology, Pennsylvania State Coll., 1937–39; faculty member, Dept. of Sociology, Yale Univ. (instructor, 1939–42; assistant professor, 1942–47; associate professor, 1947–52; full professor, 1956–62); sociologist, Laboratory of Applied Physiology (later the Center of Alcohol Studies), Yale Univ.,

1943–62; director, Yale Univ. Center of Alcohol Studies, 1950–62; director, Yale Univ. Summer Sch. of Alcohol Studies, 1950–62; professor, Dept. of Sociology, Rutgers University, 1962–75; director, Rutgers Univ. Center of Alcohol Studies, 1962–75; professor emeritus, Rutgers Univ., beginning 1975.

In the years after the repeal of National Prohibition, no single group did more to revive professional and lay interest in drinking-related questions (especially the conception of alcoholism as a disease) than the researchers at the Yale University Center of Alcohol Studies. Of these individuals, one of the most prominent was sociologist Selden D. Bacon, whose career in alcohol studies has spanned five decades. Indeed, the Bacon family has long had an interest in the American "liquor question": Selden's great-grandfather was Leonard Bacon,* an early antebellum foe of the traffic, while his father (also Selden) earned considerable recognition as a constitutional lawyer fighting the Eighteenth Amendment. While completing his graduate education at Yale University, Bacon performed research in Pennsylvania on that state's police forces (he also served as editor of the *State Chiefs of Police Bulletin*). After earning his doctorate, however, he joined the faculty of his alma mater in 1939 and four years later became affiliated with the alcohol-related research then underway at the Laboratory of Applied Physiology. The laboratory, which soon emerged as the Yale Center of Alcohol Studies, became the young sociologist's permanent academic home. His work focused on a wide variety of sociological aspects of alcohol use in America and contributed in great measure to producing some of the nation's first accurate data on drinking patterns among youth as well as disproving the "skid-row" stereotype of alcoholism. Rather, Bacon's research (along with that of other center faculty) found problem drinking prevalent in all socioeconomic strata. In addition, he became active civically in a number of anti-alcoholism efforts. Between the 1940s and 1960s he served on the Connecticut Commission on Alcoholism, sat on various medical and governmental panels concerned with problem drinking (including the national Cooperative Commission on Alcoholism), and helped Marty Mann* launch the organization which became the National Council on Alcoholism. Bacon had emerged, in fact, as one of those most responsible for reestablishing alcohol-related issues (previously tainted, in much of the popular mind, by the Prohibition controversy) as a legitimate public question.

In 1950, Bacon succeeded E. M. Jellinek* as director of the Yale Center. He spent the following decade in managing its research and publication programs, as well as expanding the institution's faculty. At the same time, he served as director of the (by then) nationally recognized Yale Summer School of Alcohol Studies, which the center had conducted annually since 1943. The later 1950s, however, proved difficult years for both the center and its director. Factions within the administration of Yale University, in reviewing the institution's long-term academic goals, began a lingering debate over future support of the center's operations. While Bacon anticipated a favorable outcome for the alcohol research programs, he also led a search for a more hospitable academic environment, which ultimately resulted in the center moving to the New Brunswick, New Jersey, campus of Rutgers University in 1962. It was at Rutgers that Bacon saw the largest expansion of the center's activities, especially during the later 1960s, when the federal government significantly increased its funding of alcohol-related research. (The Center of Alcohol Studies became, in fact, a major recipient of this federal effort.) With his institution now a central part of a national alcoholism research effort, Bacon was a frequent consultant on the subject with various private and governmental agencies and a speaker highly regarded both in lay and professional circles. His direct personal involvement in basic research lessened over the years as his administrative responsibilities grew (the Rutgers Center staff numbered approximately one hundred people by the early 1970s), but he continued to publish in a more theoretical vein, notably on various aspects of alcohol beverage control and alcoholism prevention policies. Bacon retired as director in 1975 (and from the Rutgers faculty in 1980) at age sixty-five, turning the center's reins over to psychologist John A. Carpenter (who had also made the move from Yale to Rutgers). Yet after leaving the post he had held for so many years, Bacon has retained an active interest in the alcohol studies field— thus maintaining the old family connection with the subject handed down from Leonard Bacon of Temperance Movement fame.

**Bibliography:**

A. "Inebriety, Social Integration, and Marriage," *Quarterly Journal of Studies on Alcohol* 5 (1944): 86–125, 303–39; with Robert Straus, "Alcoholism and Social Stability: A Study of Occupational Integration in 2,023 Male Clinic Patients," *Quarterly Journal of Studies on Alcohol* 12 (1951): 230–60; with Robert Straus, *Drinking in College* (New Haven, CT, 1953); ed., "Understanding Alcoholism," *Annals of the American Academy of Political and Social Science* 315 (1961); ed., "The Process of Addiction to Alcohol: Social Aspects," *Quarterly Journal of Studies on Alcohol* 34 (1973): 1–27; "Research and the Center of Alcohol Studies," *Annals of the New York Academy of Science* 273 (1976): 81–86; "On the Prevention of Alcohol Problems and Alcoholism," *Journal of Studies on Alcohol* 39 (1978): 1125–47.

B. *American Men and Women of Science: The Social and Behavioral Sciences,* 13th ed. (New York, 1978); *Current Biography, 1952* (New York, 1952), 32–34; *Directory of American Scholars,* 2nd ed. (Lancaster, PA, 1951), 34; *Who's Who in American Education,* vol. 14 (Nashville, TN, 1950); *Who's Who in the World,* 2nd ed. (Chicago, 1973), 58.

**BAILEY, Hannah Johnston**    (5 July 1839, Cornwall-on-the-Hudson, NY— 23 October 1923, Portland, ME). *Career:* schoolteacher, near Plattekill, NY, 1858–67; active social reform work with WCTU and other groups, 1883–1916.

Hannah Johnston Bailey was the daughter of a Quaker minister and received a major portion of her education at a Friends' boarding school. She was devout in her faith, and pacifism, one of its central tenets, became a theme closely woven through the story of her temperance work. Independently wealthy after the death of her manufacturer husband in 1882, she dedicated the rest of her life to religion and to reform causes. She took an active role in Quaker affairs, particularly the support of foreign mission work; and although little is known of her specific interest in alcohol problems (beyond the fact that many Quakers avoided liquor on religious grounds), she joined the Maine WCTU in 1883, probably finding it the most convenient avenue to reform efforts outside of her denomination. Working with fellow Maine reformer Lillian M.N.A. Stevens,* she pursued such goals as the construction of a separate state women's reformatory and women's suffrage. In this last field she assumed genuine prominence, serving as president of the Maine Woman Suffrage Association between 1891 and 1897 and as treasurer of the National Council of Women between 1895 and 1899. Her energy and dedication won her the respect of WCTU president Frances Willard,* who saw Bailey's efforts as fitting justification of the union's "Do Everything" approach to reform.

In 1887, with the powerful encouragement of Willard, Bailey agreed to head the new WCTU Department of Peace and International Arbitration. This work became a passion, and she launched what one source termed "the greatest women's peace movement of the nineteenth and early twentieth centuries." Her primary object was the abolition of war, and with this in view her department published a wealth of literature while she personally sponsored and gave lectures, travelled the world and held forth with international leaders, and campaigned in the cause of opposition to all forms of violence. In conjunction with other WCTU leaders, she frequently addressed petitions and letters to Congress and to President Benjamin Harrison on behalf of arbitration and world peace, and she lodged a sharp protest when America threatened to become militarily involved in the Chilean crisis of 1892. Her crusade extended to arguments against the draft, military drill in youth organizations, capital punishment, lynching, boxing, and military toys. Her commitment to peace never faltered, and after she retired as department superintendent in 1916, she was crestfallen when the WCTU endorsed American entry into World War I the following year.

**Bibliography:**

A. *Reminiscences of a Christian Life* (Portland, ME, 1884); National WCTU, Department of Peace and International Arbitration Reports, *Minutes* (1888–1916).

B. NAW 1, 83–85; NCAB 10, 421–422; SEAP 1, 255–56; Merle Curti, *Peace or War: The American Struggle, 1636–1936* (New York, 1936); Mary Earheart, *Frances Willard: From Prayers to Politics* (Chicago, 1944); Frances E. Willard and Mary Livermore, eds., *A Woman of the Century* (New York, 1893).

**BAIN, George Washington**    (24 September 1840, Lexington, KY—28 March 1927, Lexington, KY). *Career*: editor, *Riverside Weekly*, 1873–77; organizer and officer, Independent Order of Good Templars, 1870–79; Chautauqua and lyceum lecturer, 1880–1927.

A committed Methodist since he was thirteen years old, George Bain became active in the Temperance Movement early in life and remained a staunch and articulate champion of the cause as long as he lived. After a brief editorial career, Bain became deeply involved with the Independent Order of Good Templars in the early 1870s. The Order of Good Templars was one of the largest of a number of fraternal organizations that grew in the wake of the Washingtonian Movement in the 1840s. Created to foster temperance among members, they assumed many of the social attributes of such later fraternal lodges as the Elks or Moose—and many of them also became active politically in the temperance cause. In 1871 Bain was elected grand councilor of the Kentucky Good Templars, and while the head of the order (he was grand worthy chief templar between 1872 and 1879) he supervised the effective petitioning of the legislature to secure a state prohibitory act. Although the lawmakers passed a local option bill instead of total prohibition, Bain's leadership was acclaimed. After this, he went on to campaign in most of the local option contests in Kentucky. During his time with the order Bain also edited *The Good Templar's Advocate* for five years, and before his resignation from the group in 1874 he was instrumental in building the Kentucky Templars to about 24,000 members.

Bain's work with the Good Templars and on behalf of prohibitory legislation garnered him considerable national recognition. With this increasing celebrity came a number of requests that he seek some national or state political office. He had joined the Prohibition Party in 1876 and remained faithful to it throughout his career; but he refused to allow himself to be nominated for any political position. Instead, he drew upon his natural gift for oratory—and launched a successful career on the Chautauqua and lyceum lecture circuit. Temperance, not surprisingly, was his major theme; and even when speaking on other issues he generally managed to put in a word for the antiliquor cause. It was on the speaker's platform, he claimed, and not in politics, that he could do the most good, and he may have been right: He proved an effective lecturer nationally and took active roles in campaigns for constitutional prohibition in Kansas, South Dakota, Pennsylvania, Iowa, Michigan, Tennessee, and Ohio. At his death he was esteemed as one of the "elder statesmen" of the Temperance Movement.

**Bibliography:**

A. *Wit, Humor, Reason, Rhetoric, Prose, Poetry and Story Woven Into Eight Popular Lectures* (Louisville, KY, 1915).

B. SEAP 1, 256–57; WW 1, 45.

**BAIRD, Robert**    (6 October 1798, near Pittsburgh, PA—15 March 1863, Yonkers, NY). *Education*: studied at Acad. of Uniontown, PA, circa 1813–15; studied at Washington and Jefferson Coll., circa 1815–19; B.A., Princeton Theological Sem., 1822. *Career*: principal, Princeton Acad., 1822–27; agent, American Bible Society, 1827–29; agent, American Sunday School Union, 1829–34;

agent in Europe, French Association (later called the Foreign Evangelical Society, and then the Foreign Christian Union), 1834–63.

There are three major elements in the record of Robert Baird's career. First, chronologically, was his effort on behalf of the common school system in New Jersey; second, his leadership of the nationwide movement to establish Sunday schools; and third, his work for temperance in the countries of Northern Europe. He was a Presbyterian minister, and his commitment to an ideal of Christian piety was the common denominator in his threefold mission. In this commitment, he represented one of the most fundamental impulses in the whole development of American society and particularly in the flowering of reformism that took place during the nineteenth century. Baird was fortunate enough to see most of his labors yield considerable fruit. After completing his education and serving for five years as the principal of a private academy in Princeton, New Jersey, he became an effective lobbyist for public school legislation in the state. He is generally credited with giving considerable force to legislative developments that by 1838 made New Jersey's school system a model for other states. He then combined his interests in religion and education, serving successively as an agent for the American Bible Society and the American Sunday School Union. He dramatically improved the finances of the union, founded thousands of Sunday schools all over the nation, wrote voluminously on religious topics, and firmly established his reputation as a reform organizer.

This reputation, plus his longstanding commitment to moral causes, led to his involvement with temperance work. In 1834, a group of Americans interested in fostering Protestantism in France formed the French Association and hired Baird as their agent. He was to live in Paris and had instructions to survey the tenor of religious affairs on the continent. His zeal for moral reform, however, carried him beyond his original mission. He developed an intense interest in problem drinking in Europe, and he began to investigate the prospects of founding a European organization modeled on the American Temperance Society. The U.S. ambassador in Paris encouraged him, and Baird subsequently authored a major history of the American Temperance Movement in French, *Histoire des sociétés de tempérance des Etats Unis d'Amérique* (1836), in order to popularize the dry cause. He then took to the road to spread his dry gospel. It became a life-long work: his proselytizing took him on a journey of almost three decades and some 300,000 miles over the face of Northern Europe, from Belgium, France, Scandinavia, and Switzerland to Prussia and Russia. Behind him, the reformer left a trail of temperance societies, often established with the blessings of local heads of state. His greatest successes, however, appear to have been in Scandinavia, where Baird provided key leadership in building enduring dry organizations, launching antiliquor publications and securing the support of influential social leaders (including the King and Queen of Sweden). During his years of temperance work, Baird remained the agent of the French Association (and its successor groups) and died in its service in 1863 while on a return trip to his native America.

**Bibliography:**

A. *A View of the Mississippi Valley* (Philadelphia, 1832); *Histoire des sociétés de tempérance des Etats Unis d'Amérique* (Paris, 1836); *Visit to Northern Europe in Sketches, Descriptive, Historical, Political and Moral of Denmark, Norway, Sweden and Finland, and the Free Cities of Hamburg and Lubeck* (New York, 1841); *Religion in the United States of America* (Edinburgh, 1843); *Sketches of Protestantism in Italy Past and Present, Including a Notice of the Origin, History and Present State of the Waldenses* (Boston, 1845; 2d ed., 1847); *The Christian Retrospect and Register: A Summary of the Scientific, Moral and Religious Progress of the First Half of the 19th Century* (New York, 1851).
B. DAB 1, 511–12; DARB, 24–25; SEAP 1, 257; WW 1, 77; Henry Martyn Baird, *The Life of the Rev. Robert Baird, D.D.* (New York, 1866); John F. Hageman, *History of Princeton and Its Institutions* (Philadelphia, 1879); John MacLean, *History of the College of New Jersey*, vol. 2 (Philadelphia, 1877).

**BAKER, Purley Albert**  (10 April 1858, Jackson Co., OH—30 March 1924, Westerville, OH). *Education*: local and normal schools, Jackson and Green cos., Ohio; D.D. (honorary), Ohio Wesleyan Univ., 1907. *Career*: public school-teacher, 1882–83; ordained in Methodist Episcopal Church, 1883; served various pastorates in Ohio, 1884–95; headed Cleveland District, Anti-Saloon League of Ohio, 1896; state superintendent, Anti-Saloon League of Ohio, 1897–1903; general superintendent, Anti-Saloon League of America, 1903–24.

Legal liquor never knew a more implacable foe than Purley Albert Baker. A devoutly religious man, Baker apparently drew his initial motivation from his Methodist faith, a creed which had long stood in the forefront of dry reform. Thus inspired, he launched his long and eventful temperance career alone, apart from any dry organization. After two years of teaching school, he was ordained in 1883, and as a young clergyman riding between a number of Ohio pastorates he made total abstinence a central facet of his preaching. Baker's revivalist style and vociferous advocacy of the antiliquor cause brought him considerable local notoriety as well as impressive results. Scores took the pledge upon hearing him, and when he assumed the Methodist pulpit at Gallipolis, Ohio, his activities became still more dramatic. In a town with many saloons and powerful proliquor elements, the pastor won many to the temperance banner, including a saloon owner who joined the church and publicly dumped his "wet goods" into the gutter. Baker's ability to whip up dry sentiment was such that proliquor forces soon feared him and once even tried to jail him through a trumped up misdemeanor charge. The case was absurd—Baker stood accused of illegally posting notices of a church meeting—and the incident rebounded to further discredit the minister's enemies. Indeed, Baker's renown as a dry champion consequently grew, and organized temperance groups, notably the newly founded Anti-Saloon League, began urging him to take a larger role in the antiliquor fight. For a time he stood aloof, preferring his solitary crusade; but in the mid-1890s, by which time he led a larger congregation in Columbus, Ohio, Baker was becoming a crusader of national reputation whether he liked it or not.

He became a truly national figure upon joining the Anti-Saloon League in 1896. He had finally become convinced that only carefully managed, mass national groups would ever win the war against liquor; and once committed to the league, his zeal never faltered. By 1897 he was Ohio state superintendent and led a difficult drive to enforce local and state dry laws. Ohio had considerable dry support, but there were still some pockets of resistance, especially in the larger urban areas. Baker, however, proved a master of organization and effectively marshalled religious and civic support in favor of strict enforcement. Wet opposition crumbled in the face of the attack; Baker and his co-workers effectively "dried out" even such urban areas as Cincinnati, Cleveland, and Toledo within five years. He was so successful that other temperance leaders urged the application of his methods on a national scale; and in 1903, when league founder Howard Hyde Russell* resigned as general superintendent to take direct charge of temperance work in New York, Baker replaced him as the organization's national leader. Thereafter, his talent for management and for rallying others to his position (even wet leaders admired his abilities on these counts) shone to full advantage. He was instrumental in building league strength (particularly in the South, where it was initially weak), planning league political victories in state after state, and uniting all temperance groups—with the league in the van— in the final push for National Prohibition. A Republican in politics, Baker strove successfully to cultivate dry support in the major parties rather than linking temperance fortunes to the small Prohibition Party. His crusading zeal won him a great number of tributes, including an honoray D.D. degree from Ohio Wesleyan University and the vice presidency of the World League Against Alcoholism. At his death in 1924, he had the satisfaction of having presided over his beloved league as it climbed to the heights of national influence.

**Bibliography:**

A. "As General Superintendent Baker Saw the Situation in Maine One Week Before the Vote Was Taken," *American Issue* 19, No. 9 (1911): 4–5; "Endorsement of Anti-Saloon League by Methodists," *American Issue* 20, No. 6 (1912), 19, 1.

B. SEAP 1, 258–60; *American Issue* (Indiana ed.), June 11, 1912; E. H. Cherrington, *History of the Anti-Saloon League* (Westerville, OH, 1913); Peter H. Odegard, *Pressure Politics: The Story of the Anti-Saloon League* (New York, 1928).

**BAMBERGER, Simon**  (27 February 1847, Darmstadt, Germany—6 October 1926, Salt Lake City, UT). *Career*: storekeeper, wholesaler, miner, MO and WY, 1860s; hotel business, mining, banking, utility and railroad interests, 1869–1926; member, Utah Senate, 1903–7; governor of Utah, 1917–21.

Simon Bamberger's career offers a prime example of the fusion of Progressivism and temperance. He arrived in Utah in 1869 via a somewhat roundabout route: a Jewish immigrant from Germany, he arrived in the United States in 1861. After pursuing a number of fruitless business ventures in the Midwest and Wyoming, he finally started a successful hotel operation in Salt Lake City. Later he built up highly lucrative investments in mining properties, the profits from which subsequently established him in railroads, banking, and utilities as well. From near poverty, then, Bamberger had risen to Utah's economic elite. His success brought him not only public recognition but also a personal sense of pride in his adopted state. Becoming involved in civil affairs, he served five years on the Salt Lake City School Board; his performance brought him public acclaim and opened the door to higher office. Elected to the State Senate in 1903 (as a Democrat), he quickly established a reputation as a Progressive reformer, including a strident support for prohibition, and as a spokesman for the economic interests of the region. When he ended his term in 1907 and returned to private life, he had a solid reputation for integrity and leadership. Although a Jew (one of the most prominent of the relatively small Utah Jewish community), his conduct, plus the example of his own lifestyle of hard work and civic concern, brought him enormous popularity with the state's large Mormon majority. When he returned to the political lists in 1916 to run for the governorship, he won with the largest plurality of any candidate in Utah history. His administration launched a highly diverse Progressive program, and Bamberger had the satisfaction of presiding over the enactment of reform legislation on the care of the mentally ill, utilities regulation, workmen's compensation, public education, prison reform, public health, and aid for the handicapped. Employing his keen fiscal acumen, he did it all while changing a state treasury deficit into a surplus.

While pursuing his other reform interests, Governor Bamberger singled out temperance for special attention. He was a personal abstainer from alcohol and tobacco, which fit the preferences of his numerous Mormon constituents. In addition, Bamberger's views on the matter were in full accord with many other businessmen and Progressives: Alcohol abuse and the liquor traffic were productive not only of personal tragedies to drinkers but of economic waste and social disruption. He therefore wasted no time in attacking the problem. His initial message to the legislature, in January 1917, included a forceful call for a strict prohibition law and, following that, for a prohibition amendment to the Utah State Constitution. Such action, he declared, was "the first duty of the Legislature," a "covenant with the people of Utah." Nor did the governor want to wait for the law. The mandate of the people was clear, he insisted, and he expected the dry laws to be in effect no later than August of 1917. Putting the full prestige of his office behind the measure, Bamberger saw the law clear the legislature by February, and it was indeed operative by August. In an administration studded with solid accomplishments, the governor considered the Utah dry laws one of his finest achievements. Perhaps fortunately, however, he left office before popular sentiment turned against the Temperance Movement. Seventy-one years old when elected, he chose not to seek a second term and turned to active direction of his business interests. At his death in 1926, National Prohibition was the law of the land and the Utah Constitution was bone dry.

**Bibliography:**

B. SEAP 1, 262–63; WW 1, 52; Juanita Brooks, *The History of the Jews in Utah and Idaho* (Salt Lake City, UT, 1973); S. George Ellsworth, ed., "Simon Bamberger: Governor of Utah," *Western State Jewish Historical Quarterly* 5, No. 4 (1973); David T. Golden, "Simon Bamberger," *Universal Jewish Encyclopedia*, vol. 2 (New York, 1940); Frank Thomas Morn, "Simon Bamberger: A Jew in a Mormon Commonwealth" (M.S. thesis, Brigham Young University, 1966); Leon L. Watters, *The Pioneer Jews of Utah* (New York, 1952).

**BANKS, Louis Albert**    (12 November 1855, Corvallis, OR—17 June 1933, Roseburg, OR?). *Education*: studied at Philomath Coll. and Boston Univ., 1870s; D.D., Mt. Union Coll., 1891; LLD., Philomath Coll., 1918. *Career*: ordained in Methodist Church, 1879; temperance and religious author and publisher, 1880 to late 1920s; pastorates in Boston, New York, Kansas City, MO, and Seattle, WA, 1870s–1890s; lecturer, Anti-Saloon League of New York State, 1894–95; evangelistic preaching, 1895 to circa 1911; lecturer, National Anti-Saloon League, 1913 to 1920s.

Like many other ministers of his generation, Louis Banks used the pulpit as a powerful agent on behalf of the Temperance Movement. His career, however, was especially notable in that he concentrated his gospel on America's city populations, and with a good deal of success. Indeed, his urban crusade offers an interesting balance to the hoary characterizations of the Temperance Movement as a chiefly rural phenomenon hostile to the city. After a Methodist ordination in 1879, Banks had congregations in a number of major industrial centers ranging from Boston and New York in the East to Seattle in the far West. In all of these pastorates, he hammered away at the liquor traffic in his preaching and sought ways to put the urban temperance voice on a permanent footing. In 1880, for example, he founded the *Pacific Censor* (Vancouver, Washington), the first dry newspaper in the state, and launched such a heated barrage against drink that he became one of the most controversial drys in the region. His first book, *Censor Echoes* (1881), was largely a collection of his editorials and further enhanced his reputation as a firebrand. So great was wet hatred for Banks that he became a literal casualty in the war against alcohol: speaking during a Washington State campaign in 1881, an enraged Vancouver tavernkeeper put a bullet into him. It was a futile act. The wound was not serious and served only to spur Banks's already considerable enthusiasm.

As his temperance commitment increased, Banks became active in agitation for a national prohibition amendment. His efforts in that contest took a number of directions. At first, like many others of his mind, he became convinced that neither of the major political parties would make such an amendment a priority. Consequently, he joined the Prohibition Party and in 1893 stood as its candidate for governor of Massachusetts (he had a Boston pastorate at the time). Later, however, as the political impotence of that party became clear, he affiliated with the rising Anti-Saloon League. The league, with its bipartisan approach to the Republicans and Democrats, offered better results, and Banks quickly emerged as one of its most vigorous workers. He served first as a lecturer for the New York State League, maintaining his focus on urban populations, and after several years of evangelical preaching went to work for the National League (1913). He then ranged the country on behalf of Prohibition, developing one of the most effective platform styles in the league arsenal. When the World Prohibition League grew out of national temperance activities, Banks, without hesitation, promptly worked appearances for the new organization into his already busy schedule. In addition to his oratory, he was also a formidable reform author— at least if measured in terms of sheer production. Over his long career, he wrote more than fifty titles, usually on temperance, but on other religious and reform topics as well. In sum, Banks was the epitome of the reformer who built the league to the height of its power and a clear example of the movement's ability to capture the life-long dedication of its followers.

**Bibliography:**

A. *Censor Echoes* (Vancouver, WA, 1881); *The Saloon-keeper's Ledger* (Westerville, OH, 1896); *Seven Times Around Jericho* (Westerville, OH, 1897); *The Great Sinners of the Bible* (1899); *Ammunition for the Final Drive on Booze* (Westerville, OH, 1917); *The Lincoln Legion* (Westerville, OH, 1917).

B. SEAP 1, 271–72; WW 1, 54.

**BARKER, Helen Morton**    (7 or 8 December 1834, Rickville, NY—6 May 1910, ?). *Education*: studied at Gouverneur Wesleyan Sem., late 1840s? *Career*: taught school, Oswego, NY, 1850s?; organizer, lecturer, and local officer, New York State WCTU, 1870s; president, Dakota Terr. WCTU, 1884–89; president, South Dakota State WCTU, 1889–93?; treasurer, National WCTU, 1893–1900?

Helen Barker made a near lifetime career of the Woman's Christian Temperance Union. A career of such strength and longevity as Mrs. Barker's was a remarkably familiar story in WCTU annals, and it represented not only part of an important agency in the national expansion of the Temperance Movement but also in the advancement of women generally toward greater participation in civil affairs. Deeply religious (she was married to a minister), like many of her sister stalwarts she moved easily from church attendance to temperance meetings in her native New York State, and then on to a thoroughgoing absorption in dry evangelism. Barker (then Helen Morton) had been a schoolteacher for a number of years in the 1850s, but once she started as a reformer, no other vocation stood in her way. She joined the WCTU as soon as it was organized in her area and became president of the Allegheny County, New York, chapter in 1877. While serving in this capacity, she became an organizer and lecturer for the state union and travelled extensively throughout the region promoting the movement. When the family moved (for reasons unknown) to Dakota Territory in the early 1880s, she continued her temperance work with the same old zeal. Elected president of the territorial union in 1884, she then led the South Dakota chapter when the Territory split between the states of North and South Dakota in 1889. Under her steady hand (and with the aid of hundreds of other women), temperance became as much a part of the "Wild West" as other social activities and played its part in bringing stability to the area. In 1892, Barker was named as one of the women managers of the Columbian Exposition in Chicago, a position that brought her a measure of national prominence. Indeed, her clear leadership abilities, including her fine WCTU record in New York and Dakota, saw her elected National WCTU treasurer shortly thereafter. Mrs. Barker held this position for a number of terms until she retired in the face of failing health.

**Bibliography:**

B. SEAP 1, 274–75; WW 1, 56; Ruth Bordin, *Woman and Temperance: The Quest for Power and Liberty, 1873–1900* (Philadelphia, 1981).

**BARKLEY, Alben William**    (24 November 1877, Grover Co., KY—30 April 1956, Lexington, KY). *Education*: A.B., Marvin Coll., 1897; studied at Emory Coll., 1897–98; studied at Univ. of Virginia Law Sch., 1902; at various dates over his career: LLD. (honorary), Univ. of Louisville, Univ. of Kentucky, Center Coll., National Univ., Emory Univ., Kentucky Wesleyan Coll., Michigan State Coll., DePauw Univ., Westminster Coll., Rider Coll.; DHL. (honorary), Univ. of Florida, Dropsie Coll. for Hebrew and Cognate Learning; M.S., Bryant Coll. *Career*: admitted to bar, KY, 1901; prosecutor, McCracken Co., KY, 1905–9; judge, McCracken Co., 1909–13; member, U.S. House of Representatives, 1913–27; member, U.S. Senate, 1927–49, 1954–56; vice president of the United States, 1949–53.

Alben Barkley's political career ranks among the most successful of any elected official of the twentieth century. He is best remembered as Harry S Truman's vice president and, before that, as Senate majority leader under Franklin Roosevelt during the difficult years of the Great Depression and World War II. These high positions, however, came only after a long political apprenticeship. He was admitted to the Kentucky bar in 1901 and by 1909 had won election as county prosecutor (1905) and then as county judge. Soon after (1913), he ran successfully for Congress, and he represented the First Kentucky District in the House until 1927. Over these eventful years his stance on national issues mirrored the views of his state constituents, a fact which dictated a strong antiliquor stance on Barkley's part in the battle for National Prohibition. Despite its large distilling industry, Kentucky was one of the most enthusiastically dry states, and Congressman Barkley took full advantage of the opportunities the temperance cause afforded. He lent his support to any number of local dry campaigns both in Kentucky and neighboring states, and he became an effective scourge of the liquor traffic on the floor of the House. Perhaps his most noted effort in this capacity was the Sheppard-Barkley bill, which put Washington, D.C., in the dry camp. He also voted for the Eighteenth Amendment, campaigned vigorously for state ratification, and then sponsored a number of measures—some considered extreme even by other drys—to implement its enforcement (one of his bills would have prohibited the use of any foodstuff in the manufacture of any kind of intoxicating beverage).

But the congressman was nothing if not an astute politician. When the tide of popular opinion shifted against Prohibition, Barkley chose not to defend it with his former energy. He won election to the Senate in 1927, by which time the deficiencies of the dry experiment were becoming increasingly apparent. His position on the Eighteenth Amendment in that chamber gradually came to reflect the majority stance of the Democratic Party, a stance which finally saw the party openly hostile to the dry cause. With the victory of Roosevelt (an acknowledged wet) in 1932 and Repeal in 1933, Barkley quickly came to terms with the new administration and had few regrets about leaving his days as a Prohibition advocate behind him. The man who had been a hero to many temperance workers in the 1920s was, by the 1930s, only too glad to end his associations with the discredited dry cause. The inability of the prohibitionists to hold men like Barkley in the ranks of the crusade was indicative of the Temperance Movement's final decline as a significant political force. Barkley, however, put to good use the political acumen he had sharpened while fighting the temperance wars. He assumed a major role in shaping New Deal legislation and rose to great stature in the Senate and the Democratic Party. He was majority leader for over a decade (1936–47), minority leader from 1947 to 1949 during the brief Republican ascendancy in the Senate, and vice president under Truman from 1949 to 1953. The veteran Kentuckian then returned to the Senate in 1955, where he sat until his death in 1956. He was honored as few other politicians of his day, receiving a host of honorary degrees and public and private awards, including a gold medal by act of Congress.

**Bibliography:**

A. *The Reasons for Prohibition* (Washington, DC, 1925); *Domestic Stability, National Defense, and Prosecution of World War Two* (Washington, DC, 1942); *That Reminds Me* (Garden City, NY, 1954).

B. BDAC, 553; SEAP 1, 275–76; WW 3, 49–50.

**BARNES, Albert**   (1 December 1789, Rome, NY—24 December 1870, Philadelphia, PA). *Education*: B.A., Hamilton Coll., 1820; graduated from Princeton Sem., 1824. *Career*: Presbyterian minister, Morristown, NJ, 1825–30; minister, First Presbyterian Church, Philadelphia, 1830–67; retirement, 1867–70.

Albert Barnes typified the historical connection between religious revivalism and the growth of the Temperance Movement throughout the nineteenth century. A Presbyterian clergyman, Barnes's deep concern for social reform—he was active in the abolitionist crusade and the Sunday school movement as well as with antiliquor forces—flowed almost naturally from his religious beliefs. From the late 1820s, he was a leading proponent of the New School side of the theological disputes that rocked orthodox Calvinism during the Second Great Awakening. He denied the doctrine of original sin and held that men were open to salvation and sinful only through their own willful actions. They were thus free to atone for their transgressions, and those who accepted God's grace, Barnes argued, could be saved. God, in other words, had not predestined certain individuals to redemption and others to damnation. Men and women were responsible for their own fates in the eyes of the Lord. Barnes, over the 1830s, defended these views doggedly against the attacks of more conservative Presbyterians who adamantly rejected the idea that unregenerate man could alter his chance of salvation. The struggle ultimately split the denomination, leaving a breach that failed to heal until 1870. (In the interim, Barnes also worked to bring about a reconciliation of the liberal and conservative factions.) While embroiled in theology, however, whether maintaining his own position or working to restore the unity of the church, he still found time to lead congregations, first in Morristown, New Jersey, and then in Philadelphia, as well as assuming an active role in the governance of Union Theological Seminary. He was, then, by any accounting, one of the central figures of his generation in Presbyterian affairs.

Barnes brought the same intensity to social reform that characterized his religious concerns. Indeed, in many respects his reform efforts mirrored his theological positions. In urging his congregations, and Americans in general, to labor on behalf of temperance and other causes, he was, in effect, urging them to acts of personal and social atonement—acts fully consonant with a willful striving for salvation. And Barnes was more than a preacher, setting a high-toned example himself. In Morristown, he rallied the local populace so effectively against "the traffic" that he almost eliminated illegal sales. He insisted as well that the church take a strong stand on the liquor question, including support for prohibitory legislation. In demanding prohibition, Barnes helped lead the movement away from its initial reliance on "moral suasion" as a means of dealing with drinking problems. "You may go far into the temperance question by moral suasion," he wrote at one point, "but it has failed in removing the evil, and, from the nature of the case, must always fail," as long as government allowed the existence of any legal liquor. He continued to speak out on behalf of prohibition for almost fifty years and had the satisfaction of seeing the rest of the Temperance Movement adopt his views on the need for legal action. Nor did he hesitate to maintain his position on the church's responsibility in leading the fight—an argument that generated some heated criticisms from fellow Presbyterians. To the end of his career, the old crusader never flagged, and his nearly life-long pursuit of religious truth and the good society offered a telling illustration of the power of the pulpit in the nineteenth-century struggle for social reform.

### Bibliography:

A. *Notes Explanatory and Practical on the Scriptures*, 11 vols. (Philadelphia, 1832–53); *Sermons on Revivals* (Philadelphia, 1841); *An Inquiry Into the Scrip-*

*tural Views of Slavery* (Philadelphia, 1855); *The Atonement* (Philadelphia, 1859); *Lectures on the Evidences of Christianity in the Nineteenth Century* (New York, 1868).

B. DAB 1, 627-29; DARB, 30–31; NYT, Dec. 27, 1870; SEAP 1, 277–78.

**BARNES, Frances Julia Allis** (14 April 1846, Skaneateles, NY—?). *Education*: studied at Packer Collegiate Inst., 1860s. *Career*: temperance organizing with Frances Willard, 1874–79; superintendent, National Youth WCTU, 1880.

The career of Frances Barnes enlightens an aspect of the Temperance Movement which, over time, assumed an importance fully equal to the assault on the liquor traffic itself and certainly proved more enduring over later generations. This was the crusade's encouragement of women to take an increasingly active role in American public affairs generally. To be sure, the antiliquor reform in many respects went hand in hand with the struggle for women's rights, but the full implications of this union were not always obvious at first. They took time to surface, sometimes only as young women who learned the skills of leadership and organization in temperance ranks later applied their talents in other quarters. And it was Frances Barnes, as much as any other temperance leader, who worked to give women just such initial leadership opportunities. Married to a New York attorney in 1871, Barnes was fully aware of national temperance activities, although she failed to become involved immediately. The trigger for her participation came in 1874, when she sat in on an antiliquor meeting during a visit to Chicago. In charge of the meeting was Frances Willard,* soon to be president of the newly formed Woman's Christian Temperance Union, and Barnes, as one temperance account put it, "at once enlisted in the service" for the "battle against the saloon." If nothing else, her action served to demonstrate the energizing impact of Willard. Indeed, Barnes was soon one of Willard's closest aides, becoming her travelling companion and secretary over many years of crusading efforts. As early as 1875, however, Barnes's personal leadership qualities became evident to union officials, and in need of good organizers, they gave her a mission of her own. It was the start of one of the most distinguished careers of any WCTU leader.

The union directed Mrs. Barnes toward work with young women, a task which revealed her as a genuine humanitarian. She first organized girls in New York and Illinois (1875–79) to support the activities of the senior WCTU, and did so well that the 1880 convention of the union named her superintendent of a permanent national department, the Young Woman's Christian Temperance Union (YWCTU). While holding this new position, however, she continued her work in New York, where she was extremely successful in drawing youth to the dry banner in their own young people's organizations. As she became familiar with the urban areas of the state, though, Barnes expressed concern about the well-being of children generally and devoted some of her attention to alleviating the plight of poor youth in New York City. Among other things, she established a number of free reading rooms as well as a lecture series geared to the needs of young men. In 1890, she served as an American delegate to the annual convention of the British Women's Temperance Association and convinced that organization to add a YWCTU to its departments (Lady Henry Somerset, a close friend of Willard's, took charge of the new effort.) The following year, Barnes was elected secretary of the World's YWCTU, which, although never becoming an important international movement, was at least an expression of the desire to spread the dry message as universally as possible (she did attend a World Convention in 1910 in Scotland). After this, however, her health began to fail, and in her later years she was unable to sustain her old pace. By this time, the WCTU was having increasing difficulty in recruiting young women anyway (more were joining suffrage groups than dry organizations), and Barnes gradually let go of her duties. She retired as one of the most respected leaders of the movement.

**Bibliography:**

B. SEAP 1, 278; WW 1, 56; Ruth Bordin, *Woman and Temperance: The Quest for Power and Liberty, 1873–1900* (Philadelphia, 1981).

**BARNUM, Phineas Taylor**    (5 July 1810, Bethel, CT—7 April 1891, Bridgeport, CT). *Career*: show business promoter, beginning 1830s; member, Connecticut legislature, circa 1867–69; mayor, Bridgeport, CT, 1875–78; co-founder (with J. A. Bailey), Barnum and Bailey Circus, 1881–91; philanthropic, business, and writing activities, to 1891.

P. T. Barnum was the great American showman of the nineteenth century, known mainly for "the Greatest Show on Earth," his circus, menagerie, and collection of freaks. At the age of forty, after having established himself in show business, he began to suffer fears that, like many prominent men of his time, he might fall victim to alcoholism. It had ruined others, the great promoter noted, and he went on to ask, "What guarantee is there that I may not become a drunkard?" He began to limit his drinking to wine; but three years later, at the inspiration of a lecture by E. H. Chapin (whom Barnum had invited to speak in his home city of Bridgeport, Connecticut), he smashed all his champagne bottles and took the total abstinence pledge. Not satisfied with halfway measures, he then went on to become an extremely popular temperance lecturer himself. At times, he even featured the antiliquor message in his stage productions. In 1849, for example, when he managed the successful American tour of Swedish singer Jenny Lind, Barnum often lectured in the concert hall on nights when Miss Lind did not perform. He claimed never to have felt a deeper commitment to any cause than temperance; and although theatrics were part of Barnum's personality, he may have been sincere in this instance. Indeed, when he served in the state legislature and as mayor of Bridgeport (from the late 1860s to the mid-1870s), he did take steps to advance temperance laws, and his personal abstinence lent further credence to his claim.

There appears to have been no real personal basis for Barnum's fear of liquor, since he had never been an especially heavy drinker. He professed having been moved by Chapin's call to be an example to others. There seems, however, also to have been something in Barnum that recoiled from any threat to his emotional stability and equilibrium, his mental and physical efficiency, even of brief duration. "How many good opportunities have passed," he once asked, "never to return again, while a man was sipping a social glass with his friend!" This was not quite the same kind of threat he usually talked about in his lectures. In those lectures it was the wider dangers of alcohol he inveighed against, the long-term threat to getting ahead in life, to the family (he was devoted to his own), and to the security of the nation from crime and poverty. These were staple values of the temperance crusade, but they surely took on special meaning when expounded by so great a financial success and public a personality as Barnum. Expounded by him they also lost most of their Puritanical stigma, for here was a man who epitomized the pragmatic approach to life, whose offerings of often dubious wonders proclaimed the right of the common man to make his own judgements in his own self-interest. Like Barnum's grotesques, temperance also invoked the sometimes pseudoscientific language which could be expected to appeal to an industrializing nation—to citizens who were coming to hold scientific vocabulary and judgement as part of the democratic domain. Still, there was something in Barnum's fear of drink as a releaser of emotion that stood at odds with his vocation as an entertainer, but it was precisely this tension which the circus was intended to sublimate harmlessly. Barnum connected the extremes of temperance oratory—even its humbug or fraud—with a principle of showmanship which at one and the same time served as his personal offensive against one of the chief social problems of the day and as a rallying cry for others which, he hoped, would enlist them against the repressiveness of drink as well. To him the whole enterprise of living was showmanship, admittedly sometimes deceitful, but tending ultimately—unlike indulgence in drink—to the happiness of the participants, showmen and audience alike.

**Bibliography:**

A. *The Liquor Business: Its Effects Upon the Minds, Morals and Pockets of Our People* (New York, 1854?); *Struggles and Triumphs* (1869; New York, 1920); *The Story of My Life...* (San Francisco, 1886); *Thirty Years of Hustling...* (Rutland, IL, 1890); *The Swindlers of America...* (New York, 1903); *Lion Jack: A Story of Perilous Adventure...* (New York, 1904).

B. SEAP 1, 279–80; Raymond Fitzsimmons, *Barnum in London* (New York, 1970); Irving Wallace, *The Fabulous Showman: The Life and Times of P. T. Barnum* (Boston, 1973); Morris Robert Werner, *Barnum* (New York, 1924).

**BARTON, Arthur James**  (2 February 1867, near Jamesboro, AR—19 July 1942, Wilmington, NC). *Education*: A.B., Union Univ., 1891; D.D., Union Univ., 1897; D.D., Baylor Univ., 1903; LLD. (honorary), Union Univ., 1927. *Career*: ordained Baptist minister, 1888; principal, Gadsden (TN) Male and Female Acad., 1891–92; president, Lexington (TN) Baptist Coll., 1892–94; minister, various country churches (TN), to 1894; minister, Edgefield Church,

Nashville, TN, 1894–96; service on church missionary boards and editor of Baptist publications, 1896–1905; minister, pastorates in AR, TX, LA, 1906–1924; superintendent, Missouri Baptist General Association, 1924–26; general director, Cooperative Program of the Southern Baptist Convention, 1926–27; minister, Temple Baptist Church, Wilmington, NC, 1930–42.

James Barton spent his adult life immersed in the affairs of his beloved Baptist Church and in the war against liquor. After his ordination in 1888, he took charge of a large number of pastorates stretching from Tennessee to Texas, and he became thoroughly versed in the skills of church organization and management. Indeed, at various times he held leadership positions on boards overseeing Baptist missionary work and took a leading role in editing church publications. By the 1920s the denomination had called on Barton several times to direct the operations of its regional administrative efforts, and he emerged as one of the leading church spokesmen of his day. It was no surprise, then, when church officials selected him for a seat on the executive committee of the National Baptist Conference in Washington, D.C. (1911). Barton was delighted with his new post. It not only established him as a clerical leader of national stature, but put him in a position to lobby Congress on behalf of church-supported legislation. And during this period that meant working on behalf of prohibition, a cause long dear to the Baptist reverend. Indeed, Barton had used his pulpit frequently to pummel "the traffic," and in Washington he was able to follow his conscience to much greater practical effect. Under his leadership, the conference drafted what became known as the Sheppard-Kenyon bill. Similar to the later (1913) Webb-Kenyon bill, the measure called for the abolition of interstate liquor shipments whenever such traffic would result in the illegal sale of beverage alcohol in dry areas. Barton's performance on behalf of the proposed law revealed him as a hard-working and tenacious lobbyist.

The 1911 Baptist Conference was the start of a major temperance career for Barton. He also took part in the next conference (1912), which was largely devoted to pressing dry measures in Congress. Five years later, he also helped draw up the Sheppard-Hobson resolution, which called for a National Prohibition amendment to the Constitution (and which later became the Eighteenth Amendment). In the meantime, the reverend had substantially expanded his antiliquor role. He attended the first meeting of the International Congress on Alcoholism in Milan, Italy, in 1913, as an official American delegate and represented the United States again at the 1921 congress in Lausanne, Switzerland. Back home, his efforts received local recognition as well. He was elected superintendent of the Texas Anti-Saloon League in 1915 (at the time, he had a pastorate in Waco), and he bent every effort to rally support for National Prohibition in the Lone Star State. He also served at various times with a number of other temperance organizations, both locally and nationally. During these years of labor, Barton remained active in other areas as well: His participation in church affairs never flagged, for example, and he sat on the National Council of the Boy Scouts of

America. Yet his place in the public mind was as the temperance leader par excellence. It was a recognition he had fully earned.

**Bibliography:**

B. SEAP 1, 282; WW 1, 48.

**BASCOM, John**  (1 May 1827, Genoa, NY—2 October 1911, Williamstown, MA). *Eduction*: A.B., Williams Coll., 1849; A.M., Williams Coll., 1852; graduated from Andover Theological Sem., 1855; LLD. (honorary), Amherst Coll., 1873, Williams Coll., 1897, Univ. of Wisconsin, 1905; D.D. (honorary), Iowa Coll., 1880. *Career*: professor of rhetoric, Williams Coll., 1855–74; president, Univ. of Wisconsin, 1874–87; lecturer in sociology, Williams Coll., 1887–91, 1901–3; professor of political science, Williams Coll., 1891–1901; retirement, 1903–1911.

John Bascom held perhaps as impressive an array of intellectual interests and credentials as anyone ever connected with the Temperance Movement. The master of several academic disciplines and one-time president of the University of Wisconsin, Bascom nevertheless always found time to devote to the antiliquor reform. From his student days onward, and during his distinguished professional career, he compiled a steady record of involvement in the cause and of regular public pronouncements against drink. His commitment was such that, in 1880, he broke his long affiliation with the Republicans (he had voted with the Liberty and Free Soil parties prior to that) and joined the Prohibitionists. His major contribution to the temperance reform, however, was not in politics. Rather, it would seem to be his efforts to give prohibition a firm and rigorous philosophical rationale. His writings in psychology, ethics, religion, and social theory are frequently threaded with implications, if not overt statements, against the use of alcohol, not to speak of the actual liquor traffic itself. More directly to the point, his *Philosophy of Prohibition* (1885) gave one of the single most intellectually sophisticated expositions of that topic. While temperance workers certainly appreciated Professor Bascom's work, it apparently suffered in popularity from the usual handicaps of philosophical writings, mainly their sophistication and complexity. Bascom, however, even at his most sophisticated, generally was unable to free himself from a relatively heavy-handed religious perspective on reform issues. Thus a high degree of moralizing was evident in his writings on temperance. There is of course no telling what effect a greater degree of intellectual disinterestedness might have had on his argument for prohibition, although in any case his high standing in academic circles helped lend considerable credence to his views among many of the more thoughtful dry adherents.

**Bibliography:**

A. *An Appeal to Young Men on the Use of Tobacco* (New York, 185-?); *Aesthetics, or the Science of Beauty* (New York, 1875); *The Philosophy of*

*Prohibition* (New York, 1885); *Prohibition and Common Sense* (New York, 1885); *Science, Philosophy and Religion* (New York, 1885); *Woman Suffrage* (Madison, WI?, 188–?).

B. SEAP 1, 282–83; WW 1, 66.

**BATEHAM, Josephine Abiah Penfield Cushman**    (1 November 1829, Alden, NY—15 March 1901, Oberlin, OH). *Education*: graduated from Oberlin Coll., 1847. *Career*: schoolteacher, Oberlin, OH, 1847–48; missionary work in Haiti, 1848; editor, then contributor, *Ohio Cultivator*, 1850–54?; delegate, International Peace Congress, London, 1851; president, State Temperance Society of the Women of Ohio, 1853; fruit farming and housewife in Painesville, OH, 1864–74; leader of Painesville, OH, temperance crusade, 1874; participant in state and national WCTU activities, 1874–84; superintendent, National WCTU Department for Suppression of Sabbath Desecration, 1884–96; retirement, 1897–1901.

Josephine Bateham was raised in an atmosphere of religion and reform (her father was a minister and her mother one of the leading founders of the State Temperance Society of the Women of Ohio), and it seemed only natural that she would later become deeply involved with reform work and the cause of temperance in particular. In 1874, when she did indeed contribute her organizational abilities as well as her dedication and insight to the newly formed Woman's Christian Temperance Union, the crusade found in her a leader whose efforts and devotion were of crucial significance to its growth. She married the Reverend Richard Cushman soon after her graduation from Oberlin College (a hotbed of antebellum reform activity) in 1847, but he died less than a year later in Haiti, where the couple were serving as missionaries. She returned to Oberlin and in 1850 married Michael Bateham, a leading figure in Ohio agriculture and founder, editor, and publisher of the *Ohio Cultivator*. Mrs. Bateham became editor of the women's section of her husband's paper and contributed numerous articles on topics ranging from women's rights, education, and peace to housekeeping and flower gardening. Her work on the *Cultivator* revealed a woman who was at once knowledgeable, articulate, and deeply sensitive to the broad variety of reform movements then sweeping the nation. Both she and her husband became involved in several of these efforts, especially the peace movement, and when the International Peace Congress was held in London in 1851, the couple went as United States delegates. (The British barred female delegates, however, and a disappointed Mrs. Bateham had to watch the proceedings from the gallery.) By this time the Temperance Movement was taking root in Ohio, and the Batehams became active participants. In 1852, Mrs. Bateham was elected president of the Temperance Society of the Women of Ohio a year after its formation (by her mother among others), and she took an active leadership role when the "Woman's Crusade" erupted in her hometown of Painesville. By the time the WCTU gained momentum in 1874, she was one of its staunchest supporters and its leading spokeswomen in Painesville.

After her husband's death in 1880, Mrs. Bateham became increasingly active in both the state and national branches of the WCTU. From 1884 to 1896 she was superintendent of the union's Department for the Suppression of Sabbath Desecration. Her work for the union centered around this issue, and she travelled widely, once giving over three hundred lectures in one year, besides publishing leaflets and a *Sabbath Observance Manual* (1892). When Senator Henry Blair* of New Hampshire introduced a Sunday rest bill, which called for the prohibition of all secular work on the Sabbath within federal territories, she gave the proposed law her wholehearted support. She testified on behalf of the measure before a Senate hearing and then organized the circulation of the WCTU's huge petition endorsing the bill. Blair's initiative, however, which would have barred the movement of the mails and interstate commerce on Sunday as well, failed to reach a vote. Undaunted, Bateham continued to work for Sunday closing laws, and it was largely through her unyielding efforts that the union was able to insure a Sunday closing requirement at the World's Columbian Exposition in 1893, an important initial victory despite its later being circumvented. After years of service, she retired from active crusading and went to live near two of her children in Norwalk, Ohio. She died on a visit to Oberlin at age seventy-one in 1901.

**Bibliography:**

A. *Sabbath Observance Manual* (Evanston, IL?, 1892).

B. NAW 1, 110–11; Frances E. Willard and Mary A. Livermore, eds., *A Woman of the Century* (New York, 1893).

**BEAUCHAMP, Lou Jenks**    (14 February 1851, Cincinnati, OH—4 June 1920, Medford, IA). *Career*: telegraph editor, *Cincinnati Star*, circa 1870s; wrote poems and sketches for New York newspapers; managing editor, *Fort Wayne Gazette*, circa 1877; lecturer and author, 1877–1920.

The reformed drinker was often a celebrity on the temperance lecture circuit. Speakers like John B. Gough,* for instance, held audiences spellbound with their firsthand stories of delirium tremens, the craving for drink, and dramatic battles for recovery. Such a lecturer was Lou Jenks Beauchamp. He was a humorist, writer, and for seven years a heavy drinker—probably an alcoholic. Unable to end his "indulgence in drink" by himself, Jenks reformed with the aid of one Millie Gardner, whom he subsequently married (1877). Sober for the first time in years, he turned his talent for humor to the cause of temperance. In his new dedication to the antiliquor crusade, he was typical of a great many indulgers who finally took the pledge and joined their voices—telling and retelling the horrors of drink—in the growing evangelical spirit of the movement in the latter half of the nineteenth century. Joining a dry fraternal lodge (perhaps to help maintain his own sobriety), he rose to the rank of deputy supreme templar in the Order of Good Templars; and like numerous other converts who took to the speaker's platform, he helped, by virtue of his talent, in transforming the character of that organization and of the movement in general from private and local assistance into a genuinely national crusade. Beauchamp published sketches and poems on many humorous and temperance themes and addressed large audiences in Canada, England, and Scotland as well as all over the United States. He probably gave some ten thousand speeches on temperance and other subjects over the course of his career, from which he derived a secure income. The effectiveness of his platform efforts and his biting wit may be measured by reports that he personally induced over 400,000 persons to pledge total abstinence and that his life was threatened more than once by partisans of the liquor interest. While he never reached the stature of a Gough, Beauchamp was nevertheless one of the most notable figures on the stump for temperance, and his career offered a good illustration of the subject's appeal to mass popular audiences.

**Bibliography:**

A. *Sunshine* (Hamilton, OH, 1879); *This, That and the Other* (Hamilton, OH, 1882); *What the Duchess and I Saw in Europe* (Hamilton, OH, 1896).
B. SEAP 1, 289; WW 1, 75.

**BEAVER, James Addams**    (21 October 1837, Millerstown, PA—31 January 1914, Bellefonte, PA). *Education*: graduated from Jefferson Coll., 1856; LLD. (honorary), Dickinson Coll., 1889, Hanover Coll., 1889, Univ. of Edinburgh, Scotland, 1889. *Career*: admitted to bar, PA, 1859; law practice, 1859–61; Union army (rose to brigadier general), 1861–64; law practice, 1864–87; business interest in nail factory, 1880s; governor of Pennsylvania, 1887–91; law practice, 1891–95; judge, Pennsylvania Superior Court, 1895–1914.

The Civil War was a catalyst in the careers of many nineteenth-century Americans, and James Beaver first climbed to public prominence in the Union army. He was a Republican in politics and was convinced that war would follow the election of Abraham Lincoln in 1860. When fighting indeed broke out, he entered service as a lieutenant in 1861 and saw almost constant duty until late 1864. In between, leading troops from his native Pennsylvania, Beaver took part in some of the toughest actions of the war. He fought at Fredericksburg, Chancellorsville, Gettysburg, the Wilderness, Cold Harbor, and Ream's Station (where he was severely wounded in the leg). Cited for gallantry more than once, he received a brevet promotion to brigadier general in November 1864 and mustered out in December due to medical incapacity. Thereafter, he prospered as a lawyer and businessman and became active in state politics. His prestige at the bar and his fine war record made him an attractive candidate, and in 1882 he ran for governor. He lost by only some forty thousand votes and, encouraged by his strong race, ran again successfully in 1886. In office (1887–91), Beaver displayed qualities commonly associated with many early Republicans—namely, a keen interest in social reform legislation and governmental sponsorship of internal improvements. His administration was noted for its attention to road and waterway construction, educational reforms, forest conservation, and—with the special interest of the governor—temperance.

Beaver's personal commitment to temperance reform was quite sincere (although the origins of his enthusiasm are unclear). His pursuit of prohibitory legislation, however, proved frustrating, as he could never marshal sufficient political strength to carry such a measure. Yet it was not for want of trying. In 1887, at the beginning of Beaver's term, popular feeling on the liquor question in Pennsylvania was running quite high. With the governor's blessing, the legislature wrote a prohibition amendment to the state constitution, which it then placed on the ballot for a popular referendum. At the same time, however, it passed another measure, the so-called Brooks High License Law, which had the dual effect of raising state revenue through license fees and driving many of the worst saloons out of business (they were either refused licenses or could not afford the fees). Intended as a reform bill, the Brooks Law ironically helped kill the prohibitory amendment. With revenues up and the worst saloons gone, public anger with the traffic relaxed and support for prohibition waned. Beaver, probably sensing the measure was in trouble but unable to delay the referendum, set the election for June 18, 1889, when the antiliquor forces suffered a stunning popular defeat. The amendment lost by over 188,000 votes and dry politics in the state remained in disarray for years afterward. Beaver himself—still a temperance man—chose not to run again and returned to his legal practice in 1891. He ended his long and distinguished career with almost two decades of service as a state superior court judge.

**Bibliography:**

B. DAB 2, 112–13; WW 1, 76–77; Harry Macholm Chalfant, *Father Penn and John Barleycorn* (Harrisburg, PA, 1925); John B. Linn, *History of Center and Clinton Counties* (1883).

**BEECHER, Lyman**    (12 October 1775, New Haven, CT—10 January 1863, Brooklyn, NY). *Education*: B.A., Yale Coll., 1797; M.A., Yale Coll., 1798. *Career*: ordained as Presbyterian minister, 1799; minister, Presbyterian Church, East Hampton, Long Island, 1799–1810; minister, Congregational Church, Litchfield, CT, 1810–26; minister, Hanover Street Congregational Church, Boston, 1826–32; minister, Second Presbyterian Church, Cincinnati, OH, 1833–43; president, Lane Theological Sem., Cincinnati, OH, 1832–50; active retirement as writer and lecturer, 1851–63.

Abandoning the family tradition of blacksmithing, Lyman Beecher enrolled at Yale College when he was eighteen years old. At Yale he was profoundly influenced by Timothy Dwight, who became president of the college when Beecher was a sophomore, and he decided to remain in school after graduation as a student of divinity. He received an M.A. in 1798 and two years later was ordained by the Presbyterian Church. His first pulpit was at East Hampton, Long Island, where the meager salary of three hundred dollars a year plus firewood made him long for a better situation. In 1810 the call came from the Congregational Church in Litchfield, Connecticut, and he moved his family there. At Litchfield, Beecher launched a nonstop revivalism by giving sermons twice on Sundays and weekdays in various public buildings and private homes. The force and enthusiasm of Beecher's preaching soon swept many of the staid congregations of New England off their feet. By 1826, Boston orthodoxy, in recognition of the new religious feeling, set about establishing a new church based on the free doctrines espoused by Beecher. He was installed as the minister of the Hanover Street Church, and in little over six years he made it one of the most successful in New England. Meanwhile, he had found time to play a prominent role in establishing the foundations of the organized Temperance Movement in New England, a Domestic Missionary Society to educate young men for the ministry, and the American Bible Society. There was, however, a strain of intolerance and demagoguery in Beecher's preaching, and its anti-Catholic flavor is held largely responsible for the attack in 1831 on the Ursuline convent in Charlestown, Massachusetts, which was burned to the ground.

When Lane Theological Seminary was founded in Cincinnati in 1832, Beecher was appointed its first president. The climate in the Midwest, however, was not as salubrious as it had been in the Northeast. His liberal views were not welcomed by many conservative Presbyterians, who charged Beecher with heresy, slander, and hypocrisy. Essentially, the charges revolved around the New Englander's emphasis on free will rather than orthodox predestination, his claim to have substantial support for his position within the church, and his insistence that Scripture adequately buttressed his ideas. Beecher was acquitted of the charges, and although his opponents pursued a three-year appeal to the General Assembly, their objections proved unavailing. Although he was to remain at Lane for eighteen years, the controversy smoldered on, eventually resulting in the secession of a portion of the Presbyterian Church (with Beecher remaining with the more liberal faction). Beecher resigned in 1850, returning to Boston in hopes of continuing his work there, but a stroke left him paralyzed, and he spent his remaining years at the home of his son, Henry Ward Beecher.

Beecher was very prominent in the early years of the Temperance Movement in America. As early as 1808 he had become an implacable foe of hard liquor by observing the effect it had on the Montauk Indians, who were supplied with whiskey by unscrupulous whites. He wrote later, "It was horrible, horrible...I swore a deep oath in my mind that it shouldn't be so." In Litchfield, he found a report by a committee of the Connecticut General Association of Congregational Churches assigned the task of determining, "How can drunkenness be prevented?" weak and inconsequential. Its conclusion was that little could be done to solve the problem. Enraged, Beecher moved to have the committee discharged and a new one appointed. It was, and he was made chairman. Only a day later he delivered his own report, which was succinct and to the point. It urged the General Association to recommend that all ministers discuss the problem before their congregations, that church members abstain from drink, that parents stop drinking at home, that employers provide more healthful beverages for their employees, and that voluntary associations be formed to help governmental officials enforce temperance statutes. It concluded with a peroration on the need of prompt and vigilant action, equating the evils of drink with that of a foreign invasion. His recommendations were adopted and became the basis of the first large-scale organized assault on drink in American history. Later on, Beecher followed up his initial blast against the traffic with his famous *Six Sermons on the Nature, Occasions, Signs, Evils and Remedy of Intemperance* (1826), which was instantly acclaimed as a classic polemic on behalf of total abstinence. After moving back to Massachusetts in the 1850s, he also championed the cause of the Maine Law and was applauded as a dry hero when the Bay State enacted its own prohibitory statute. His death in 1863 at the age of eighty-five brought to a close one of the earliest and most effective careers in American temperance history.

**Bibliography:**

A. *Six Sermons on the Nature, Occasions, Signs, Evils and Remedy of Intemperance* (1826; New York, 1827); *A Plea for the West* (Cincinnati, OH, 1832); *Views on Theology* (Cincinnati, OH, 1836); *Works*, 3 vols. (Boston, 1852–53); *Autobiography, Correspondence, etc., of Lyman Beecher, D.D.*, ed., Charles Beecher, 2 vols. (New York, 1864–65).

B. DAB 2, 135–36; NYT, Jan. 12, 1863; WW H, 117–18; Stuart C. Henry, *Unvanquished Puritan: A Portrait of Lyman Beecher* (Grand Rapids, MI, 1973); Charles R. Keller, *The Second Great Awakening in Connecticut* (New Haven, CT, 1942); Lyman B. Stowe, *Saints, Sinners, and Beechers* (New York, 1934).

**BENEZET, Anthony**   (31 January 1713, St. Quentin, France—3 May 1784, Philadelphia, PA). *Career*: teacher, Germantown (PA) Acad., 1739–42; teacher, Friends' English Public Sch., 1742–54; teacher and principal, private women's sch., Philadelphia, 1755–66, 1768–84.

Born to a Huguenot family in 1713, young Anthony Benezet did not grow up in his native France. Since the repeal of the Edict of Nantes in 1685, French Protestants had found their freedom to worship increasingly restricted, and in 1715 the Benezets left for a more sympathetic religious climate. They went first to Holland, then moved on to London, where the family spent sixteen years. In the British capital, Anthony was attracted to the Society of Friends, and he became a Quaker at the age of fourteen. In 1731 the Benezets moved again, this time to Philadelphia, where Anthony joined his brothers in the importing business. A career in commerce, however, did not prove to his liking, and Benezet soon felt a call to teach. He began with a position at Germantown Academy, just outside of Philadelphia, and then, moving on to other schools, made teaching his life's work. Benezet was an innovative educator, and he introduced some new departures in the field. In 1755, for example, he founded a girl's school to remedy what he believed to be the serious neglect of female education. A budding friendship with John Woolman brought him into contact with the still small antislavery movement in the United States, at this time almost exclusively a Quaker preserve. Benezet wrote extensively on the question of black slavery, and some of his work, notably, *A Caution and Warning to Great Britain and Her Colonies in a Short Representation of the Calamitous State of the Enslaved Negroes* (1766), and *Some Historical Account of Guinea, with an Inquiry Into the Rise and Progress of the Slave Trade* (1771), gained him a modest public reputation. Practicing what he preached, Benezet founded a school for black children in Philadelphia, leaving his modest estate at his death to support what was later called Benezet House.

Benezet's reform interests however, went beyond education and antislavery. He was also an early advocate of temperance. He first became interested at a Quaker meeting when a young man urged society members to cease manufacturing or using distilled beverages. Two years later, in 1774, Benezet produced a powerful tract entitled *The Mighty Destroyer Displayed* (1774). It is regarded as one of the first major publications on temperance produced in America. Speaking of the "dreadful havock" of alcoholic drinks, the pamphlet sought to present the best medical knowledge then available on the subject, and to present it in an objective and noninflammatory manner. Quoting one Dr. Hoffman, Benezet listed the "many fatal diseases" brought on by overindulgence in alcohol, among them "hectic fevers, jaundices, dropsies," and so on. Autopsies of alcoholics, he claimed, revealed the damage done to vital organs, liver, stomach, and bowels, by strong liquor. Again quoting medical opinion, Benezet suggested that those who lacked the strength of will to abstain ought at least to water their drinks, decreasing the quantity of alcohol regularly until only small amounts were with the water. Alcohol was never intended for human consumption, anyway, he insisted, but was strictly for medicinal purposes. Alcoholic beverages were poisons, no less, and should be treated as such. They produced fevers, inflammation of the brain, and ultimately death, the Quaker warned. The immediate impact of Benezet's temperance writings was slight, although there is little doubt that they had some influence on the later work of Benjamin Rush.*

**Bibliography:**

A. *A Caution and Warning . . . of the Calamitous State of the Enslaved Negroes* (Philadelphia, 1766); *An Historical Account of Guinea . . .* (Philadelphia, 1771); *The Mighty Destroyer Displayed* (1774; Trenton, NJ, 1779); *Short Account of the People Called Quakers* (Philadelphia, 1780); *Some Observations on the Situation, Disposition and Character of the Indian Natives of This Continent* (Philadelphia, 1784).

B. DAB 2, 177–78; DARB, 43–44; SEAP 1, 323–29; Wilson Armstead, *Anthony Benezet* (1859; Freeport, NY, 1971); Robert Vaux, *Memories of the Life of Anthony Benezet* (Philadelphia, 1817).

**BENNETT, William Wirt**   (10 October 1869, Oregon, IL—15 April 1932, Rockford, IL). *Education*: attended Univ. of Illinois, 1880s. *Career*: admitted to bar, IL, 1896; partner in securities investment business and legal practice, beginning 1896; mayor, Rockford, IL, 1911–23.

William Bennett, born in the same year as the founding of the Prohibition Party, possessed at least two of the most prominent chracteristics shared by many of his antiliquor contemporaries: He loved his church and he loved the law. And if the first gave him a basis for moral indignation against the liquor traffic, the second gave him a means of fighting it effectively. Admitted to the bar in 1896, Bennett established a successful legal practice and business career in Rockford, Illinois, where he also became a pillar of the local Congregational Church. Indeed, his church activity was constant over the years, and he served two terms (1923 and 1924) as moderator of the state Congregational Conference. His position in the community was such that his election as mayor in 1911 was no real surprise, an evident popularity confirmed by two additional successful races for the office. It was during his years as mayor, however, that Bennett's position on the liquor question came before the public. Until then he had not participated in antiliquor activity; but once in office, he emerged as a tenacious and skillful opponent of drink in general and of the license system in particular. Rockford, a city of some fifty thousand people, had lived with liquor licenses for years. Technically, the licenses were supposed to police the saloons, limit their number, and enable local authorities (through license revocations) to close objectionable establishments. Bennett found that the opposite was true: Illegal saloons—called "blind pigs"—flourished; and even legal bars often ignored control laws. In a sweeping crackdown, he pinpointed the location of Rockford's "blind pigs" and forced them out of business. The entire affair, as far as Bennett was concerned, demonstrated the futility of licensing as a means of controlling alcohol problems.

Bennett's campaign soon brought him national attention in temperance circles. He used the Rockford experience as an argument for prohibition as the only effective way to combat the traffic, and his message reached major audiences at such forums as the National Anti-Saloon League Convention of 1911. Back home, the mayor continued to wage his personal war against liquor. Under his leadership, the city voted itself dry in 1912, a fact which also enhanced Bennett's public recognition as a dry spokesman. And he clearly enjoyed the role. Indeed, his identification with the cause of national prohibition became such that he devoted considerable time to regional temperance efforts. He served as treasurer of the Illinois Anti-Saloon League in 1911, and then as president from 1918 to 1926. With Prohibition the law of the land, Bennett became active on the lecture circuit as well, promoting the enforcement of the antiliquor laws throughout the Midwest. Yet while temperance work was a major focus in his life, he was also active in other civic affairs. At one point he was president of the Illinois Mayor's Association as well as a trustee of Rockford College. Indeed, he was one of the first citizens of his community, and his commitment to its welfare clearly accounted for much of his temperance outlook. For Bennett, who fully reflected the attitudes of millions of other Americans of the day, "the demon" and the saloon—with their legion of attendant problems—simply had no place in decent communities.

**Bibliography:**

B. SEAP 1, 332; WW 1, 84–85.

**BENTLEY, Charles Eugene**    (30 April 1841, Warner's, NY—4 February 1905, Lincoln, NB?). *Education*: studied at Monroe Collegiate Inst. and Oneida Conference Sem., 1850s. *Career*: farmer in NY, IA, NB, 1860s to 1890; Baptist minister, Surprise, NB, 1880–?; temperance worker and political candidate of Prohibition and Liberty parties, 1886–1900.

Charles Eugene Bentley was a firm believer in the largely Republican politics of his adopted (1878) state of Nebraska until the presidential election of 1880. Until then, the small-town Baptist preacher hoped that the GOP would face up to the "liquor question" and outlaw beverage alcohol as part of its larger political program. He accordingly voted for Garfield and the rest of the Republican ticket that year, only to find later that his faith had been misplaced. The GOP, he gradually realized, would not make prohibition a central issue in the state, and Bentley became convinced that only a separate party with a focus on temperance would carry the day for the dry reform. He joined the small Nebraska Prohibition Party and quickly became one of its most active voices. He was presiding officer at its first convention in 1884, and he heartily approved of the endorsement it gave to former GOP Kansas Governor John P. St. John* as the dry candidate for president. The same convention nominated Bentley for the state legislature, his initial foray into the political lists. Although he lost (along with the rest of the ticket), he and the party doggedly pursued electoral office on behalf of their cause. Two years later, Bentley set his sights even higher, running for Congress; he then took over as chairman of the Nebraska Prohibition Party Executive Committee in 1890. In that office he led a tough campaign for a dry amendment to the state constitution.

The peak of Bentley's political career as a Prohibitionist came in the 1890s. He ran successively for governor and U.S. senator, amassing a respectable (for a Prohibitionist candidate) 25,000 votes in the latter bid. In 1896, however, he was caught up in a bitter factional struggle within the party. The argument centered on the Free Silver issue, which had become a major national concern over the 1890s. When the dominant wing of the Prohibition Party failed to endorse Free Silver at its 1896 convention, a minority group, including Bentley, bolted the gathering in protest. In actuality, the split reflected even broader differences among Prohibitionists. Older leaders wanted a narrow focus on temperance work, while others, "broad-gaugers," to use the term of historian Jack Blocker, wanted a sweeping reform program. Bentley stood with the "broad-gaugers," seeking a party responsive to the wider needs of the nation and with greater voter appeal. Thus, while the parent, single-issue party nominated Joshua Levering* of Maryland for president, the bolted faction, meeting as the newly organized National Party (also called the Liberty Party) chose Bentley as their standard bearer. For the Nebraska crusader it was an honor, but one more symbolic than real. As the election heated up, most of the National Party membership deserted to the campaign of Democrat and Populist William Jennings Bryan.* Yet Bentley faced his predicament without recriminations and after the election returned to the leadership of the Nebraska party, where he remained an effective campaigner and administrator. Thus the Prohibition Party, while never a national power, was at least enduring, a true legacy of men like Charles Bentley.

**Bibliography:**

B. SEAP 1, 333–34; WW 1, 86; Jack S. Blocker, Jr., *Retreat from Reform: The Prohibition Movement in the United States, 1890–1913* (Westport, CT, 1976).

**BERRY, Joseph Flintoft**   (13 May 1856, Aylmer, Canada—11 February 1931, Binghamton, NY). *Education*: studied at Milton Acad., Ontario, 1870s; D.D., Lawrence Univ., 1898; LLD. (honorary), Cornell Coll., IA, 1904; Syracuse Univ., 1905. *Career*: ordained in Methodist Church, 1874; served various Michigan pastorates, 1876 to 1880s; associate editor, *Michigan Christian Advocate*, 1884–90; editor, *Epworth Herald*, 1890–94; elected bishop, 1904.

Throughout his life as a minister and editor, Joseph Berry always stood squarely against legal liquor. A sickly youth, he completed his education only after a valiant personal struggle to overcome his health problems. Ordained in 1874, his first charges were pastorates in small Michigan towns; and had it not been for editorial opportunities arising, it is entirely likely that Berry would have passed his years as a relatively obscure country parson. In 1884, however, while leading the congregation at Mt. Clemens, Michigan, he was asked to help edit the Methodist *Michigan Christian Advocate*—and it was as a religious editor that he made his first mark in life. He stayed with the *Advocate* until 1890, compiling a reputation for efficiency and skill as well as a forceful pen on behalf of Methodist moral positions. When the church established the *Epworth Herald*, the official publication of the Epworth League (the Methodist organization for young people), it called on Berry to assume the editor's job. In his four years in the position (1890–94), he vastly expanded the *Herald's* circulation and at the same time built up the membership of the Epworth League itself. Speaking with the voice of the league, Berry also used the *Herald* as a platform for the temperance crusade. Berry was in full sympathy with the dry stances of the Methodist Church from the beginning of his career and made the cause a central part of Epworth activity. In a typical editorial, he spurred on league members "in the name of God and righteousness and of besotted men and suffering women and starving children, we call upon you to get ready!" The liquor traffic was the enemy, he warned, and "This means *war*." It was not enough, Berry proclaimed, just to be sympathetic toward the dry cause. The age demanded action, and he wanted Methodists to work actively to topple the evil—and if necessary, even to be "martyrs" for the final victory. In recognition of his service, the Methodist General Conference elected him a bishop in 1904, helping to assure the continued dominance of the antiliquor position within the church hierarchy.

**Bibliography:**

B. SEAP 1, 337–38; WW 1, 89.

**BIDWELL, John**    (5 August 1819, Ripley Hills, NY—4 April 1900, Chico, CA). *Education*: studied at Kingsville Acad., Ashtabula, OH, 1836. *Career*: principal, Kingsville Acad., 1837; schoolteacher, Darke Co., OH, 1838; farming and teaching, near Weston, MO, 1839–40; work at Sutter's Fort, CA, 1841–45; served against Mexico in California rebellions, 1845–46; gold prospector, 1849; established Rancho Chico, 1849 (farmer until 1900); member, California Senate, 1849; member, U.S. House of Representatives, 1865–67; active in California political and civil affairs, 1867–1900.

A streak of luck ran through the career of John Bidwell. An eager young man, he tried his hand at teaching and farming before immigrating to California in 1841 via one of the first wagon trains to arrive from the East in that Pacific coast territory. He was naturalized as a citizen of the Mexican province in 1844, but then took part in the Bear Flag revolt in 1846. He ended up a major in that brief struggle, which saw California finally become part of the United States. Already a man of some public note then, his notoriety soared when during the Gold Rush of 1849 Bidwell struck it rich along the Feather River near Sutter's Fort. Suddenly a wealthy man, he bought a 22,000-acre homestead—Rancho Chico—which he steadily built into one of the most productive ranches in the state. By the early 1850s he had a reputation as California's most prominent agriculturalist, and Rancho Chico, skillfully managed, had established Bidwell as one of the state's richest men by his early thirties. He also became one of the most active politically. A Democrat, he served in the State Senate, taking a major role in party affairs. During the Civil War, however, he was staunchly pro-Federal (he was briefly a major general of militia, probably the result of his opposition to California secessionists), supported Lincoln, and was elected to Congress as a Unionist in 1864. He refused renomination in 1866, but returned home with a keen sense of public duty. Indeed, Bidwell came back a reformer with an evident desire to cleanse his home state of corruption and social evils—just as the war had cleansed the nation of secession and human slavery.

To Bidwell, signs of social "decay and corruption" in California were all too obvious. He saw an entire array of evils threatening stability and democratic institutions. The unrestricted immigration of Chinese, the growth of business monopolies, and "the great liquor power" seemed, in his mind, to directly imperil the republic, and he spent his postbellum years campaigning actively against them all. He ran unsuccessfully for governor in 1875 at the head of an Anti-Monopoly Party, sat in an anti-Chinese convention in 1886, and joined the

Prohibition Party in 1890. In his attachment to temperance he had the zealous support of his wife, Annie Ellicott Bidwell, who had a local reputation as an antiliquor crusader herself. John stood once as the Prohibitionist candidate for governor (1890), and in 1892 headed the ticket for president. Upon accepting the nomination, he declared that the dry party was the only political group "organized at this time to save the country." With Annie campaigning tirelessly at his side, he gained over 264,000 votes, one of the best showings of any Prohibition Party candidate. The 1892 election, however, was his last. He retired to Rancho Chico, although he continued his interest in public affairs (he had, while pursuing his political fortunes, served as a University of California regent and donated land for the construction of a state college). Upon his death in 1900 he was one of the most respected men in the state.

**Bibliography:**

A. *Addresses, Reminiscences, etc. of Gen. John Bidwell*, comp. C. C. Royce (Chico, CA, 1907); *A Journey to California...* (San Francisco, 1937); *In California Before the Gold Rush* (Los Angeles, 1948); *Echoes of the Past: An Account of the First Immigration to California...* (Chico, CA, 19—?).

B. DAB 2, 247–48; SEAP 1, 343–44; WW H, 123; Rockwell Denis Hunt, *John Bidwell: Prince of California Pioneers* (Caldwell, IN, 1942).

**BITTENBENDER, Ada Matilda Cole**    (3 August 1848, Macedonia, PA—15 December 1925, Lincoln, NB). *Education*: graduated from Lowell's Commercial Coll., 1869; studied at Pennsylvania Normal Sch., 1874–75; studied at Frobel Normal Inst., 1876–77. *Career*: editor, *Osceola Record*, Osceola, NB, 1879–81; editor, local Farmers' Alliance journal, 1881; delegate, Nebraska State Board of Agriculture, 1881; founder and president, Nebraska Woman Suffrage Association, 1881–82; admitted to bar, NB, 1882; temperance organizing and legal work for WCTU, 1882–92; private legal practice, 1892 to circa 1920; writing on philosophical subjects, circa 1911 to 1920s.

Ada Bittenbender (born Cole) fit the classic mold of the nineteenth-century broad-based reformer. Well educated and articulate, she was in early sympathy with both the Temperance and women's suffrage movements; and she was further encouraged toward reform by her marriage in 1878 to attorney Henry Clay Bittenbender, an ardent dry and later an official in the Prohibition Party. The same year, she and her husband moved from their native Pennsylvania to Nebraska, where she began her career in earnest. Using her literary talents, she edited agricultural journals for a few years, gaining enough recognition to be named the first woman member of the State Board of Agriculture. She also developed a strong commitment to feminism and emerged as a regional champion of women's rights. Helping to found the Nebraska State Woman Suffrage Association, she served as its president in 1882 and in the same year (after reading law with her husband) broke new ground for her sex by being the first woman admitted to the state bar. The most promising outlet for her reform enthusiasm was the Nebraska chapter of the Woman's Christian Temperance Union, in which she quickly established herself as a dominant voice. Joining in 1882, by 1883 she had become state superintendent of temperance legislation (a position she held until 1889) and had begun to barrage the legislature with proposed bills. She successfully urged the passage of measures giving women equal rights to the guardianship of their children, building an institution for delinquent women, introducing temperance education in the public schools, and abolishing tobacco sales to minors. And while she was never able to secure an actual prohibition law, her track record was good enough to propel her to greater responsibility within the WCTU.

Her rise to national prominence came in 1887, when she was chosen National WCTU superintendent of legislation and petitions. To this she quickly added duties as an attorney for the National Union, with her office in Washington, D.C. There, her legal and lobbying talents reached full flower. She became a familiar figure before congressional committees, where she frequently testified on legal aspects of temperance legislation. Mrs. Bittenbender also won admission to practice before the Supreme Court, only the third woman in American history to gain this distinction. (The temperance crusade, in this case, clearly served as a vehicle in advancing her legal career). On all platforms, however, she was noted as an elegant and persuasive advocate of her cause. While she strongly urged the passage of a national prohibition amendment during her Washington years, she seems to have realized that the time was not yet right for such a measure. She reserved her chief disappointment for the failure of a series of proposals which would have forbidden the sale of liquor in the District of Columbia and the federal territories. And perhaps ultimately frustrated at the slow pace of reform, she slowly cut her ties with the WCTU. She returned to Nebraska in 1890, sought no more union offices, and instead joined the Prohibition Party. She received almost 5 percent of the vote when she ran as its candidate for a seat on the State Supreme Court in 1891. Yet this was her last major reform effort; tired by years of temperance work, she returned first to her legal practice and then to writing. She apparently showed little public interest as the dry crusade rolled toward the National Prohibition she once sought with such skill and dedication.

## Bibliography:

A. *Woman Suffrage Campaign Song Book* (Lincoln, NB, 1882); *The National Prohibitory Amendment Guide* (Chicago, 1889); *History of the Nebraska W.C.T.U. Department of Legislation and Petitions* (Lincoln, NB, 1893); *Tedos and Tisod: A Temperance Story* (Lincoln, NB, 1911); "History of the Woman's Christian Temperance Union in Nebraska" (unpublished manuscript, Nebraska State Historical Society).

B. *Lincoln* (NB) *Star*, Dec. 15, 1925; NAW 1, 153–54; SEAP 1, 348–49; B. V. Austin, ed., *The Temperance Leaders of America* (1896); Frances E. Willard and Mary A. Livermore, eds., *A Woman of the Century* (New York, 1893).

**BLACK, James**   (23 September 1823, Lewisburg, PA—19 December 1893, Lancaster, PA). *Education*: studied at Lewisburg Acad., 1840–43. *Career*: admitted to bar, PA, 1846; organized Conestoga (PA) division of Sons of Temperance, 1846; grand worthy chief templar, Pennsylvania Independent Order of Good Templars, 1858; right grand worthy councilor, Lancaster Lodge of Good Templars, 1864; founder, Prohibition Party, 1869; Prohibition Party activities, to 1893; railroad and financial interests, to 1893.

Not satisfied with the progress of the Temperance Movement in the years immediately following the Civil War, James Black, a lawyer and longtime temperance advocate, became convinced of the need to move the antiliquor crusade into the middle of the national political arena. His struggle toward this end earned him recognition as a founder of the Prohibition Party and, in temperance circles, fame as its first presidential candidate Black, as he later related the story, became a temperance man at age sixteen. While employed as a mule driver on a Pennsylvania canal construction project, older workers supposedly forced him to join them in a binge. Recovering from his drunken stupor, the young Black pledged himself never to touch another drop and to do what he could to save others from alcholism. Shortly afterward, he joined (in 1840) a local Washingtonian society—an offshoot of the Washingtonian temperance revival of the period—and six years later helped organize the Conestoga division of the Sons of Temperance. Participation in the fraternal lodge no doubt served to assuage his personal fears of drink, but Black had set his sights on the liquor question considerably higher. In the early 1850s he began his first serious prohibitionist political activity, serving as chairman of the Lancaster County Prohibition Commmittee. He had high hopes of securing a "Maine Law" to dry out Pennsylvania. In this he failed, but there is little doubt that his campaign stimulated considerable interest in the measure and that the committtee rallied enough support to elect two dry candidates to the state legislature. His interest in fraternal temperance groups also remained high, and in 1857 he was a cofounder of a local lodge of the International Order of Good Templars (modeled generally after the Freemasons), in which he took an active leadership role. During this period Black showed himself to be utterly uncompromising on the matter of total abstinence: He persuaded the Templars to reject even cider drinkers from membership and during the Civil War called on President Lincoln to end whiskey rations in the army. Thus, with the possible exceptions of Neal Dow* and Lyman Beecher*, it is doubtful that the antebellum period produced a more strident opponent of "the demon".

After the war, Black acted forcefully to revitalize the reform crusade, which had lost considerable momentum during the conflict. At the 1865 National Temperance Convention in Saratoga, New York, he took the first major step in this direction. He secured approval of an ambitious plan calling for a dry National Publication House, a financial seed of $100,000, and James Black to manage the entire operation. He then worked to foster support for an independent political party based on the prohibition issue. In early 1867, under the auspices of the state Good Templars, a convention met in Harrisburg, Pennsylvania, to consider the political implications of the matter (with Black in the chair). This convention, meeting in subsequent years, finally emerged as the separate Prohibition Party in 1869, and it was no surprise that Black received its first presidential nomination in 1872 (although the party did consider other names, such as Benjamin F. Butler* and Horace Greeley*). He tallied only some 5,600 votes in the general election, but the party at least was launched, and Black remained a central voice in its affairs until his death. Nor did he confine his activities to politics. He was a prominent Methodist layman and generously supported his church (over the years, Black had done well in railroad and other business investments), and as an avid reader, he compiled the most complete temperance library of his generation. With his passing in 1893, the antiliquor cause—as well as its opponents—acknowledged the loss of one of the most accomplished reformers of the century.

**Bibliography:**

A. *The Cider Question* (Chicago, 1862); *Is There a Necessity for a Prohibition Party?* (New York, 1876); *Brief History of Prohibition* (NewYork, 1880); *History of the National Prohibition Party* (New York, 1885).
B. DAB 2, 310; SEAP 1, 351; WW H, 126.

**BLAIR, HENRY WILLIAM**    (6 December 1834, Campton, NH—14 March 1920, Washington, DC). *Education*: A.M. (honorary), Dartmouth Coll., 1873. *Career*: admitted to bar, NH, 1859; appointed solicitor, Grafton Co., NH, 1860; Union army officer (rose to lieutenant colonel), 1862–65; legal practice, 1865 to 1870s; member, New Hampshire Assembly, 1866; member, New Hampshire Senate, 1867–69; member, U.S. House of Representatives, 1875–79, 1903–5; member, U.S. Senate, 1879–91; legal practice, 1895–1920.

Over his long tenure in public office, including twelve years in the U.S. Senate, Henry Blair combined orthodox Republican concerns on trade and economic policies with an enthusiasm for social reform that at times bordered on the zealous. After completing his legal training and compiling an impressive record as an infantry commander during the Civil War, he plunged into a life of public service that rapidly carried him to national recognition. He was elected to Congress for the first time in 1875 (after serving a political apprenticeship in the New Hampshire legislature) and served in either the House or the Senate for most of the next two decades. Blair quickly emerged as a man of multiple interests—the epitome of the broad-based reformer. He pioneered efforts to support public education with federal funds, fought hard for women's suffrage (on several occasions he introduced unsuccessful suffrage amendments to the Constitution), championed the rights of labor (creation of the Department of Labor was, in great measure, due to his efforts), and argued at length in favor of temperance, veterans' pension benefits, the rights of blacks, conservation, and other causes. Many of Blair's positions marked him as a man ahead of his time and did not fare well in Congress. Yet legislative success was not his yardstick of a measure's worth. For governing Blair's activities was an intense sense of religious mission: The great advances in American history, he claimed, came through the power of the pulpit, and following its lead, to labor in the cause of reform was doing God's work.

Central to the senator's reform efforts, however, was his commitment to the antiliquor crusade. He argued at length that the abolition of the liquor traffic was as noble a goal as the abolition of slavery—indeed, that it would save mankind from slavery to drink. Moreover, he was convinced that temperance lay at the root of many other social evils and that the elimination of "the demon" would make other reform struggles that much easier. Thus in 1876 he offered a resolution in the House of Representatives calling for a prohibitory amendment to the Constitution. Compared with the later Eighteenth Amendment, Blair's was a fairly moderate proposal. It would have banned the manufacture and sales of beverage alcohol after 1900, allowing time to compensate the liquor business and educate the public on the need for the measure. Blair's amendment never generated major support, but it was the first attempt at a constitutional solution to the temperance question. And as Blair predicted, when national prohibition finally did become the law of the land in 1920, it came under a much harder law than his. Despite this defeat, however, the New Hampshire crusader remained a leading spokesman for the cause. He constantly urged the church to champion prohibition, and, in his monumental history of *The Temperance Movement* (1888), predicted that civilization would rise or fall on the liquor issue (he foresaw, however, a dry victory in the end). His interest in public affairs extended beyond his retirement from the Senate (1891), and he was a familiar figure around Washington, D.C., where he moved in 1895. Turning down a federal judgeship, he accepted the post of ambassador to China, but the Chinese government refused to accept him, a result of his vote, while a senator, to exclude Chinese immigrants from the United States. He finished his years as a private attorney and was recognized as one of the deans of American reform.

**Bibliography:**

A. *The Temperance Movement: Or, the Conflict Between Man and Alcohol* (Boston, 1888).

B. *Congressional Record*, 52nd Cong., 1st sess., 3151 ff.; DAB 2, 334–35; SEAP 1, 354–55; WW 1, 103; Ezra S. Stearns, *History of Plymouth, New Hampshire* (1906).

**BLOOMER, Amelia Jenks**    (27 May 1818, Homer, NY—30 December 1894, Council Bluffs, IA). *Career*: schoolteacher, Seneca Co., NY, circa 1835; governess and tutor, Waterloo, NY, 1837–40; contributor to local newspapers, NY, 1840s; deputy postmaster, Seneca Falls, NY, 1849–53; founder and editor, *Lily*, 1849–55; active reform and suffrage writer, lecturer, and organizer, beginning 1850s.

Amelia Jenks Bloomer was long sympathetic to reform causes, but it was not until after her marriage that she became actively involved in the crusading ferment of antebellum America. Indeed, when Dexter Bloomer—a successful Quaker lawyer, antislavery advocate, and joint editor of a Whig newspaper—offered his wife encouragement in her interests, she responded by launching one of the most notable reform careers of her generation. As was fairly typical of the period, Mrs. Bloomer first became a public figure through her work for the Temperance Movement. She began by writing short articles for her husband's newspaper on "social, moral, and political questions" and then started contributing to a number of New York temperance and reform journals, including the *Temperance Star*, the *Free Soil Union*, and the *Water Bucket*. Her commitment to the dry cause stemmed at least in part from her interest in the Washingtonian Movement, which swept a good deal of the country in the mid-1840s and generally increased popular consciousness of the liquor question. The dangers alcoholism posed to the stability of the home, and thus to the social position of many nineteenth-century women, particularly caught public attention. By 1840, Amelia had helped organize a Ladies Temperance Society in her home town of Seneca Falls, and in January of 1849 she began publishing the *Lily*, intended as a small antiliquor newspaper. The *Lily*, one of the first papers in the nation (if not the first) to be founded and operated by a woman, steadily proved a financial success, and its notoriety grew as Bloomer's own interests began to expand. In 1848, she had attended—though only as a spectator—the famous Seneca Falls meeting on women's rights (she did not sign the women's Declaration of Independence). But as publisher of the *Lily*, her reform activities soon included the women's rights and suffrage movements, and the journal's lively pages soon included the writings of Susan B. Anthony,* Elizabeth Cady Stanton, and other suffrage advocates. Thus temperance, for Bloomer, proved a springboard to broader reform goals.

Increasing public recognition as a feminist brought fame to both Amelia and to the *Lily*. It also brought a certain amount of controversy: For a number of years she advocated (but did not invent) the wearing of billowing, Turkish-style pantaloons now called (after her) bloomers. She dropped the fad, however, when it threatened to divert attention from what she considered serious reform. And in this regard, Bloomer always stayed close to the temperance cause. She continued to lecture widely on the subject, even urging women to divorce drunken husbands. Fraternal temperance groups were also a favorite activity: She was a member of the Independent Order of Good Templars in both New York (where she held office as deputy grand chief templar of the state lodge) and in Ohio, where the Bloomers moved in 1853. Mrs. Bloomer insisted, however, on equality for women in the fight against liquor; and when a New York City dry convention (1853) refused to seat females, she took part in a walkout and the organization of a rival Whole World's Temperance Convention. In 1855, the Bloomers moved again, this time to Council Bluffs, Iowa (Dexter Bloomer, it seems, had developed a passion for living on the frontier), where Amelia found it uneconomical to continue publishing the *Lily*. (It folded in 1856, a year after she sold it.) But she kept up her own personal crusading, helping to organize temperance and suffrage groups and churches in her adopted state, as well as performing relief work for soldiers during the Civil War. She was in failing health in her later years, although she never lost interest in public affairs or her personal identification with what she considered the noblest causes of her era.

**Bibliography:**

A. ed., *Lily: A Ladies Journal Devoted to Temperance and Literature*, 1849–55.

B. DAB 2, 385; NAW 1, 179–81; WW H, 129; Dexter C. Bloomer, *Life and Writings of Amelia Bloomer* (1895; New York, 1975); Charles Neilson Gattey, *The Bloomer Girls* (London, 1967); Margaret Farrand Thorp, *Female Persuasion* (New Haven, CT, 1949).

**BOK, Edward William**   (9 October 1863, Helder, Netherlands—9 January 1930, Lake Wales, FL). *Education*: Brooklyn, NY, public schools; LLD. (honorary), conferred by Pope Pius X, 1907, Rutgers Univ., 1923, Tufts Univ., 1923, Williams Coll., 1926. *Career*: stenographer, 1884–88; conducted Bok Syndicate, 1886–91; editor-in-chief, *Ladies Home Journal*, 1889–1919; philanthropist and author, 1920–30.

Edward Bok is an interesting example of American values. The way in which his role as a man of letters and philanthropist merged with his temperance bias says much of how the finest American sensibilities of reform and the public good could unite with the dry crusade. Bok immigrated from Holland at six years of age in 1870, son of an impoverished but distinguished family (the Bok line had included admirals, high government officials, and justices). He started school without knowing any English, but he proved a quick study and by his teens and early twenties had mastered the language well enough to land several jobs as a stenographer and editor (notably, he wrote for the *Brooklyn Eagle* at age nineteen). He rose subsequently to editor of advertising at Charles Scribner's Sons in 1887, the proprietor of the Bok Syndicate Press beginning in 1886, and editor-in-chief of the *Ladies Home Journal* in 1889. He remained with the *Journal* until 1919 and during his long affiliation with the magazine established a reputation for editorial excellence and innovation, reform sentiments, and integrity. He brought such talent as Bret Harte, Mark Twain, Rudyard Kipling, and William Deans Howells to the pages of the *Journal*, plus articles on home and child care, religion, art, public affairs, and women's personal problems. The *Journal* also offered a forum for Bok's personal views on issues of the day. He editorialized on behalf of temperance, women's suffrage, political reform, environmental protection, and public safety. Under his care, the magazine was a major financial success with the loyalty of millions of readers.

Throughout his life, Bok's interests in reform were genuine and unwavering. He was one of the first to discuss the issue of venereal disease in the popular press, and he fought hard on a number of conservation questions (including protecting Niagara Falls from power interests). After World War I he was also one of the country's leading advocates of international peace. Yet in all of his efforts, Bok's approach was that of a rational individual who sought to lead through reason, not fanaticism. So it was in his advocacy of temperance. Many of his arguments against liquor were identical to those of the formal temperance organizations, but he never led a chapter of any dry society and his voice was never shrill. In one article, he noted that he based his personal abstinence in part on the fact that alcohol had ruined some of the best minds he had ever known. "A clear mind," he warned, "and liquor do not go together." It was his wish that good citizens lead by example, that they give up alcohol so that others would follow their lead out of a sense of doing the right and intelligent thing. As calm and reasoned as his reforming style was, however, Bok still took great pride in his antiliquor work. In his Pulitzer–Prize–winning autobiography, *The Americanization of Edward Bok* (1921), he devoted considerable space to temperance activities, which he thought were necessary in the accomplishment of other reform goals (a view also shared by many other temperance workers). The coming of the 1920s, though, lessened his antiliquor pursuits. He retired from the *Ladies Home Journal*, and his time became increasingly spent on his peace campaign and his various philanthropic enterprises (he was a major bene- factor, for example, of the Philadelphia Symphony Orchestra). Yet his career had amply demonstrated the appeal of the dry reform to Americans of humane and liberal persuasions, as well as the power of the popular press in fostering the cause.

**Bibliography:**

A. *Henry Ward Beecher Memorial* (privately printed, 1887); *Before He Is Twenty* (Philadelphia, 1894); *The Young Man and the Church* (Philadelphia, 1894); *Successward: A Young Man's Book for Young Men* (New York, 1895); *The Americanization of Edward Bok: The Autobiography of a Dutch Boy Fifty Years After* (New York, 1921); *Twice Thirty: Some Short and Simple Annals of the Road* (New York, 1925).

B. DAB Supp. 1, 91–93; NYT, Jan. 10, 1930; SEAP 1, 36; *Ladies Home Journal* (March 1930; *Publishers' Weekly*, Jan. 18, 1930.

**BOLTON, Sarah Knowles**  (15 September 1841, Farmington, CT—21 February 1916, Cleveland, OH). *Education*: graduated from Hartford Female Sem., 1860. *Career*: teacher, Natchez, MI, 1860; author, beginning 1860s; associate editor, *The Congregationalist*, 1878–81; temperance activities, beginning 1873; work for the American Humane Society, 1900s to 1916.

An active reformer for most of her adult life, Sarah Bolton was first drawn into the Temperance Movement after her marriage to Charles Edward Bolton in 1866. Charles was a man of generous humanitarian sentiments, and it was not long before husband and wife were deeply committed to the cause. They became active in local temperance activities, and in 1874 both took a prominent role in the Woman's Crusade in Ohio, which intensified her hatred of the liquor traffic. With the founding of the WCTU in the aftermath of the crusade, Mrs. Bolton quickly became an ardent member of the new organization. She had acquired a modest literary reputation before her reforming days (as a poet and novelist), and she showed no hesitation in writing for the movement. She wrote a short book for the cause, *The Present Problem* (1874), but it proved of little impact, selling only some 250 copies. But Sarah continued in the crusade undiscouraged, ultimately rising to a leadership position. For several years she served as assistant corresponding secretary of the national group, working closely with WCTU President Frances E. Willard.* She also returned to the literary war against liquor. The failure of her first dry title behind her, she employed her energetic pen and considerable talents for turning a phrase on behalf of the cause once more, and she authored a number of additional volumes and tracts on alcohol-related issues.

Mrs. Bolton was as devoted to writing as she was to reform, and while working for the WCTU and the Women's Christian Association she wrote prolifically, producing two volumes of poetry, several novels, and a series of successful biographical works designed to assist in popular education. Written with enthusiasm and vigorous narrative, their titles accurately reflect their character: *Poor Boys Who Became Famous* (1885), *Girls Who Became Famous* (1886), and *Famous American Statesmen* (1888). Her reform interests, as was true of many reformists of the WCTU, were as diversified as the different genres she utilized in her writing, for they encompassed issues ranging from temperance and women's rights to the working conditions of laborers and animal welfare. She wrote an imressive and influential paper on the former subject, having spent two years in Europe studying methods used to upgrade working conditions, which she read before the American Science Association in Saratoga, New York. Though perhaps not one of the more outstanding figures of the Temperance Movement, she was certainly as committed and loyal to the dry crusade as any of its leading spokesmen, and her career typified the dedication and broad range of talents which made the WCTU the successful organization it was in the late nineteenth century.

### Bibliography:

A. *The Present Problem: A Temperance Story* (New York, 1874); *Famous American Authors* (New York, 1887); *Lives of Girls Who Became Famous* (New York, 1895); *A Country Idyl, and Other Stories* (New York, 1898); *Sarah K. Bolton: Pages from an Intimate Autobiography*, ed. Charles K. Bolton (Boston, 1923).

B. DAB 2, 423–24; WW 1, 114; Charles K. Bolton, *The Boltons in Old and New England* (Boston, 1890).

**BOOLE, Ella Alexander**   (26 July 1858, Van Wert, OH—13 March 1952, New York, NY). *Education*: A.B., Coll. of Wooster, OH, 1878; A.M., Coll.

of Wooster, 1881; Ph.D., Coll. of Wooster, 1895; LLD. (honorary), Coll. of Wooster, 1938. *Career*: various leadership positions in U.S. and international temperance organizations, 1885–1903, 1909–52.

Ella Boole dated the birth of her sympathies for the temperance cause from the Woman's Crusade of the early 1870s, when she was still a teenager. The convictions awakened in the young girl led to one of the longest and most distinguished records of accomplishment in the annals of the Temperance Movement. Her active service began with her marriage (1883) to Methodist Reverend William H. Boole, a co-founder of the Prohibition Party; he soon took a pastorate near the New York City Bowery, and the Booles were active in mission work among the area's many alcoholics. At the same time, she earned a reputation as one of New York State's most dedicated temperance leaders. She had become state WCTU corresponding secretary as early as 1886 and had risen to the presidency of the group by 1898. An accomplished speaker and a good organizer, she used the WCTU as a means to further not only temperance but a host of other reforms as well. Taking the challenge of National WCTU President Frances Willard* to "Do Everything" to heart, Boole worked on behalf of child labor reform, women's suffrage, international peace, and related causes. Still concerned with temperance, she left the WCTU in 1903 for a position with the Women's Board of Home Missions of the Presbyterian Church; but she returned in 1909 to lead the New York Union as president. From that point on, her stature in temperance circles grew steadily. In 1914, after participating in National WCTU affairs, Mrs. Boole won election as a national vice president; and in this capacity she took a leading role in rallying support among women's groups for constitutional prohibition. In 1920, with Prohibition an accomplished fact, she became treasurer of the World WCTU (although she retained the National WCTU office), and ran for the Senate on the Prohibition Party ticket. (She had even campaigned vigorously, if unsuccessfully, for the Republican nomination.) By the mid-1920s, few WCTU women could boast of having contributed as much to what at the time seemed the victory of the dry cause.

When Boole assumed the presidency of the National WCTU in 1925, she saw her mission as contributing to the effective enforcement of the Volstead Act. She soon emerged as one of the most vigorous and uncompromising defenders of Prohibition; speaking before WCTU gatherings and political groups, she urged Americans to support the dry laws and to oppose any modifications in enforcement measures. With the courage of her convictions, she forcefully defended her positions before congressional committees—even to the point of tongue-lashing them when she considered them hostile or uncooperative. She poured her hopes for the Eighteenth Amendment into her book, *Give Prohibition Its Chance* (1929), which the dry faithful bought by the thousands; she was unable, however, to counter the declining public support for the temperance cause, which had become fully evident by the time the book was published. On the defensive, she dug in her heels and refused to condone changes in the Volstead Act—an obstinacy which drew fire not only from wets but from drys who feared that all would be lost unless compromises were reached. By 1930 the situation had deteriorated to such an extent that she was ridiculed during an appearance at the Women's National Republican Club—all of which seemed mild enough compared with the devastating blows the dry cause suffered in the election of 1932 and the coming of Repeal in 1933. Mrs. Boole took some consolation in the fact that temperance workers still held her in high regard. She served as president of the World WCTU between 1931 and 1947 and retained emeritus status after that. But there was no denying her disappointment over the losing struggle for Prohibition at home: Rather than presiding over the WCTU as its goal of total abstinence became a permanent reality, she instead endured the humiliation of defeat while leading an increasingly unpopular cause.

**Bibliography:**

A. *Give Prohibition Its Chance* (Evanston, IL, 1926); "Should the Sale of Liquor Be Legalized?" *Congressional Digest*, Jan. 12, 1933.

B. DAB Supp. 5, 79–80; NYT, March 14, 1952; SEAP 2, 366; WW 3, 89; Helen E. Tyler, *Where Prayer and Purpose Meet* (Evanston, IL, 1949); S. Walker, "With Ella in the Desert," *Outlook*, April 9, 1930.

**BOOTH, Evangeline Cory**  (25 December 1865, London—17 July 1950, Hartsdale, NY). *Education*: privately educated at home; M.A. (honorary), Tufts Coll., 1921; LLD. (honorary), Columbia Univ., 1939. *Career*: commanded Salvation Army operations in London area, 1891–96; Salvation Army command in Canada, 1896–1904; U.S. command, 1904–34; generalship of the Salvation Army, 1934–39; active retirement.

Evangeline Booth was the daughter of General William Booth, founder of the Salvation Army. Under the tutelage of her parents, she developed the religious faith and sense of dedication to the poor and rich that has marked the Salvation Army since its birth. As a youth she worked in London, where her acts of charity and help earned her the name "White Angel of the Slums." A good organizer and speaker, she rose quickly to the command of London area operations and took control of the army's international training facilities. Evangeline also developed a reputation as a problem solver, and General Booth frequently called on her talents whenever a situation demanded a diplomat or a troubleshooter. Her abilities in this regeard resulted in her first trip to the United States, in an effort to smooth difficulties between her father and brother, who commanded the army in America. Then, after commanding in Canada since 1896, she assumed the leadership in America herself in 1904 and began actively broadening the denomination's work on behalf of reform causes, relief efforts, and social services. The army established a network of homes for working women, administered disaster assistance, and arranged aid for the unemployed, released convicts, unwed mothers, and American troops overseas in World War I. This last effort in particular created a wave of popularity for the army and for Booth personally (she was awarded the Distinguished Service Medal in 1919).

This popularity stood her in good stead when she worked on behalf of Prohibition. She had long believed in temperance as a means of combatting poverty and maintaining the stability of home life; and her acquaintance with WCTU President Frances Willard* had familiarized her with the American dry crusade even before she took her post in the United States. Booth was a persuasive advocate for the cause, and she spoke widely on the subject. Unlike many other temperance workers, she was able to amass considerable information on the direct results of excessive drinking from the Salvation Army's national social work operations—all of which gave her arguments particular force. With the coming of Prohibition, Miss Booth was initially pleased with the results, and she reported a variety of improvements in the lives of the urban poor as a consequence. While she never argued that all drinking had ended or that the Eighteenth Amendment was on its way to eliminating poverty altogether (a promise some of the most extreme drys had made), she did insist that army field workers saw less drunkenness, less family violence, more money spent on family necessities, and a general improvement in the lives of those the army served. On this limited basis, she urged the nation to continue its dry experiment and lent her voice against Repeal. In 1934, however, she was called away from the temperance fight (which by then had been lost anyway) and back to London when she was elected the fourth general of her denomination. The end of her five-year generalship in 1939 marked the final tenure in that office for a Booth and the shift to a more corporate leadership in the Salvation Army. Miss Booth herself then returned to the United States, where she had become a citizen in 1923.

**Bibliography:**

A. *Love Is All* (New York, 1908); with Grace Livingston Hill, *The War Romance of the Salvation Army* (Philadelphia, 1919); *Prohibition and Its Early Results* (London, 1920); *Some Have Stopped Drinking* (Westerville OH, 1928); *Toward a Better World* (Garden City, NY, 1928).

B. NAW 1, 204–7; NYT, July 18, 1950; SEAP 1, 368; Sallie Chesham, *Born to Battle: The Salvation Army in America* (Chicago, 1965); Philip Whitwell Wilson, *General Evangeline Booth of the Salvation Army* (New York, 1948); Herbert A. Wisbey, Jr., *Soldiers Without Swords: A History of the Salvation Army in the United States* (New York, 1955).

**BOREMAN, Jacob Smith**    (4 August 1831, Middlebourne, VA—7 October 1919, Ogden, UT). *Education*: A.B., Washington and Jefferson Coll., 1853; studied law, Univ. of Virginia, 1853–55. *Career*: legal practice, Parkersburg, VA, 1855–58, and Kansas City, MO, 1858–61; city attorney, Kansas City, MO, 1861–62; judge, Jackson Co., MO, and Kansas City Criminal Court, 1862–68; member, Missouri House of Representatives, 1869; editor, *Kansas City Bulletin*, 1870; associate justice, Supreme Court of Utah, 1873–80, 1885–89; Utah commissioner of schools, 1889–94; legal practice, Ogden, UT, 1889–1919.

Judge Jacob Boreman combined a long career as a tough man of the law with an equally intense hatred of the liquor traffic. He was not affiliated with the prohibitionist cause in his early years, which he devoted primarily to legal activities. The future judge joined the Virginia bar in 1855 and practiced in that state for a number of years (with his brother Ingraham Boreman, later governor of West Virginia). Moving to Missouri in 1858, he quickly established an excellent reputation in his adopted Kansas City, where he won election as city attorney in 1861. Boreman's interest in public affairs subsequently brought him greater responsibilities. Over the next several years he worked hard to hold slaveholding Missouri for the Union during the Civil War, and while still sitting on the bench he served with the Kansas City Guards and on recruiting drives for other outfits of the Missouri militia. As a justice he worked and sat in both county and city courts until 1869, when he ran successfully for a seat in the state House of Representatives. He came to national prominence when, in 1873, he accepted a federal appointment to the Utah judiciary. (Utah was then a territory.) Boreman wasted no time in building a reputation as a stern and aggressive justice. He pushed the prosecution of Mormon leader Brigham Young on polygamy charges, as well as the arrest of the leader of a Mormon band that had massacred an immigrant train in the 1850s. His bold stands established him as one of the most respected (although by no means beloved) lawmen in the territory.

Utah saw Boreman's antiliquor sentiments take concrete form. As a devout and active Methodist, he shared his church's opposition to the liquor traffic, and he gave the enforcement of alcohol beverage laws a high priority while on the bench. In Mormon Utah, despite his other difficulties with the denomination, his dry stand brought him considerable respect. He spread his base of influence in state society through work with the Good Templars Order (of which he was a member), the Betterment League (a dry organization urging enforcement of liquor control statutes), and the local Prohibition Alliance. Temperance workers credited his efforts with greatly assisting the battle against illegal sales. In 1900, Boreman (by then back in private legal practice) elected to focus his political energies entirely on the temperance crusade. He was a founder of the Utah branch of the Prohibition Party and became active in organizing for the new organization at the grassroots level around the state. The same year, he stood unsuccessfully for the governorship as the party's first standard bearer. And while the Prohibitionists of Utah (like those elsewhere) never became a major political influence, the rise of their party and their ability to attract the likes of Jacob Boreman was testimony to the developing power of temperance in the popular mind.

**Bibliography:**

B. SEAP 1, 372; WW 1, 103.

**BOWERSOCK, Justin Dewitt**   (19 September 1842, New Alexander, OH— 27 October 1922, Lawrence, KS). *Education*: Ohio public schools. *Career*:

various manufacturing and business interests (including banking), Lawrence, KS, 1877–1922; mayor, Lawrence, KS, 1881–85; member, U.S. House of Representatives, 1899–1907.

Like many other businessmen of his period, Justin Dewitt Bowersock became involved early in life with the Temperance Movement. He began his career in manufacturing in Lawrence, Kansas, in 1877, when he dammed the Kansas River to power a textile plant. Over the following years, the immigrant from Ohio proved a business prodigy and through a series of astute investments became established as a successful merchant, banker, and partner in an ironworks and power company. At the same time, he began an equally dedicated affiliation with the antiliquor movement. He joined the local Sons of Temperance lodge and subsequently served in a number of leadership positions. Abstinence, for the young businessman, went hand in hand with thrift and efficiency, and while building his own career he was on the public record as a convinced prohibitionist. As his economic fortunes and social standing grew, Bowersock moved easily into civic participation. He assumed the presidency of the Lawrence Chamber of Commerce and the Lawrence Clearing House Association, both positions lasting many years. His first political triumph came in 1881, when he won election as mayor, and he then moved on to terms in the Kansas House of Representatives and Senate. In 1890 he won a seat in Congress, where he served for four terms (he was defeated in a race for the Senate in 1903). In office, Bowersock drew heavily on his temperance background and proved a ready ally of antiliquor measures. He also entered several pieces of legislation himself on behalf of the dry crusade, and he scored a number of successes. The most notable in this regard was the so-called Bowersock Bill, or the "Anti-Army Canteen Bill," which dried out military post canteens. The passage of this statute was part of a quickening tide of temperance activity in Congress during these years, and it ultimately led to further legislation banning the sale of alcohol at U.S immigrant stations.

**Bibliography:**

B. SEAP 1, 386; WW 1, 122.

**BOWMAN, Karl Murdock**    (4 November 1888, Topeka, KS—4 March 1973, San Francisco, CA). *Education*: A.B., Washburn Coll., 1909; M.D., Univ. of California at Berkeley, 1913; D.Sc., Washburn Coll., 1953; LLD., Univ. of California at Berkeley, 1964. *Career*: internships in hospitals in Los Angeles and New York State, 1913–21; captain, Army Medical Corps, 1917–19; psychiatrist (practice, research, and teaching positions) at hospitals and universities (including Harvard, New York Univ., Univ. of California Sch. of Medicine), 1921-73; professor emeritus, Univ. of California Sch. of Medicine, 1956–73; Alaska commissioner of mental health and superintendent, Alaska Psychiatric Inst., Anchorage, 1964–67; medical consultant, U.S. government and United Nations, 1940 to 1970s.

The career of psychiatrist Karl Bowman marked a growing scientific interest in alcohol problems after the end of National Prohibition. Bowman's early medical practice began with an internship at Children's Hospital in Los Angeles in 1913, from which he moved on to hospitals in New York City and Boston, where he was chief medical officer of Boston Psychopathic Hospital from 1921 to 1936. During this period he also taught psychiatry at Harvard Medical School. He received considerable recognition in his field and upon leaving Boston held important posts in a number of mental health institutions from New York to California and Alaska until his retirement in 1967. Respect for his work was such that he became a much sought-after expert witness in court trials involving questions of the mental capacity of the accused. The most celebrated instance was his testimony in the dramatic Leopold–Loeb murder trial in 1924. Throughout his long and distinguished career, Bowman remained actively involved in research, and much of his work was notable. He pioneered insulin and shock therapy in mental illness, did work on the ductless glands, revived psychiatric interest in alcoholism, and, in the early 1950s, served as director of the California Sexual Deviation Research Project.

The modern field of alcohol studies and treatment owes him a special debt. His attention helped restore scientific and professional credibility to a subject which many doctors and laymen considered too tainted by Prohibition to warrant serious study. Along with alcohol studies pioneer E. M. Jellinek,* Bowman produced a (for its day) classic review of the alcoholism treatment literature, "Alcohol Addiction and Its Treatment" (1941), which served to stimulate further research in the area. His work helped foster the revival of the idea (long held by medical authorities before Prohibition) that alcoholism was a medical problem fully deserving the attention of the treatment community. He also served in an advisory role to the *Quarterly Journal of Studies on Alcohol*, the only major scholarly publication then devoted to the subject. He was honored with many professional awards and society memberships, including a term as president of the American Psychiatric Association in the 1940s.

**Bibliography:**

A. *Personal Problems for Men and Women* (New York, 1931); "Psychoses Due to Drugs or Other Exogenous Poisons," 349–91, in G. Blumer, ed., *The Practitioner's Library of Medicine and Surgery*, vol. 9 (New York, 1936); "The Treatment of Acute Deliria," *Virginia Medical Monthly* 67 (1940): 724–32; with E. M. Jellinek, "Alcohol Addiction and Its Treatment," *Quarterly Journal of Studies on Alcohol* 2 (1941): 312–90; with N. S. Solomon and J. Wortis, "Review of Psychiatric Progress, 1943: Alcohol, Neurosyphilis, Physiological Therapy," *American Journal of Psychiatry* 100 (1944): 537–41.

B. *Contemporary Authors*, vols. 41–44, 1st rev. (Detroit, MI, 1979), 86–87; NYT, March 4, 1973; WW 5, 78.

**BOYNTON, Melbourne Parker**    (6 November 1867, Lynn, MA—16 June 1942, Shelby, MI). *Education*: studied at California Coll. and Univ. of Chicago

Divinity Sch.; D.D. (honorary), Des Moines Coll., 1911. *Career*: minister, First Baptist Church, San Francisco, 1894–97; Woodlawn Baptist Church, Chicago, 1897–1937, minister emeritus, 1937–42.

Boynton combined two careers, those of Baptist clergyman and temperance organizer, to promote his life-long crusade for the abolition of the liquor traffic. Ordained in 1892, he led a San Francisco pastorate for several years before taking a Chicago church in 1897, where he remained until his retirement. He proved an excellent administrator, and he successfully placed his parish on a sound financial footing. His fine reputation gave him a leading voice in Chicago religious councils, and he was active in a number of city pastoral associations. He also took a serious interest in civil affairs, serving on a number of local governmental panels as well as directing the Better Government Association of Chicago. In his personal preaching and civil positions, Boynton fully reflected his denomination's (and his own) opposition to legal liquor. He chaired the Illinois Baptist State Convention's Committee on Temperance and helped organize the Illinois Anti-Saloon League. For years he served on its board of directors, as well as holding other offices. He became an active platform speaker against "the demon" as well, spreading his activities beyond the Chicago area. He spoke in a number of Prohibition campaigns around the state and wrote on behalf of the dry position in various periodicals. In the decade before National Prohibition, Boynton had emerged clearly as one of the premier dry champions in the Midwest.

As the political influence of the league increased in the state, the reverend also became caught up in the electoral process. His most serious involvement in politics came in the election of 1916, when he secured the Republican nomination for Congress from his Chicago district. His Democratic opponent was incumbent James R. Mann, minority leader in the House. Mann had incurred the particular wrath of the Anti-Saloon League (and of the dry reform in general) in his guise as a leading opponent of Richard Hobson's* National Prohibition amendment. Public sentiment was building toward a constitutional assault on alcohol, and in posing Boynton against Mann, the league hoped to break the back of wet resistance once and for all. In this case, while the wets won the electoral battle, they came out of the contest too scarred to win the war. Boynton lost, but Mann had to fight hard to hold on; and elsewhere in Congress the drys swept to a resounding victory. Their comfortable majority after the 1916 elections allowed them to pass a dry amendment (the Eighteenth) easily in 1917. Boynton remained committed to that amendment to the end. In 1933, in his last foray into temperance electoral politics, he won a seat in the state convention called to ratify the Twenty-First Amendment (Repeal). He fought a stubborn rear-guard action for the dry cause; at the finish, however, he could take comfort not in carrying the day but only in having followed the dictates of his conscience.

**Bibliography:**

B. SEAP 1, 390; WW 1, 74.

**BREHM, Marie Caroline**    (30 June 1859, Sandusky, OH—26 January 1926, Long Beach, CA). *Education*: educated privately and in Ohio public schools, 1860s–1870s. *Career*: temperance worker, including offices with WCTU, 1891–1926.

The career of Marie Brehm was a classic illustration of the organizational talents and reforming zeal that launched the Temperance Movement to national influence. She was not a healthy child, and after an Ohio public school education, illness prevented her going on to college or assuming an active role in public affairs as a young woman. But a program of home study and a devout Presbyterian faith inclined her nevertheless to an interest in civic activities and social movements; and when she finally ventured into public life at age thirty-two, she made the most of her opportunities. Joining the Illinois WCTU, she quickly gained a reputation as a fiery lecturer on both temperance and woman's suffrage. Between 1891 and 1896 she held a number of state and local WCTU posts, while in 1896 her interest in the suffrage question led her to the superintendency of the National WCTU Franchise Department. Brehm also served as president of the Illinois Union from 1901 to 1906. In all of these positions she proved a tireless and devoted worker; never marrying, she poured virtually all her time into her temperance career. She represented a number of antiliquor groups at international and national conferences, served on national Presbyterian boards concerned with the alcohol question, and was respectively appointed by Presidents William Howard Taft and Woodrow Wilson as an American delegate to the Twelfth, Thirteenth, and Fourteenth International Congresses Against Alcoholism in 1909, 1911, and 1913. Brehm was a workhorse of her cause, and her record of service was one of the most impressive in the ranks of the antiliquor reform.

As a reformer, Brehm also illustrated the broad social interests of many temperance workers. In 1889, she represented the National WCTU at the International Conference of Reformers in Buffalo, New York; and her efforts on behalf of church work, Sunday schools, woman's suffrage, and education, while secondary to her temperance work, were still considerable. She never completely abandoned these related causes, even after much of the antiliquor crusade followed the Anti-Saloon League into a narrow emphasis on prohibition in the early 1900s. In fact, while most of the movement pursued prohibitionist goals through majority-party politics, Brehm remained a partisan of the Prohibition Party, which retained a measure of the broad-based reforming spirit. She chaired the National Committee of the Prohibition Party in 1920, served on the National Committee as a California delegate in the 1920s, and in 1924 was put forward as a Prohibitionist nominee for vice president. Brehm declined the nomination, but her activities in the party were testimony to her own linking of the temperance and other reforms and of the Prohibition Party's willingness to include women in the political process.

**Bibliography:**

B. SEAP 1, 399; WW 1, 134.

**BRIGGS, Arthur Hislop**    (1858, San Francisco, CA—29 October 1934, Los Gatos, CA). *Education*: A.B., Northwestern Univ., 1881; A.M., Northwestern Univ., 1883; STB., Boston Univ. Sch. of Theology, 1887; studied at Univ. of Berlin and London Library, 1880s; D.D., Northwestern Univ., 1899. *Career*: ordained in Methodist Church, 1887; pastorates in San Francisco, Vallejo, and San Jose, CA, and Denver, CO, 1887–97; president, Iliff Sch. of Theology, Denver, CO, 1897–1900; pastor, Central Church, San Francisco, 1901–4; organizing and administrative work with California Anti-Saloon League, from 1910.

Well educated and articulate, as well as a devout Methodist pastor, Arthur Briggs proved an able champion of temperance in his native California throughout the late nineteenth and early twentieth centuries. Early in his career, ministerial duties prevented his assuming any direct role in the antiliquor struggle. He led a number of California congregations after being ordained in 1887, and after his marriage to Edna Iliff (1897) of Denver, Colorado, for three years took on the presidency of her family's Iliff School of Theology. But despite his lack of any dry organizational affiliation, Briggs's Methodism early confirmed him in his opposition to drink (his father also had been a staunch dry). The temperance message was always a central part of his preaching, and when he finally joined the California Anti-Saloon League in 1910, his zeal led him steadily up the ladder of dry leadership. He served first in a number of league organizational positions, helping to run its state headquarters and manage field operations in San Francisco (1914–16). He was quite successful and league work came to dominate his career. He won election as state league president in 1916 (a largely ceremonial post he held until 1919) and simultaneously assumed responsibilities as superintendent of the Northern California League. Briggs, quite clearly, had emerged as one of the most prominent antiliquor crusaders of the West.

During his years at the head of the league, Briggs tried to ally the Temperance Movement with Progressive social reform activity and politics. In this, he followed the lead of his friend Daniel M. Gandier, state superintendent of the entire California League. Together, they worked closely with cooperative factions of both the Republican and Democratic parties, and by 1918 had established the league as one of the most influential forces in state politics. The effect brought considerable national recognition to Briggs, and his stature rose still further after 1919, when he began to edit the dry *California Liberator*. With Gandier's death in 1920, the zealous parson replaced his mentor as state superintendent. In accepting the state's highest dry office, however, Briggs overreached himself. He was not really happy in the top spot (he apparently was more comfortable in a subordinate role), and Prohibition, ratified the year he took office, proved inordinately hard to enforce in California. This fact was due less to his leadership—for he did well enough in maintaining the league's political power—than to declining popular support for dry policies over time and the inability to keep bootleggers away from the state's vast coasts and borders. At any rate, the league could not hold off disenchantment with the Eighteenth Amendment, nor the resurgence of the wets. Briggs held the superintendent's post until his death in 1934, by which time he suffered the pain of seeing not only Repeal but the league itself reduced itself to a shadow of its former strength.

**Bibliography:**

B. WW 1, 138; Gilman M. Ostrander, *The Prohibition Movement in California, 1848–1933* (Berkeley, CA, 1957).

**BRIGGS, George Nixon**   (12 April 1796, Adams, MA—12 September 1861, Pittsfield, MA). *Career*: admitted to bar, MA, 1818; town clerk, Lanesboro, MA, 1824; registrar of deeds, Berkshire Co., MA, 1824–31; member, U.S. House of Representatives, 1831–43; governor of Massachusetts, 1844–51; judge, Massachusetts Court of Common Pleas, 1853–58.

On September 12, 1861, shortly before he was to leave on a special diplomatic mission to New Granada, George Nixon Briggs died tragically in a shooting accident. His death meant the loss of one of the more promising politicians of his day and certainly the passing of one of the most devoted advocates of the Temperance Movement. Coming from simple roots and lacking a formal education, Briggs first came to public attention as a lawyer in 1827, when he successfully defended an Indian accused of murder. After a political apprenticeship in local offices, he won election to Congress in 1830 as a Whig, where he emerged as a quiet but dedicated foe of slavery. He brought this conviction back to his native Massachusetts in 1844, when he returned as governor; indeed, he used the office to sponsor one of the broadest reform programs of any antebellum state administration. He stood strongly for temperance, opposed the Mexican War and the annexation of Texas on the grounds that they would aid the spread of slavery, and, always conscious of his own lack of schooling, worked hard on behalf of public education. In fact, he was proud of his reputation as a supporter of Massachusetts colleges, the policies of Horace Mann,* and the extension of state educational facilities. Briggs was also an active Baptist layman and served his church with the same honest and hardworking sense of duty he offered the state. Upon leaving the governorship, he returned to private legal practice and was then appointed to the bench in 1853.

Briggs's stature as a reformer and political leader made him invaluable to Massachusetts temperance forces. He was an active dry throughout his public career, and he frequently took the lead in organizing antiliquor groups. While in the House, he assisted in founding the Congressional Temperance Society and for a time sat as its president. In its early days, the society was moderationist in tone, but Briggs soon came down on the side of total abstinence. In 1836, he took his arguments before the National Temperance Convention, held at Saratoga, New York, and played a leading role in the debate that eventually made abstinence the official policy of the crusade. Later on (1842), in addressing a reformed—on completely dry lines—Congressional Society, he noted that the earlier moderationist organization had "died. . . with a bottle in one hand and a pledge in the other.'' It was a view that mirrored the rest of the movement's stance on moderation by this time. As governor, Briggs remained equally committed to the cause. He spoke widely (and, at times, heatedly) on the subject, and in 1844 led twenty thousand Bostonians in a parade supporting the Washingtonians. Five years later, he took the lead in welcoming Father Mathew* when the Irish priest brought his temperance crusade to the state capital. While hopeful that "moral suasion" would reduce alcohol problems, Briggs still favored prohibition legislation; and when Maine succeeded in passing its famous prohibitory statute (the Maine Law), the governor took part in a public celebration in Boston in honor of the event. In 1856 he became president of the American Temperance Union, a post he held until his untimely death.

### Bibliography:

A. *Legislative Temperance Meeting: Governor Briggs' Speech* (Boston?, 1844); *Is Temperate Drinking Safe?* (Philadelphia, 1850?); *Popular Education: A Lecture...* (Providence, RI, 1851).

B. DAB 3, 41–42; SEAP 1, 416–17; WW H, 142; S. Briggs, *Archives of the Briggs Family* (1880); Williams C. Richards, *Great in Goodness: A Memoir of Geo. N. Briggs, Governor of the Commonwealth of Massachusetts, from 1844 to 1851* (Boston, 1866).

**BROWN, Martha McClellan**    (16 April 1838, Baltimore, MD—31 August 1916, Cincinnati, OH). *Education*: graduated from Pittsburg Female Coll., 1862; Ph.D. and LLD. (both honorary), Waynesburg (PA) Presbyterian Coll. *Career*: organizational and administrative work with International Order of Good Templars, 1860s–1880s; editor, *The Temperance Visitor* and the *Alliance Monitor*, 1870s; headed National Prohibition Alliance, 1881; National Executive Committee, Prohibition Party, 1876–96; vice president and professor, Cincinnati Wesleyan Woman's Coll., 1882–92; president, Woman's Rotary Club of Cincinnati, OH, 1914–15.

In 1896 the Prohibition Party national convention adopted a single-plank platform which, for the first time in the party's history, excluded a commitment to other reform issues, notably woman's suffrage. The convention at this point witnessed the departure of Martha McClellan Brown, who had served three terms on the National Executive Committee, and thus simultaneously the end of an outstanding thirty-five-year contribution to the Temperance Movement. Mrs. Brown's prominence in the movement's activities had begun with a shift in her budding lecture career from patriotic to temperance topics following the Civil War and had eventually included positions in the national organizations of the Good Templars and the Woman's Christian Temperance Union as well as the Prohibition Party. She had been instrumental in the formation of both the two latter groups. In Ohio, in February 1874, she had inspired the formation of the country's first woman's state temperance organization, and that summer, according to no less an authority than Frances Willard,* she provided the same kind of originating impulse for the National WCTU, which was to become one of the strongest and most enduring temperance organizations in American history. Already in early 1869 she had assisted in the formation of Ohio's Prohibition Party, and later that year, as grand vice templar of the Ohio Independent Order of Good Templars, attended the Grand Lodge meeting in Oswego, New York, out of which the national Prohibition Party eventually emerged. She had served as vice president and a member of the platform committee at the first party convention in 1876 (in addition to her appointment on the Executive Committee), and in 1877 had helped to bring about a rapprochement between the party and the WCTU. She also wrote temperance lessons for the Sunday school quarterly of the Methodist Episcopal Church. In these many ways she played a role of the highest importance in the growth of the movement from a relatively primitive, evangelical stage through its full-fledged national politicization. Bearing especially in mind the mobilization of women in general which she helped to bring about, the decision of the 1896 convention to ignore the suffrage issue must have seemed a singularly, not to say absurdly, ungrateful gesture to Brown.

It was not her first disappointment, however. Sources suggest that Mattie (as she was called) may have hoped for the first presidency of the WCTU after her significant effort in founding it, but apparently the new organization wished to dissociate itself from the fervency of the Good Templars. She had no further formal connection with the WCTU, and in 1876 she separated from the Good Templars as well when they refused to admit blacks. By the time of her break with the Prohibition Party she had begun to draw away from the Temperance Movement altogether, and although late in life she lectured and toured again for the Good Templars, her main involvements were academic—art, literature, and philosophy—and civic. One may imagine that having lived as many as five years apart from her husband (a Methodist minister) and six children during her active prohibitionist days—not to speak of disappointments along the way—she may have found some relief in narrowing the scope of her ambition to things either intellectual or local.

### Bibliography:

A. *Biographical Sketch of Rev. H. A. Thompson* (New York, 1880); *Accident of Sex* (New York, 1881).

B. NAW 1, 254–56; NYT, Feb. 27, 1882; SEAP 1, 433–34; I. Newton Pierce, *The History of the Independent Order of Good Templars* (1869); Frances E. Willard, *Woman and Temperance* (Hartford, CT, 1883).

**BROWNLOW, William Gannaway**   (29 August 1805, Wythe Co., VA—29 April 1877, Knoxville, TN). *Career*: Methodist minister, 1826–36; editor, *Tennessee Whig*, 1838–61; pro-Union political activity, TN, 1861–64; governor of Tennessee, 1865–69; member, U.S. Senate, 1869–75; owner and editor, *Knoxville Whig*, 1875–77.

A tradition of rhetoric in both oratory and written prose runs deep in the

Temperance Movement. It is, to a great degree, the movement's very historical substance—and it surely offers one of the most obvious explanations of its considerable duration and success. However, few if any of the figures in this tradition brought such a talent for personal derisiveness and tactless candor as Bill Brownlow, "the Fighting Parson." Parson Brownlow also partook of another major strain in the reform tradition: the Methodist doctrine of human perfectibility. Here again, Brownlow wrought the materials of his tradition with a vehemence uniquely his own—a vehemence so thoroughgoing, it should be added, that it suggests a certain self-conscious humor which strips much of his writing of any genuine bitterness. The historical meaning of Brownlow's career may be interpreted in the light of these two critical features, his rhetorical power and his Methodism, and their combustion under the heat and pressure of the War Between the States.

Having begun as a carpenter in the culturally isolated region of eastern Tennessee, Brownlow educated himself and qualified for the Methodist ministry in 1826 at the age of twenty-one. His native intelligence and ambition, however, soon outgrew the medium of itinerant preaching and moved him to political writing. He retired from active ministry in 1836 and by 1838 had established himself as an important journalistic exponent of the Whig Party. That he should have inferred from Methodism that the Union must stand seems explicable, since a cohesive federal system, it could be argued, offered the greatest likelihood of far-reaching social reform. His defense of slavery, on the other hand, and particularly the method of that defense—arguing mainly from the master–slave metaphorics of the Old and New Testaments—undoubtedly subverts the consistency of any reformist posture. This Brownlow himself seems to have recognized in later years, when his opinion about slavery changed. But despite this early paradox—indeed heightening it—Brownlow devoted his twenty-two-year career as editor of the influential *Knoxville Whig* to opposing secession and was eventually shut down and even imprisoned by the Confederacy as a result. He later became governor of Tennessee and then U.S. senator. Throughout his career—as preacher, journalist, and legislator—his cutting style slashed vigorously against liquor (and tobacco as well). In addition, he organized the Sons of Temperance and the Cadets of Temperance (for children) throughout east Tennessee and is credited with having gotten local option into the Whig Party platform of 1855. As governor he initiated legislation ultimately leading to the famous Four-Mile Law, which forbid the sale of liquor within four miles of any Tennessee educational institution that lay outside city limits. He especially dwelt upon the relation between alcohol and crime. Avid in all things, he could hardly have been satisfied with anything less than total national prohibition, which he called for at almost every conceivable opportunity. His vigor was sadly impaired when shortly before his second term as governor he was stricken with palsy. He was nonetheless returned to office, but as his condition worsened, particularly through a pitiable term as senator, the poignancy of such a fate for such a character deepened.

**Bibliography:**

A. *A Political Register* (Jonesboro, TN, 1844); *Americanism Contrasted with Foreignism, Romanism and Bogus Democracy* (Nashville, TN, 1856); *Ought American Slavery to Be Perpetuated?* (Philadelphia, 1858); *Brownlow, the Patriot and Martyr, Showing His Faith and Works, as Reported by Himself* (Philadelphia, 1862); *Sketches of the Rise, Progress, and Decline of Secession* (Philadelphia, 1862).

B. DAB 3, 177–78; SEAP 1, 434; WW H, 149; E. M. Coulter, *William G. Brownlow: Fighting Parson of the Southern Highland* (Chapel Hill, NC, 1937); James Welch Patton, *Unionism and Reconstruction in Tennessee, 1860–1869* (Chapel Hill, NC, 1934).

**BRYAN, William Jennings**   (19 March 1860, Salem, IL—26 July 1925, Miami, FL). *Education*: A.B., Illinois Coll., 1881; A.M., Illinois Coll., 1884; LLB., Union Coll. of Law, 1883; LLD. (honorary), Univ. of Nebraska, Univ. of Maryland, and Univ. of Arizona, at various dates. *Career*: practiced law in Jacksonville, IL, 1883–87; practiced law in Lincoln, NB, 1887–90; member, U.S. House of Representatives, 1890–94; editor-in-chief, *Omaha World-Herald*, 1894; Democratic Party candidate for president, 1896; colonel during Spanish-American War (saw no action), 1898; Democratic candidate for president, 1900; editor, *Commoner*, 1901; Democratic candidate for president, 1908; secretary of state under Wilson, 1913–15; president, National Dry Federation, 1918.

As speaker and writer, William Jennings Bryan was possessed of one of the most influential voices the United States has ever known. He was unarguably the leader of the Democratic Party from 1896 to 1916, and arguably its leading spokesman for ten years afterward. His seemingly inexhaustible verbal energy played an important part in securing the major Progressive reforms of his era: the popular election of senators, an income tax, the requirements of publication of ownership and circulation of newspapers, the creation of a Department of Labor, national prohibition, and woman suffrage. Somewhat paradoxically, he spent the latter portion of his life fighting the theories of evolution, which he felt were both a cause and symptom of contemporary godlessness, and in advocating a literal interpretation of the Bible. He was the Democratic candidate for president three times (1896, 1900, and 1908), and secretary of state under President Wilson from 1913 to 1915. In 1921 he moved to Florida because of his wife's ill health, profited from the real estate boom, and became a millionaire. He died just a few days after the famous Scopes trial, in which he had assisted in prosecuting a Tennessee schoolteacher for teaching evolution. Although the prosecution was successful, Bryan had undergone an embarrassing cross-examination by Clarence Darrow. Bryan was not capable, by temperament or education, of making an argument in the terms of science. He believed in the necessity of religious emotion and felt that the ascendancy of biological language threatened the possibility of evoking such emotion. His reputation as a figure of intellectual history has suffered immeasurably and ironically from his resistance to the tide of progress on the point of evolution, though quite possibly he was not the simple fool historians (and contemporary opponents) have sometimes alleged. His approach to life was rhetorical—whether simple-mindedly or otherwise must be left for deeper analyses. But undoubtedly Bryan felt that the quality of life turned upon the tone of the language in which it was expressed, and his consistency at this level of tone superseded to some extent his intellectual consistency.

Bryan found an apt medium for his rhetoric in the National Prohibition movement. Always an abstainer, he began politically as a supporter of local option, and as early as 1910 he was on the stump against the saloon in his home state of Nebraska. With his normal eloquence, he branded the traffic both "an outlaw and a nuisance" and thundered for the people's right to control or abolish it. By 1920 he was to be found pressing (unsuccessfully) for a dry plank in the Democratic platform. He subsequently refused the nomination of the Prohibition Party for president (although some Prohibitionists had supported him in 1896), though by now he was firmly converted to the prohibitionist cause and would come to be regarded as one of its main heroes. In 1913, upon his nomination as secretary of state, he had appealed to President Wilson for, and had been granted, the right to serve only nonalcoholic drinks at his official table. His style in discussing the matter of drink was as usual a highly listenable movement from conversational usage and rhythm into more formal and grander constructions, keeping always the touch of a master evangelist upon the pulse of his audience. In his telling, the struggle against drink was a divinely ordained battle for emancipation from an "enemy that has made victims of men throughout the ages." The "driving of intoxicating drinks off the earth," he intoned, ranked with the "abolition of war everywhere" as "the two greatest reforms for which the world waits." It was this kind of spellbinding style that made Bryan invaluable to the Temperance Movement. He could "command a hearing for the cause," wrote one dry author, "from thousands of men who would not go near the ordinary temperance meeting." Until his death during the heyday of National Prohibition in 1925, the "Great Commoner" was firm in his dry belief, and one of the last organizations he consented to lead was the National Dry Federation.

### Bibliography:

A. *The First Battle: A Story of the Campaign of 1896...* (Chicago, 1896); *Speeches of William Jennings Bryan, Revised and Arranged by Himself* (New York, 1913); *Prohibition* (Washington, DC, 1916); *The Bible and Its Enemies* (Chicago, 1921); *The Menace of Darwinism* (Chicago, 1921); *Memoirs* (Philadelphia, 1926).

B. DAB 3, 196–97; SEAP 1, 440–42; Paul W. Glad, *McKinley, Bryan and the People* (Philadelphia, 1964); Paul W. Glad, *The Trumpet Soundeth: William Jennings Bryan and His Democracy, 1896–1912* (Lincoln, NB, 1960); Paul W.

Glad, *William Jennings Bryan: A Profile* (New York, 1968); Louis William Koenig, *Bryan: A Political Biography of William Jennings Bryan* (New York, 1971).


**BUCKINGHAM, William Alfred**    (28 May 1804, Norwich, CT—3 February 1875, Norwich, CT). *Career*: dry goods business, 1826–48; carpet manufacturing, 1830–48; organizer and treasurer, Haywood Rubber Co., Colchester, CT, beginning 1848; mayor, Norwich, CT, 1849–50, 1856–57; governor of Connecticut, 1858–66; member, U.S. Senate, 1869–75.

William Alfred Buckingham was one of those enterprising men of the middle 1800s whose compelling drive and initiative lifted them from success to success in business (first dry goods, then carpets, then rubber) and ultimately into high political office. These qualities were as useful in the Temperance Movement as anywhere else, and Buckingham worked for that cause with the same tireless efficiency that had won his reputation in business and government. This reputation was perhaps most enhanced by his role as one of Abraham Lincoln's war governors. He was among that elite group of governors the president came to depend upon for counsel and emergency materiel and men; his most famous accomplishment in this context was quickly (and without legal authority) raising a regiment of volunteers to meet Connecticut's first Civil War quota and eventually a state contingent of 55,000 without using the draft. His popularity with Connecticut citizens was on a plane with the respect accorded him by Lincoln, and he was reelected governor seven consecutive times for a period of eight years, until he finally refused renomination in 1866. In 1868 he was elected to the U.S. Senate, where by available reports he distinguished himself further as a member of the Commerce Committee and as chairman of the Committee on Indian Affairs. He died shortly before the end of his term.

Like many other Republicans, Buckingham had a lively interest in religious and social reform. He was active in his own Congregational church, a benefactor of Yale Divinity School, and a noted temperance enthusiast. From 1862 he was president of the American Temperance Union, and in that year in connection with his government function of supplying war materiel to the Union forces, he helped initiate a movement to abolish the navy's spirit ration. His speech at the twenty-fifth anniversary of the American Temperance Union (May 25, 1863) continued in this view, arguing that American soldiers and sailors should be protected from the traffic while in the ranks. Buckingham's efforts in this direction ultimately came to little—armies are seldom noted as paragons of sobriety, and the Union army was no exception. But during a period when the War Between the States overshadowed other national concerns—and helped send the Temperance Movement into hiatus—the labors of the Connecticut governor did much to keep the dry spark alive so that it could rekindle after Appomattox. A bronze statue of Buckingham stands in the state capitol in Hartford.

**Bibliography:**

A. *The Currency* (Washington, DC, 1870); *The Currency-Specie Payments* (Washington, DC, 1873); *The Covenant and Duty of Church Members* (n.p., n.d.).

B. DAB 2, 228–29; SEAP 2, 445; WW H, 151; S. G. Buckingham, *The Life of Wm. A. Buckingham* (Springfield, MA, 1894); F. W. Chapman, *The Buckingham Family* (Hartford, CT, 1872); *For President U.S. Grant, for Vice President Wm. Alfred Buckingham* (1868?).

**BUELL, Caroline Brown**    (24 October 1843, Marlboro, MA—13 October 1927, East Hampton, CT). *Career*: temperance organizer and WCTU official, 1873 to circa 1926.

At the age of twenty-two, Caroline Buell was widowed when her husband, Lieutenant F.W.H. Buell, was killed in action at the Battle of Chapin's Farm, Virginia, in 1865. She never remarried, but thereafter, until her death in 1927, she devoted all of her not inconsiderable energies to the cause of temperance. In 1872 she joined the Good Templar Order, a fraternal organization dedicated chiefly to promoting abstinence among its members. Craving a more active role, Mrs. Buell joined the Woman's Christian Temperance Union upon its founding in 1874. She at once embarked upon the sort of activity that was henceforth to characterize her work in liquor reform, that of organizer. From 1876 to 1883, Mrs. Buell served on the publication committee of three which was responsible for putting out the official journal of the WCTU, *Our Union*, as well as holding positions as assistant recording secretary (1878–80), corresponding secretary (1880–93), and superintendent of the Department of Christian Citizenship (1898–1902). Sensing the need to impress upon the young the evils of drink, Mrs. Buell organized the Loyal Temperance Legion, the children's auxiliary of the WCTU. In addition, she worked diligently for the professionalization of the WCTU. On this premise, she founded the first school to train WCTU workers in the proper methods and practices that would make the WCTU a more efficient and businesslike organization. Appropriately, Mrs. Buell served as the director of the Mountain Park Lake, Maryland, facility for twelve years after its founding as a training school. At the age of sixty, in 1903, she gave up her posts in the National WCTU, but she was not yet ready to give up entirely in her campaigns against drink. In 1906 she was elected to the presidency of the Connecticut WCTU, a position she held until shortly before her death. Thus for Caroline Buell the temperance cause was actually a career, and her beloved WCTU enjoyed in her membership the aid and dedication of considerably more than a volunteer. Buell, in fact, was the epitome of the temperance professional.

**Bibliography:**

A. *The Helping Hand, or, the ABC of Organizing a W.C.T.U.* (Chicago, 1887).

B. SEAP 1, 446–47; WW 1, 162.

**BULLOCK, Helen Louise**    (29 April 1836, Norwich, NY—?). *Career*: piano teacher, 1855–86; lecturer and organizer, New York State WCTU, 1886; lecturer and organizer, National WCTU, 1886–1918.

The conjunction of feminism and temperance was not an uncommon aspect of the antiliquor movement of the nineteenth century, and it was certainly evident in the career of Helen Bullock. Although her initial interest was music, and she taught piano from 1855 to 1886, as early as age fifteen Bullock became involved in the temperance cause when she joined the Independent Order of Good Templars. She worked in behalf of the fraternal group for many years, and with the founding of the Woman's Christian Temperance Union, she became a charter member. In 1886, she was lecturing and organizing actively for the WCTU in New York State, and the experience opened her eyes to other reforms. Shortly thereafter, some of these additional causes attracted Bullock's interest, and she pursued them with the same vigor she had shown in her initial reform commitment. Taking advantage of Frances Willard's* "Do Everything" policy, she became superintendent of the WCTU's Department of Anti-Narcotics in 1888 and helped get passage of an anticigarette law through the New York legislature. In 1898, Bullock became increasingly involved in the problems of women. That year she was apponted national superintendent of the Purity Department of the WCTU, as well as serving as the head of Rescue Work for Girls in New York. Sensing the truth that practical education was the surest way to assure the rise of women, she organized the Anchorage, a rescue home for women at Elmira, New York, that combined shelter as well as industrial training for disadvantaged women. The new institution flourished, and Bullock's reputation in social work grew accordingly. Her preeminence in this field was recognized when the name of the facility was changed in 1907 to the Helen L. Bullock Industrial Training School for Girls. When she retired from active service (after thirty-two years in the Temperance Movement), Bullock could take satisfaction in knowing that through her efforts over forty thousand new members had joined the WCTU, and scores of women had become self-supporting and self-reliant members of their communities. And not least, a small beginning had been made toward the goal of making women the full social partners of men.

**Bibliography:**

B. SEAP 1, 449–50.

**BURLEIGH, William Henry**    (2 February 1812, Woodstock, CT—18 March 1871, Brooklyn, NY). *Career*: printer, *Stonington* (CT) *Phoenix*, 1830–32; printer and contributor, *Schenectady* (NY) *Cabinet*, 1831–33; assistant editor, *Unionist*, 1833–37; lecturer, American Anti-Slavery Society, 1836–43; editor, *Literary Journal*, 1836–37; editor, *Christian Freeman*, 1843–49; editor, *Prohibitionist*, 1849–55; lecturer, New York State Temperance Society, 1849–55; harbor master, Port of New York, 1855–70.

As was characteristic of many antebellum temperance advocates, William

Henry Burleigh expressed his humanitarian concerns through the pursuit of a variety of social reforms. At various times he lent his efforts on behalf of antislavery, women's rights, and the campaign against beverage alcohol. A printer and journalist by trade, Burleigh's first encounter with reform activity came in 1833, when his brother asked him to help edit the *Unionist*, a Connecticut paper established to publicize and support Prudence Crandall's school for black children. The experience had a marked impact on the young printer, who subsequently became staunchly attached to the abolitionist cause. He taught briefly at the Crandall school and then became a regular lecturer for the American Anti-Slavery Society until 1843. He was never one to mince words on the issue, and several years later his views almost got him killed: he publicly condemned the Mexican War as a plot to extend slavery and narrowly escaped lynching by an enraged mob. And while he never provoked another such violent response, the same depth of commitment marked Burleigh's other crusades. When he began working for the New York State Temperance Society in 1849, for example, he blasted the demon rum with identical editorial and rhetorical verve. He roamed the state for six years as the society's lecturer, while at the same time managing the operations of the group's journal, the *Prohibitionist*. But for all of his zeal, his active crusading came to an end in 1855, when Burleigh took a job as harbor master for the Port of New York (even reformers find they need steady incomes at some point). He continued to write, however, and his columns showed a man still on the side of reform. Yet Burleigh's pen was not directed totally against social problems. Indeed, his style developed over the years, and during the 1840s he also emerged as a poet of some distinction. His verse was generally quiet and studious in tone, which one biographer thought was a reflection of the life Burleigh really longed to lead—but which was denied him by "his goading conscience." Still, the reformer broke through occasionally even in poetry, as evidenced in a volume of popular antiliquor verse, *The Rum Fiend and Other Poems* (1871). At the end of his years, he was respected both for his work as a reformer and as an author; indeed, for Burleigh the two always had been related fields anyway.

### Bibliography:

A. *The Tyranny of Intemperance* (New Haven, CT, 1845); *The Devil and the Grog-Seller: A Ditty for the Times* (Philadelphia, 1848); *The Freeman's Weapon* (Albany, NY, 185-?); ed., *The Republic Pocket Pistol...* (New York, 1860); *Poems by William H. Burleigh, with a Sketch of His Life* (New York, 1871); *The Rum Fiend and Other Poems* (New York, 1871).

B. DAB 3, 286; NYT, March 19, 1871; WW 1, 77; Charles Burleigh, *The Geneology of the Burley or Burleigh Family of America* (1880).

**BURRELL, David James**   (1 August 1844, Mt. Pleasant, PA—5 December 1926, Madison, NJ). *Education*: A.B., Yale Univ., 1867; graduated from Union Theological Sem., 1870; D.D. (honorary), Parsons Coll., 1883, Rutgers Coll.,

1916; LLD. (honorary), Hope Coll., 1900. *Career*: ordained in Presbyterian Church, 1872; missionary, Chicago, 1872–76; minister, Second Church, Dubuque, IA, 1876–87; minister, Westminster Church, Minneapolis, MN, 1887–91; minister, Marble Collegiate Church, New York City, 1891–1926.

A prohibitionist since his early college days, David Burrell was known for his eloquence in speech, his persuasive oratory, and his implacable opposition to the liquor traffic. After ordination (1872) he served for a number of years in urban missionary work in Chicago and in pastorates in Dubuque, Iowa, and Minneapolis, Minnesota. He was effective with his city congregations, both of them growing dramatically under his leadership, and Burrell acquired a reputation for stirring and powerful sermons. His message was inbred heavily with the social gospel of the period, and since his earliest ministry he preached against intemperance, moral corruption, Sabbath breaking, and the degradation of life in the city. When he was still in Dubuque, he was already active in the Temperance Movement, and he campaigned actively for prohibitionist candidates in the late 1870s. Later, he served as a member of the Board of Managers of the American Temperance Society. He brought this strong background of reform with him in 1891, when he accepted a call to the famous Marble Collegiate Church (Dutch Reformed) in New York City (where he remained, in one capacity or another, for the rest of his life).

It was in New York that he reached his highest stature as a cleric. He ran his new church effectively and agreed at various times to edit denominational publications (1909–13) and to teaching assignments at Princeton Theological Seminary (beginning in 1903). The pastorate also offered the greatest challenge in urban temperance activity Burrell had ever faced, and he met it head on. His sermons, including powerful statements on the liquor question, were reprinted frequently and widely discussed. He was convinced that the movement could effectively rally urban electoral support as well, and he therefore combined his preaching with dry politics. He was one of seven incorporators of the Anti-Saloon League of New York, and he served ably in the positions of executive director from 1905 to 1924 and president from 1921 to 1923. The prominence of Marble Collegiate and his active governance of the New York League soon brought Burrell national recognition from temperance workers. He sat for a number of years as a vice president of the National Anti-Saloon League, where his experience in urban organizing and problems helped enable the organization to build significant strength among city-dwellers. Indeed, it would be difficult to cite a better example than Burrell of the league's success in marshalling the church against the traffic.

**Bibliography:**

A. *The Religions of the World: An Outline of the Great Religious Systems* (Philadelphia, 1902); *Christ and Progress: A Discussion of Problems of Our Time* (New York, 1903); *The Evolution of a Christian* (New York, 1906); *Why*

*I Believe the Bible* (New York, 1917); *The Laughter of God, and Other Sermons* (New York, 1918).

B. DAB 3, 324–25; NYT, Dec. 6, 1926; SEAP 1, 465–66; WW 1, 172.

**BUTLER, Benjamin Franklin** (5 November 1818, Deerfield, NH—11 January 1893, Washington, DC). *Education*: graduated from Waterbury Coll., 1838. *Career*: admitted to bar, MA, 1840; legal practice, 1840–61; member, Massachusetts House of Representatives, 1853; member, Massachusetts Senate, 1859–61; general, Union army, 1861–65; member, U.S. House of Representatives, 1866–75, 1877–79; governor of Massachusetts, 1882; legal practice and political activity with Greenback and Anti-Monopoly parties.

Few men of his generation stirred as much controversy as Benjamin F. Butler. As Union commandant of captured New Orleans, the Confederacy decried him as "Beast Butler" and declared him an "outlaw"; Northern reformers applauded his ideals; while fellow army officers frequently denounced him as a tactical incompetent who kept his command only through his considerable political influence. It seems that no one who knew the man was neutral—they loved or hated him. His background was that of a successful lawyer whose undeniable personal ambition and political acumen had established him as a leading light in Massachusetts Democratic politics. In the 1850s he sat in both the state House and Senate, where he was noted (unlike many other Democrats) for his outspoken abolitionism (a stance which did him no harm politically in largely antislavery Massachusetts). He came to national prominence at the Democratic Convention of 1860, when he fought the nomination of Stephen A. Douglass and threatened a walkout by Massachusetts delegates. With the start of the war, he remained firmly loyal and took a commission as brigadier general of militia. And once in federal service, his conduct was such as to fascinate historians of the conflict ever since. His years of active command finally ended under a cloud in 1864 (Grant, among others, was disgusted with Butler's lackluster leadership, especially his performance in the Bermuda Hundred, Virginia, area and at Fort Fisher), but his personal popularity and political reputation remained high in his home state. He subsequently served a number of terms in Congress and one as governor of Massachusetts (and ran twice for the presidency), affiliated variously with the Republicans, Democrats, Greenbackers, and Anti-Monopolists.

Like many other reform-minded Americans of the age, Butler included temperance in his wide variety of social and political concerns. While he never became a prominent leader of the antiliquor movement, his position is interesting nevertheless as representative of a particular variety of reform thought. The future general became active in the movement in the early 1830s, when he served as vice president of a local temperance society and attended a number of conferences on the liquor question. It was a period of transition for the cause: The moderationists' position, which deplored drinking to excess and the use of distilled liquor (and which previously had been dominant), was slowly giving way to an orthodoxy of total abstinence. Butler was a moderationist man and as such stingingly denounced drunkenness and hard liquor—but he refused to extend condemnation to all drinking or to endorse prohibition. As the movement as a whole shifted to the harder line, however, Butler became less and less active. By the later 1840s he had largely severed his relationship with the crusade, although he still spoke out on occasion. In 1849, at the thirteenth annual meeting of the American Temperance Union, he called for strict legislation to control illegal alcohol sales; and while he still would not take a total abstinence stand, he lauded the spread of temperance sentiment throughout the nation. The rise of the antislavery controversy, however, soon diverted Butler from most other reform activities, and he never seriously again pursued the dry banner.

## Bibliography:

A. *Opening Argument of Mr. Butler, of Massachusetts, One of the Managers on the Impeachment of the President* (Washington, DC, 1868); *The Present Relations of Parties, Duties of the Republican Party. . .* (Lowell, MA, 1870); *Butler's Book: Autobiography and Personal Reminiscences of Major-General Benjamin F. Butler* (Boston, 1892); *The Private and Official Correspondence of Gen. Benjamin F. Butler, during the Period of the Civil War*, 5 vols. (Norwich, MA, 1917).

B. Robert S. Holzman, *Stormy Ben Butler* (New York, 1954); Henry Norman Hudson, *A Chaplain's Campaign with Ben Butler* (New York, 1868); Howard Pervear Nash, *Stormy Petrel: The Life and Times of General Benjamin F. Butler, 1818–1893* (Rutherford, NJ, 1969); Hans Louis Trefousse, *Ben Butler: The South Called Him Beast* (New York, 1957); Nathan Weiss, "The Political Theory and Practice of General Benjamin Franklin Butler" (Ph.D. diss., New York University, 1961); Richard Sedgewick West, *Lincoln's Scapegoat General: A Life of Benjamin F. Butler, 1818–1893* (Boston, 1965).

# C

CANNON, James, Jr. (13 November 1864, Salisbury, MO—6 September 1944, Chicago, IL). *Education*: A.B., Randolph-Macon Coll., 1884; A.M., Princeton Univ., 1889; B.D., Princeton Theological Sem., 1888; D.D, Randolph-Macon Coll., 1903. *Career*: Methodist minister, South Portsmouth, VA, 1884–94; president, Blackstone Coll. for Girls, 1894–1911, 1914–18; editor, *Christian Advocate*, 1904–18; superintendent, Anti-Saloon League of Virginia, 1910–19; chairman, National Legislative Committee, Anti-Saloon League, beginning 1914; elected Methodist bishop, 1918; member of numerous church and temperance boards and committees, 1900s–1930s; retirement, 1938–1944.

James Cannon has been described as the most effective Anti-Saloon League lobbyist in the nation's capital during the years immediately prior to the enactment of the Eighteenth Amendment. As was typical of many temperance leaders, he grew up steeped in the antiliquor traditions of the Methodist Church, and he built his career on passionate commitments both to the denomination itself and to Prohibition. Well educated, Cannon showed considerable talent in his first pastorate in Virginia, and by 1894 had become president of a denominational women's school (Blackstone), which he built into a thriving small college. Ambitious for himself and for Methodism, he also led the fight to tighten church control over other educational institutions as well (notably Randolph-Macon College), to strengthen church administration generally, and to increase the impact of Methodism via the religious press (in 1904 he assumed the editorship of the *Baltimore and Richmond Christian Advocate*). In all of his activities he moved aggressively and was often caustic and abrasive; yet he had a reputation for getting things done, and by 1909 he was clearly one of the central religious figures of his region. Further recognition of the fact came in 1911, when he was named superintendent of a major Methodist educational and recreational facility near Wayneville, North Carolina—which, with his usual organizational talent, he turned into a financial success for the church. His church record was genuinely impressive, and the Methodists, to no one's real surprise, elected him bishop in 1918.

Cannon was never an original theological thinker, and on most religious issues he was a conservative. In politics, however, he was willing to face social reform squarely at times. He embraced Prohibition because he honestly felt it would bring about a better society—one in which he fully expected his moral values would predominate, but also one with greatly reduced drunkenness, poverty, crime, corruption, and disease. His political methods, however, evinced a tough pragmatism, a willingness to engage in relentless legislative battles, and the same attention to organization and detail that characterized his handling of church affairs. His impact on the national antiliquor struggle was profound, although his first efforts on behalf of the dry cursade were in Virginia (where he had worked with the Anti-Saloon League since 1902). In 1910, he founded the *Richmond Virginian*, a temperance newspaper which he used to blister the traffic and to call for a statewide referendum on a prohibitory law. The same year, he became superintendent of the Virginia League, and over the next several years he orchestrated a successful drive for the vote he had called for editorially. It resulted in an overwhelming prohibitionist triumph. His Virginia success led to increased responsibilities as chairman of the National League's Legislative Committee. He soon made his mark in Washington, D.C., as the Temperance Movement's most tenacious spokesman, and his efforts were acknowledged as instrumental in the framing and ratification of National Prohibition during Woodrow Wilson's administration. Cannon, in temperance circles, had emerged as a giant and, as a leader of the dry lobby, one of the most powerful men in American public life as the dry experiment began in 1920.

Powerful men, however, make enemies, and Cannon was no exception. If he was respected (and, in some quarters, feared), he was rarely loved, even among his allies. Rather, he was cold and aloof, and his singular zeal and dedication gave him a reputation for combativeness and even for political viciousness. Indeed, his defense of the Eighteenth Amendment over the 1920s seemed to confirm these views and made him one of the most hated men alive among wets. Although a Democrat, for example, in 1928 he led a brutal (but effective) campaign against his party's nominee for president, wet Governor Alfred E. Smith of New York. The bishop urged fellow Democrats to vote for Republican Herbert Hoover and resorted to smear tactics against Smith which made his Catholic religion a campaign issue. Cannon claimed too much credit for Hoover's victory, but his stock among drys was never higher. Yet his opponents burned for revenge, and they had only months to wait. In 1929, the press and Senator Carter Glass (of Cannon's own Virginia) leveled a damning series of charges against the antiliquor champion, ranging from gambling in stocks and hoarding flour during World War I to adultery. A five-year furor ensued, including civil litigation and church investigations, and Cannon ultimately was cleared of all charges. His standing as a moral and political leader, however, never recovered: Thousands continued to believe him guilty, and in any case the repeal of Prohibition took away his major issue. He faded quickly from public view, and his death in 1944 (while attending an Anti-Saloon League conference in Chicago) excited little public comment.

### Bibliography:

A. *Temperance Reform in the United States of America* (Westerville, OH, 1921); *Prohibition in the United States* (Westerville, OH, 1923); *We're Going

*Dry to Stay* (Westerville, OH, 1926); *The Present Day Whisky Rebellion and How to Meet It* (Washington, DC, 1932); *Bishop Cannon's Own Story*, ed. Richard L. Watson (New York, 1955).

B. DAB Supp. 3, 131–32; SEAP 2, 506–7; WW 2, 100–101; Thomas M. Coffey, *The Long Thirst: Prohibition in America, 1920–1933* (New York, 1975); Virginius Dabney, *Dry Messiah: The Life of Bishop Cannon* (New York, 1949).

**CAPPER, Arthur**     (14 July 1865, Garnett, KS—19 December 1951, Topeka, KS). *Career*: compositor, *Topeka Daily Capital*, 1884; reporter, editor, *Topeka Daily Capital*, 1880s to 1891; correspondent, *New York Tribune*, 1891–93; publisher, various Kansas and Midwestern newspapers and periodicals (including *North Topeka Mail* and *Topeka Daily Capital*), 1893–1951; governor of Kansas, 1915–19; member, U.S. Senate, 1919–49.

After an education in Kansas public schools, Arthur Capper first entered the newspaper business in 1884 as a compositor on the *Topeka Daily Capital*. The young typesetter, however, proved a talented writer himself and quickly rose through the ranks on the *Capital*, serving successively as a reporter and then city editor. In 1891 he was hired by the *New York Tribune* as its Washington, D.C., correspondent. Yet he missed his native Kansas, and after saving enough from his salary he returned home and bought the *North Topeka Mail*, a weekly paper. A committed Republican, Capper used the *Mail* to buck the rising Populist tide in Kansas, and he built the paper into a solid financial success. By 1904 he had acquired a second paper, the *Topeka Daily Capital*, with which he had first started, and then continued securing new publications. Over the course of the years Capper would own twenty-seven papers in all, twelve of them at one time. Many of these were small farm journals, which he referred to as his Farm Press. With journalistic success, Capper began to dabble in politics. He ran for governor of Kansas in 1912 and lost by only twenty-nine votes. It was his first and only loss; thereafter, he won sixteen consecutive electoral contests. By 1915 he was governor; by 1919 he was U.S. senator from Kansas, the first of five terms in the upper house of Congress. His political career was certainly long enough, but not an especially noteworthy one. Few pieces of significant legislation are attached to his name, although the Capper-Volstead Acts of 1922 and 1926 and the Capper-Ketcham Act of 1928 were of some prominence in their day. The first two provided government aid to farm cooperatives and the last supported 4-H Clubs. Neither, however, made a lasting impact.

Capper's association with the Temperance Movement began with his earliest days in the newspaper business. While an editor on the *Daily Capital* in the 1880s, his prohibitionist sentiments became a matter of public record, and his entry into Kansas politics saw him emerge as an effective and committed dry champion. While governor of the state, Caper made a practice of addressing church congregations from the pulpit in support of prohibition, and he threw his full support behind a successful effort to pass a Kansas "bone-dry" law in 1917. Thereafter, he publicly defended the effectiveness of the statute—an effort which garnered him considerable national attention—and also travelled to neighboring

Nebraska to campaign for temperance laws there. When that state went dry, the Nebraska Dry Federation gave Capper a major share of the credit for the victory. Upon his election to the Senate, the Kansas reformer continued to work on behalf of the cause he had made an integral part of his political career. One temperance source cited him as "among the staunchest of dry leaders in the Senate," even though he had little reputation in Washington as a forceful orator. After repeal, however, Capper's public support for the antiliquor crusade faded, and he shifted his activities to New Deal politics (which, as a Republican, created something of a stir among many of his constituents). While holding office, however, the senator also kept in close touch with his business interests. His newspaper empire continued to grow, so that by the time he died in 1951 its total circulation had risen to some five million. Most of his estate, by Capper's specific wish, was used to create the Capper Foundation for Crippled Children.

**Bibliography:**

A. *The Agricultural Bloc* (New York, 1922); ed., *Citizenship* (New York, 1933); with Earl C. Michener, *The Congress* (Chicago, 1933); *Addresses and Messages...* (Topeka, KS, 19-?).

B. Byron M. Crowley, "The Public Career of Arthur Capper Prior to His Senatorial Service" (M.A. thesis, Kansas State Coll. of Pittsburgh, 1938); *Journal of the West* (Oct. 1974): 26–39; Homer E. Socolofsky, *Arthur Capper: Publisher, Politician, Philanthropist* (Lawrence, KS, 1962).

**CARSE, Matilda Bradley**    (19 November 1835, Saintfield, Ireland—3 June 1917, New York, NY). *Career*: president, Chicago Central Woman's Christian Temperance Union, 1878–1917; president, Woman's Temperance Publishing Association (publisher of *Union Signal*), 1880–98; active retirement, 1913–1917.

We know little of the early years of Matilda Carse (born Bradley), only that she was educated in her native Ireland before immigrating to the United States in 1858. She married a successful railroad manager, Thomas Carse, in 1861. Thomas, however, died of tuberculosis in 1870, leaving Matilda financially secure but with three children to raise alone. She settled in Chicago and became active in local charity work. Her involvement with the Temperance Movement stemmed partly from a tragedy: In 1874 her youngest son was run down and killed by an intoxicated cart driver, and Mrs. Carse subsequently decided to devote her life to the war against drink. She joined the Chicago Central WCTU at this point and won election as president in 1878 (a position she held until her death in 1917). Carse established a reputation as an energetic and effective organizer with a broad range of interests. In this, she reflected the influence of National WCTU President Frances E. Willard,* whose "Do Everything" reform policy sought to ally temperance with a host of other social causes. Under Mrs. Carse, the Chicago Central Union was notably successful in this regard, founding the Bethesda Day Nursery (Chicago's first day-care center for children of working mothers), several kindergartens, an employment agency, and a temperance reading room for men. In addition, the local union directed other charity efforts, a full range of "gospel temperance" meetings, and the introduction of matrons for female prisoners in Chicago police stations. All of those activities had the benefit of Carse's genuine business acumen. She raised most of the necessary finances by herself, managed expenditures, and planned all budgets. In fact, her management skills quickly made her a major asset to the National Union.

Her greatest business contribution to the WCTU came in publishing. The organization had always understood the need for an effective media effort in spreading the dry message, although the WCTU literary presence had not been great during the 1870s. In 1880, however, Carse moved to correct the situation. She founded (and became president of) the Woman's Temperance Publishing Association, a publications clearinghouse for WCTU literature. The company was staffed entirely by women and issued a wide variety of tracts and booklets on social reform, the *Signal*, the official organ of the Illinois Union, and later the national *Union Signal*. By 1890, over one hundred women worked for the association and were issuing more than 125 million pages annually. Like many other businesses of the era, however, the association was hit hard by the depression of the mid-1890s, and its operations consequently suffered. Mrs. Carse resigned in 1898 and the association itself folded in 1903. But the effort had proven that women could manage an extensive business, and the *Union Signal*, at least, continued to publish. Carse's resignation, moreover, was not due fully to the association's reverses. Rather, she was pursuing even bigger game. In 1887, she had launched a building effort for the "Woman's Temple" in downtown Chicago, an office structure that would provide a headquarters for the National Union as well as rental income. She had progressively devoted more of her time to this project, and when the depression threatened its financial success (it was just completed when the economic collapse came in 1893), she decided to turn all her efforts to saving it. It was a losing battle, with what to do about the situation causing considerable strife within the union. At last, after the death of Willard in 1898, and over Carse's objections, the WCTU annual convention voted to sell out at a loss. Although disappointed, Carse tried to restore unity to the organization, acting as a mediator in later years between the adherents of Willard's "Do Everything" policy and a growing faction which sought a narrower focus on prohibition.

**Bibliography:**

B. NAW 1, 292–93; SEAP 2, 524; WW 1, 199; Clara C. Chapin, ed., *Thumb-Nail Sketches of White Ribbon Women* (Evanston, IL?, 1895).

**CARSKADON, Thomas Rosabaum**    (17 May 1837, Sheetz's Mill, VA—21 January 1905, Keyser, WV). *Career*: farmer, Keyser, WV, beginning 1858.

A farmer by profession, Thomas Carskadon came by his reformist tendencies naturally. Born in Virginia, Carskadon was strongly influenced by his father's determination to end involuntary servitude in his home state. Although a slaveholder himself, the elder Carskadon, a delegate to the Virginia House of Burgesses for six years, was among those who had sought to get the legislature to abolish slavery in the two decades prior to the Civil War. This effort failed, but his father's actions had a profound effect on young Thomas. All his life he would maintain a strong opposition to servitude in any form, including enslavement to drink. Indeed, because the liquor industry flourished in the years after the Civil War, his judgement on the conflict was that the real victor was drink. Like his father, Thomas Carskadon took an active interest in politics and was, like many other Southerners in the antebellum South, originally a Whig. And like many Whigs he was opposed to secession, so much so that when Virginia voted to secede, Carskadon left his party and his state. He joined the Republican Party and took an active part in detaching the western counties of Virginia to form the new state of West Virginia. Carskadon was appointed U.S. assessor for the Second West Virginia District by both Presidents Lincoln and Johnson. The latter, however, removed him on account of his sympathies with the Radical Republicans, who were at the time strongly opposed to Johnson's mild Reconstruction policy. Carskadon's last official acts in the Republican Party were to serve as electors for both Grant and Hayes. In 1884 he broke with the GOP over the liquor issue, as indeed did many temperance advocates. If his political principles would not let him tolerate secession, neither would they allow compromise on the liquor question. Accordingly, he became one of the founders of the West Virginia Prohibition Party and was its first candidate for the governorship of West Virginia in 1888. For the rest of his life, Carskadon devoted himself to the welfare of the Prohibition Party, chiefly as fund-raiser and local organizer. He pursued politics, however, without neglecting his farming interests, out of which he wrote *Silos and Ensilage*, a book that was standard in its field for the time.

**Bibliography:**

B. SEAP 2, 524–25.

**CARY, Samuel Fenton**   (18 February 1814, Cincinnati, OH—27 September 1900, College Hill, OH). *Education*: graduated from Miami Univ. (OH), 1835; graduated from Cincinnati Law Sch., 1837; LLD. (honorary), Miami Univ., 1840s? *Career*: legal practice, Cincinnati, OH, 1837–45; farmer, College Hill area, near Cincinnati, OH, beginning 1845; active temperance organizing, lecturing, editing, beginning 1845; paymaster general for Ohio troops during Mexican War, 1845–46; editor, *Ohio Temperance Organ*, 1852–53; editor, *Crusader*, 1856–57; recruiting for the Union army in Ohio, 1861–65; member, U.S. House of Representatives, 1867–69; active retirement and political activity with Greenback Party, 1870s to 1900.

The antebellum Midwest proved fertile ground for the growing Temperance Movement, and the crusade was able to attract some of the region's most notable citizens. In Ohio, the leading advocate of the antiliquor cause was Samuel Fenton

Cary, one of the leading residents of the Cincinnati area, and certainly one of the state's more interesting sons. Cary's family had settled in the region (then on the frontier) in 1813, the year before he was born, and established itself over Samuel's youth as one of the wealthiest in the city. Samuel himself emerged as something of a prodigy: After completing his education (1837), he launched a brilliant legal career. Still in his twenties, he won acclaim as one of the ablest lawyers in the state. This fine reputation, plus his work on behalf of William Henry Harrison's presidential campaign, resulted in Cary's election to the Ohio Supreme Court at the age of twenty-six—an honor he declined in favor of the private practice that was making him rich. By 1845 he was indeed rich, a fact which made his action of that year all the more stunning: For motives not precisely known, the successful lawyer gave up his career and announced his intention to devote his life to the temperance crusade. For the next fifteen years, he was Ohio's premier dry leader. Acting first as the driving force in the organization of the state Sons of Temperance lodges, in 1848 Cary was elected most worthy patriarch of the National Sons Division. An eloquent lecturer, the reformer spoke on tours across the nation and throughout the British Isles. He also edited a number of antiliquor publications, which further enhanced his national reputation. As the 1850s dawned, "General" Cary (he kept the title by courtesy after serving as paymaster general of Ohio troops during the Mexican War) was one of the best-known drys in the country.

The "General" was also one of the nation's most active political prohibitionists. Over the 1840s, and into the early 1850s, many Ohioans had become increasingly perplexed at a number of social changes then shaping the state. While there was economic prosperity, many established citizens were also alarmed at the arrival of thousands of German and Irish immigrants and the rapid urbanization of parts of Ohio. Concern eventually focused on a visible manifestation of urban and immigrant life, drinking; and as historian Jed Dannenbaum has noted, the Temperance Movement grew accordingly among native-born Ohioans. The result was a hard fought campaign in 1853, with Cary leading the drys, to pass an Ohio version of the prohibitory Maine Law. While there were hopes that prohibition would restore a measure of social order, many temperance voters, including General Cary, sincerely hoped the dry statute would alleviate the poverty, crime, and other social ills that had accompanied the industrialization of the state. When it came, however, the popular vote on the law proved a stunning defeat for temperance workers. The Democrats, who professed support for personal temperance but opposed legal prohibition, maintained a party loyalty at the polls that overwhelmed the less organized friends of the proposed law. The Ohio Temperance Movement never fully recovered until the dry resurgence of the 1870s. Cary himself did the best he could to keep remaining antiliquor spirits high, but with the coming of the Civil War he shifted his attention to Union army recruiting activities. Following the conflict he served a term in Congress as an independent, where his old humanitarian sentiments shone through in efforts on behalf of labor (he was a champion of the eight-hour day) and monetary reform. In fact, his concern over currency issues finally led him to the Greenback Party, which nominated him for vice president in 1876. That was his last quest for office, however, and Cary spent his remaining years as a familiar and respected pillar of Cincinnati society.

**Bibliography:**

A. *Cary's Appeal to the People of Ohio...* (Cincinnati, OH, 1847); ed., *The National Temperance Offering and Sons and Daughters of Temperance Gift* (New York, 1850); with others, *License or No License, That Is the Question* (Cincinnati, OH? 1852).

B. SEAP 2, 529; *Biographical Encyclopedia of Ohio of the Nineteenth Century* (Cincinnati, OH, 1876); Jed Dannenbaum, "The Crusader: Samuel Cary and Cincinnati Temperance," *Cincinnati Historical Society Bulletin* 31 (1975): 136–51; Jed Dannenbaum, "Drink and Disorder: Temperance Reform in Cincinnati, 1841–1874" (Ph.D. diss., Univ. of California, Davis, 1980); Charles T. Greve, *Centennial History of Cincinnati and Representative Citizens*, vol 2 (Chicago, 1904); P.R.L. Pierce, *A History of the Introduction and Progress of the Order of the Sons of Temperance in the State of Ohio* (Cincinnati, OH, 1849).

**CASS, Lewis**  (9 October 1782, Exeter, NH—17 June 1866, Detroit, MI). *Education*: studied at acad. in Exeter, NH, 1792–99; studied law under Governor Miegs of Ohio in Marietta, circa 1800–1802. *Career*: teacher, Wilmington, DE, 1799; admitted to bar, OH, 1802; member, Ohio legislature, 1806; U.S. marshall for Ohio, 1807–12; army officer, 1812–13; governor of Michigan Territory, 1813–31; secretary of war, 1831–36; U.S. minister to France, 1836; member, U.S. Senate, 1845–48, 1849–57; secretary of state, 1857–60; active retirement, 1860–66.

A strong personal commitment to temperance was an integral part of the distinguished career of Lewis Cass as a soldier, politician, and statesman. He apparently grew up a teetotaler, claiming at one point, "I have never tasted ardent spirits, nor have I, at any time during my life, been in the habit of drinking wine." While he never explained his motives for his early stance against alcoholic beverages, he always insisted over his career "that I have done well enough without them." Indeed he did, as his progress through life was marked by an almost unbroken string of successes. A lawyer by trade, his skills at the bar brought him a public stature that led to a seat in the Ohio legislature (1806) at age twenty-four. He became a noted Jeffersonian and nationalist, and with the coming of the War of 1812 he survived the American debacle at Detroit and went on to establish an impressive record of command. He was a major general when the conflict ended. A devoted Democrat thereafter, he served successively as governor of Michigan Territory, secretary of war under President Andrew Jackson, minister to France, senator from Michigan, and secretary of state in the cabinet of James Buchanan. He had an influential voice in party affairs and almost won the presidency as his party's nominee in 1848. Cass never really relented in his hatred of Great Britain, and he had a reputation as an expansionist in foreign policy and as a hard-liner when American rights were concerned, especially when dealing with the English. In domestic affairs, he was generally a firm Jacksonian; he advocated compromise and "squatter sovereignty" on the slavery question but championed the Union when the South seceded. In addition, Cass displayed genuine literary talents and frequently wrote on historical, diplomatic, and political subjects.

Throughout his years in public service, Cass sought to popularize his ideas on temperance and to mold policy on the question whenever he could. Although he never became involved with major dry organizations, he made no secret of his aversion to the liquor traffic, and the Temperance Movement looked o him as an ally. During his years of military service, for instance, he was appalled at the drunkenness among his men, which made a lasting impression on him. He argued for abstinence while in ranks—an example he set personally—and later, while secretary of war, promulgated regulations replacing the army spirits ration with coffee. He also took measures to control liquor sales to the troops by civilians, although the practical effects of these efforts are open to question. Still, they fully reflected Cass's personal view that drink only interrupted efficiency and good order. This also extended, as far as he was concerned, to negotiations with the Indians. While governor of Michigan, he shared the Jacksonian view that the Indians had to be removed from the East, but he did urge a humane approach to resettling the tribes in the West. Accordingly, he refused to ply them with alcohol—standard practice for many whites—during treaty discussions, a practice adhered to while dealing with the Indians in his later federal posts. Cass was also the first president of the Congressional Temperance Society in the 1830s, when it was founded by members of Congress and other governmental officials. Thus, while he was by no means a zealous reformer, the Michigan Democrat was certainly consistent in his views, was willing to lead by example, and within the powers of the offices he held, was a proponent of using government to control drinking excesses.

### Bibliography:

A. *Considerations on the Present State of the Indians...* (Boston, 1828); *Speeches, etc.*, 31 pamphlets (Washington, DC, 1836–52); *France: Its King, Court, and Government* (New York, 1848); *Three Hours at St. Cloud, by an American* (n.p., 184-?).

B. DAB 3, 562–64; SEAP 2, 530–31; WW H, 167; Andrew C. McLaughlin, *Lewis Cass* (Boston, 1899); W.L.G. Smith, *Fifty Years of Public Life: The Life and Times of Lewis Cass* (New York, 1856); William T. Young, *Sketch of the Life and Public Services of Gen. Lewis Cass...* (Detroit, 1852).

**CHAFETZ, Morris Edward**    (20 April 1924, Worcester, MA— ). *Education*: B.S., Tufts Univ., 1944; M.D., Tufts Univ., 1948. *Career*: intern, Marine Hosp., Detoit, MI, 1948–49; resident in psychiatry, State Hosp., Howard, RI,

1949–51; fellow in neurophysiology, Instituto Nacional de Cardiologia, Mexico, 1951–52; director, Alcohol Clinic, Massachusetts General Hosp., 1957–68; director, Clinical Psychiatric Service, Massachusetts General Hosp., 1968–70; acting director, Division of Alcohol Abuse and Alcoholism, National Inst. of Mental Health, 1970–71; director, National Inst. on Alcohol Abuse and Alcoholism, 1971–75; principal research scientist, Johns Hopkins Univ., beginning 1975; president, Health Education Foundation, Washington, DC, beginning 1976; chairman of the board, Health Inst., Washington, DC, beginning 1977.

Trained as a psychiatrist, Chafetz emerged as one of the most articulate and influential public advocates of the medical treatment of alcohol-related disorders. While practicing at a number of psychiatrically oriented centers (notably those of the Massachusetts General Hospital, where Chafetz served in various administrative capacities between 1957 and 1970), and during his teaching (he was on the faculty of the Harvard University Medical School from 1954 to 1970), he focused considerable effort on the problem. His research involved the development of alcoholism treatment programs, and as director of the Alcohol Clinic at Massachusetts General (1957–68), he was able to apply them in a clinical setting. His writings on the subject established him as a national authority in the field, and Chafetz steadily rose as a spokesman for the cause of public action to deal with alcohol problems. (At the same time, it should be noted that Chafetz also made important contributions to the study of psychological factors at work in Parkinson's disease.) By the early 1960s, Chafetz was a consultant on alcoholism to the National Institute of Mental Health (NIMH) and had made a survey of alcohol problems and treatment approaches in Eastern Europe (where he travelled extensively). When the federal government established a division of NIMH to deal with alcoholism, Chafetz led its activities, and when further legislation created the National Institute on Alcohol Abuse and Alcoholism (NIAAA) as a separate agency, the Massachusetts psychiatrist was named as its first director in 1971.

In office, he emphasized that the institute was not opposed to drinking, that alcoholism—not liquor—was the problem. He urged a program of creating ''responsible'' drinking patterns in the country, as well as major federal involvement in the funding of treatment, education, and prevention efforts. Over his tenure, he successfully built a considerable popular constituency for the federal alcoholism programs (including much of the liquor industry) and, by virtue of his position, shaped much of the early national effort until his resigantion in 1975. Chafetz, however, never felt obligated to adopt any doctrinaire positions on alcohol problems. After leaving office (when he became deeply involved in health education activities), he differed publicly with others in the field, and NIAAA itself, on such issues as ''responsible drinking'' (Chafetz retained his belief in the idea while others felt it might encourage drinking problems) and the controversial ''Rand Report,'' which suggested that some alcoholics might be able to return to controlled drinking (Chafetz defended the study). In any event, Chafetz has remained an active participant in the alcoholism field, and his career with NIMH and NIAAA served as a telling illustration of the growth of federal participation in health-related areas during the 1960s and 1970s.

**Bibliography:**

A. with Harold W. Demone, Jr., *Alcoholism and Society* (New York, 1962); *Liquor: The Servant of Man* (Boston: 1965); with Howard T. Blane and Marjorie J. Hill, eds., *Frontiers of Alcoholism* (New York, 1970); *Why Drinking Can Be Good for You* (Briarcliff Manor, NY, 1976).

B. *American Men and Women of Science*, 13th ed., vol. 1 (New York, 1976), 675; *Who's Who in America*, 41st ed., vol. 1 (Chicago, 1980–81), 585; Carolyn L. Wiener, *The Politics of Alcoholism: Building an Arena Around a Social Problem* (New Brunswick, NJ, 1981).

**CHAFIN, Eugene Wilder**    (1 November 1852, East Troy, WI—30 November 1920, Long Beach, CA). *Education*: LLB., Univ. of Wisconsin, 1875. *Career*: private legal practice, Waukesha, WI, 1876–1900; superintendent, Washingtonian Home for Inebriates, Chicago, 1901–4; political and lecturing work with Prohibition Party, 1904 to circa 1913.

A keen sense of law and order, social justice, and public duty characterized the distinguished temperance career of Eugene Chafin. After completing his education, he practiced law in Waukesha, Wisconsin, for almost twenty-five years, during which time he pursued an active interest in civil affairs and social reform. He served in a number of local positions, including a seat on the board of education, president of the county agricultural society, member of the library board, police court magistrate, and justice of the peace. He was also a dedicated member of the Methodist Epworth League (sitting twice as Wisconsin state president), which added a deeply religious dimension to his perceptions of public service. His reform interests focused largely on the Temperance Movement, his first active involvement coming at age fourteen when he joined the Independent Order of Good Templars. Over the years, he undertook an increasing range of responsibilities on behalf of the order, and in the early 1900s he sat as his state's representative in the International Supreme Lodge of Good Templars. Chafin's concern over assisting the alcoholic, which was part of his experience with the Good Templars, took even more concrete expression in 1901, when he became superintendent of the Chicago Washingtonian Home for Inebriates. The institution, one of the pioneer American alcoholism rehabilitation centers, combined both medical and spiritual treatment approaches and was generally prosperous under the Wisconsin reformer's leadership (1901–4). While involved with these activities, however, Chafin gradually drifted toward a total commitment to yet another field—dry politics.

Chafin originally had been a Republican, but in 1881 he joined the Prohibition Party. Almost immediately he plunged into electoral contests, running the following year for Congress. Four years later (1886) he ran for state attorney general (and twice more, in 1901 and in 1904), and in 1898 for governor. While never elected, he emerged as a vigorous campaigner and became a familiar figure in Wisconsin politics. Somewhat curiously, although an ardent dry, in these early contests he never had much faith in statutory prohibition (including a National Prohibition amendment). "The scheme to destroy the liquor traffic by constitutional provision," he later remarked, "has always been and always will be a huge farce." Yet he labored with the Prohibitionists as a means of forming public sentiment against the traffic, enforcing regulatory laws, and ultimately ending the liquor evil (in all of its forms) through turning citizens away from the saloon. Chafin also considered the party the only true reform group then in politics and hoped it would prove a vehicle to further other Progressive era legislation. In 1908 and 1912 he received the Prohibition nomination for the presidency, and he conducted his usual spirited campaign. He retained a fairly broad reform orientation on the stump, including a commitment to civil rights. Indeed, during the 1908 contest he risked his life to stop the lynching of a black man by an Illinois mob. With the approach of National Prohibition, Chafin's opposition to statutory measures apparently slackened; he made a number of speaking tours on its behalf and then turned to an interest in international dry efforts. He lectured in both Australia and New Zealand before his death at home in Long Beach, California (where he had moved in the 1900s), in 1920.

**Bibliography:**

A. *The Voters' Handbook...* (Waukesha, WI, 1876); *Chafin's Lives of the Presidents of the United States of America* (Waukesha, WI, 1896); *Lincoln: The Man of Sorrow* (Chicago, 1908); *The Church and School...* (Chicago? 1911); *The Master Method of the Great Reform: Speeches of Eugene W. Chafin...* (Chicago, 1913).

B. *Chicago Tribune*, Dec. 1, 1920; DAB 3, 590–91; SEAP 2, 544–45; WW 1, 206; Jack S. Blocker, Jr., *Retreat from Reform: The Prohibition Movement in the United States, 1890–1913* (Westport, CT, 1976).

**CHALFANT, Harry Malcolm** (26 June 1869, Coal Center, PA—10 November 1932, Narberth, PA). *Education*: graduated from California (PA) State Normal Sch., 1886; A.B., Washington and Jefferson Coll., 1892; A.M., Washington and Jefferson Coll., 1895; D.D. (honorary), Washington and Jefferson Coll., 1922. *Career*: ordained in Methodist Church, 1893; minister, local Pennsylvania pastorates, 1893–1909; editor, *Pittsburgh Christian Advocate*, 1902–8; editor, *Keystone Citizen*, 1909–10; editor, *American Issue* (Pennsylvania ed.), 1910–32; district superintendent, Anti-Saloon League of Pennsylvania, 1932.

There was never any shortage of those using a pen on behalf of the temperance crusade. Few, however, focused their antiliquor careers so completely on literary pursuits as Harry Chalfant. He began as Methodist minister and in all of his local pulpits stressed the evils of the liquor traffic. His first editorial duties came in 1902, when he agreed to help bring out the *Pittsburgh Christian Advocate*, a church-related antiliquor publication. He enjoyed the work and in 1909 gave up his work on the *Advocate*, as well as the ministry, to undertake the editorship of the *Keystone Citizen*. Chalfant's management of the *Citizen* and his hard-hitting attacks on the Pennsylvania liquor traffic were well received by temperance workers and won the special recognition of the state Anti-Saloon League. The following year, the league in fact adopted the *Citizen* (with Chalfant as editor), making it the Pennsylvania edition of the *American Issue*. As editor, the former minister emerged as a prolific author himself, who took a special liking to exposing false or fraudulent claims on the part of his wet counterparts. He also undertook several major books, notably a history of the antiliquor struggle in his native state, *Father Penn and John Barleycorn* (1920). As a speaker, Chalfant served the league long and well, stumping the state for years on behalf of dry candidates and Prohibition. Even as Repeal loomed, he remained steadfast in the cause. He kept dry publications functioning in Pennsylvania, sat as a member of the National Anti-Saloon League Executive Committee, and, in 1932, assumed the duties of a district superintendent with the Pennsylvania League. And even though he had relinquished his ministerial duties in 1909, Chalfant always remained an avid churchman, taking part, whenever his duties allowed, in Methodist affairs (in 1920, for example, he was a delegate to the Methodist General Conference). He fought for his cause until the end and died in 1932, a year before the demise of the "noble experiment" itself.

**Bibliography:**

A. *An Exercise for Sunday Schools on World's Temperance Studies* (Philadelphia, 1915); *Father Penn and John Barleycorn* (Harrisburg, PA, 1920); *Paying the Fiddler* (Philadelphia, 1929); *These Agitators and Their Idea* (Nashville, TN, 1931).

B. SEAP 2, 545–46; WW 1, 206.

**CHAMBERS, John** (19 December 1797, Stewartstown, Co. Tyrone, Ireland—22 September 1875, Philadelphia, PA). *Career*: ordained Presbyterian minister, 1825; minister, Ninth Associate Reformed Church, Philadelphia, 1825–75.

Reformation of the habitual drinker was a central aspect of the Temperance Movement. Another was prevention, an entire series of efforts to stop the young from acquiring the habit to begin with. It was in this latter aspect that John Chambers excelled. A native of Ireland who came to America at an early age, Chambers studied privately for the ministry of the Presbyterian Church while living in Baltimore, Maryland. In 1825 he was ordained and made pastor of the Ninth Associate Reform Church in Philadelphia, where he remained for the rest of his life. Such was the power of his teaching and influence that a number of his congregation went on to become ministers themselves, and one, the later great merchant John Wanamaker, founded the celebrated Bethany Sunday School. From the start, Chambers took temperance as his chief mission, especially the task of keeping the young from forming the liquor habit. He organized a Youth's

Temperance Society, which became the forum for his not inconsiderable talent as an orator. Chambers made a special practice of indicting the liquor trade for subverting youth, and his savage attacks on saloonkeepers, brewers, and distillers earned him their fiercest obloquy, and sometimes even more. On several occasions he was verbally and physically assaulted on the streets of the City of Brotherly Love by the outraged recipients of his scorn. But he met them either by icy indifference or a mild turning of the other cheek. Chambers had a unique way of bringing his temperance message home to others. He refused to officiate at any funeral service where liquor was served and once compelled the mourners to bring the remains of the deceased to him for the obsequies rather than enter premises where spiritous beverages were consumed. When he died in 1875 the Philadelphia Presbytery honored his memory by naming the new church at Broad and Sansom streets the Chambers Presbyterian Church.

**Bibliography:**

B. SEAP 2, 547–48.

**CHANNING, William Ellery**   (7 April 1780, Newport, RI—2 October 1842, Bennington, VT). *Education*: graduated from Harvard Coll., 1789; studied theology, Cambridge, MA, 1801–2. *Career*: tutor, Richmond, VA, 1798–1800; minister, Federal Street Congregational Church, Boston, 1803–42.

Over decades of crusading, the Temperance Movement ultimately moved away from the moral-suasionist, rationalist idea that individuals would voluntarily give up strong drink out of any personal or social motives. And the triumph of the prohibitionist (''legal suasionist'') position has often obscured the fact that the less strident approach also had some articulate supporters. One of the most eloquent of these was William Ellery Channing. Spiritual leader, liberal theologian, and influential author, Channing came from impeccable New England Calvinist stock, the first Channing having arrived in America in 1711. After graduating from Harvard College in 1798, he tutored briefly in Virginia and returned to Boston to study theology, to which he applied himself with such dedication and enthusiasm that he gradually undermined his health by long and arduous hours of study. In 1803, Channing was ordained in the Congregational Church and was elected minister of the Federal Street Church in Boston, where he remained until his death in 1842. It was while serving in the pulpit that Channing became embroiled in the religious controversy surrounding Calvinism, and especially Congregationalism, in the late eighteenth and early nineteenth centuries in New England. Many of the more liberal theologians were rejecting the harsh Calvinism of their forebears, a Calvinism that featured a stern and unforgiving God, and arguing for a more liberal interpretation of the Scriptures. Channing took his stand with them and, stressing the goodness of God, the freedom of the human will, and the perfectability of man, became the focal point for the origins of Unitarianism. Channing, however, had no real interest in founding a new church or a new denomination. Not doctrine, but individual freedom was his true aim. He was even uncomfortable with the name "Unitarian," not wishing to see the new ideas frozen into institutionalized form.

Out of Channing's religious ideas came significant social ideas. Among them was the distinctly modern notion that society had obligations for the regeneration of the individual. Indeed, Channing seems to have anticipated modern social theory in that he saw the problem of individual evil inherent in the evils of society. The individual must not be held solely accountable for his shortcomings, nor is he to be left to seek his salvation unaided. Social conditions and attitudes are just as responsible for an individual's fate as his own failures. So far had Channing come from the faith of his fathers. These ideas are reflected in Channing's views on temperance. He understood the evils of drink and attacked them in his *Thoughts on Temperance* in 1834. But aggressive and powerful as was his attack on contemporary social evils, he was opposed to coercive morality. The law is but a weak reed to lean upon, he argued, in the reformation of the individual. Rather, he favored the reformation of social institutions, including the elimination of the saloon through an "enlightened and vigorous public sentiment" (that is, through society-wide moral suasion). Prohibition had no place in Channing's solution to the problem of drink. Frail health forced Channing from the pulpit into writing, and over the course of his life he wrote extensively on literature, politics, history, and philosophy as well as on social and moral questions. His influence on Emerson, Bryant, Longfellow, Lowell, and Holmes is now clearly acknowledged by literary historians. The base of Channing's statue in the Public Garden of Boston bears the inscription: "He breathed into theology a humane spirit." He tried to do no less for temperance; and although the movement adopted the legislative approach to reform that Channing warned against, many antiliquor crusaders still acknowledged him as an "aggressive and powerful" enemy of the "prevalent evils of his day."

## Bibliography:

A. *Discourses, Reviews and Miscellanies* (Boston, 1830); *Discourses* (Boston, 1832); *Slavery* (Boston, 1835); *An Address on Temperance . . .* (Boston, 1837, and subsequent editions); *Poems* (Boston, 1847); *The Works of William E. Channing, D.D.*, 8th ed., 6 vols., (Boston, 1848).

B. DAB 4, 4–7; SEAP 2, 553–54; John W. Chadwick, *William Ellery Channing* (Boston, 1903); William H. Channing, *Memoir of William Ellery Channing, with Extracts from his Correspondence and Manuscripts*, 3 vols. (Boston, 1848); David P. Edgell, *William Ellery Channing* (Boston, 1955); Jack Mendelsohn, *Channing the Reluctant Radical* (Boston, 1971); Robert L. Patterson, *The Philosophy of William Ellery Channing* (New York, 1952).

**CHAPIN, Sarah (Sallie) Flournoy Moore**    (14 March 1830? Charleston, SC— 19 April 1896, Charleston, SC). *Career*: civic charity work, Charleston, SC (primarily with YMCA and Ladies Christian Association), 1860s–1870s; WCTU organizer and lecturer, 1880–96.

It was a common pattern in the lives of the nineteenth-century women temperance workers that their full-time involvement came only with widowhood. The career of Sarah Chapin fits the pattern perfectly. Married at seventeen to Leonard Chapin, who had left Massachusetts for the more salubrious climate of South Carolina, Sarah Chapin devoted herself up to the Civil War largely to the life of what she herself described as a "literary scribbler." During the Civil War, in which her husband served in the Confederate cavalry, Mrs. Chapin got her first taste of organizational work as president of both the Soldiers' Relief Society and the Ladies' Auxiliary Christian Association of Charleston. But it was only after the death of her husband in 1878 that Mrs. Chapin found her true vocation, and it came about by one of those happy accidents that so often change lives. Attending a temperance convention in Ocean City, New Jersey, in 1879, Chapin was called upon to speak extemporaneously. Not only did she impress her audience with her eloquence, but she also discovered a hitherto unsuspected life's work. Her energy, intensity, and fiery dedication brought her to the attention of Frances Willard,* who was looking for someone to organize the southern branch of the newly founded Woman's Christian Temperance Union. This Chapin did, not only for South Carolina (where she was elected president of the state union in 1883), but eventually for the entire South, where she travelled as much as twenty thousand miles a year, often giving a speech a night. No wonder Willard caller her "that great-hearted and intrepid leader of the South." During the 1870s and 1880s, when reunion and reconciliation between the sections were taking place, Chapin's work for temperance, both in the North and the South, was regarded by many of her contemporaries as a significant contribution toward healing the wounds of the Civil War.

Chapin was at first hesitant to pursue Willard's broad-based approach to reform, fearing that WCTU endorsements of other reforms would drive a wedge in the Temperance Movement and cost it outside support. This was especially true with woman's suffrage, which she at first saw as too divisive an issue to link with the fortunes of the union. Yet as women increasingly took the initiative in the antiliquor struggle, Chapin came to see the necessity and logic of female suffrage—it would vastly enhance the impact of women in reform work—and she gave it her unstinting support beginning in 1891. After this, she embraced other causes as well. She launched a campaign for better educational opportunities for South Carolina women, and her efforts led ultimately to the founding of Winthrop College for Women. Another reform for which she labored succeeded in 1895, when the new state constitution raised the age of consent for girls from ten to sixteen. Still, the antiliquor crusade remained her chief interest, and she was a tireless champion of state and national prohibition legislation. And although she was unable to get full prohibition in South Carolina (her lobbying efforts, however, came close to success), she at least had the satisfaction of seeing the saloons closed in 1893 and the liquor trade taken out of the hands of individual entrepreneurs and made a state monopoly. Indefatigable, stalwart, and eloquent, Sarah Chapin was one of the undeniable bulwarks of the Temperance Movement in the late nineteenth-century American South, to which the monument raised over her grave in Charleston, paid for by money collected from all over the United States, gives ample testimony.

**Bibliography:**

A. *Fitz-Hugh St. Clair, the South Carolina Rebel Boy; or, It Is No Crime to Be Born a Gentleman* (Charleston, SC, 1872).
B. NAW 1, 321–22; SEAP 2, 554.

**CHEEVER, George Barrell**    (6 February 1814, Hallowell, ME—1 October 1890, Englewood, NJ). *Education*: graduated from Bowdoin Coll., 1825; graduated from Andover Sem., 1830. *Career*: ordained in Congregational Church, 1833; minister, Howard Street Congregational Church, Salem, MA, 1833–38; minister, Allen Street Presbyterian Church, New York City, 1838–44; minister, Church of Puritans, New York City, 1846–67; active literary work, 1867–90.

The decades of antebellum social reform activity produced more than a few fiery polemicists. Not many reformers, however, generated as much controversy in so many fields as did George Barrell Cheever. Strident in almost everything he did, Cheever began his public career as a Congregationalist minister, a role which soon found him embroiled in theological disputes. He attacked Unitarians for their literary tastes, hurled barbs at Episcopalians for their use of ritual, and later denounced the Catholic Church when he thought it was trying to outlaw Bible reading in the public schools. Withal, he was a popular preacher with his own congregations, for whatever else he was, he was seldom boring. Like many Americans of his age, Cheever firmly believed that it was the church's responsibility to define both private and public mores and to denounce sin in all of its guises. That being the case, he never lacked for subject matter. His sermons and his enormous literary output over the years rang with attacks on intemperance, Sabbath breaking (Cheever considered it outrageous, for example, to run trains on Sundays), alleged theological errors, opponents of capital punishment (he zealously defended the practice on Scriptural grounds), slavery, and other evils. The impassioned preacher was especially combative on the slavery question, arguing that society owed blacks more than emancipation; they also deserved full citizenship and education (in this regard, at his death he left his own substantial library to Howard University). In sum, George Cheever approached the archetypical antebellum reformer.

His first major exposure to public controversy, however, at least as a national figure, came as an antiliquor crusader. Only two years after his ordination, he penned a scathing satire on the involvement of church officials with the liquor business, "The True History of Deacon Giles' Distillery," which appeared in the *Salem* (MA) *Landmark* of February 1835. The story was an allegory, depicting a distillery run by a deacon who also sold Bibles; and although Cheever gave the distiller a fictitious name, the situation matched reality in Salem fairly closely. Indeed, the real "Deacon Giles," a Salem man named Stone, unsurprisingly took umbrage and sued Cheever for libel. In a case that won a celebrated niche in dry tradition, Deacon Stone won a judgement, although that was hardly the end of the matter. "The True History" had aroused so much hostility that the foreman of the distillery physically attacked the author, and the *Landmark*'s press was destroyed by a mob. Stone won a thousand dollars and the satisfaction of seeing Cheever jailed for a month. The minister, though, had his own supporters, who made him as comfortable as possible in jail, gave him a rousing reception upon his release, and applauded when he subsequently (and stubbornly) published yet another blast at Stone entitled "Deacon Jones' Brewery: or the Distiller Turned Brewer." This time, Cheever had considerable popular backing and no legal action resulted. While the zealous parson never lessened his hatred of the traffic, his polemics against Deacons Giles and Jones were his greatest contributions to temperance literature, and they remained favorites of drys for years. Yet in retrospect, they were just an early part of Cheever's remarkable literary career: At his death, his collected works came to over twenty-three bound volumes and some fifty pamphlets and other shorter titles.

### Bibliography:

A. *The American Commonplace Book of Prose* (Boston, 1828, and later editions); *The American Commonplace Book of Poetry* (Boston, 1829, and later editions); *Wanderings of a Pilgrim in the Shadow of Mt. Blanc* (New York, 1845); *God Against Slavery; and the Freedom and Duty of the Pulpit to Rebuke It as a Sin Against God* (New York, 1857); *The Dream, or the True History of Deacon Giles' Distillery, and Deacon Jones' Brewery* (New York, 1859); *The Guilt of Slavery and the Crime of Slaveholding, Demonstrated from the Hebrew and Greek Scriptures* (New York, 1860).

B. DAB 4, 48–49; SEAP 2, 563–64; WW H, 172; H. T. Cheever, ed., *Memorabilia of Geo. B. Cheever* (New York, 1891); H. T. Cheever, *Memorial Address . . . Upon the Life, Character and Influence of Dr. Geo. Barrell Cheever* (Washington, DC, 1892); *Congregational Yearbook* (1891).

**CHERRINGTON, Ernest Hurst**   (24 November 1877, Hamden, OH—13 March 1850, Worthington, OH). *Education*: studied at Ohio Wesleyan Univ., 1893–97; LLD. (honorary), Ohio Wesleyan Univ., 1920; D.L. (honorary), Otterbein Coll., 1922. *Career*: teacher, Ross Co., OH, circa 1897–1900; editor, *Kingston* (OH) *Tribune*, 1900–1; superintendent, Canton District, Anti-Saloon League of Ohio, 1902–3; assistant superintendent, Anti-Saloon League of Ohio, 1903–5; state superintendent, Anti-Saloon League of Washington, 1905–8; assistant editor, *American Issue*, 1908; editor, *American Issue*, beginning 1909; general manager of Anti-Saloon League publishing interests, beginning 1910; founder and general secretary, World League Against Alcoholism, 1919; executive secretary, Board of Temperance of the Methodist Church, 1936–48; retirement, 1948–50.

In his autobiography, Bishop James Cannon,* one of the most influential temperance leaders in American history, credited Ernest Cherrington with being the man most responsible for the passage of the National Prohibition amendment to the Constitution. The remark was (in true Cannon fashion) an overstatement; but it was also a tribute to a man with a rare blend of literary and managerial gifts and an abiding dedication to the antiliquor cause. Though a moderate in comparison with many other temperance advocates, Cherrington, who had become affiliated with the Anti-Saloon League in the early 1890s, devoted most of his productive career to the cause. He began as a league speaker in Ross County, Ohio, but climbed steadily through the organization's administrative ranks as his reputation for effectiveness grew. While serving in his various managerial posts, however, Cherrington also took an active interest in editing dry publications (beginning with the Washington State League's *Citizen* in 1905.) His performance was such that the National League called him to Chicago in 1908 to serve as assistant editor of the group's new official organ, *American Issue*. Within two years he was editor and also had assumed responsibility for all of the league's other publications. He subsequently established and headed the American Issue Press in Westerville, Ohio, which gave the league a major publishing capacity. Running the publication effort was a critical role, as the league placed great emphasis on the effective use of the media in publicizing its cause, and Cherrington rapidly became one of the most influential voices in league circles (although often without major public recognition). He also emerged as a central figure in organizational fund-raising efforts and financial management and in developing an active league speakers bureau. In addition, Cherrington wrote voluminously on behalf of the crusade. His many editorials, pamphlets, articles, and books established him as one of the most learned of the movement's leaders, and his editorship of the six-volume *Standard Encyclopedia of the Alcohol Problem* (1925–30) was, by any measure, a monumental accomplishment.

While his chief claim to recognition grew from his literary and managerial talents, Cherrington was also active in other areas. He was a frequent lecturer and he spearheaded league efforts to found the World League Against Alcoholism. He served as the general secretary of the new group from 1919 on and was repeatedly an American representative to the world organization's international congress abroad down to 1923. Cherrington also worked with temperance groups other than the Anti-Saloon League, as well as taking an active role as a lay leader of the Methodist Church. When, after Repeal, the fortunes of the Temperance Movement in general and the league in particular went into decline, Cherrington worked hard to revitalize the crusade and in 1936 moved to Washington, D.C., to head the Methodist Board of Temperance. And although the movement itself could not be salvaged, he was able to keep some dry publications solvent and reduce the debt of the board. Even in adversity the tireless editor showed an openness to new ideas not often shared by other drys. He cooperated, for example, with the early efforts of the Yale University Summer School of Alcohol Studies (which sought to lift discussion of alcohol-related issues out of an exclusively wet–dry context) and displayed a reasonableness in debate that belied the frequently zealous image of antiliquor argument. He was a true scholar and statesman of his cause and probably its most effective literary voice.

**Bibliography:**

A. *History of the Anti-Saloon League* (Westerville, OH, 1913); *The Evolution of Prohibition in America* (Westerville, OH, 1920); *America and the World Liquor Problem* (Westerville, OH, 1922); with William Eugene Johnson and Cora Frances Stoddard, eds., *Standard Encyclopedia of the Alcohol Problem*, 6 vols. (Westerville, OH, 1925–30).

B. DAB Supp. 4, 160–61; SEAP 2, 565–66; Norman H. Clark, *The Dry Years: Prohibition and Social Change in Washington* (Seattle, WA, 1965); Peter Odegard, *Pressure Politics: The Story of the Anti-Saloon League* (New York, 1928); Richard L. Watson, ed., *Bishop Cannon's Own Story* (New York, 1955).

**CLARK, Myron Holley** (23 October 1806, Naples, NY—23 August 1892, Canadaigua, NY). *Career*: sheriff, Ontario Co., NY, 1837; hardware business, 1840s–?; village president, Canadaigua, NY, 1850–51; member, New York Senate, 1853–54; governor of New York, 1855–57; collector, U.S. Internal Revenue Service, 1862–68; active retirement, 1868–92.

Myron Holley Clark was one of the Temperance Movement's most successful antebellum representatives in electoral politics. Certainly he did as much as anyone to politicize the antiliquor question in New York State. Clark reflected a major part of the reform politics of his era, standing as an avowed radical on the slavery and temperance issues and gaining a wide public reputation as an uncompromising champion of his pet causes. He filled a number of local offices to the satisfaction of his constituents, but his chance to have a significant political impact came in 1852, when he won election (he was a Whig) to the New York State Senate. He took his seat as a professed supporter of Maine Law legislation (Neal Dow's victory in that state had helped inspire him), and he lost no time in pursuing his antiliquor goal. At the same time, however, he displayed his penchant for reform in other areas as well. He played an effective role, for instance, in framing a series of needed railroad reforms. His greatest triumph, however, came in 1854 when the Senate and Assembly approved a "Bill for the Suppression of Intemperance." In effect, it was a New York Maine Law, which would have secured legal prohibition in the state. Clark justifiably received a major share of credit for the measure, and he was outraged when Governor Horatio Seymour vetoed it. Yet that hardly ended the matter, as Clark, having come so close, was not about to give up. Indeed, his counterattack was to cost Seymour and the Democrats dearly. For in New York, if only briefly, an antiliquor wave was about to crest.

The confrontation over the prohibition law was the catalyst for a general reform awakening in New York politics. At the request of a number of dry groups, Clark agreed to run against Seymour for governor in 1854. At the same time, antislavery organizations, including some Democrats and the Anti-Nebraska Party, and the Whigs lent their support; Clark thus was able to campaign as the leader of a broad coalition of reform-oriented groups. (Clark himself thereafter maintained that the coalition was the origin of the state Republican Party.) The contest was bitter and close, and the dry candidate won by a mere 309 votes. Yet upon taking office he urged the prompt passage of a prohibition statute, and a friendly legislature complied. While the law had considerable popular support, the new governor was still destined to see it frustrated. He was able to enforce it, at least partially, for eight months, with hotly debated results. At that point, however, the New York Supreme Court declared the statute unconstitutional, and Clark was not able to wring another measure out of the legislature in his term. But Clark still breathed the same temperance fire, and it cost him renomination. As the nation's sectional crisis deepened, public interest in temperance lessened, and political leaders felt that Clark, so heavily committed to the issue, could not win. He later accepted an appointment from the Lincoln administration as collector of Internal Revenue, and although he did run as the Prohibition Party candidate for governor in 1874, he remained largely out of politics for the rest of his life.

**Bibliography:**

B. DAB 4, 138; SEAP 2, 625–26; WW H, 177; Charles Z. Lincoln, ed., *State of New York: Messages from the Governors*, vol. 4 (Albany, NY, 1909); *Myron H. Clark's Prohibitory Liquor Law and Governor Seymour's Veto* (New York, 1854).

**CLEARY, James Mathew**    (8 September 1849, Dedham, MA—?). *Education*: studied at St. Lawrence Coll., Calvary, WI, and St. Francis Sem. and Coll., Milwaukee, WI. *Career*: ordained in Roman Catholic Church, 1872; priest, archdiocese of Milwaukee, WI, 1872–92; priest, Church of St. Charles, Minneapolis, MN, 1892–1909; priest and organizer, Parish of the Incarnation, Minneapolis, MN, 1909–?.

James Mathew Cleary was apparently sympathetic to the Temperance Movement since boyhood but did not become active in the crusade until after his ordination as a Catholic priest in 1872. (He was ordained a year before the minimum normal age with a special dispensation from Rome.) From the start of his religious career, however, he made temperance a central part of his pastoral message. He was an active priest for twenty years in the Milwaukee, Wisconsin, archdiocese, and during those years worked almost constantly (since 1873) with the Catholic Total Abstinence Union of America. He became president of the Wisconsin Union in 1880 and for twelve years (over the 1880s and 1890s) was president of the national organization. As such, Father Cleary became a noted temperance speaker on the Chautauqua and popular lecture circuit. In 1887 and 1888 he devoted considerable time to duties as a national lecturer and organizer for the CTAU and on a tour to various parts of the country gave the total abstinence pledge to over one hundred thousand Catholics. He worked closely over the years with Bishop John Ireland* (for many years the guiding hand of the CTAU), and it was on his urging that Cleary moved to Minneapolis in 1892 in order to establish a new pastorate. The new location did nothing to dampen his dry enthusiasm, and the crusading priest emerged as an articulate national voice for the dry cause, respected beyond his fellow Catholics. Indeed, his reputation was such that he served (in the early 1900s) as a first vice president of the Anti-Saloon League. While active with the ardently prohibitionist league, however, he always remained conscious of his position as a Catholic leader. Privately, Cleary was in favor of prohibitory legislation, and publically he spoke out frequently against Catholic involvement in the liquor traffic. Like Bishop Ireland, he saw temperance activity as a means of breaking down old Protestant prejudices against Catholics. But Cleary never insisted that the church itself endorse National Prohibition, and he always remained committed to church authority. Still, over his tenure as head of the Total Abstinence Union, he helped advance dry sentiments with both the laity and hierarchy of the church and broadened the popular base of the movement itself. If, as some historians have noted, temperance was largely a Protestant crusade, Cleary and his co-workers gave it a substantial Catholic and Irish leavening.

**Bibliography:**

A. SEAP 2, 628; WW 4, 180; Sr. Joan Bland, *Hibernian Crusade: The Story of the Catholic Total Abstinence Union of America* (Washington, DC, 1951).

**COCKE, John Hartwell**    (19 September 1780, Surry Co., VA—1 July 1866, Fluvanna Co., VA). *Education*: graduated from Coll. of William and Mary, 1798. *Career*: planter, Bremo plantation, Fluvanna Co., VA, 1803–66; brigadier general, Virginia militia, 1814–15; active reform interests in agriculture, education, temperance, and slavery, beginning circa 1815.

A man of deep religious piety and a strong devotion to the betterment of mankind, John Hartwell Cocke's career was in many respects typical of other antebellum social reformers. Well educated and quite wealthy, Cocke settled in 1803 at Bremo, his estate in Fluvanna County, Virginia, to enjoy life as a planter. Yet an active mind and a keen interest in civil affairs assured that Cocke would not devote all of his time to the plantation. He emerged as an agricultural innovator, decrying Virginia's dependence on tobacco, and assisted in founding new agricultural societies to promote better cultivation methods and crops in the state. His concern for agriculture also led him to question slavery, which he came to believe was both unjust and a bane to farming. As a result, Cocke developed a life-long interest in the American Colonization Society, which sought to end slavery gradually by resettling blacks in Africa and compensating their owners. His interest in temperance stemmed, apparently, from his service in the War of 1812. Cocke ultimately rose to brigadier general of militia in command of defenses around Richmond; and while on duty he reportedly was appalled at the impact of drunkenness on the troops. He brought it under control among his own men through stern discipline, but the experience left a lasting impression on the planter–general. Thereafter he spoke out endlessly against the evil and took a temperance pledge himself (reserving, however, his right to use wine in moderation). By the 1830s, Cocke was Virginia's leading temperance voice, and he increasingly leaned toward a prohibitory solution to the abuse of ardent spirits. In 1834 he sat as president of the first state temperance convention, and in 1836—although still a moderationist—he was elected president of the national American Temperance Union. In that position, he challenged other antiliquor crusaders to demand legislative action "to discourage and finally break up the nurseries of crime, the distilleries and the licensed grog-shops." But he noted that "above all" they had "to appeal to public opinion, which is, at last, the governing principle in all the great moral reforms of a free people."

For Cocke, temperance was part of a galaxy of reforms he believed necessary in building a more humane and just society. The "appeal to public opinion" was vital, in his view, if the republic was to fulfill its promise in any number of areas; and he did his best to guide popular opinion along paths he thought best for all. He set a high moral example in his personal conduct, and in refusing civil honors (including a nomination for governor) as a reward for public service, established a model for disinterested and selfless citizenship. Cocke also worked hard on behalf of religious causes, including the American Bible and Sunday School societies, and for the establishment of a sound Virginia educational system. He played an influential role (although without the visibility of Thomas Jefferson) in establishing the University of Virginia and served for over thirty years on its Board of Visitors. Not all of Cocke's fellow Virginians agreed with his stands, but he was widely respected, and even critics of his causes seemingly admired his courage and high motives. His temperance convictions offered a promiment example in this regard: Cocke was far in advance of popular opinion on the subject in Virginia, and the antebellum dry movement never did gain a mass following in the South. But there was little doubt that its gentleman champion had the best interests of his society at heart—and he usually received credit for that. Indeed, some historians have felt that only Cocke's genuine personal modesty and aversion to public honors kept him from recognition as one of the great Virginians of his age.

## Bibliography:

A. *Letters from Professor Stuart, of Andover, Lucias M. Sargent, Esq., of Boston, Ge. Cocke, of Virginia, and Rev. Justin Edwards, D.D., on the Maine Liquor Law...* (New York, 1851); *Tobacco, the Bane of Virginia Husbandry* (Richmond, VA, 1860); *Temperance Essays and Selections from Different Authors...Also a Treatise on Tobacco, by Gen. John H. Cocke*, ed. Edward C. Delavan (Albany, NY, 1865); *The Idol of Two Hundred Millions...* (Fitchburg, VA, 187-?).

B. DAB 4, 253–54; SEAP 2, 638; WW H, 182; Philip A. Bruce, *History of the University of Virginia*, vol. 1 (New York, 1920); Charles Chilton Pearson and J. Edwin Hendricks, *Liquor and Anti-Liquor in Virginia, 1619–1919* (Durham, NC, 1967).

**COFFIN, Lorenzo Sweet**   (9 April, 1823, Alton, NH—17 January 1915, Fort Dodge, IA). *Education*: studied at Oberlin Coll., 1840s. *Career*: teacher, Geauga (OH) Sem., 1840s; farmer on land claim near Ft. Dodge, IA, 1840s–1860s; soldier in Union army, 1861–65; itinerant minister on Iowa frontier, Freewill Baptist Church, 1866 to 1880s; member, Iowa State Board of Railroad Commissioners, 1883–1888; continuing philanthropic work for disabled railroad workers, convicts, and railroad-affiliated temperance groups, until 1915.

Lorenzo Coffin's early years ran in no fixed career channel, and few would have predicted his eventual rise as a temperance champion and philanthropist. He tried his hand successively at teaching (at Geauga Seminary in Ohio, where both future President and Mrs. James A. Garfield were his students) and farming before the Civil War without distinction in either field. During the sectional conflict he served as an enlisted man in an Iowa regiment, finally becoming chaplain (without any religious training or ordination) of the Thirty-second Iowa Infantry. With the coming of peace, Coffin chose to pursue his newly acquired ministerial calling, and he obtained ordination as a Freewill Baptist. Over the next sixteen years he became a familiar part of the frontier Iowa scene as he preached among the prairie settlements. He carried the Gospel anywhere he found a forum, without pay and without a permanent church. The itinerant developed a public reputation as a reform-minded humanitarian, and in 1883, during years of intense interest in railroad regulation on the prairies, Coffin was named to the State Board of Railroad Commissioners at the age of sixty. To this new position Coffin brought a ministerial concern for what might be termed his new parishioners, the riders and workmen of the railroads who had been long without an official advocate. The preacher-turned-regulator immediately addressed the pressing issue of safety on the job, and for a man lacking previous governmental experience he proved remarkably effective. Coffin devised and successfully lobbied for state and national legislation mandating railroad safety devices which were credited with saving many lives over the years. Moveover, as Coffin saw it, the railroad safety movement went hand in hand with the Temperance Movement—a reform the Baptist minister had long since adopted in his preaching.

By the late nineteenth century, many American railroad companies had already taken a firm stand on the liquor question. Regulations generally forbid drinking on the job, often under penalty of dismissal. Building upon the existing sentiment against "the demon," in 1893 Coffin organized the "White Button" temperance movement among railroad workers in an effort to keep them dry (and thus employed) and safe on the job. Soon thereafter, in an expansion of this work, he became president of the Railroad Temperance Association. Coffin's career, then, exemplified the profound interrelationships of the period between growing industrial concerns over the consequences of alcohol abuse, temperance and humanitarian reform, and the crusading impulses of the emerging "social gospel" (of which Coffin's labors were certainly an example). By the early 1900s, although no longer a commissioner, this network of interests had become a powerful web of influence for Coffin: Organized temperance, he concluded, was a keystone of reform in general, and he took up the cause with typical zeal. In 1907 the Iowa Prohibition Party chose him as its candidate for governor, while the following year he was the United Christian Party nominee for vice president of the United States. He also served for a time as president of the state Anti-Saloon League. Coffin's Progressive instincts ranged even more widely without losing sight of his temperance goals: He played a leading role in establishing the Home for Disabled Railroad Men near Chicago; and on his farm near Fort Dodge he opened a home for discharged convicts, "Hope Hall," where they could stay until they found means of support. In Lorenzo Coffin, then, temperance found one of its most humanitarian spokesmen.

**Bibliography:**

B. SEAP 2, 643; WW 1, 238.

**COLMAN, Julia**   (16 February 1828, near Troy, NY—10 January 1909, Brooklyn, NY). *Education*: studied at Lawrence Coll., Appleton, WI, 1849–51; graduated from Cazenovia Sem., Cazenovia, NY, 1855. *Career*: teacher, various elementary schools in WI; editorial work and writer, Methodist Sunday-School Union and Tract Society, NY, 1856–67; free-lance author and lecturer, 1867–75; editorial and administrative positions, National WCTU, 1876–1909.

Colman's interests in scientific and medical issues, possibly stimulated by concern over her own frail health, were the hallmarks of her career. While on the staff of the Methodist Sunday-School Union she authored a column for children in the Union's publication which reflected her concerns over health-related issues. She campaigned, for example, against smoking among the young. But Miss Colman refrained from active reform efforts until she left the Methodist organization in 1867 (she had apparently become frustrated over her lack of advancement). She then prepared a number of lectures on diet, temperance, tobacco, and other medical issues and entered the public lecture circuit. She also helped to support herself by writing a variety of antiliquor and antismoking tracts. To sharpen her skills, Colman attended courses in a number of medical schools, and, combining her acquired knowledge with her literary skills, authored some highly successful pamphlets. In 1875 she organized a summer "temperance school," which brought her considerable praise from the fledgling WCTU. Thus without any formal affiliation with the Temperance Movement, Colman had become established as a respected spokeswoman for the dry cause.

Her independent work ended in 1876, when she began writing a children's page for the WCTU's *Our Union* and became chairwoman of the union's "leaflet" committee. A hard and effective worker, Colman became superintendent of the new (1880) WCTU Department of Temperance Literature, which over the next decade produced a barrage of literature aimed at all segments of the American public. These publications were intended to provide "scientific" arguments against alcohol, and in this regard Colman herself wrote a widely used school text, *Alcohol and Hygiene*, and a host of shorter items. She also assumed direction of the WCTU's Health Department. Her apparent success, however, did not lead to personal tranquility. For years, she had issued many of her own articles and tracts through publishers other than the Woman's Temperance Publishing Association, an organization headed by Matilda Carse* and strongly supported by others in the WCTU. This led to considerable bitterness within the union, and in 1891 Colman lost a power struggle to Carse, who replaced her as head of the Department of Temperance Literature. Saddened at this rebuff, Colman remained loyal to the WCTU nevertheless and continued with her other duties—although until her death she continued to write for other organizations. A committed reformer, she willed her small estate to a Southern school for blacks.

### Bibliography:

A. *Catechisms on Alcohol and Tobacco* (1872, and many later editions); *Alcohol and Hygiene* (Chicago, 1880); *The Juvenile Temperance Manual for Teachers* (New York, 1885).

B. NAW 1, 363–64; SEAP 1, 653; Frances E. Willard, *Woman and Temperance* (Hartford, CT, 1883); Frances E. Willard and Mary A. Livermore, eds., *A Woman of the Century* (New York, 1893).

**COLQUITT, Alfred Holt**    (20 April 1824, Waltor Co., GA—26 March 1894, Washington, DC). *Education*: graduated from Princeton Coll., 1844. *Career*: admitted to bar, GA, 1845; major, U.S. army during Mexican War, 1846–48; member, U.S. House of Representatives, 1853–55; private legal practice, 1855–59; member, Georgia legislature, 1859; officer, Confederate army (rose to major general), 1861–65; lawyer and farmer, 1865–76; governor of Georgia, 1876–82; member, U.S. Senate, 1883–94.

Alfred Colquitt is a veritable character out of the mythology of the Old South. Courtly, brave, and a superb orator, he commanded the elements of the Southern ideal with the authority of a genuine heir; his stature as a spokesman for the South only might be surpassed by his father, Walter T. Colquitt, one of the great politicians of antebellum Georgia. The son spent a career as Georgia's leading politician, first a member of Congress, then a Georgia legislator, governor, and finally senator. His public history was compounded of ardent secessionism in 1860, a Confederate generalship, Methodist religion, and a vehement prohibitionism. He was, like his father, a licensed Methodist preacher, and it was this facet of his character that probably determined his attitude toward drink most directly. Indeed, if anything subverted the harmony of his personality, it was his intense religiosity and moralism, which colored his outlook on social issues, politics, and his own strong sense of personal honor. He was a passionate defender of the South (and slavery) before the Civil War, served with distinction in the Southern army during the conflict (he won an impressive victory at the Battle of Olustee in 1864), and was a bitter opponent of Georgia's Reconstruction government after the Confederate defeat. With the end of Reconstruction, however, he resumed his political career and in 1876 was elected governor by the widest margin in Georgia history. His tenure in office was tumultuous: He proved an able administrator and, although apparently honest, was accused of shady political compromises to advance his career. Outraged at the charges, he sought and won a second term (1880) in order to vindicate himself. After 1883 he served in the Senate until his death in 1894.

Throughout his public career Colquitt was a zealous champion of the antiliquor crusade. Even before the War Between the States, when temperance was at a low ebb in the South (too many temperance workers were also abolitionists for Southern tastes), the future governor was a convinced dry. After the war, when temperance workers began to make steady gains in the former Confederacy, Colquitt had a sympathetic hearing for his views, and his personal reputation also helped to enhance the status of the cause. While governor, his advocacy of prohibition won him the intense enmity of liquor interests in the state, and he listed them among his most virulent enemies while in office. As a senator, one of his first legislative initiatives was an attempt to dry out the District of Columbia. In this he failed, but he garnered the applause of the growing Temperance Movement and went on to become a popular antiliquor lecturer. He spoke on the subject frequently in the Northern states, where the sight of a Southern Democrat espousing the dry position generated considerable publicity. To the end, Colquitt was noted for his fiery style on the platform and his combativeness on behalf of any cause he advocated.

**Bibliography:**

A. *Relations Between the Senate and Executive Departments . . .* (Washington, DC, 1886); *The Weight of the Tariff on American Homes and American Farmers . . .* (Washington, DC, 1890).

B. DAB 4, 315–16; SEAP 2, 659–60; WW H, 185; *Atlanta Constitution*, March 26, 27, 1894; I. W. Avery, *History of the State of Georgia from 1850 to 1881* (Atlanta, GA, 1881); H. A. Scomp, *King Alcohol in the Realm of King Cotton* (Chicago, 1888).

**COLVIN, David Leigh**    (28 January 1880, South Charleston, OH—7 September 1959, Yonkers, NY). *Education*: studied at American Temperance Univ., Harriman, TN; A.B., Ohio Wesleyan Univ., 1900; graduate study at Univ. of California and Univ. of Chicago; Ph.D., Columbia Univ., 1913. *Career*: temperance organizer, lecturer, author, and politician, 1899–1959.

Few individuals gave more of themselves to the dry crusade than David Colvin. Even before leaving college (part of which he attended at the ardently antiliquor American Temperance University), Colvin was a Prohibitionist of considerable note, having risen to president of the National Intercollegiate Prohibition Association. He became a national organizer for this group upon graduation in 1900, and within a year had helped raise the number of such campus groups from 12 to 150. While pursuing his graduate education he remained active in temperance work, holding offices in a number of organizations and maintaining a focus on bringing the dry message to college students. His hope was to persuade as many future social, political, and economic leaders as possible of the virtues of temperance, and to this end he worked to form student discussion groups on the liquor question and to foster the inclusion of formal alcohol-related courses in college curricula. His passion for the cause was evident in his marriage as well: In 1906 he wed Mamie White, an influential Prohibitionist in her own right (she had been active in the IPA and a vice president of the New York WCTU), and as Mamie Colvin* she became his life-long companion in the movement.

The approach and ratification of National Prohibition gave Colvin's life even greater focus. During the effort to pass the Eighteenth Amendment he helped lead a number of politically active groups and served a term as vice president of the World Prohibition Federation. The same motive also prompted him to run for the Senate and the New York mayoralty under the Prohibition Party banner in 1916 and 1917. He was a tireless speaker as well. Commissioned as a captain during World War I, he spoke to the troops on temperance and patriotism, and after the war he lectured widely at universities in Britain and Western Europe. Colvin stressed that Prohibition could succeed only through active enforcement, and he worked selflessly in a variety of capacities to aid enforcement efforts. In this regard, he took a leading role in trying to rekindle temperance spirit when the Eighteenth Amendment finally came under effective attack. To save Prohibition, he ran unsuccessfully for senator again in 1932 and for president in 1936 after Repeal. He continued staunchly in the cause long after the decline of the Temperance Movement as a potent social and political force; and he could point to an almost unrivalled record of service (indeed, it was virtually a career) on behalf of the dry reform.

**Bibliography:**

A. *The Bicameral Principle in the New York Legislature* (New York, 1913); *Prohibition in the United States: A History of the Prohibition Party and of the Prohibition Movement* (New York, 1926).

B. SEAP 2, 661; WW 3, 175; Jack S. Blocker, Jr., *Retreat from Reform: The Prohibition Movement in the United States, 1890–1913* (Westport, CT, 1976).

**COLVIN, Mamie White**   (12 June 1883, Westview, OH—30 October 1955, Clearwater, FL). *Education*: A.B., Wheaton Coll., 1905; studied at Columbia Univ., 1906–7, 1909–10; Doctor of Art of Oratory, Staley Coll. of the Spoken Word (Boston), 1937; LLD., Houghton Coll., 1946; LLD. (honorary), Wheaton Coll., 1947; LHD. (honorary), Southwestern Univ., 1948. *Career*: president,

New York Co. WCTU, 1916–21; vice president, New York State WCTU, 1921–26; president, New York State WCTU, 1926–44; vice president, National WCTU, 1933–44; president, National WCTU, 1944–53.

Mamie White Colvin's was a life dedicated to prohibition. She grew up in a staunchly dry family where the Temperance Movement was a daily fact of life. At ten years old she joined a "Band of Hope," an antiliquor children's group and a forerunner of the WCTU's Loyal Temperance Legion. Her constant affiliation with dry organizations continued even after leaving home. While at college, she was a member of the Intercollegiate Prohibition Association, in which she met her future husband, David Leigh Colvin,* at that time the president of the association. After briefly doing postgraduate work at Columbia University in political philosophy, she began devoting her entire energies to the prohibition Movement. In 1910, both Colvins were members of the U.S. delegation to the Woman's Christian Temperance Union convention in Glasgow, Scotland. Upon their return they settled in Fort Washington, New York, where Mrs. Colvin (she preferred "Mrs. David Leigh Colvin" publicly) promptly organized the local branch of the WCTU, and from then on she rose rapidly through the ranks of the organization. In 1914 she was county recording secretary of the New York WCTU, in 1921 state vice president, in 1926 state president, in 1933 national vice president, and in 1944, national president. If the Temperance Movement can be said to have offered a certain upward mobility to women, Colvin certainly offers one of the best examples of the phenomenon.

Mrs. Colvin's great strength as a temperance advocate was her oratorical ability. While at Wheaton she took part in the Intercollegiate Prohibition Association's oratorical contests and won college, state, and interstate contests, placing second in the national competition. Her powerful voice was raised in support of National Prohibition, rejecting any compromise in favor of moderation with the frequent observation—even after Repeal—that "alcohol is no respecter of moderate drinkers." Palliatives such as medical and psychiatric treatment of alcoholics, she argued, were merely self-serving devices aimed at solving "the problems of drunkenness by curing the alcoholics and allowing the business to continue." Despite this view, she did attend the Yale University Summer School of Alcohol Studies in 1944 because she wished to convey her sympathy with alcoholics and their problems without, however, endorsing the sociological, medical, and psychological approach of the Yale School. Even the failure of the Eighteenth Amendment did not discourage her, and she argued that the experiences of World War II in rationing would have made it a success had those methods been used earlier. While temperance fortunes were clearly in retreat over the 1940s, Colvin's efforts kept some vibrancy in the WCTU, and the organization felt her loss in 1953 when she left owing to ill health. Her husband also continued his association with temperance, mainly in politics. He sought the mayoralty in New York City in 1917, ran for vice president in 1920, for senator in 1932, and for president in 1936, each time on the Prohibition Party ticket. And through all of his campaigns, Mrs. Colvin remained his most tireless and dedicated supporter. At her death in 1955, she was arguably America's "first lady" of the receding antiliquor crusade.

**Bibliography:**

B. *Current Biography* (1944): 104–6; NYT, Oct. 31, 1955; WW 3, 175; Fred D. L. Squires, "Mrs. D. Leigh (Mamie White) Colvin," *Union Signal* 81 (1955): 378–80.

**COMSTOCK, Elizabeth Leslie Rous**    (30 October 1815, Maidenhead, Berkshire, England—3 August 1891, Union Springs, NY). *Education*: attended English Quaker schools, Islington and Croyden, England. *Career*: taught school, Quaker schools, England, circa late 1830s–1840s; storekeeper, Bakewell, Derbyshire, England, and Belleville, Ontario, Canada, 1850s; minister, Society of Friends, Belleville, Ontario, Canada, 1854; minister, Society of Friends, Rollin, MI, 1858–85; travelled as reformer under Quaker auspices for antislavery, temperance, women's rights, prison reform, and hospital work during Civil War, 1850s–1880s.

During the mid-nineteenth century, Quakerism began a dramatic evangelical revival. In keeping with the activist reform spirit of the times, many young members of the Society of Friends emerged who set aside the traditional quietism of their faith (or at least tried to moderate it) and threw themselves wholeheartedly into the social turmoil of the antebellum years. One of those who best illustrated this aspect of Quakerism was Elizabeth Comstock, who combined a devotion to personally ministering to the suffering with strong organizational powers for marshalling material and moral aid for them. She was the daughter of a scholarly English Quaker family, and after her first husband died in 1849, she finally immigrated to Canada with her child in 1854. She started to preach in her new home in Belleville, Ontario, and became noted for her deep spirituality and fine style of oratory. In 1858 she married John T. Comstock and moved with him to the frontier Quaker community of Rollin, Michigan, where her full powers as a minister came into flower. It was in Rollin that Comstock also became involved in social crusading. The town was a "station" on the Underground Railroad, and the Quaker preacher became zealously devoted to the abolitionist cause. Antislavery, in fact, became a highlight in her speaking (which was in demand throughout the Western states by this time), as well as pleas for other causes such as temperance, education, peace, prison reform, and women's rights. She became noted for her visits to prisons and spiritual work with inmates— including thousands of prisoners of war during the Civil War—and she appears to have had a considerable knack for evoking the consolations of religion for the suffering. Besides the many prisoners who testified to her comforting powers, President Lincoln was once moved to pray with her.

While Mrs. Comstock was best known for her work with blacks and with prisoners, she also saw temperance as a crucial reform. It was linked, she noted, with other evils. The majority of men she spoke to in jail, for example, were behind bars "either directly or indirectly through liquor." After the end of the war, she allied herself with the upsurge in women's temperance activity that swept the nation. The 1870s saw her speaking in a number of Eastern urban centers on behalf of the new Woman's Christian Temperance Union, and she reportedly drew enthusiastic responses. Shortly thereafter, she worked closely with Kansas Govenor John P. St. John* in the settlement of former slaves in his state. The association with the fiery dry St. John (as well as with the crusaders of the WCTU) seems to have made a lasting impression on Comstock. As she grew older, she increasingly made the Temperance Movement a more important part of her message, and even after failing health forced her to cut back on her public appearances in the 1880s, she still spoke out against the evils of the traffic. Her reforming zeal and her deeply humanitarian instincts made her one of the most eminent Quakers of her age, and her passing in 1891 (in Union Springs, New York, where she had moved after her husband died in the 1880s) was mourned in her adopted America and native England.

**Bibliography:**

A. *Life and Letters of Elizabeth L. Comstock*, comp. C[atherine] Hare (London, 1895).

B. DAB 4, 331–32; NAW 1, 369–70; NCAB 22, 456–57; WW H, 186; Rufus M. Jones, *The Later Periods of Quakerism* (London, 1921); Frances E. Willard, *Woman and Temperance* (Philadelphia, 1883).

**CONWELL, Russell Herman**    (15 February 1843, Worthington, MA—6 December 1925, Philadelphia, PA). *Education*: studied at Yale Coll., 1860–62; LLB., Sch. of Law, Albany Univ. (NY), 1865; D.D. (honorary), Temple Univ., 1898; LLD. (honorary), Temple Univ., 1900. *Career*: officer (promoted to lieutenant colonel), Union army, 1862–65; legal practice, Minneapolis, MN, 1865–67; immigration agent for Minnesota in Germany, 1867–71; reporter and editor (*Boston Traveller*), legal practice, lecturer, author, Boston, 1871–80; ordained in Baptist Church, 1879; minister, Lexington, MA, 1880–82; minister, Grace Baptist Church, Philadelphia, 1882–1925; president, Temple Univ., 1888–1925.

Russell Conwell was Philadelphia's Baptist preacher of material success, and he opposed alcoholic beverages as one of the ways men divert themselves from the "acres of diamonds" he claimed were under everybody's nose. "Acres of Diamonds" was the title of what has been called the most successful lecture ever delivered, and Conwell delivered it some six thousand times. The message that anyone, especially Christians, could get rich, coming as it did from the pastor of one of the largest congregations in America, held considerable appeal for thousands (if not millions) of Americans. While he was a preacher of undeniable stature, however, Conwell's formative years had given little evidence of his future career. In fact, he had been a professed atheist in college, and religion apparently had no appeal for the young lawyer until he was badly wounded in action at the Battle of Kenesaw Mountain in 1864, a feeling which deepened with the shock of his wife's death in 1872. Thereafter, Conwell moved steadily toward religious involvement. During the 1870s, as a successful businessman in Boston, he was active in Bible study and work with youth groups, and after a Baptist ordination in 1879 he energetically rebuilt a failing congregation in Lexington, Massachusetts. His subsequent move to Philadelphia and the pulpit of Grace Baptist Church (1882) marked the beginning of his emergence as a national figure. While he was never known as a dynamic speaker, his message of self-help and personal upward mobility was widely appreciated in its day. Seeking to aid the industrious in their passage to success, Conwell opened night-school classes in the Grace Church basement, which by 1888 had evolved into Temple University. The institution helped many poorer students get professional training and a higher education, and there is no doubt that the Baptist pastor's idea had blossomed into a major community asset. He remained president of Temple until his death.

Conwell's gospel of worldly success had no room for drink. Preaching that advocated thrift, hard work, sobriety, and the will to triumph over hardship found the bottle to be its very antithesis: Drunkenness was the personification (in this view) of waste, sloth, and possible failure. Thus the influential minister was personally a temperance man, and during the initial years of his tenure in the pulpit he went to considerable lengths to denounce the liquor traffic and its associated evils. The only solution, he claimed, was personal abstinence for individuals and prohibitory legislation for government. Conwell himself had joined the Independent Order of Good Templars in 1866 and maintained his membership thereafter. As his fame and duties at Grace Church expanded, he never ceased his denunciations of "the demon," but they became a less frequent part of his message. He was simply too involved in other areas (notably as president of Temple) to devote the major block of his time to the dry cause that characterized the work of some other pastors of the era. He never took an active role with any organized temperance society, although he approved of the enactment of National Prohibition. For Temperance Movement stalwarts, this was evidently good enough; for if Conwell never formally joined them (aside from his affiliation with the fraternal Good Templars), they were happy to publicize his dry sympathies, as if linking the crusade to a major success story. In that many temperance arguments on the nature of the good life were similar to his, Conwell was apparently happy to oblige.

**Bibliography:**

A. *Woman and the Law* (Philadelphia, 1876); *Acres of Diamonds: How Men and Women May Become Rich* (Philadelphia, 1890, and subsequent editions); *Observation* (New York, 1917); *What You Can Do with Your Will Power* (New York, 1917); *Effective Prayer* (New York, 1921); *Unused Powers* (New York, 1922).

B. DAB 4, 367–68; NYT, Dec. 7, 1925; SEAP 2, 709–10; WW 1, 253;

Agnes R. Burr, *Russell H. Conwell and His Work* (Philadelphia, 1917; rev. ed., 1926); Albert H. Smith, *The Life of Russell H. Conwell* (Boston, 1899).

**COTTERILL, George Fletcher**    (18 November 1865, Oxford, England—1949, Seattle, WA). *Education*: studied civil engineering with James Owen, Essex Co., NJ, 1881–83. *Career*: landscape engineer, Hudson Co., NJ, 1883–84; various engineering positions, Seattle, WA, 1884 to 1940s; assistant city engineer, Seattle, WA, 1892–1900; member, Washington State Irrigation Comm., 1903–5; member, Seattle City Planning Comm., 1926–28; member, Washinton State Highway Dept., 1916–19; member, Washington State Senate, 1907–11; mayor, Seattle, WA, 1912–14; engineering consultant to various federal agencies, 1930s; supervisor, U.S. Works Progress Admin., Island Co., WA, 1940–41; active work with Independent Order of Good Templars, 1884 to 1940s.

Before moving to the United States from his native England in 1872, young George Cotterill was already developing his faith in the Temperance Movement. His parents were total abstainers and had been dry activists with the British antiliquor crusade. George himself had joined a "Band of Hope," a youth temperance group, run by his mother. Settling later in Montclair, New Jersey, the Cotterill family retained their interest in the cause, with the son, then in his teens, serving as an officer in another dry youth organization numbering hundreds of members. Trained as a civil engineer, he moved in 1884 to Seattle, Washington, where over the years, and in a variety of private and public capacities, he established a distinguished professional reputation. He was especially noted for his work in city planning, landscape design, and highway engineering. Yet he never ceased his antiliquor activity. Upon moving to the city he joined the Order of Good Templars and rose to grand secretary of the Washington Grand Lodge within five years (1885). He held a succession of other major posts with the Templars through the years and was finally elected as the first national chief templar in 1905; he filled that office until 1913. Beginning in 1908, he was also involved in international Templar activities and for many years held office as an international counselor. Without question Cotterill was one of the most celebrated and committed Good Templars in the history of the order. He was also one of the most adept at using his positions within the lodge to further the cause of prohibition. The hard-working engineer tirelessly rallied lodge and public support for dry candidates and legislative measures throughout the 1880s and 1890s, even editing several dry newspapers. With a number of friends, he founded *The American Issue* (not the later Anti-Saloon League publication of the same name), which he used to support the Prohibitionist presidential candidacy of John Bidwell* in 1892—and which he considered making a permanent journal until it succumbed financially shortly later. He was probably as dedicated a reformer as his region could boast.

Perhaps the most interesting side of Cotterill's career, however, was the deep commitment to Progressivism that shone through it from beginning to end. Over the years, he linked his work for the temperance crusade with other reforms including women's suffrage (he wrote the suffrage amendment to the Washington constitution), municipal administrative reform, campaigns against prostitution in Seattle, and direct primaries for U.S. senators. A Democrat, he ran for local and national office (both the House and Senate) several times, and served in the State Senate (1907–1911) and as mayor of Seattle (1912–14) as well as in a large number of appointive positions. In all of his posts he acquired a reputation for solid probity and intelligent management. He also saw his offices as opportunities to pursue dry goals. In the State Senate, he was instrumental in the passage of the Washington local-option law, and worked hand in hand with the local Anti-Saloon League (which he had helped found in the early 1900s) in the unsuccessful drive for state prohibition in 1914. The league also endorsed Cotterill when he ran for mayor in 1912 and maintained close ties with the reformer in his temperance efforts down to the 1920s. Cotterill's sense of propriety, however, finally led him to break with the Anti-Saloon organization. In the mid-1920s, after a heated argument, he claimed that the league improperly placed his name in nomination for governor (while he was attending a dry convention out of state), and although there was something of a rapprochement when he actually did run in 1928, the relationship was never the same. At no time, though, did his temperance enthusiasm ever dim. His voice was heard nationally on dry issues (at various times he made speaking or campaign tours in Oklahoma, Maine, and New York), and he continued to act according to the dictates of his conscience. In 1928, for example, he broke with his party over the nomination of Alfred E. Smith. Rather than vote for the wet New Yorker, Cotterill endorsed Herbert Hoover. It was typical of the man: The reformer-engineer uniformly tried to place principle before politics.

### Bibliography:

A. *Puget Sound: The Mediterranean of the Pacific* (Seattle, WA, 1927); *The Climax of a World Quest* (Seattle, WA, 1928); the George F. Cotterill Papers are in the University of Washington Library, Seattle.

B. SEAP 2, 722–23; WW 5, 153; Norman H. Clark, *The Dry Years: Prohibition and Social Change in Washington* (Seattle, WA, 1965).

**CRAFTS, Wilbur Fisk**    (12 January 1850, Fryeburg, ME—27 December 1922, Washington, DC). *Education*: A.B., Wesleyan Univ., 1869; A.M., Wesleyan Univ., 1871; B.D., Boston Univ. Sch. of Theology, 1871; Ph.D. (honorary), Marietta Coll., 1896. *Career*: minister, various Presbyterian and Congregational pastorates in Stoneham, Havesill, and New Bedford, MA, Dover, NH, Chicago, and Brooklyn and New York, NY, 1870s–1900s; reform lobbying and writing, Washington, DC, 1900s to 1922.

Although ordained in the Methodist Church, young Reverend Crafts served throughout his pastoral career in Presbyterian and Congregational pulpits. Little is known, however, of his local activities as a minister; rather, Wilbur Crafts made his mark as a reform worker on the national level. He first went on record against the liquor traffic while in college, when he emerged as a vigorous temperance lecturer. He wrote and spoke on behalf of the dry cause for the rest of his life, but he soon became involved in other causes as well. Most notably, Crafts established himself as a driving force in the Sunday school movement and in efforts to make the Sabbath a legally enforced day of rest. Over the 1880s he promoted Sunday schools as a means of instilling "Christian citizenship" in the nation's youth and vainly sought congressional assistance in his movement. He had better luck with the American Sabbath Union, which he founded in 1889, and as the head of the Reform Bureau, established in 1895. As the leader of these groups, Crafts proved instrumental in the framing of national legislation placing limits on Sunday travel, curtailing liquor sales on military posts, and regulating the sale of alcohol, firearms, and opium on American-owned Pacific Islands. Upon moving to Washington, D.C., Crafts left the pulpit and devoted himself full time to lobbying and writing efforts, and he developed as a rather prolific author on temperance and other reform topics.

We should also note that he did not work alone. Over his long years in the service of reform, Crafts had the ardent support of his wife, Sara Jane Crafts (born Timanus), whom he had married in 1874. She worked closely with him on behalf of the Sunday-School Union and antiliquor organizing and in authoring reform tracts. Indeed, so great was her involvement in the dry crusade that Reverend Crafts often found her away from home on missions for the WCTU (she was superintendent of the World's WCTU Sunday School Department for twenty-five years) and on speaking tours that took her as far afield as Iceland, Italy, Norway, the Orient, Holland, and Switzerland. Thus in many respects, theirs was a marriage built around their dedication to the dry movement. After Wilbur's death in 1922, Sara carried on until age forced a limitation of her activities. She finished her years with a solid reputation in her own right, and one suspects that no one would have been more pleased with the fact than Reverend Crafts.

## Bibliography:

A. "The Responsibilities of Christian Citizenship," 164–70, in *Centennial Temperance Volume: A Memorial of the International Temperance Conference...* (New York, 1877); with Sara Jane Crafts, Mary Leitch, and Margaret W. Leitch, *Protection of Native Races Against Intoxicants and Opium* (Chicago, 1900); with Sara Jane Crafts, *Intoxicants and Opium* (New York? 1908); with Sara Jane Crafts, *World Book of Temperance* (New York? 1908).

B. SEAP 2, 727–28; WW 5, 156; "Pioneer Worker for Prohibition—Dr. Wilbur F. Crafts...," *Union Signal* 49, No. 1 (1923): 9.

**CRANFILL, James Britton**   (12 September 1858, Parker Co., TX—28 December 1942, Dallas, TX). *Education*: M.D., Texas Medical Board, 1879; LLD. (honorary), Simmons Coll., Baylor Univ., 1900, 1920. *Career*: medical practice, 1879–82; editor, *Turnersville* (TX) *Effort*, 1881–82; editor, *Gatesville* (TX)

*Advance*, 1882–87; editor, *Waco* (TX) *Advance*, 1887–92; financial secretary, Baylor Univ., beginning 1889; superintendent, Baptist missionary work, TX, 1889–92; ordained, Baptist Church, 1890; editor, various Baptist and Prohibitionist publications (including the *Baptist Standard*), 1892 to 1920s.

Physician, editor, author, and reformer, James Cranfill was one of the most active members of the Prohibition Party in Texas in the late nineteenth and early twentieth centuries. A devout Baptist, he turned increasingly to church-related work after initially pursuing careers in medicine and publishing. In charge of Baptist missionary work in Texas from 1889 to 1892, he was ordained in 1890, after which he wrote and spoke widely on denominational subjects for the rest of his life. He also wrote or edited some three dozen books, ranging from Biblical interpretation and inspirational stories for the young to tracts on various reform and medical questions of the day. Some of this literary outpouring focused on prohibition, a cause Cranfill advocated with tireless enthusiasm. In this stance, he reflected the position of many of his fellow Missionary Baptists, who constituted one of the most important elements of regional support for the Temperance Movement. His dry sentiments were also learned at home as a boy. While his father drank moderately, his mother taught him "that there was nothing good in whiskey from any standpoint whatsoever." The crusading editor fought the "saloon crowd" at every turn, even becoming a lecturer for the United Friends of Temperance. He was effective enough to provoke a heated reaction from wets, including a threat on his life. Active in state Democratic politics, Cranfill tried to move the party toward a prohibitionist position, and in 1884 he sponsored an antiliquor resolution at the party convention in Houston. When the convention tabled it and the Democrats showed no subsequent interest in the measure over the following two years, Cranfill bolted the party. Joining the Prohibition Party in 1886, he helped build the dry political organization at the grassroots level, and it polled some nineteen thousand votes in its first state general election. The reforming Baptist served for years on the party's state and national executive committees, positions which brought him a measure of recognition in reform circles across the country.

Cranfill always placed a major emphasis on his work with the party and for many years sought ways to increase its influence on popular opinion. He was not willing, however, to soften its stress on the prohibition question by embracing other reform causes in order to attract votes. The Texan was a "single-issue" man, as opposed to other members who sought to broaden the base of the party through endorsements of labor reform, women's suffrage, and other causes. Yet, with some exceptions, his unquestioned dedication made him one of the most popular men in the Prohibitionist organization. Accordingly, the 1892 national convention of the Prohibition Party (meeting in Cincinnati) nominated him for vice president. They dry electoral defeat was not discouraging as Cranfill had no expectation of winning, and he worked steadily over the years to shore up Prohibitionist finances, oversee party publications, and manage its relations with other antiliquor groups. He also lent a hand in the campaign that ultimately saw

National Prohibition ratified in his native Texas. During this struggle, he added service as a reporter for the Associated Prohibition Press to his list of other duties. Although disappointed in later years at the Repeal of the Eighteenth Amendment, Cranfill remined active to the end in Texas religious, civic, and educational affairs.

**Bibliography:**

A. *Dr. J. B. Cranfill's Chronicle: A Story of Life in Texas* (New York, 1916); *From Memory: Reminiscences, Recitals, and Gleanings from a Bustling and Busy Life* (Nashville, TN, 1937).

B. SEAP 1, 728–29; WW 2, 133; Jack S. Blocker, Jr., *Retreat from Reform: The Prohibition Movement in the United States, 1890–1913* (Westport, CT, 1976).

**CROSBY, Howard**    (21 February 1826, New York—29 March 1891, New York, NY). *Education*: graduated from Univ. of City of New York, 1844; D.D. (honorary), Harvard Univ., 1859; LLD. (honorary), Columbia Univ., 1871. *Career*: professor of Greek, Univ. of City of New York, 1851–59; professor of Greek, Rutgers Univ., 1859; ordained, Presbyterian Church, 1861; minister, Fourth Avenue Presbyterian Church, New York City, 1863–91; chancellor, Univ. of City of New York, 1870–81.

Throughout his professional career, Howard Crosby, distinguished educator and Presbyterian clergyman, classed himself a firm stalwart of temperance. Most leaders of the dry movement, however, werc not so sure. For Crosby's thinking on the liquor question was indeed out of step with most antidrink voices in the late nineteench century, and in many ways he represented one of the last articulate remnants of an earlier temperance credo—moderation. In his mind temperance was the avoidance of extremes, and if he believed the drink trade to be productive of poverty, crime, waste, and misery, he was just as sure that total abstinence and prohibition would lead only to social discord and disrespect for the law and in the end make alcohol problems worse instead of better. A careful scholar and a well-read theologian, he concluded that scriptural arguments against all drinking—arguments that were standard Temperance Movement weapons—were rubbish. He fully conceded that distilled spirits were harmful and urged his readers away from them with a conviction worthy of a teetotaler. Even lighter drinks, including wines, were dangerous when used to excess. But Crosby saw nothing harmful in wine consumed in moderation. "Jesus and his disciples used wine;" he noted once, "hence I do not hesitate to use it." The influential minister was equally skeptical of prohibitionists. While he publicly applauded their motives as "praiseworthy" and their zeal for reform as "commendable," he insisted that legal prohibition could never be enforced and would "only exasperate men of good repute and enkindle opposition to all reform." Limit the traffic, Crosby argued, restrict its sales, and monitor its licenses carefully; but to try to ban it was a fool's errand. His stances, and his forceful and eloquent statements of them, enraged and baffled teetotalers and prohibitionists. They castigated him for encouraging false hopes on the safety of moderate drinking, while other ministers denounced his deviation from the orthodox temperance position, holding that Christ and the Bible condoned only unfermented grape juice. No less a reform voice than Wendell Phillips* blasted the New York clergyman more than once. Still, Crosby never budged and learned to live fighting the excesses of the liquor traffic on one hand and what he saw as the excesses of extremist reformers on the other.

Even Crosby's detractors, however, admitted that he was a man of great talents and conviction. He was a respected professor of Greek, a hard-working pastor, and a dedicated supporter of the University of the City of New York, his alma mater. He served the institution for years as a trustee and for more than a decade as chancellor. Crosby was also a reformer. He did good service in organizing the New York Young Men's Christian Association (and served a term as its president), taught Bible classes, pioneered international copyright laws, headed the Society for the Prevention of Crime, and wrote widely on reform subjects. In light of all of this, it is not difficult to speculate that more than Crosby's specific views on the antiliquor question bothered the Temperance Movement: It was also the fact that someone of his stature held those views. Crosby's reputation was such that the more extreme reformers could not simply dismiss him—and that rankled. Nevertheless, Crosby fought the good fight as he saw it. With the help of his son, Ernest Howard Crosby, he proved one of the most influential advocates of high-license laws in the state. He also urged effective local measures against illegal New York City saloons. Such contributions, even from a moderationist, could not be ignored. "Notwithstanding his views on temperance," one dry conceded, "there can be little doubt that Crosby exercised considerable influence on legislation in New York with regard to the regulation of intemperance and crime." That was more than could be said of the bulk of even the most ardent prohibitionists.

### Bibliography:

A. *Lands of the Moslem* (New York, 1851); *Bible Companion* (New York, 1870); *Jesus: His Life and Work* (New York, 1871); *A Calm View of the Temperance Question* (Boston, 1881); *Moderation vs. Total Abstinence* (New York, 1881); *Commentary on the New Testament* (New York, 1885); "Anti-Prohibition," in *The Cyclopedia of Temperance and Prohibition* (New York, 1891).

B. DAB 4, 567–68; NYT, March 30, 1891; SEAP 1, 734–35; WW H, 197; J. L. Chamberlain, ed., *Universities and Their Sons: New York University* (New York, 1901); *Christian Advocate*, April 2, 1891; *New York Tribune*, March 30, 1891; J. M. Van Buren, *Gospel Temperance: A New Principle* (New York, 1883).

**CROTHERS, Thomas Davidson** (21 September 1842, Charlton, NY—12 January 1918, Hartford, CT). *Education*: M.D., Albany Medical Coll., 1865.

*Career*: private medical practice in NY, 1866–70; assistant professor of the practice of medicine, Albany Medical Coll., 1871–74; assistant physician, New York State Inebriate Asylum, Binghamton, 1875–78; superintendent, Walnut Hill Asylum, Hartford, CT, 1878–80; president and superintendent, Walnut Lodge Hosp., Hartford, CT, 1880–1918; editor, *Quarterly Journal of Inebriety* (later the *Journal of Inebriety*), 1876–1914.

Throughout the late nineteenth and early twentieth centuries, Crothers was in the forefront of an international effort to win medical recognition of "inebriety"—addiction to alcohol and other drugs—as a distinct disease. Belief that addiction, particularly alcoholism, was an illness had been gaining since the late eighteenth century, but Crothers sought to refine the disease conception and to put it on a scientific footing. By the 1870s, he and others were arguing that inebriety (the result of long-term drug or alcohol use) had clear characteristics: It was an addiction, with the body becoming physically and psychologically dependent on the drug for normal functioning. This dependence developed in phases, which were progressive and predictable. They included a physical "craving" for the drug and an inability to stop using (or drinking) it once started; the condition ultimately caused the degeneration of nerve and brain cells, leading in turn to insanity or death. Crothers was convinced that his ideas conformed to clinical reality, and during his long career he amassed data on thousands of alcoholics and other addicts in order to buttress his claims. In the 1860s he served on the medical staff of the nation's first "inebriate asylum" in Binghamton, New York, and thereafter he headed a similar institution in Connecticut. In these capacities, Crothers probably had as much experience with such patients as any practitioner of the period.

Crothers's interests, however, lay beyond clinical practice alone; he was also an active missionary for the disease conception among professionals and laymen. From the 1870s until his death he was an officer of the Association for the Study and Cure of Inebriety, the leading organizational exponent of the disease concept as well as of the construction of special asylums for inebriate care. He edited the association's *Journal of Inebriety* until it ceased publication in 1914, and he wrote voluminously on the subject for a variety of other professional journals, including the *Journal of the American Medical Association*. It is likely that the modern disease conception of alcoholism adopted a number of the ideas articulated by Crothers and his co-workers. Crothers was particularly concerned with the legal aspects of inebriety as well, and argued before many professional forums that society would be better served by mandating treatment for alcoholics and addicts rather than punishing them. He carried his message to nonprofessionals with equal vigor, and he won many friends among temperance workers. Antiliquor reformers felt that Crothers's ideas lent scientific credence to their own warnings on the dangers of drink, while the doctor in turn looked favorably on the WCTU's "scientific temperance" educational efforts. Although cool toward actual prohibition at first—he thought that medicine offered a better solution to alcohol problems—Crothers finally supported the idea, viewing it as a preventive measure in the fight against inebriety.

**Bibliography:**

A. "Are Inebriates Curable?" *Journal of the American Medical Association* 17 (1891): 923–27; ed., *The Disease of Inebriety* (New York, 1893); "Historic Address on the *Journal of Inebriety*, Its Birth and Growth," *Journal of Inebriety* 19 (1897): 19–29; "A History of Text-Book Teachings of Alcohol and Narcotics in Common Schools," *Journal of Inebriety* 24 (1902): 43–52; *Inebriety: A Clinical Treatise on the Etiology, Lymptomology, Neurosis, Psychosis and Treatment and the Medico-Legal Relations* (Cincinnati, OH, 1911); "A Review of the History and Literature of Inebriety: The First Journal and Its Work up to the Present," *Journal of Inebriety* 33 (1912): 139–51.

B. SEAP 2, 735–36; WW 1, 280; Leonard Blumberg, "The American Association for the Study and Cure of Inebriety," *Alcoholism: Clinical and Experimental Research* 2 (1978): 235–40; E. M. Jellinek, *The Disease Concept of Alcoholism* (New Haven, CT, 1970); Mark Edward Lender, "Jellinek's Typology of Alcoholism: Some Historical Antecedents," *Journal of Studies on Alcohol* 40 (1979): 361–75; T. L. Mason, "Anniversary Address," *Journal of Inebriety* 1 (1876): 1–24.

**CUNNEEN, John Francis**   (21 May 1868, Limerick, Ireland—?). *Career*: machinist, Chicago mining and railroad companies, 1886–19—?

At its heart, the American Temperance Movement was largely Protestant and antipluralist. Yet it was never exclusively so; for over its long history, either for reasons of its own or in response to other groups, the movement did make genuine efforts to broaden its base of support among Catholics, immigrants, and the working class. The career of John Cunneen was a key example in this regard. When he was one year old his parents immigrated from their native Ireland to Cleveland, Ohio, where John attended Catholic parochial schools. He became a skilled worker, practicing the trade of machinist in Chicago, where he moved when he was eighteen. (He gained some modest recognition by inventing an automatic rocking grate for steam boilers.) The basis of his interest in temperance is unknown, but Cunneen apparenly had been an abstainer, and in 1900, when he was thirty-two, the Irish machinist joined the Annunciation Total Abstinence Society of Chicago (a branch of the Catholic Total Abstinence Union). It was the first step in a long period of dedication to the Temperance Movement within the Catholic Church during which he held a wide variety of offices, including the presidency of the Annunciation Society for ten years. Cunneen spent his evening hours after work talking to working men about the evils of drink and generously contributed a part of his wages to the antiliquor cause. Over time his total contributions would come to $2,500, no mean sum for those times, especially from a worker. In 1908 he became an Anti-Saloon League lecturer and was especially noted for his efforts in carrying the dry message to working men in the Midwest (although he also took speaking engagements in the East). At one point, in a reflection of industrial support for the crusade, his employer (the Chicago and Northwestern Railroad) granted him a leave of absence to go on a lecture tour. He was fond of remarking to audiences that, in his work against the traffic, he was spending the same time and money on a noble cause that others were spending on drink—but that he was benefiting while drinkers were losing both health and wealth. Cunneen was also a member of the Prohibition Party and worked on its behalf for some sixteen years. With Repeal, however, he faded from the public scene, and little is known of his latter years.

## Bibliography:

A. with Father C. P. Baron, comp., *What Some Great Catholic Leaders Think of Liquor and Prohibition...* (Westerville, OH, 1918).
B. SEAP 2, 743–44; *The American Issue* (Illinois ed.), Jan. 1, 1909.

**CUYLER, Theodore Ledyard**     (10 January 1822, Aurora, NY—26 February 1909, Brooklyn, NY). *Education*: graduated from Princeton Univ., 1841; graduated from Princeton Theological Sem., 1846; D.D. and LLD. (both honorary), Princeton Univ. *Career*: ordained, Presbyterian Church, 1848; minister, Burlington, NJ, 1848–49; minister, Third Presbyterian Church, Trenton, NJ, 1849–53; minister, Market Street Dutch Reformed Church, NY, 1853–60; minister, Lafayette Avenue Presbyterian Church, Brooklyn, NY, 1860–90; pastor emeritus and active writing and lecturing, 1890–1909.

The Reverend Cuyler once remarked that he considered preaching "spiritual gunnery," and by all accounts of his career his voice was indeed a potent weapon on behalf of both religion and reform. In fact, there are few better examples than Cuyler of the alliance between the two areas in nineteenth-century America. After a thorough education for the ministry, he held three pastorates in New Jersey and New York between 1848 and 1860, in which he emerged as an eloquent and forceful preacher. He was a leader of the 1858 religious revival in the New York area, and although a theological conservative, the young pastor was zealous in urging salvation on his fellow Christians. His long and widely lauded tenure in the Brooklyn pulpit of the Lafayette Street Presbyterian Church began in 1860; and it was there, over the next three decades, that Cuyler rose to national attention. Under his leadership, the congregation grew from several hundred to several thousand members, becoming one of the largest Protestant churches in the region. Cuyler himself, while attending to normal pastoral duties, began writing what eventually grew into a veritable tidal wave of publications for the reform and religious press (including his fascinating and highly readable autobiography, *Recollections of a Long Life* [1902]). One historian's tabulation notes four thousand articles to his credit at his death, some of which were translated into other languages, as well as twenty-two books. In addition to his writing, Cuyler was also a popular speaker and never tired of bringing his usually devotional messages to a variety of audiences. In an era noted for its dynamic clergy, then, Theodore Cuyler was one of the nation's most active clergymen.

The Brooklyn minister's wide range of interests drew his attention to any number of reform causes and philanthropies, most of which received some good word from his pen or pulpit. But his special concern was for the Temperance Movement, which he saw as pursuing the Lord's work. As such, he insisted that the church lend its unqualified support to the reform. "If Jesus Christ established his church for the very purpose of saving human society from its sins," he wrote in 1876, "then surely the largest sin that curses society [the liquor traffic] should command the church's foremost attention." It certainly had Cuyler's attention, and over the years he lost no opportunity to denounce drink as "the chiefest enemy of Christ, of Christianity, and of our country." He urged his congregations to total abstinence, rejoiced at the temperance crusade of Father Mathew in the 1840s, and welcomed the rising tide of temperance sentiment in his own state of New York during the 1850s. While he felt that prohibitory legislation was a social necessity, he warned that such a body of law would become "a farce" unless supported by the public conscience. Nevertheless, his was a leading voice raised in protest in the mid-1850s when Governor Horatio Seymour vetoed a New York prohibition statute. The outraged clergyman then took part in a campaign that elected prohibitionist Governor Myron Clark.* Cuyler also lent his influence to efforts aimed at employing full-time local "missionaries" to spread the dry gospel in New York churches, to convince ministers to make temperance an integral part of their Sunday messages, and to introduce antiliquor lessons into American Sunday schools. To the end of his days, the forthright reverend expounded his belief that alcohol was a dire threat to the nation itself, a source of inefficiency and waste, and that the Temperance Movement was nothing less than a divinely inspired instrument of national salvation.

## Bibliography:

A. *Intellect, and How to Use It* (Newark, NJ, 1863); "A Knock at the Door of Christ's Church," 11–50, in *Centennial Temperance Volume: A Memorial of the International Temperance Conference...* (New York, 1877); *Lafayette Avenue Church: Its History and Commemorative Services* (New York, 1885); *Recollections of a Long Life: An Autobiography* (New York, 1902); *Our Christmas Tides* (New York, 1904).

B. DAB 5, 18–19; NYT, Feb. 27, 1909; SEAP 2, 748–49; WW 1, 290.

# D

**DAGGETT, David** (31 December 1764, Attleboro, MA—12 April 1851, New Haven, CT). *Education*: graduated from Yale Coll., 1783; LLD., Yale Coll., 1827. *Career*: admitted to bar, CT, 1786; member, Connecticut legislature, 1791–97, 1805–9; member, State Council, 1797–1803, 1809–13; member, U.S. Senate, 1813–19; associate justice, Connecticut Superior Court, 1826–28; Kent professor of law, Yale Univ., 1826–48; mayor, New Haven, CT, 1828–30; chief justice, Connecticut Supreme Court of Errors, 1832–34.

In Connecticut justice and politician David Daggett we observe a real bastion of New England Federalism. Educated for the law, Daggett rose quickly as a lawyer and state legislator highly regarded for his skill and eloquence in debate. Holding either elective or judicial office for most of his career, he was one of the most influential state leaders of his generation—and one of the most implacably conservative. Like other Federalists of the period, the rise of Jeffersonian democracy appalled him, and he employed all of his rhetorical and literary skills to resist the swelling popular tide. Daggett stoutly defended the established church, the restricted franchise, and the existing social order, while deploring all forms of social turmoil and the expansionist and nationalist tendencies of the Jefferson administration. His outlook on society ultimately took on something of a siege mentality as Federalism steadily lost ground over the 1800s. Convinced that America's republican institutions were under assault and in grave danger, the dedicated conservative took up the gauntlet for the old order at almost every opportunity. As a judge, for example, he became a strict constructionist, opposed to the extension of national governmental powers; he also tried to keep Connecticut society closed to new groups. In this regard, he presided at the trial that convicted Prudence Crandall of teaching school for free black children (1833); it was generally conceded that the conviction came as a result of Daggett's charge to the jury to the effect that even free blacks were not citizens. It was indicative of his mistrust of social change generally.

It was this same aversion to change and disorder that motivated Daggett's interest in the Temperance Movement. He saw drunkenness as a source of major societal instability and thus to be eliminated for the sake of national preservation. Unlike other dry reformers, he was not interested in building a new society but in maintaining an environment in which his morality held sway and his norms dominated social relationships. Not for Daggett the later sentiments that linked the dry cause to abolitionism, women's rights, or labor law reform. Yet on his own terms he was an effective antagonist of "the demon." With his usual eloquence, he blasted "the grog-shops and tippling-houses" as the "outer chambers of hell," microcosms of the dissolution and anarchy he saw in liberal politics generally, and urged the public to brand their owners as no better than "thieves and counterfeiters." Only then, he went on, would the "virtue. . .essential to a republican government" survive among the citizenry. Beyond oratory, however, Daggett was also an organizer. He was one of the most vigorous leaders of the Connecticut Temperance Society and for a considerable length of time the president of the local temperance society in New Haven. His reputation as a dry champion was such that the American Temperance Society made him an honorary member, an honor in which he placed a great deal of pride. On the bench, Justice Daggett was equally consistent: He did his best to create a favorable legal climate for temperance legislation and thus opened the door to increasing dry reliance on the legislative approach to reform. In the career of David Daggett, then, temperance was not so much a vision of the future as it was a pillar of the established order.

**Bibliography:**

A. *Count the Cost. . .* (Hartford, CT, 1804; Tarrytown, NY, 1922); *Steady Habits Indicated. . .* (Hartford, CT, 1805); *Motion* (Washington, DC, 1814).

B. DAB 5, 26–27; SEAP 2, 753; WW H, 202; F. B. Dexter, *Biographical Sketches of Graduates of Yale College*, vol. 4 (New Haven, CT, 1907); Frederick Charles Hick, *Yale Law School: The Founders Collection* (New Haven, CT, 1935); Dwight Loomis and J. Gilbert Calhoun, *Judicial and Civil History of Connecticut* (Hartford, CT, 1895).

**DANIELS, Josephus**  (18 May 1862, Washington, NC—15 January 1948, Raleigh, NC). *Education*: studied at Wilson Collegiate Inst. (NC) and Univ. of North Carolina; Litt. D. (honorary), Washington and Lee Univ.; LLD. degrees (honorary), Univ. of North Carolina, Davidson Coll., Ohio Wesleyan Univ., Rutgers Univ., Univ. of Maryland, Dickensen Coll., Pennsylvania Military Acad. *Career*: editor, *Wilson* (NC) *Advance*, circa 1880; admitted to bar, NC, 1885 (did not practice); editor, *Raleigh* (NC) *State Chronicle*, beginning 1885 (later merged the *Chronicle* with other publications); North Carolina state printer, 1887–93; chief clerk, Department of the Interior, 1893–95; secretary of the navy, 1913–21; U.S. ambassador to Mexico, 1933–42; work on Woodrow Wilson and Franklin D. Roosevelt foundations and on Jefferson Memorial Commission, 1930s–1940s.

The career of Josephus Daniels furnished a clear example of the links between Progressivism and the temperance reform. Indeed, it was not as a prohibitionist but as a cabinet member in the administration of Progressive Democrat Woodrow Wilson that the North Carolinian first rose to national reputation. Although educated to the law, young Josephus chose instead to enter the newspaper business and soon established himself as a power in the regional press. After becoming editor of the *Raleigh State Chronicle* in 1885, he merged the paper with a number of other journals over the years, and his editorial voice had considerable reach. A life-long Democrat, Daniels's journalistic endorsements (including those favoring the antiliquor cause) and personal activities gradually saw him identified with the Progressive wing of the party. For years he served on the Democratic National Committee (1896–1916) and, using his skills as a publicist to the fullest, directed press relations for the presidential campaigns of William Jennings Bryan* and Woodrow Wilson. During the Wilson administration, Daniels served for eight years as secretary of the navy, and it was in this post that he came to public notice as a major temperance figure. Once in office, he quickly issued General Order 99, which barred beverage alcohol (for other than medicinal uses) from all navy vessels and shore facilities after July 1, 1914. The order caused grumbles of discontent from the fleet, but the Temperance Movement sang the praises of the secretary. Later on, during World War I, he tightened the dry grip on the service by establishing prohibition zones around locales under navy jurisdiction. Clearly, Secretary Daniels saw nothing funny in the proverbial drunken sailor.

In his effort to bring the virtues of temperance to the fleet, Daniels assured himself of a position as a major spokesman of the dry cause. He openly endorsed the National Prohibition amendment, which many other Democrats, including President Wilson, had not clearly embraced. The measure, he claimed, "was a deliberate expression of a great people, moving forward first from township to county, then from county to state, and then from state to the entire country from ocean to ocean." In 1920, the Fifteenth International Congress Against Alcoholism, held in Washington, D.C., elected Daniels an honorary president, at which time he called on the group to spread the message of Prohibition to the corners of the earth. America, he said, was dry to stay, and he asked that the convention consider what might be done to halt the international liquor traffic under the covenant of the proposed League of Nations. It was a challenge for man, he intoned, "worthy of the high mission for which his Maker intended him." In this request, however, Daniels was doomed to disappointment. The United States refused to join the league and in the years after the navy secretary left office began a retreat from the Eighteenth Amendment itself. During these difficult years, the North Carolina Democrat stood by Prohibition, defending it especially in the face of a growing opposition in his own party's rank and file. When Franklin D. Roosevelt made actual Repeal a campaign pledge in 1932, Daniels urged caution but remained loyal to the party. He liked Roosevelt personally, and although pained at the demise of the "noble experiment," he staunchly supported the president during his long tenure in office. He served as ambassador to Mexico from 1933 to 1942, and he spent his later years engaged in philanthropic activities and in writing; he was particularly proud of his several volumes on the life of Woodrow Wilson.

**Bibliography:**

A. "Welcome Address," in Ernest Hurst Cherrington, ed., *Proceedings of the Fifteenth International Congress Against Alcoholism* (Washington, DC, 1921);

*Our Navy at War* . . . (Washington, DC, 1922); *The Life of Woodrow Wilson, 1856–1924* (1924; Westport, CT, 1981); *The Wilson Era: The Years of War and After, 1917–1923* (Chapel Hill, NC, 1946); *Shirt-Sleeve Diplomat* (Chapel Hill, NC, 1947); *The Cabinet Diaries of Josephus Daniels, 1913–1921*, ed. E. David Cronon (Lincoln, NB, 1963).

B. SEAP 2, 756–57; WW 2, 143; Jonathan Daniels, *The End of Innocence* (Philadelphia, 1954); Carroll Kilpatrick, ed., *Roosevelt and Daniels: A Friendship in Politics* (Chapel Hill, NC, 1952); Joseph L. Morrison, *Josephus Daniels: The Small-d Democrat* (Chapel Hill, NC, 1962); Joseph L. Morrison, *Josephus Daniels Says* . . . (Chapel Hill, NC, 1962).

**DAVIS, Edith Smith**    (20 January 1859, Milton, WI—19 March 1917, Milwaukee, WI). *Education*: A.B., Lawrence Univ., 1879; A.M., Lawrence Univ., 1882; LHD, Lawrence Univ., 1907; postgraduate study at Wellesley Coll. *Career*: instructor of English literature, Clark Univ., Atlanta, GA, 1881–84; temperance activities with WCTU, beginning 1884.

Articulate and well educated, Edith Smith Davis epitomized the careers of many late nineteenth-century American women who found the Temperance Movement a convenient door to social participation. We know relatively little of Edith Smith's early background—only that she grew up in rural Wisconsin in a family well enough off to provide her with an excellent formal education and that she was sufficiently accomplished to launch an independent career as a professor of English literature at Clark University in Atlanta, Georgia. She taught there from 1881 to 1884, when she left teaching after her marriage that year to Methodist minister John Scott Davis. There is scant evidence, however, as to why she plunged actively into temperance activities at the same time. Her husband's Methodism may have had something to do with her decision (the denomination produced many antiliquor champions), although she may also have been attracted to the managerial opportunities presented to talented women by the expanding Woman's Christian Temperance Union. At any rate, Davis joined the WCTU and quickly came to the attention of its president, Frances Willard.* Her abilities to communicate and to organize effectively made her a valuable aid to Willard, who relied on her in conducting White Cross and "social purity" campaigns among young women. At the same time, Davis developed a reputation as an effective administrator, and her responsibilities within the union began to grow accordingly. She served effectively as president of the local WCTU chapter in Milwaukee, Wisconsin, where she had moved with Reverend Davis, and assumed the leadership of a number of National WCTU departments. She placed considerable stress on her duties as superintendent of the Bureau of Scientific Temperance Investigation and of the Department of Scientific Temperance Instruction in Public Schools and Colleges. Under her authority, these WCTU divisions tried to marshall scientific data to support temperance arguments against bevarage alcohol, to have these views taught in classrooms around the nation, and to provide both students and teachers with instructional materials. She wrote some of this herself, and her *Compendium of Temperance Truth* (1916) offered a convenient summary of WCTU positions on most aspects of the liquor question. She was a frequent lecturer for teachers' groups and in 1907 founded and edited the *Temperance Education Quarterly*. In addition to her work with the National WCTU, Davis was also a member of the World's WCTU.

**Bibliography:**

A. *Compendium of Temperance Truth* (Evanston, IL, 1916).
B. SEAP 2, 763; WW 1, 300.

**DAVIS, Nathan Smith** (9 January 1817, Greene, NY—16 June 1904, Chicago, IL). *Education*: studied at Cazenovia Sem., NY; graduated from the Coll. of Physicians and Surgeons, Fairfield, NY, 1837; A.M. (honorary), Northwestern Univ.; LLD. (honorary), Illinois Wesleyan Univ. *Career*: medical practice, Vienna and Binghamton, NY, 1837–47, New York City, 1847–49, Chicago, after 1849; professor, Rush Medical Coll., 1849–59; founder, professor, dean of faculty, Chicago Medical Coll. (now part of Northwestern Univ.), 1859–98; editor, *Chicago Medical Journal*, 1855–59; editor, *Chicago Medical Examiner*, 1860–73; editor, *Journal of the American Medical Association*, 1883–89; active in Chicago area civic and philanthropic causes.

Born and raised in rural New York State, Nathan Smith Davis emerged as one of America's most influential medical men of the nineteenth century. Throughout his long and distinguished career, he combined a love of his profession with an intense interest in civil affairs and reform work. Indeed, he began making a name for himself quite early. While serving as president of the Broome County (NY) Medical Society, he attended a convention of the state medical society at which he offered a resolution calling for improvements in medical education. The resulting activities led to the founding of the American Medical Association, of which Davis was remembered ever after as the symbolic "father." After two years of practice at the College of Physicians and Surgeons in New York City, he joined the faculty of Rush Medical College in Chicago, where he worked for ten years. It was in Chicago that his civic and reform interests came to the fore. After a cholera epidemic, Davis led a campaign for public sanitation and in 1850 induced the city to construct modern sewage facilities. The same year he also took the lead in founding Mercy Hospital, the first such public establishment in the growing metropolis. His chief reform passion, however, remained medical education, and in this field lay perhaps his greatest contributions. With a number of other doctors (also from Rush), he founded a medical department in small Lind University (1859), which soon became Chicago Medical College (which in turn was the basis for the medical school of Northwestern University). The venture quickly became a major success, and Davis, both as professor and dean of the faculty, was free to institute his ideas on the proper training of doctors. Along with the school, Davis's reputation grew as he served on any number of medical and civil boards and societies; he helped found the

Illinois and Chicago medical societies, Union College of Law, Northwestern University, the Chicago Historical Society, and other organizations. He also wrote extensively on medical subjects and at various times was editor of a number of medical journals.

One of those journals was the *American Medical Temperance Quarterly*, of which Davis had charge at the turn of the century. This task was a direct result of the doctor's intense interest in the Temperance Movement. His commitment was longstanding, and he gave his time and talents freely on behalf of the cause. Davis believed, along with many of the better-educated physicians of his generation, that alcoholism was an addiction and a disease and was thus a concern of the medical community. In fact, he was one of the nation's first physicians to take major steps to rehabilitate the inebriate. In the aftermath of the Washingtonian temperance revival in the late 1840s, he helped found the Washingtonian Home for the Reformation of Inebriates. The home had a largely spiritual treatment regimen, but Davis saw to it that patients got adequate medical attention and that the staff compiled case study data for clinical purposes. In order to stimulate further inquiry on the problem, the Chicago physician later founded the Medical Temperance Society, which met annually during the conventions of the American Medical Association. The group called for the serious scientific study of alcohol problems and heatedly denounced the frequent medicinal use of alcohol by physicians. Davis also argued that evidence holding alcohol to be a food was wrong, stating instead that it had virtually no value for the human system. As interest in the issue mounted over the late nineteenth and early twentieth centuries, Davis's organization eventually merged with the larger, but similar, American Association for the Study and Cure of Inebriety; and there is little doubt that Davis's reputation enhanced the status of the resulting new group, the American Association for the Study of Alcohol and Other Narcotics. (This merger also combined the *Medical Temperance Quarterly* with the association's *Quarterly Journal of Inebriety*.) The medical front, however, was not the limit of Davis's efforts. He was also a firm prohibitionist. In the antebellum years, he served as chairman of the executive committee of the Illinois Maine Law Alliance and in 1855 led an effort to pass prohibitory legislation in the state. During the postwar reform movement, he did his best to cooperate with dry leaders, lending scientific support to their arguments against drink whenever he could. In great measure, then, his career was illustrative of the dry crusade's faith that the weight of medical evidence supported its case against "the demon."

**Bibliography:**

A. *History of the American Medical Association* (Philadelphia, 1855); *Contributions to the History of Medical Education and Institutions in the United States* (Washington, DC; 1877); "Inebriate Asylums: The Principles that Should Govern Us in the Treatment of Inebriates, and the Institutions Needed to Aid in Their Restoration," *Quarterly Journal of Inebriety* 2 (1877): 80–88; *Verdict of Science Concerning the Effects of Alcohol on Man* (London, 187-?); *Influence of Alcohol on the Human System*... (New York, 1895); *History of Medicine, with the Code of Medical Ethics* (Chicago, 1903).

B. DAB 5, 139; SEAP 2, 765; WW 1, 302; I. F. Danforth, *Life of Nathan Smith Davis* (Chicago, 1907); Arnold Jaffe, *Addiction Reform in the Progressive Age: Scientific and Social Responses to Drug Dependence in the United States, 1870–1930* (New York, 1971); Albert Ernest Wilkerson, "A History of the Disease Concept of Alcoholism" (DSW diss., Univ. of Pennsylvania, 1967).

**DAVIS, Noah**    (10 September 1818, Haverhill, NH—20 March 1902, New York, NY). *Education*: studied at seminary in Lima, NY; private study of law. *Career*: admitted to bar, NY, 1841; legal practice in Gaines, Buffalo, Albion, NY, 1841–57; justice, New York Supreme Court, 1857–68, 1872–87; member, U.S. House of Representatives, 1869–70; U.S. attorney for the Southern District of New York, 1870–72; private practice, New York City, 1887–1901; retirement, 1901.

Social leaders and reformers have called attention to the connections between addiction and crime in America on an almost constant basis since the nineteenth century. Certainly the rise of the Temperance Movement brought the issue into bold relief: Dry workers repeatedly claimed that alcohol problems lay at the root of most crime and violence in the United States and that prohibitory legislation would vastly reduce the nation's law enforcement burdens if adequately enforced. In advancing these arguments, antiliquor crusaders often used their own statistics, which wets frequently challenged. Yet there were those within the judiciary and law enforcement agencies of the country who made the same case, and one of the most prominent of these was Judge Noah Davis of New York State. While never an outright prohibitionist, Davis was described as a "temperance advocate," and his allegations regarding the relationships of criminality and intemperance offered more zealous drys some potent ammunition. The judge himself was one of the most distinguished members of the New York judiciary. Beginning in private practice in the late 1840s, he received an appointment to the State Supreme Court in 1857 and over the course of his career served a number of terms on that high tribunal. After a term in the U.S. House of Representatives (he was a staunch Republican, and, although a reformer, he was also a close friend and personal lawyer of President Ulysses S. Grant), he was for two years U.S. attorney for the Southern District of New York. Returning to the Supreme Court in 1872, he presided at the famous trials of Edward Stokes and William M. ("Boss") Tweed. It was Davis, in fact, who sent Tweed to jail. His years on the bench, however, convinced the noted judge that most cases coming before the courts had their origins in beverage alcohol. His only literary contribution, a small volume entitled *Intemperance and Crime* (1883), dealt with the subject in detail. In it, Davis claimed that some three-fourths of all crime and poverty in America was due to drink, and he especially decried the existence of the saloons (which were, in Davis's period, indeed frequently centers of corruption and various criminal activities). In 1890, he was a leading member of a group of public figures who called for a national congress to consider the social disruption attributed to the liquor traffic (the congress met on June 11–12 of that year in New York City). The stature of the man was such that his arguments on the liquor question could not easily be disregarded, and temperance authorities made considerable use of his information. Davis died in 1902 after having returned to private life.

**Bibliography:**

A. *Intemperance and Crime* (New York, 1883).
B. DAB 5, 140; NYT, March 21, 1902; SEAP 2, 765; WW 1, 302.

**DAY, Albert**   (6 October 1812, Wells, ME—27 April 1894, Melrose Highlands, MA). *Education*: graduated from Harvard Medical Coll., circa late 1830s. *Career*: medical practice, including work with alcoholics, Boston, 1840s–1850s; member, Massachusetts legislature, 1856; superintendent, Washingtonian Home for Inebriates, Boston, 1857–67; superintendent, New York State Inebriate Asylum, Binghamton, 1867–70; operated private alcoholism asylum, Greenwood, MA, 1870–73; superintendent, Washingtonian Home for Inebriates, 1873–1893; operated private inebriate asylum, Melrose Highlands, MA, 1893–94.

In the career of Dr. Albert Day, we find the work of one of America's earliest specialists in the medical treatment of drinking-related problems. Day's interest in rehabilitation stemmed from involvement as a young man with the Temperance Movement. He was an abstainer, and he was fascinated with the success, however temporary, of the Washingtonian temperance revival in drying out thousands of drunkards in the 1840s. Thereafter, he paid special attention to alcohol problems in his medical practice and worked in a number of asylums offering temporary shelter to inebriates in the Boston area. In 1856, Day won election to the Massachusetts legislature (although we know little of his politics or the basis of his campaign), and he used his brief term to press for public support of alcoholism treatment facilities. The result was state incorporation of the Washingtonian Home for Inebriates in Boston, and Day became superintendent in 1857. The Washingtonian Home was intended as a spiritually oriented shelter for alcoholics, but the new superintendent instituted medical care and began collecting clinical data on problem drinkers. Day's reputation as a specialist in alcoholism treatment grew accordingly, and in 1867 he received a call to take over the troubled New York State Inebriate Asylum at Binghamton. Three years later, however, after leaving the financially ailing New York institution, Day returned to Massachusetts, where he opened a private inebriate asylum in Greenwood. He remained closely identified with the Washingtonian Home, however, and in 1873 (after the Greenwood home burned) the institution's directors asked him to come back to Boston. He did and remained for another two decades. During those years he became a leading national spokesman for the medical treatment of alcohol-related problems. He also made the Boston asylum a major source of clinical information, as tens of thousands of patients passed through its doors over the late nineteenth century.

While a widely recognized clinician, Day was never an original or innovative thinker. Other physicians pioneered the ideas he tried to put into practice. Yet Day's contributions were notable in that he did as much as anyone to popularize the disease conception of alcoholism. He was among the charter members of the American Association for the Study and Cure of Inebriety and for several years served as president of the organization. He lectured and wrote on alcoholism treatment widely and at times cooperated with Temperance Movement spokesmen in efforts to warn youth away from alcohol. Day's one book, a slim volume entitled *Methomania* (1867), summarized his experiences with problem drinkers and enjoyed a respectable circulation for books of its type. He also had a number of articles published in the *Journal of Inebriety*. As chief of the Washingtonian Home, Day proved effective over his long tenure in office. The institution was relatively stable financially and Day treated (or supervised the treatment of) some thirty thousand patients. When he finally resigned in ill health in 1893, he had led the asylum for thirty years, and his leaving brought expressions of regret from much of the alcoholism treatment community of the era. The aged doctor, however, never fully retired. Moving to the Boston suburb of Melrose Highlands, he opened a small private asylum and began accepting a limited number of patients. Before the new venture could establish itself, however, Day succumbed to a heart attack. At his death, his professional colleagues recognized him as "the oldest pioneer worker" in the alcoholism field.

**Bibliography:**

A. *Methomania* (Boston, 1867).

B. SEAP 2, 767; T. D. Crothers, "The Late Dr. Albert Day—a Biographical Sketch," *Quarterly Journal of Inebriety* 18 (1896): 51–55.

**DEEMS, Charles Force**    (4 December 1820, Baltimore, MD—18 November 1893, New York, NY). *Education*: graduated from Dickinson Coll., 1839; D.D., Randolph-Macon Coll., 1852; LLD. (honorary), Univ. of North Carolina, 1877. *Career*: Methodist minster, New Jersey circuit, 1839–40; agent, American Bible Society, NC, 1840–42; professor of humanistic studies, Univ. of North Carolina, 1842–48; professor of natural sciences, Randolph-Macon Coll., 1849; president, Greensville (NC) Female Coll., 1850–54; boarding school director, Wilson, NC, 1859–60; founder and editor, *The Watchman* (New York City), beginning 1865; founder and minister of nondenominational Church of the Strangers, 1866–92.

The devout and pious son of equally religious parents, Charles Deems apparently dedicated his life to the ministry as early as age thirteen. The boy, barely into his teens, reportedly raised a small stone altar and began preaching to friends—and set a pattern that carried him through an active life in the ministry. This boyhood "gospel" also launched his reform career, as some of his early "sermons" were temperance orations. Like his love of preaching, his dedication to the antiliquor crusade became a personal hallmark over the years. After completing his undergraduate education, he spoke in a number of New Jersey pulpits for a year before moving to North Carolina as an agent for the American Bible Society in 1840. Deems liked the South and his career flourished there. While continuing to preach and becoming active in the hierarchy of the regional Methodist conference, he also taught at and headed a number of educational institutions. His pen was active as well, and the fervent reverend developed a modest reputation as a commentator on social and religious issues. Deems was a moderate during the growing sectional crisis and opposed secession as against the best interests of his adopted state. When war broke out, however, he supported the Southern cause and suffered the pain of losing a son in the fighting. With the defeat of the Confederacy, perhaps seeking relief from the memories of the war and his lost son, he moved in late 1865 to New York City, where he began a new chapter in his career.

It was in New York that Deems rose to his full stature as a national figure. He founded and began editing a religious publication, *The Watchman*, and, unable to avoid the lure of the pulpit, rented a hall in which he began preaching. Still an orthodox Methodist (at one point in 1866 he was considered for a bishopric back in the South), his new message was nondenominational. From these beginnings, he established the Church of the Strangers, which reached out to all, regardless of specific denomination. The church became one of the most popular in the city (and it's minister one of the best known in the region). By 1870, Deems's fame was such that Cornelius Vanderbilt, who had shunned philanthropy previously, donated a building for the church; in turn, a grateful Deems played a crucial role in raising the funds to found the Vanderbilt University (1873). Throughout his New York tenure, the pious cleric made temperance preaching an important part of his message. His arguments on the subject were not especially novel: He thundered against the traffic and against politicians and voters who allowed it to exist. But his voice was influential and could hardly be ignored as the antiliquor crusade heated up in the latter part of the nineteenth century. Indeed, in 1890, Deems was a popular choice to preside over a major national temperance congress held in New York in June of that year. The pulpit, Deems always insisted, belonged in the vanguard of the struggle against drink. His activities, however, never focused on any single issue. He continued to edit, write, and speak on many religious and social topics, as well as tour Europe and the Holy Land. Illness curtailed his active schedule only during his final year, and he is remembered through the Deems Lectureship of Philosophy at the City University of New York.

**Bibliography:**

A. *Jesus* (New York, 1872); *Mr. Deems's Sermons* (New York, 1885); *Scotch Verdict in re Evolution* (New York, 1885); *Autobiography and Memoir by His Sons* (New York, 1897).

B. DAB 5, 192–93; SEAP 2, 777–78; WW H, 211.

**DELAVAN, Edward Cornelius**    (6 January 1793, Westchester Co., NY—15 January 1871, Schenectady, NY). *Career*: apprenticed to printer, Albany, NY, circa 1809–1814; importing agent in Britain, circa 1814–21; wine merchant, New York City, 1821–26; active temperance work, 1829–71.

Irony has always offered one of the more interesting elements in history, and the Temperance Movement certainly had its share. Consider, as a prime example, the career of Edward C. Delavan of New York State. He was a most improbable temperance man: He spent some of his most productive years in the liquor traffic, actually amassing a fortune as a wine merchant, and was a drinker himself for many years. Yet he ultimately turned against his former business (with a vengeance) and emerged as one of the giants of antebellum reform—indeed, as one of the greatest leaders and benefactors the antiliquor crusade ever found. With little formal education, young Delavan worked first for a printer and then kept a store (which expanded to a thriving retail business) along with his brother in Albany, New York. During these years he was a fairly constant drinker, although later in life he claimed to have mustered the will to avoid slipping into actual intemperance. (He added, however, perhaps to dramatize his own story, that of his fifty drinking companions, no less than forty-four went to besotted ends.) Following the War of 1812 he went abroad as his firm's agent in Europe, and after seven years returned to open his own business in New York City as a wine merchant. He prospered in the traffic, but in the mid-1820s (by then quite wealthy) he suddenly gave it all up and returned to Albany. He subsequently explained that a friend, one Peter Remsen, persuaded him that liquor men usually failed as a result of drink. Delavan was so impressed by the plea that he resolved to devote the rest of his life to the battle against his own former trade (Remsen, then near death, further encouraged his friend with a gift of a thousand dollars to assist the cause). It was the start of a momentous temperance career.

Delavan began his activities in Albany and gained his first public recognition there. In 1829, along with the Reverend Eliphalet Nott* (another major figure in the early Temperance Movement), he founded the New York State Temperance Society and worked diligently to build its membership. He was also generous with his own funds. Several years after establishing the society, he became so impressed with the temperance preaching of the Albany minister, Nathaniel Hewitt,* that he financed a European speaking tour for the man. In an effort to marshall significant endorsements for the developing Temperance Movement (which had not yet become a total abstinence crusade), he prevailed upon Justin Edwards* to circulate a petition denouncing the use of distilled spirits. Eventually, it received the signatures of Presidents (or ex-Presidents) Madison, John Quincy Adams, Tyler, Fillmore, Pierce, Jackson, Van Buren, Taylor, Polk, Buchanan, Lincoln, and Johnson. It was a major publicity coup for the reformers. Delavan's most notorious effort, however, came in 1835, when he published an exposé of Albany brewers. He claimed they were using water drawn from sources polluted by (among other things) offal from local slaughterhouses, and the charges created a sensation. The brewers sued Delavan for $300,000, while temperance forces rallied to the New York reformer. Inherent in the entire controversy was a growing movement away from the moderationist position of many reformers (who still claimed that beer and wine were acceptable beverages): If the brewers could be discredited, then so would moderation. The trial was delayed for five years, when Delavan was acquitted. In the meantime, he was recognized widely as New York's premier dry leader and became chairman of the executive committee of the national American Temperance Union when it was organized in 1836 (he also donated $10,000 to its treasury).

Besides his other efforts, Delavan was a critical force behind the publishing activities of the antebellum movement (an interest that continued after the war as well). He directed the publication of two Albany-based journals, the *American Temperance Intelligencer* and the *Temperance Recorder*, conducted an extensive literary campaign on the Bible-wine question, and donated another seven thousand dollars to distribute some 150,000 copies of the Sewall plates on the effects of drinking on the stomach (and other dry titles). Managing the affairs of a thriving temperance press in Albany for over twenty years, Delavan was ultimately responsible (directly or indirectly) for the international distribution of over 13.6 million temperance books, pamphlets, graphics, and tracts of various kinds. By any measure, it was a prodigious undertaking. Delavan's personal fame spread along with the literature, and he even made a tour of Europe to urge the dry cause on national leaders there. (He even persuaded King Louis Philippe of France to sign a declaration against habitual drinking.) Later in life, financial reverses forced the ardent reformer to reduce his donations of both time and money to the cause (he also spent an increasing amount of time on the management of Union College, of which he was a board member). Nor did Delavan place much faith in prohibition, preferring instead moral suasion. Yet to the end he was as stalwart a foe of drink as America ever produced.

### Bibliography:

A. *Defense of Dr. Sewall's Work on the Pathology of Drunkenness, and His Drawings of the Stomach, as Affected by the Use of Alcoholic Drinks. . .* (Albany, NY, 1843); *Letter to the Bishops of the Episcopal Church on the Adulteration of Liquors. . .* (Albany, NY, 1859); *Temperance and Wine Countries* (New York, 1860); *Prohibition: A Letter from E. C. Delavan. . .* (New York, 1867); ed., *Temperance Essays, and Selections from Different Authors* (New York, 1869).

B. SEAP 2, 779; "Edward C. Delavan," *The American Temperance Magazine and Sons of Temperance Offering* (1851): 30–41; Mark Edward Lender and James Kirby Martin, *Drinking in America: A History* (New York, 1982); Alice Felt Tyler, *Freedom's Ferment: Phases of American Social History from the Colonial Period to the Outbreak of the Civil War* (1944; New York, 1962).

**DEXTER, Samuel**    (14 May 1761, Boston, MA—4 May 1816, Athens, NY). *Education*: graduated from Harvard Coll., 1781; studied law with Levi Lincoln, Worcester, MA, 1780s; LLD. (honorary), Harvard Coll., 1813. *Career*: admitted to bar, 1784; private legal practice, beginning 1784; member, Massachusetts House of Representatives, 1788–90; member, U.S. House of Representatives, 1793–95; member, U.S. Senate, 1799–1800; secretary of war, 1800; secretary of the treasury, 1801–2; private legal and political activities, to 1816.

Possessed of one of the most brilliant legal careers in nineteenth-century Massachusetts, Samuel Dexter rose quickly as a man of public affairs. At the same time, his activities admirably demonstrated the reform concerns of much of the contemporary New England social elite. After completing his undergraduate education at Harvard with "highest honors," he read law for several years before admission to the bar and establishment of his own practice. Settling in Charleston in 1788, he won election (as a Federalist) the same year to the state legislature, where he quickly made his mark. Dexter's careful arguments and sound judgement won him considerable respect as well as political support, which later carried him successively to the national government as a congressman (1793–95) and senator (1799–1800). During the presidency of John Adams he also served terms as secretary of war and of the treasury (where his tenure carried briefly into the administration of Thomas Jefferson). Between electoral offices, and after leaving government in 1802, Dexter won acclaim as a lawyer, and clients actively sought his services. While not ranked as a major legal thinker by many who knew him, Dexter's tactical skills and eloquence were first-rate, and he won a number of highly controversial trials in his years before the bar. With a secure income and a respected place in Massachusetts society, he felt free to follow an active interest in social reform and political positions occasionally at odds with Federalist orthodoxy. For example, while he opposed most of the policies of President James Madison, Dexter strongly endorsed America's declaration of war against Great Britain in 1812. While he declined an offered diplomatic post from Madison in 1815, the national administration retained its respect for the Bay State lawyer.

Dexter was also a pioneer temperance reformer. Long before most of his fellow citizens became interested in the liquor question, the noted Federalist was helping to lay the foundation of a successful mass movement devoted to the issue. In 1813, he was elected the first president of the new Massachusetts Society for the Suppression of Intemperance. The group was the first organization in the state to address temperance issues, and Dexter's emergence as its leader was indicative of his concerns over both drinking problems and the social disruption attributed to them. Drinking, he feared, was reaching astronomical heights in the United States and was imperiling the nation's youth both physically and spiritually. As president of the society, he wrote a number of tracts on temperance personally and worked to generate a broad base of popular support for the budding movement. Like many other reformers of the period, however, Dexter saw intemperance more as a moral than a legal problem. He declined to use his public offices or legal skills to legislate against the liquor traffic, and he preferred to attack the problem through a reform of public morality. His death, in 1816, came before either the society or the Temperance Movement generally had reached any position of major social or political influence—and thus the early reformer never had to face the later movement controversies over moral versus legal suasion and moderation versus total abstinence (Dexter himself was a moderationist). Yet Dexter's social prestige lent credence to the cause, and his early organizational work established a firm base upon which later crusaders built.

**Bibliography:**

A. *Circular Addressed to the Members of the Massachusetts Society for the Suppression of Intemperance* (Boston, 1814); *Mr. Dexter's Address to the Electors of Massachusetts...* (Boston, 1814).

B. DAB 5, 280–81; SEAP 2, 797–98; WW H, 217; O. P. Dexter, *Dexter Genealogy, 1642–1904* (1904); Sigma [Lucius Manlius Sargent], *Reminiscences of Samuel Dexter* (Boston, 1814).


**DE YO, Anna Marden**    (18 October 1868, Glasgow, IL—4 March 1953, San Francisco, CA). *Education*: studied at Univ. of California, 1918. *Career*: active in various WCTU groups on the state (CA) and national levels, 1911–53.

We know very little of Anna De Yo's (born Marden) early years—only that she grew up in Illinois, where she finished high school, and then moved to California with her husband Palmer George De Yo (whom she married in 1885). The picture is equally cloudy on why she became involved with the Temperance Movement at all, much less at forty-three years old, but when she did, she devoted herself to the cause with an enthusiasm matched by few others. De Yo joined the California WCTU in 1911, a time when the movement for National Prohibition was clearly gaining momentum. She served as an organizer and lecturer for three years and then won election to the office of corresponding secretary, a post she held until 1927. She was active on behalf of prohibitionist efforts in the state, and her energy and efficiency as an administrator finally brought her some much-deserved recognition from the National WCTU. By the late 1920s, with Prohibition increasingly coming under effective wet fire, the national organization needed capable officers to maintain support for the flagging crusade. Thus in 1927 De Yo took office as corresponding secretary of the National WCTU, headquartered in Evanston, Illinois. From that position she helped wage the losing dry battle against Repeal, and even after this defeat her faith in the antiliquor cause held firm. She remained in office until 1942, when she returned to California. There, she was active in the local WCTU chapter of Fresno County and was a familiar figure in the state's dwindling temperance ranks until her death in 1953, twenty years after the demise of Prohibition. While temperance had provided a career for Mrs. De Yo, she always had found time for other pursuits as well. She belonged to a number of groups devoted to women's rights and to the League of Women Voters and was a devout Methodist.

The dry crusade had always been proud of the dedication and sense of civic duty in its membership, and thus in Anna De Yo it found one of its best.

**Bibliography:**

B. WW 3, 226.

**DICKIE, Samuel**   (6 June 1851, Oxford Co., Canada—5 November 1925, Albion, MI). *Education*: B.S., Albion Coll., 1872; M.S., Albion Coll., 1877; LLD. (honorary), Albion Coll., 1900. *Career*: teacher and superintendent of schools, Hastings, MI, circa 1873–77; professor of astronomy, Albion Coll., 1877–87; manufacturing business, 1887–1901; mayor, Albion, MI, 1896–97; president, Albion Coll., 1901–21.

Samuel Dickie grew up in Lansing, Michigan, where he had moved with his parents from Canada in 1858. He took his undergraduate studies at small Albion College, an institution which became an integral part of Dickie's career. He subsequently earned a master's degree there (1877), served on its faculty (1877–87), and then, after more than a decade in the manufacturing business, returned to head the school as president for twenty years (1901–21). Dickie's career in education, however, distinguished as it was, brought him less national recognition than his work as a temperance crusader. Throughout his adult life he was an active foe of the liquor traffic and a zealous partisan of the small but highly motivated Prohibition Party. In 1884, the future college president chaired the party convention in Pittsburgh that nominated former Kansas Governor John P. St. John* for president. It was (of course) a losing campaign, but Dickie had an obvious thirst for dry politics, and two years later he ran for governor of Michigan at the head of the Prohibition ticket. In 1887 he orchestrated a drive for constitutional state prohibition in Michigan and in the same year took on additional responsibilities as chairman of the National Committee of the Prohibition Party. He held that post until 1900, although despite his considerable talents as an administrator he was unable to broaden the party's popular base (the Prohibition Party never did pose a major challenge to the two-party system). He then stepped down as chairman and took on the less demanding duties of vice chairman. While working for the party, Dickie was also active in the affairs of the Methodist Church. He was a lay delegate to every general conference from 1892 to 1916, and he used his influence to keep Methodism firmly on course in favor of temperance.

Dickie's involvement in temperance politics was remarkable in one important respect: As a member of the Prohibition Party, he was noted for his overt hostility toward the Anti-Saloon League. Dickie had always represented the faction of the party that had stood against fusion with other political groups. He had strongly opposed making common cause, for example, with the Populists. He was confirmed in his belief that the Prohibition Party alone offered the best chance for the general reform of American society and that any shift toward cooperation with other parties and their issues would constitute a perversion of the idealism that had originally motivated the anitliquor crusade. Consequently, the stalwart reformer had contempt for the nonpartisan political approach advocated by the league (and which brought it such legislative success). As a member of the Prohibitionist hierarchy, Dickie spoke against cooperation with the Anti-Saloon organization and pointedly criticized its political methods. In turn, the league, which by the turn of the century had rapidly overshadowed the small Prohibition Party in political and popular influence, wasted little effort in replying to Dickie's impassioned but largely harmless attacks. While some league officials were annoyed, most others ignored the barbs while paying their respects to the Prohibitionist standard-bearer's undeniable dedication to the fight against the traffic. They could afford to be generous, as Dickie's organization, never a major political force, had also lost the pulse of much of the Temperance Movement itself by the 1900s. While he welcomed National Prohibition, then, at his death in 1925, the old crusader remained unreconciled to the league that had done so much to achieve it.

**Bibliography:**

A. *The Anti-Saloon League: Its Methods* (Minneapolis, MN, 1912).

B. SEAP 2, 802–3; WW 3, 322; Jack S. Blocker, Jr., *Retreat from Reform: The Prohibition Movement in the United Stats, 1890–1913* (Westport, CT, 1976); *Prohibition: Is It Right? Yes! Says Samuel Dickie. No! Says D. S. Rose. Authorized Report of the Great Debate at Milwaukee . . .* (Indianapolis, IN, 1909).

**DINGLEY, Nelson**   (15 February 1832, Durham, ME—13 January 1899, Washington, DC). *Education*: studied at Waterville Coll. (now Colby Univ.), 1850s; graduated from Dartmouth Coll., 1855; LLD. (honorary), Bates Coll., 1874, Dartmouth Coll., 1894. *Career*: admitted to bar, 1856; editor and proprietor, *Lewiston* (ME) *Evening Journal*, 1856–99; member, Maine state legislature, 1862–65, 1868, 1873; governor of Maine, 1874–75; member, U.S. House of Representatives, 1881–99.

Nelson Dingley was a fervent and committed participant in the campaign for National Prohibition, and his sentiments on the matter colored all aspects of his wide-ranging career as an editor, governor, and congressman. Dingley's views on alcohol use and the Temperance Movement took shape during his boyhood in Maine. The state was in fact a battleground between wets and drys, and young Nelson was in his teens when Neal Dow* and his antiliquor allies forced the first state-wide prohibitory law in the nation through the legislature. That experience, plus the subsequent debate over enforcement efforts, found Dingley staunchly in the prohibitionist camp. Even while attending Sunday school he would lecture his classmaates on the evils of drink, a practice he continued later during his college years at Dartmouth. After graduation, the young dry prepared for a career in law; but after taking the bar (1856) he had a change of heart and decided instead on journalism. He became both proprietor and editor of the *Lewiston* (Maine) *Evening Journal*, which marked a turning point in his career.

He built the *Journal* into a highly successful newspaper and used its editorial page to voice his own social and political views. Politically, he emerged as a solid Republican (helping to advance the fortunes of the newly founded party) as well as a staunch supporter of education and the antiliquor reform. He also commented widely on religious affairs (he was a Congregationalist). Through the pages of the *Journal*, Dingley's public reputation spread steadily, and in 1861 he was elected to the state legislature. At various times he served six terms and sat as speaker in 1863 and 1864. While in office, Dingley was known for his energy and capacity for hard work, and his popularity throughout the state was well entrenched by the 1870s. Thus in 1874, when he won the first of his two terms as governor of Maine, it came as no surprise to his contemporaries.

Dingley's climb to political prominence allowed him to press for legislative action on behalf of his pet causes. As governor, he rigidly upheld Maine's prohibitory laws, although he was fully aware that many citizens opposed them and that enforcement was difficult due to loopholes. He suggested changes to make the legislation more effective, and some of these were incorporated into a dry amendment to the state constitution in 1884. Meanwhile, Dingley won election to the House of Representatives in 1881, where he served until his death almost two decades later. His years in Washington, D.C., were distinguished, and he acquired a reputation as a financial expert. He rose to the chair of the powerful Committee on Ways and Means, framed the tariff legislation that bore his name (the Dingley Tariff, passed in 1897, was the highest in American history), and was offered the position of secretary of the treasury by President McKinley (he refused in order to stay in the House). His colleagues considered him singularly impressive as a debator, and he took the floor frequently on behalf of a variety of issues. He continued to advocate temperance as a vital national reform, and the Temperance Movement gratefully acknowledged his efforts. Dingley's work against drink extended to the very Congress itself, as he lost few opportunities to praise the merits of temperance in conversations with other legislators. Indeed, during his final years in the House, the Maine lawmaker served as president of the Congressional Temperance Society. At his death, National Prohibition was still some twenty years away, but in his time, Dingley had kept the dry flame burning brightly in the national government.

## Bibliography:

A. *Prohibition and the Amendment* (New York, 1883); *The Treasury Condition. . .* (Washington, DC, 1896); *The Cotton Industry of the United States* (Washington, DC, 1898); *Maintain the National Honor* (Washington, DC, 1898); *The War Revenue Act* (Washington, DC, 1898); *Ways and Means to Meet War Expenditures* (Washington, DC, 1898).

B. DAB 5, 314–15; SEAP 2, 806; WW H, 219–20; Edward Nelson Dingley, *The Life and Times of Nelson Dingley, Jr.* (Kalamazoo, MI, 1902); Maine Writers' Research Club, *Just Maine Folks* (Lewiston, ME, 1924).

**DINWIDDIE, Edwin Courtland**   (29 September 1867, Springfield, OH—5 May 1935, Washington, DC). *Education*: studied at Wittenberg Coll. and Grove City (PA) Coll., 1880s; A.M., Grove City Coll., 1899; D.D. (honorary), Wittenberg Coll., 1922. *Career*: ordained in Evangelical Lutheran Church, 1894; secretary, Permanent Committee on Temperance, General Synod of the Evangelical Lutheran Church, 1899–1903; chairman, 1903–18; legislative superintendent, Ohio Anti-Saloon League, 1893–96; state superintendent, Pennsylvania Anti-Saloon League, 1897–99; national legislative superintendent, Anti-Saloon League, 1899–1907, 1911–20; work with Independent Order of Good Templars (including local, national, and international offices), 1890s–1920s.

Edwin Dinwiddie was one of the key architects of the Eighteenth Amendment and of efforts to enforce National Prohibition. Indeed, in one respect or another, Dinwiddie's entire adult life (and a good deal of his youth) was connected with the crusade against beverage alcohol. Ohio was a hotbed of dry activity, and as a boy he had joined the Independent Order of Good Templars, as well as local temperance societies. The young reformer then quickly moved on to membership in the Prohibition Party. He also held office in the Ohio Young Men's Prohibition League and the Ohio Prohibition Executive Committee. When he chose a career in the ministry, he also maintained his focus on the liquor question by joining the newly created Evangelical Lutheran Permanent Committee on Temperance. His work with the organization honed his administrative skills, as did his work with the Ohio chapter of the Anti-Saloon League, of which he became a member in 1893. Over the 1890s, Dinwiddie emerged as one of the most vigorous and effective temperance men in the state. He was influential in directing the affairs of the Ohio Prohibition Party and then demonstrated his commitment to the nonpartisan political approach of the league when he left the party in 1896 (he was a Republican for the rest of his life). By the turn of the century, then, Dinwiddie had risen to considerable public recognition through his efforts against the traffic in Ohio. Had he done nothing else, he would still have been accorded major plaudits as a temperance leader.

But it was on the national scene, particularly as a member of the Anti-Saloon League of America, that Dinwiddie had his greatest impact. He was in the ranks of the Ohio Anti-Saloon League almost from its inception in 1893, and the following year he headed its legislative department as legislative superintendent. In 1896 he was appointed superintendent of the Pennsylvania Anti-Saloon League. In 1899, the league's desire for national prohibitory legislation resulted in his being appointed the first national legislative superintendent, and Dinwiddie took up residence in Washington, D.C. There, he was able to maintain close contact with congressional action on temperance and liquor-related questions, and during his years in office (he served until 1907, and again from 1911 to 1920) Dinwiddie achieved notable success in getting league-endorsed bills through the Congress. Among them were the Anti-Canteen Act of 1901, which prohibited the sale of intoxicating beverages in armed service canteens; the Webb-Kenyon

Act in 1913, which prohibited the shipment of alcoholic beverages into any state in violation of that state's laws; the District of Columbia prohibition law in 1917; and a law to bar liquor advertising from the U.S. mails in states with prohibition laws. In addition, he was instrumental in getting prohibitory legislation written into numerous other laws, as well as having the major role of steering the Eighteenth Amendment through both houses of Congress in 1917. It would probably not be an exaggeration to say that almost all the laws dealing with Prohibition in one form or another enacted by Congress in the first quarter of the twentieth century were owing to Dinwiddie's work. However, he did not confine himself to the legislative work connected with the Anti-Saloon League. He held high office in the Independent Order of Good Templars for many years on the local level, and in 1905 he was elevated to national grand chief templar, the highest office in that body. Amid all this activity, Dinwiddie still found time to attend many international temperance congresses as well as to serve on numerous reform and philanthropic bodies. He died in 1935 at the age of sixty-eight, two years after Repeal, but remembered as one of the great temperance workers in American history.

**Bibliography:**

B. SEAP 2, 806–9; WW 1, 326.

**DODGE, William Earl**     (4 September 1805, Hartford, CT—9 February 1883, New York, NY). *Career*: worked in dry goods store, New York City, circa 1818–19; clerk in country store, CT, circa 1819–25; worked in father's dry goods business, New York City, 1826–33; joined firm of Phelps, Dodge & Co., beginning 1883; member, U.S. House of Representatives, 1866–67.

At the age of thirteen William Earl Dodge began one of the great careers in American business history by clerking in his father's dry goods store in New York City. When he became of age, Dodge went into the dry goods business for himself. But it was his marriage to Melissa Phelps in 1828 that enabled him to make his mark in the world of commerce. The young businessman joined his father-in-law to form the premier metals firm of Phelps, Dodge and Company in 1833. The chief business of the company was in copper and iron, but Dodge expanded his investments into a wide variety of operations, including timber and railroads. Indeed, at various times he was a major stockholder in the Erie, Jersey Central, Lackawanna and Texas Central lines. Dodge's business acumen was undeniable, and his investments made him a millionaire in relatively short order. With his financial security assured, he turned to philanthropy and soon became the benefactor of such efforts as the Young Men's Christian Association, the Evangelical Alliance, the Temperance Movement, and antislavery. Yet Dodge was never strident in his reform activities. Even though an abolitionist, for example, he still maintained friendships with business associates in the South, and he worked hard to allay sectional tensions before the Civil War. He served on the futile, last-ditch peace conference of 1861 in Washington, D.C. (although once the shooting started he helped Union recruiting drives), and favored President Andrew Johnson's antiradical Reconstruction methods while in Congress after the war (1866–67).

Of all Dodge's reform and philanthropic interests, however, the closest to his heart was the Temperance Movement. He was attached to the antiliquor cause throughout his adult life, and his views on the subject reflected those of other businessmen of the age: Drink, he believed, brought not only individual tragedy but social disorder and economic waste and inefficiency. (His father, it should be noted, set an example in this regard. The elder Dodge had prohibited liquor among his employees.) William's first public identification with the crusade came in the 1840s, when the Washingtonian temperance revival swept many of the Northern cities. Thereafter, Dodge was an enthusiastic supporter of the work of dry lecturer John B. Gough* and of the pledge-signing campaign of the Irish priest, Father Mathew.* In 1854, he allied himself with the forces that brought (if only by a small electoral margin) a prohibition law to New York State. Indeed, he was a leader of the movement, and his social status lent it considerable prestige. The New York businessman's reputation as a dry spokesman spread nationally, and other leaders of the crusade considered him one of their most effective colleagues. Seeking to impress the country with the importance of the liquor question, Dodge at one point called for a national investigation of alcohol problems. In 1865, he was elected president of the American Temperance Society, and he served in that capacity until his death in 1883. He was a crucial link, then, between the antebellum and postbellum movements, and a bulwark not only of dedication, but of civility.

**Bibliography:**

A. *Influence of the War on Our National Prosperity* (New York, 1865); *The Church and Temperance* (New York, 1892); *The Drinking Usages of Society* (New York, 18—?).

B. DAB 5, 352–53; WW H, 221–22; D. Stuart Dodge, ed., *Memorials of William E. Dodge* (New York, 1887); Richard Lowitt, *A Merchant Prince of the Nineteenth Century* (New York, 1954); Carlos Martyn, *William E. Dodge: The Christian Merchant* (New York, 1890).

**DORCHESTER, Daniel** (11 March 1827, Duxbury, MA—13 March 1907, West Roxbury, MA). *Education*: studied at Norwich Acad., 1840s; A.B., Wesleyan Univ., 1847; A.M. (honorary), Wesleyan Univ., 1856; D.D. (honorary), Wesleyan Univ., 1874. *Career*: entered ministry, Methodist Church, 1847; served pastorates (CT and MA), 1847–95; member, Connecticut Senate, 1855; member, Massachusetts legislature, 1883; superintendent, Indian Schools of the United States, 1889–93; retired from active ministry, 1895.

Three characteristic elements in the typical reform personality of the nineteenth century—religion, politics, and temperance—were combined to powerful effect in the career of Reverend Daniel Dorchester. Born into the deeply religious and reformist atmosphere of Methodism, Dorchester followed his father into the ministry in 1847, and until his retirement from it in 1895 he held over a dozen pastorates in Connecticut and Massachusetts. In the pulpit he had a reputation for eloquence and power and an insistence on addressing what he considered the pressing moral and social issues of the day. Dorchester fervently believed that Christians, both as individuals and through the organized church, had to take firm stands on important questions, even if it meant mixing religion with the affairs of state. Indeed, he led by example in this regard. In 1855, at the age of twenty-eight, he entered politics himself, winning election to the Connecticut State Senate, where he emerged as a forceful and effective champion of reform causes. He served with genuine distinction as chairman of the Senate's Committee on Idiocy, the report of which (1856) inspired ongoing research on the subject. The reverend himself acquired major repute as a sociologically oriented statistician. In 1882, having moved to Massachusetts, he became a representative in that state's legislature, and there first made his mark in the cause of temperance as chairman of the Constitutional Amendment Committee, while also serving as president of the Non-Partisan Temperance League. In 1889 President Harrison appointed him superintendent of Indian schools, in which capacity he influenced a shift in appropriations away from sectarian schools and toward industrial education. Quite clearly, then, Dorchester had emerged as a major reform figure and served as a classic demonstration of church involvement in reform politics.

In addition to his other activities, Dorchester was also a writer of considerable note in his generation. In fact, his fame as an author in some cases overshadowed his accomplishments in other fields. Generally he used his pen to demonstrate the righteousness of the various reform causes he championed over the years and to explore religious issues. His history of *Christianity in the United States* (1888), and *The Liquor Problem in All Ages* (1884), particularly demonstrated the working of a mind both scholarly in its marshalling of facts and imaginative in interpreting them. The volume on the liquor question was a contribution that remains useful to historians and offered one of the best historical justifications of the Temperance Movement ever written by a reformer. Temperance leaders were appreciative of his work, especially his call for church mobilization against the traffic. As a reform author, then, Dorchester was one of the best. Through his many publications, he penetrated the intellectual sphere with a personal energy already considerable for its effects on politics and religion, and he brought a logic to arguments against drink often lacking in the writings of other drys. Dorchester also lectured widely on the cause, and like many prominent orators of his time, his countenance and speaking voice lent powerful support to the reform he saw as so crucial for the nation's well-being.

## Bibliography:

A. *Concessions of "Liberalists" to Orthodoxy* (Boston, 1878); *The Problem of Religious Progress* (New York, 1881); *The Liquor Problem in All Ages*

(Cincinnati, OH, 1884, 1887); *The Why of Methodism* (New York, 1887); *Christianity in the United States from the First Settlement down to the Present Time* (Cincinnati, OH, 1888, 1895).

B. DAB 5, 375–76; SEAP 2, 836–37; WW 1, 333.

**DOUTHIT, Jasper L.** (10 October 1834, Shelby Co., IL—?). *Education*: studied at Wabash Coll., 1856; graduated from Meadville (PA) Theological Sem., 1867. *Career*: book and drug business, Shelbyville, IL, 1857; superintendent of public schools, Hillsboro, IL, 1858; worked in Massachusetts publishing firm, 1858–59; editor, *The Shelby Freeman*, 1860; ordained as Unitarian minister, 1862; missionary preaching, IL, until circa 1917; founder and editor, *Our Best Words*, 1880 to circa 1923; established and managed a religious camp meeting facility (later called Lithia Springs Chautauqua Association), 1890 to 1920s.

The first thirty years of Jasper Douthit's life were uneventful, except for a short-lived rebellion against his father, who did not share his son's enthusiasm for education. The split was healed, however, when the elder Douthit agreed to permit his son to enter college in return for helping to bring in one last crop on the family farm in Shelby County, Illinois. But even after this, once Jasper had made his intentions to pursue a ministerial career known, the senior Douthit objected. Jasper therefore left Wabash College, where he studied for less than a year, in 1856 and went through a succession of unremarkable jobs before finally completing his education (in theology) in 1867. While shaping his course in life, however, the young Douthit developed a strong sense of morality and public responsibility. He found an outlet in the growing abolitionist crusade in the years immediately preceding the Civil War, and he took up the cause with a passion. His outspoken advocacy of abolitionism, a view much at variance with those of his neighbors, brought him notoriety as well as the associate editorship of *The Shelby Freeman* in 1860. A medical disability kept him from military service in the Civil War, but he used his position on the newspaper to support enthusiastically the policies of President Abraham Lincoln. And he did so at some personal risk. His attacks on antiwar Democrats and the pro-Southern Knights of the Golden Circle brought him repeated threats of violence. At no time, however, did Douthit waver, and the war years seemed to move the highly religious editor further toward a life in the ministry.

Douthit described his religious upbringing as "Calvinism gone to seed," and in early manhood he joined the Unitarian Church. After preaching for some two years in his home locale, he was ordained a minister in that denomination in 1862. Douthit's radical religious views (he had completely forsaken the dogmatism of his Calvinist ancestors) kept him from many pulpits, causing him, in 1861, to build his own meeting house. He called the new place, appropriately enough, Liberty, and he launched a career of ministering to "the unchurched and mostly poor people." From the beginning, part of his message was a call for temperance. Douthit considered himself a reformed drinker who had regularly taken "a dram of whiskey each morning before breakfast," a habit which expanded into taking "a dram before each meal and then one between meals, and still oftener on stormy days and in very cold and very hot weather." When he was sixteen, although he had never heard of the Temperance Movement, Douthit "vowed to God" never to touch another drop. Seeing that many in his congregation were drunkards and saloonkeepers, he seized the opportunity, and by 1874 was devoting himself almost exclusively to temperance. He joined the Prohibition Party and even ran unsuccessfully for Congress on its ticket. One of his chief activities was the exposure of politicians who cadged votes by offering free drinks. He published their names in a monthly magazine called *Our Best Word*, which he personally edited between 1880 and 1923. In 1890, Douthit constructed a tabernacle on the family farm, where frequent encampments attracted such temperance notables as Frances Willard.* In 1905, the Lithia Springs Chautauqua Association took over the operation of the encampment. Douthit never expanded his temperance activities beyond the confines of Shelbyville and consequently never achieved the national recognition of some of the other temperance advocates. His career was thus characteristic of untold numbers who often labored in the vineyards of prohibition, building its foundations at the grassroots, but never receiving their full due.

**Bibliography:**

A. *Representative Liberal Christians and the Reformation of the Nineteenth Century* (Shelbyville, IL, 1878); *Alexander Campbell's System of Water Baptism Refuted* (Chicago, 1881); *Shelby Seminary Memorial, 1854–1869* (Shelbyville, IL, 1886); *Lithia Springs Chautauqua and Mission* (Lithia, IL, 1903); *Why I Am a Unitarian* (Shelbyville, IL, 1906); *Jasper Douthit's Story: An Autobiography. . .* (Boston, 1909).

B. SEAP 2, 840–41; WW 4, 261.

**DOW, Neal**   (20 March 1804, Portland, ME—2 October 1897, Portland, ME). *Education*: public and private elementary and secondary schols, ME, MA, to 1820. *Career*: family tanning business, beginning 1826; investments in timber, banking, real estate, and other ventures, from 1820s; temperance organizing and lecturing, 1850s; mayor, Portland, ME, 1851; officer, Union army, 1861–64; active in temperance politics and reform work, 1860s–1890s.

Neal Dow was one of the major personalities in the struggle to turn the Temperance Movement away from moral suasion and moderation toward an aggressive political quest for legal prohibition. A successful and civic-minded businessman, he was genuinely distressed over the effects of excessive drinking in his native Portland, and he had become a firm temperance man by the 1820s. While some of his associates in reform adopted moderationist views, Dow's thinking followed the total abstinence ideas of Justin Edwards* and Lyman Beecher,* so he was of little frame of mind to compromise on the liquor question. Dow also blamed the local drink trade for the alcoholism of one of his relatives, a fact which added a personal dimension to his war against booze. Making temperance his chief issue, he ran successfully for mayor of Portland in 1851 and proceeded to enforce strictly all liquor control statutes. The same year, he worked effectively with the state legislature in framing the so-called Maine Law, the nation's first state-wide prohibitory act. As the "father of the Maine Law" he quickly became a celebrity, much in demand as a speaker in the United States, Canada, and Great Britain. But the Maine Law provoked bitter opposition, and as its principal author Dow became the target of impassioned political attacks. His subsequent electoral career, which ultimately carried him to a seat in the legislature in 1858, was marked by some serious reverses and incessant controversy (including charges of corruption). Yet he never gave ground, always insisting on the merits of prohibition and hurling denunciations at its detractors. Much to his disgust, however, the Maine Law was repealed in 1855 amid claims that it was unpopular and unenforceable. A less stringent dry law replaced it in 1858; and Dow, finally aware that national enthusiasm for temperance was waning with the approach of the Civil War, seemed at least temporarily reconciled to the halfway measure. The zealous reformer had succeeded, though, in politicizing the temperance issue as never before.

Despite the cooling of prohibitionist sentiments during the sectional conflict, however, Dow remained very much in the popular eye. Like many other reformers of his generation, he was also an ardent member of the new Republican Party as well as an abolitionist. When the war came, Dow enthusiatically supported President Lincoln's appeal to arms and in 1861 joined the Union army. His still considerable political reputation gained him a commission in the Maine Volunteers, some of whom he tried to organize as "temperance regiments." In order to serve in such an outfit, a soldier had to sign an abstinence pledge. And although the dry regiments were never a major part of the army (nor, apparently, did the original such units stay dry for long), they were testimony to Dow's continuing antiliquor faith. The Maine reformer was not an especially distinguished military leader, but he rose to brigadier general before being wounded in the fighting at Port Hudson. He was captured in 1863, and after being exchanged for Confederate General Fitzhugh Lee, resigned in 1864 pleading ill health. Dow then returned to temperance work and again rose to prominence in the cause as the postwar antiliquor movement gathered momentum. He travelled the nation calling for National Prohibition, a veritable hero to a rising younger generation of dry workers. In 1880, he broke with the Republicans when it became clear that they would not adopt a clearly protemperance stance, and that same year he ran for president at the head of the Prohibition Party ticket. He also remained active in his home state of Maine, and in 1884 he had the satisfaction of witnessing the political rout of his wet opponents there: Maine adopted a prohibitory amendment to its constitution, fulfilling one of the fondest wishes of the now aging crusader. He kept a busy schedule in his later years, however; and still vigorous at eighty-six, he took a leading part in the National Temperance Congress of 1890. Late in life Dow was honored as few dry leaders ever were, and until the end younger temperance workers looked to him for advice and inspiration.

**Bibliography:**

A. "The Results of Twenty-Five Years of Temperance in Maine," 78–90, in *Centennial Temperance Volume . . .* (New York, 1877); *The Reminiscences of Neal Dow: Recollections of Eighty Years* (Portland, ME, 1898).

B. DAB 5, 411–12; SEAP 2, 842–44; Frank Loyola Byrne, *Prophet of Prohibition: Neal Dow and His Crusade* (Madison, WI, 1961); Henry S. Clubb, *The Maine Liquor Law: Its Origins, History and Results, Including a Life of Hon. Neal Dow* (New York, 1856); Alonzo A. Miner, "Neal Dow and His Life Work," *New England Magazine* 10 (1894): 397–412; Thomas W. Organ, *Biographical Sketch of General Neal Dow* (New York, 1880).

**DOYLE, Alexander Patrick**    (28 February 1857, San Francisco, CA—9 August 1912, Washington, DC). *Education*: studied at St. Ignatius Coll. and Christian Brothers Coll., 1870s; B.A., St. Mary's Coll., 1875; M.A., St. Mary's Coll., 1876; studied theology with Paulist fathers, 1875–80; LLD., Manhattan Coll., 1906. *Career*: ordained Catholic priest, 1880; domestic missionary work in Paulist Order, 1880–92; editor, *Temperance Truth*, 1892–1903; editor, *Catholic World*, 1893–1904; editor, *The Missionary*, 1896–1912; founder and secretary-treasurer, Catholic Missionary Union, beginning 1896; co-founder and rector, Apostolic Missionary House, 1902–12.

The first native-born Californian to be ordained a Catholic priest, Father Doyle, after twelve years of missionary work, enlisted in the prohibition cause as editor of *Temperance Truth* in 1892. The publication was one of a number printed by the Temperance Publishing Bureau, of which he was founder and director. Under his leadership the organization distributed a reported one million pieces of literature on behalf of the dry crusade. Father Doyle's wide publishing and editing activities extended to the management of the Paulist Press and the editorship of *Catholic World*, the chief Catholic periodical in the United States. In addition, he was the general secretary of the Catholic Total Abstinence Union of America from 1894 to 1904, and he worked tirelessly to enlist Roman Catholics in the antiliquor cause. Missionary work, however, was Father Doyle's most persistent interest. Pursuing it, however, forced him to overcome a natural disinclination for public speaking, although he ultimately became an extraordinarily popular and effective spokesman for his religious and moral views. This man, "priestly in every stepping," was ultimately to traverse the length and breadth of North America, ceaselessly urging the cause of temperance and other social reforms. In order to train missionaries on a regular basis, he helped found the Apostolic Missionary House as part of the Catholic University in Washington, D.C., where he taught until his death in 1912. To the same end, he edited yet another publication, *The Missionary*, and served as superior for American Catholic military chaplains. In the course of his work, Father Doyle made the acquaintance and enjoyed the friendship of many notable public figures of his day, including Presidents William Howard Taft and Theodore Roosevelt. In appreciation of Father Doyle's tireless efforts on behalf of the social and moral betterment of less fortunate Americans, Roosevelt paid generous tribute to him by acknowledging, in the *Catholic World*, that in his own public speeches he had drawn heavily "on the great fund of his [Doyle's] accumulated experiences."

**Bibliography:**

A. *A Truth Seeker and His Answer: What the Catholic Church Is* (New York, 19—?).

B. DAB 5, 421; SEAP 3, 845; *San Francisco Chronicle*, Aug. 10, 1912.

**DU BOSE, Horace Mellard**   (7 November 1858, Mobile, AL—15 January, 1941, Nashville, TN). *Education*: educated at Waynesboro (MI) Acad., circa 1860s–1870s; D.D. (honorary), Emory and Henry Coll., 1892. *Career*: licensed preacher, Methodist Church (South), 1876; ordained, 1879; minister, Mississippi Conference, Methodist Church, 1877–80; minister, various pastorates, TX and CA, 1881–90; editor, *Pacific Methodist Advocate*, 1890–94; editor, *Epworth Era*, 1898–1910; editor, *Methodist Quarterly Review*, 1915–18; elected bishop, Methodist Episcopal Church (South), 1918; active writing and archaeological work, 1900s–1930s.

A much-travelled ordained minister of the Methodist Episcopal Church, Du Bose found his metier in the Temperance Movement chiefly as a writer and editor. Although he served in pulpits from Tennessee and Georgia to Texas and California and held an honorary doctor of divinity degree from Emory and Henry College (1892), Du Bose did not feel that his pastoral work enabled him to cast as wide a temperance net as his writing might. Thus, he became editor of the *Epworth Era*, a religious periodical that took its name from the village of Epworth, England, where the founder of Methodism, John Wesley, was born. It was a signal publication in keeping Methodism firmly in the dry camp. Later, he was editor and book editor of the equally antiliquor *Methodist Review*. Before his editorial career, however, he did try his hand at the pulpit. After preaching for several years in Mississippi, Du Bose moved to Texas, where he led congregations in four cities over the years. The Lone Star State, where hard drinking was an almost inevitable accompaniment of hard-living ranch hands and cow punchers, became the chief focus of Du Bose's early temperance efforts (although he did not neglect other Southwestern states). Out of this interest came a temperance novel, *The Men of Sapio Ranch* (1907), which for its day and theme (the regeneration of liquor-addicted cowboys) enjoyed a wide sale. He returned to California for editorial work in 1889, went back to Texas in 1895, and finally left that state in 1896 for a series of pulpits and editorial jobs throughout the South. In 1918, his denomination elected him bishop, and he took an active part in efforts to reunite the Northern and Southern wings of Methodism. In addition, he emerged as an author of some repute, writing a number of religious and biographical titles. Continuing his interest in temperance, Du Bose found time to serve as chairman of the Headquarters Committee of the Georgia Anti-Saloon League (1913–16). He also gained some modest fame from one of his hobbies, archaeology. The reverend made some significant contributions to the field in both North America and the Holy Land. Not one of the luminaries of the Temperance Movement, then, Du Bose nevertheless carried an active spear in the battle for liquor reform in the late nineteenth and early twentieth centuries.

## Bibliography:

A. *The Men of Sapio Ranch* (Nashville, TN, 1907); *The Symbol of Methodism* (Nashville, TN, 1907); *Francis Asbury: A Biographical Study* (Nashville, TN, 1909); *History of Methodism* (Nashville, TN, 1916); *The Bible and the Ages* (New York, 1930); *Through Two Generations: A Study in Retrospect* (New York, 1934).

B. NYT, Jan. 16, 1941; SEAP 3, 865; WW 1, 343.

# E

**EDWARDS, Justin** (25 April 1787, Westhampton, MA—23 July 1853, Bath Alum Springs, VA). *Education*: graduated from Williams Coll., 1810; studied at Andover Theological Sem., 1811; D.D. (honorary), Yale Coll., 1827. *Career*: ordained, 1812; minister, Congregational Church, Andover, MA, 1812–28; temperance organizing, including founding of the American Society for the Promotion of Temperance (later called the American Temperance Society), 1820s; trustee, Andover Theological Sem., 1820–53; minister, Salem Church, Boston, 1828; agent, American Temperance Society, 1827–29; corresponding secretary and agent, American Temperance Society, 1829–36; president, Andover Theological Sem., 1836–42; president, Board of Trustees, Andover Theological Sem., 1850–53.

The early Temperance Movement was neither prohibitionist nor insistent upon total abstinence. Generally, reformers stressed moderate drinking and abstinence only from distilled liquors as the goals of their effort. Yet almost from the beginnings of organized temperance activities in the nineteenth century, some voices argued against this approach and urged instead an emphasis on total abstinence. One of the first and strongest of these was the Reverend Justin Edwards of Massachusetts. A Congregationalist minister, he began preaching sermons to his flock in 1816 on the evils of drink; and from the start, he saw no compromise with beverage alcohol. "What shall be done?" he asked at one point. "Shall this enemy be continued among us, or shall we declare a war of extermination and root it out?" His views were extreme (although Edwards never had a reputation for vituperation in debate with opponents), and they set the pattern for the rest of his reform career. Indeed, although he continued his preaching and took on other reform and civil duties over the years (he was involved, for example, in the founding of the New England Tract Society and served as a trustee of Andover Theological Seminary from 1820 to 1853, and as secretary of the American and Foreign Sabbath Union from 1842 to 1849), by the 1820s Edwards was devoting most of his time to the dry crusade. Increasingly, he denounced American drinking practices of his era, called on his countrymen to renounce all drink, and leveled a withering fire against the liquor traffic. Through his writings, in particular, the committed reverend emerged as one of the nation's most articulate foes of drink. In 1823, he published a paper decrying the drunkenness commonly associated with funeral observances, while two years later he issued a booklet that became something of a temperance classic, *The Well-Conducted Farm*. The tract had a huge circulation (178,000 copies down to 1851 alone) and was purportedly a description of a Boston farm "conducted on strict temperance principles." It was influential in curtailing the traditional practice of providing liquor rations to agricultural labor, as well as advancing the idea of abstinence generally. By the mid-1820s, then, Edwards could justifiably take considerable credit for the expanding popular current of temperance sentiments then underway in the United States.

Aside from his facile pen, however, Reverend Edwards was also an organizer. With temperance activities quickening throughout the nation, in 1826 he played a key role (along with some fifteen other men) in the founding of the American Society for the Promotion of Temperance (later called simply the American Temperance Society). It was the first national organization devoted to the liquor question, and Edwards was elected to its executive committee. The new group adopted no specific pledge, and many of its members were devoted to moderate drinking, not to total abstinence. Edwards worked hard to assure the creation of a sound administrative and financial foundation for the society, while at the same time advocating the merits of the total abstinence position. In 1827, he became the first paid agent of the organization, in charge of building local chapters, lecturing and fund raising. In fact, he became so involved with the society's affairs that he left the pulpit (he had just taken a new church in Boston), finding that he could no longer manage both positions. From 1829 to 1836, Edwards was both agent and corresponding secretary of the society and provided much of the driving force behind its success. He spoke before any number of groups, organized societies as far apart as the St. John's Temperance Society in New Brunswick, Canada, and the Congressional Temperance Society in the nation's capital (this after he had addressed a joint session of Congress). At the same time, he continued as a champion of total abstinence and was pleased when the movement gradually adopted that stance as well by the mid-1830s. All the while, he compiled copious notes on all aspects of the American liquor question and published them in the annual reports of the society. The resulting volume, *Permanent Temperance Documents of the American Temperance Society* (1835), remains a prime source of information on the progress of the dry crusade. Edwards also continued to write, and a number of his publications, notably his *Temperance Manual*, were highly successful (over 107,000 copies of the *Manual* were distributed by the American Tract Society before the Civil War). When he retired from his offices in the society in 1836, temperance leaders lauded him as they did few others. He deserved their praise: Justin Edwards had done more than most in building popular sentiments against drinking excesses into a powerful and mass-based social movement.

**Bibliography:**

A. *The Well-Conducted Farm* (Boston, 1825, and subsequent editions); *On the Immorality of the Traffic in Ardent Spirits* (Boston, 1832); *Permanent Tem-*

*perance Documents of the American Temperance Society* (Boston, 1835); *Letter to the Friends of Temperance in Massachusetts* (Boston, 1836, and subsequent editions); *A Plea for the Sabbath, Enforced by Facts* (Philadelphia, 1844); *The Temperance Manual* (New York, 1847?).

B. SEAP 3, 882; WW H, 235; *Appleton's Cyclopedia of American Biography*, vol. 2 (New York, 1887), 307; Daniel Dorchester, *The Liquor Problem in All Ages* (New York, 1888); William A. Hallock, *A Sketch of the Life . . . of the Reverend Justin Edwards* (New York, 1855); Alice Felt Tyler, *Freedom's Ferment: Phases of American Social History from the Colonial Period to the Outbreak of the Civil War* (1944; New York, 1962).

**EDWARDS, Ninian**   (17 March 1775, Montgomery Co., MD—20 July 1833, Belleville, IL). *Education*: graduated from Dickinson Coll., 1792. *Career*: admitted to bar, KY, 1798, TN, 1799; circuit court judge, KY, 1803–8; chief justice, Court of Appeals, KY, 1808–9; governor of Illinois Terr., 1809–18; member, U.S. Senate, 1818–25; governor of Illinois, 1826–30.

The career of Ninian Edwards was illustrative of how frequently the temperance issue played a role in the lives of nineteenth-century Americans, even if they never chose to become directly involved with an antiliquor organization. After completing his education at Dickinson College in Pennsylvania, young Edwards moved to the Green River area of Kentucky in 1795. Once settled, his rise to public prominence was astonishingly rapid. He was elected to the state legislature even before his twenty-first birthday. Next, he prepared for a legal career, and by 1799 Edwards had been admitted to the bar in both Kentucky and neighboring Tennessee. By 1808 he was chief justice of the Kentucky Court of Appeals and governor of Illinois Territory in 1809 (a post he held until 1818). Edwards was in fact a political prodigy, the central figure in Illinois politics for much of his generation. After Illinois was admitted to the Union, he served as one of its first senators (1818–25) and then ran successfully for the governorship once more (1826–30). In his various offices, Edwards had no special principles: He was a champion of cheap lands for settlers and of Indian removal—both positions being calculated to please his Western constituents. One the whole, his career in Washington and as governor was less than distinguished. And, as time went on, he also developed a reputation for rashness. More than once he leveled unfounded charges against political opponents, which in the end brought his career to grief. At one point, President James Monroe had appointed him ambassador to Mexico; but Edwards had to decline the office when he could not support allegations he had leveled against Secretary of the Treasury William Crawford. Even back home in Illinois, he needlessly alienated many state leaders through the same tactics. Yet he remained an influence in state electoral affairs until he finally failed in a race for Congress in 1832. A master of the political process for a time, Edwards finally fell victim to his own lack of judgement.

Yet the Midwestern lawyer was interesting beyond his involvement in politics. He also demonstrated the rise of temperance sentiment in his region, an area which became fertile ground for the antiliquor reform a generation later. Ninian Edwards was in fact a reformed "drunkard" (to use the term current in his day). Following the custom of the period, he drank heavily in his early years and accepted liquor as a normal part of social and political gatherings. But once his own drinking problem became apparent, he recoiled from alcohol, went on the wagon individually, and openly urged others to do the same. Edwards was never a prohibitionist, and his solution to society's alcohol problem was to call on other alcoholics to follow his example of personal reform. Yet he also went on record as favoring the curtailing of liquor sales to the intemperate. On the bench, he claimed that fully "half of the offenses against the penal laws usually presented by grand jurors" in Kentucky "would not have been committed were it not for intoxication." And if he often displayed a lack of any consistent political principles in office, he did denounce the prevailing use of alcohol to sway votes in the elections of the era. Plying the electorate with whiskey, he charged, was simply "corruption" and was nothing more than an "attempt to buy...votes." Edwards certainly did not put an end to the practice, but he was one of the first influential politicians of the area to try to stop it. Thus while he never belonged to any temperance organization, leaders of the later crusade would point to his statements and actions on the matter and lay claim to him as one of their ancestors in reform.

### Bibliography:

A. *The Edwards Papers...*, ed. Elihu B. Washburne (Chicago, 1884); "Executive Letter-Book of Ninian Edwards, 1826–1830," in *Collections of the Illinois State Historical Library*, ed. E. B. Greene and Clifford W. Alvord, vol. 4 (Springfield, IL, 1909).

B. DAB 5, 41; SEAP 3, 882–83; WW H, 235; Ninian Wirt Edwards, *History of Illinois, from 1778 to 1833; and Life and Times of Ninian Edwards* (Springfield, IL, 1870).

**ELLSWORTH, Elmer Ephraim**    (11 April 1837, Malta, NY—24 May 1861, Alexandria, VA). *Education*: read law privately and in the office of Abraham Lincoln, Chicago, 1850s to 1860. *Career*: worked as law clerk in Chicago legal firm; patent solicitor, Chicago, 1850s; organizer and commander, National Guard Cadets (a private volunteer military company, later called the U.S. Zouave Cadets), 1860–61; major (later colonel), Illinois National Guard, 1860; campaign staff of Abraham Lincoln, 1860; colonel, Union army, 1861.

Elmer Ellsworth was famed as the "first hero" of the Union army to fall during the Civil War. As such, temperance leaders (only after his death, we should note) deemed it well to count him as one of their own. (It never hurts to have one's cause identified with a patriot martyr.) In his lifetime, Ellsworth never belonged to any temperance society; yet there were elements in his brief career that, indeed, probably did place him in sympathy with the dry reform. From childhood, he was fascinated by the military and earnestly desired a West

Point education and an army career. Unable to get an appointment to the military academy, however, he became an enthusiast of private volunteer military outfits (which were something of a rage among American youth before the Civil War). While making only a modest living as a partner in a patent-soliciting business (and reading law at the same time), he eventually rose to national fame as commander of the U.S. Zouave Cadets, a crack drill company dressed in the loose pantaloons and tight jackets featured by a number of French army units of the era. Drill performances by Ellsworth's Zouaves were highly popular with the public, and the outfit made an extremely successful tour of Eastern cities in 1860. Discipline (while voluntarily accepted) was exacting and included adherence to Ellsworth's strictures against drunkenness and profanity. The commander, it seems, was a temperance man, although he apparently did not require total abstinence on the part of his men.

With the coming of the Civil War, Ellsworth moved quickly on to tragic fame. Commissioned a colonel in the Union army, he accompanied President-elect Lincoln to Washington, D.C., and shortly thereafter raised a regiment of Zouaves for three years' service, primarily from among New York City firemen. Leading them to Alexandria, Virginia, on May 24, 1861, he personally tore down a Confederate flag from atop a local hotel—only to be promptly shot to death by the owner of the establishment. The Southerner, in turn, went immediately to his reward at the hands of one of the colonel's escort—never knowing that his final act of marksmanship had offered his enemy's cause a "hero." Already a man of national reputation, as well as a friend of Lincoln's, the young officer's demise was widely lamented and engendered a wave of resentment against the South. Among the many other honors accorded Ellsworth's memory was the creation of the so-called Ellsworth Pledge. Thousands of men signed it throughout the army, promising not to touch liquor as long as they served in the armed forces. How long the men stuck to the pledge is anyone's guess, although the federal army was never noted as a paragon of sobriety. However, it did bespeak the fact that the Temperance Movement made a serious effort to keep the Union boys sober, and the Ellsworth Pledge received some credit in this regard (as did the "Temperance Regiments" of Neal Dow* of Maine). In that sense, then, if Ellsworth was never formally a member of the Temperance Movement, he at least became a part of its history.

## Bibliography:

A. *Complete Instructions for the Recruit . . . in the United States Zouave Cadets* (Philadelphia, 1861); *Manual of Arms for Light Infantry . . .* (Chicago, 1861); *The Zouave Drill . . .* (Philadelphia, 1861?).

B. Marcus Cunliffe, *Soldiers and Civilians: The Martial Spirit in America, 1775–1865* (Boston, 1968); Charles A. Ingraham, *Elmer E. Ellsworth and the Zouaves of '61* (Chicago, 1925); Ruth Painter Randall, *Colonel Elmer Ellsworth: A Biography of Lincoln's Friend and First Hero of the Civil War* (Boston, 1960).

**EVANS, Jervice Gaylord**    (19 December 1833, Wenona, IL—27 October 1910, Lake Bluff, IL). *Education*: studied at Peoria Wesleyan Sem., Judson Coll., Ohio Wesleyan Univ., 1840s–1850s; A.M. (honorary), Quincy Coll.; D.D. (honorary) Chaddock Coll.; LLD., Chicago Coll. of Science. *Career*: entered Methodist ministry, 1854; minister, various pastorates, IL, 1854–77; president, Hedding Coll., Abington, IL, 1872–78, 1889–98; chairman, Methodist Episcopal Church Permanent Committee on Temperance and Prohibition, 1892–1910.

The reform activities of the Reverend Jervice Evans encompassed many causes, as over the middle and late nineteenth century he lent his voice and pen against the evils of drink, slavery, and the denial of equal rights to women. Evans's zeal for reform was grounded in his piety. A deeply religious man, he served in pastorates in Illinois for almost a generation after entering the Methodist ministry in 1854. During this long tenure in the pulpit, he rose as a leading regional spokesman for his denomination, serving for seven years as secretary of the Central Illinois Conference and four years as a presiding elder. Like other Methodist parsons of the day, he was firmly of the belief that the church ought to lead in the shaping of national morality, and he seldom failed to speak his mind. He decried slavery before the Civil War and worked against it politically first in the Free Soil Party and then as a Republican. Evans labored with equal vigor on behalf of the Temperance Movement and women's rights, speaking for them from the pulpit and authoring tracts. The active reverend, it seems, was more than willing to battle sin in all its guises. Nor was he tolerant of ignorance. He was a champion of education, especially when it reinforced Christian values, and the chance to play a leading role in this regard finally enticed him from the pulpit. In 1872 he began a long period as president of Hedding College, a small religiously oriented school. His retirement from the college in 1898 found the aging reformer still energetic and still willing to wield his pen on the side of good as he saw it.

Throughout his long career, Evans clearly saw the Temperance Movement as one of the chief agents of the good society. The death of drink, he believed, would clear the way for reform progress in other areas and the triumph of Christian morality (as he saw that morality) in American life. Temperance, not surprisingly, was a familiar message in his preaching, and he leveled an especially heavy fire against the saloon. In 1880, Evans, like many other committed temperance men of the period, left the Republican Party to join the ranks of the small but highly motivated Prohibition Party. Over the following decade, he emerged as one of its true stalwarts in the Midwest, serving variously as chairman of the Illinois state party convention and as a delegate to national Prohibitionist conventions. From 1888 to 1892 he sat on the party's National Committee. His dry convictions were such that, where temperance matters were concerned, the lines between religion and politics crossed. In the midst of his work for the Prohibitionists, he also was elected chairman of the Methodist Church's Permanent Committee on Temperance and Prohibition (1892). He won reelection to the post annually until his death in 1910. Even as president of Hedding, Evans never ceased his work against the liquor traffic; indeed, his position as head of an institution of higher learning gave his voice added weight. He was noted as a "powerful" speaker when on the platform, and his impact in the battle with the traffic won the highest praise of his colleagues in reform.

**Bibliography:**

A. *Tobacco: Its History, Production, Manufacture, Properties, and Relation to Christianity* (Kawnee, IL, 1877); *The Pulpit and Politics: Or, Christianity and the State* (Chicago, 1891); *Christianity and Science Versus Evolution and Infidelity* (Galesburg, IL, 1895).

B. SEAP 3, 954–55; WW 1, 377.

**EVARTS, Jeremiah** (3 February 1781, Sunderland, VT—10 May 1831, Charleston, SC). *Education*: graduated from Yale Coll., 1805. *Career*: principal, Caledonia Co. Grammar Sch., Peacham, VT, 1803–4; admitted to bar, CT, 1806; legal practice, New Haven, CT, 1806–10; editor, *The Panoplist*, Boston, 1810–21; treasurer, American Board of Commissioners for Foreign Missions, 1811–21; editor, *Missionary Herald*, 1821–31; corresponding secretary, American Board of Commissioners for Foreign Missions, 1821–31.

Jeremiah Evarts, a staunch and committed supporter of the Temperance Movement, was typical of many of the reformers of his generation. He was interested not only in bringing an end to intemperance but in the general reform and perfection of the society in which he lived. To this end, he devoted a keen mind and a missionary zeal. Evarts started as a teacher and principal of a small public school in Vermont, but after several years the life proved too confining and he began reading law. He left the classroom behind in 1806, when he was finally admitted to the Connecticut bar and began a practice in New Haven. Yet even the law was not really satisfying, and the young lawyer was less than enthusiastic about his work. In 1810, however, Evarts found his calling: A deeply religious man since his youth (he was a Congregationalist), he followed his convictions into a life of religiously oriented reform activity. Closing his practice, he took up the editorship of *The Panoplist*, a monthly Congregationalist publication in Boston, and soon emerged as a forceful voice of reform. While under his leadership the journal not only took up religious questions but came out for temperance and Sabbath reform (he demanded, among other things, an end to Sunday postal service). The crusading editor also championed a number of humanitarian causes, some of which were far in advance of popular opinion. He spoke out with eloquence against the depredations endured by the Indians at the hands of both the federal and state governments, and he denounced the forced migration of the tribes from the South to western territories as early as the 1820s. In 1829, he wrote a series of articles on the plight of the Indians, appearing in the *New York Observer* and the *North American Review*, which garnered national attention for the Boston reformer. While he was never able to aid substantially the lot of the dispossessed tribes, he did considerably more than most social critics of his generation to stir the nation's conscience on their behalf.

Evarts's involvement with the Temperance Movement stemmed from these same humanitarian instincts. Using the pages of *The Panoplist*, and later those of the *Missionary Herald* (*The Panoplist* ceased publication, and Evarts then edited the *Herald* from 1821 until his death), he kept up a running fire against the liquor traffic. He insisted as well that the evil was too great for individuals to fight on a private basis and called for an opposition based on mass organizations. It was a bold position, coming as it did when temperance societies were still in their infancy and before the dry crusade itself had become a truly national phenomenon. Evarts, moreover, took his own advice; in addition to his powerful editorials, he also contributed his administrative skills as an early temperance organizer. In 1813, he was a co-founder of the Massachusetts Temperance Society, the first state-wide organization of its kind. Still later (in 1826), after more than a decade of increasing temperance activity, he was a founding member of the American Society for the Promotion of Temperance (later called the American Temperance Society). The reform editor had thus established himself as a national dry figure, and he remained active in the cause for years. Evarts also served prominently in other reform groups, notably the American Board of Commissioners for Foreign Missions (which he had helped found and in which he was an officer for twenty years) and the American Bible and Education Societies. He was in failing health at the end of the 1820s and suffering from consumption when he travelled to Cuba in search of a better climate in 1831. He died in South Carolina on the way back home, honored as one of the most noted philanthropists of his day.

**Bibliography:**

A. *Appeal to the Northern and Eastern Churches in Behalf of the South Western Theological Seminary...* (Maryville, TN? 1828); *The Logic and Law of Col. Johnson's Report to the Senate, on Sabbath Mails* (Utica, NY, 1829); *The Removal of the Indians...* (Boston, 1830); *Essays on the Present Crisis in the Conditions of the American Indians* (Philadelphia, 1834); *Through the South and West with Jeremiah Evarts*, ed. J. Orin Oliphant (Lewisburg, PA, 1956).

B. DAB 6, 215; SEAP 3, 955; Gardiner Spring, *A Tribute to the Life of the Late Jeremiah Evarts* (New York, 1831); E. C. Tracy, *Memoir of the Life of Jeremiah Evarts* (Boston, 1845).

**EXCELL, Edwin Othello**   (13 December 1851, Uniontown, OH—10 June 1921, Chicago, IL). *Education*: studied music privately. *Career*: gospel singer with evangelist Sam P. Jones, 1870s–1890s; hymn book publishing business, 1881–1910.

Of the legions of Americans who lent their voices to the cause of National Prohibition, few did so in quite the capacity of Edwin Othello Excell. After an education in the public schools of Pennsylvania and Ohio, Excell followed a youthful love of music down an unlikely path to financial success and major public recognition. He studied song privately and enjoyed singing during his school days, and even after moving to California to work as a mason he kept practicing his music. One day while at work (or so the story goes), Excell was singing on the job and was overheard by the prominent Georgia evangelist Sam Jones.* Jones hired him to sing in his travelling chorus, and the mason-turned-singer led the singing in the evangelist's revival meetings for the next twenty years. In the meantime, Excell became an established figure in his own right, authoring some of the most popular Protestant hymns of the day (notably the well-known "Count Your Blessings"). In 1881 he started publishing hymnals as well, and at his death he ran the largest such business in the world, with annual sales of over a million volumes. Excell, however, also had the religious convictions of his music and was active in the affairs of the Methodist Church and in the causes it supported. He was a choir director at dozens of Sunday school conventions throughout the United States and Canada and for years served as an officer (either as vice president or treasurer) in the International Sunday-School Association. (A cynic might observe that this helped sell a lot of hymn books, but he was evidently quite sincere about his spiritual commitments.) He was no less enthusiastic about the Temperance Movement. Excell took an active part in gatherings of dry organizations, including the Anti-Saloon League, and generally led the singing. (He became noted for soloing in "Down Among the Dead Men"—apparently something of a favorite among the temperance faithful.) He even edited an *Anti-Saloon League Song-Book* (191-?). The movement found him "a vital part" of its conventions, and there is little doubt that his role as a dry tunesmith helped keep the flavor of revivalism alive in much of its membership.

## Bibliography:

A. *Sacred Echoes: A Collection of Songs and Hymns for Use in Gospel Work, Camp Meetings, etc.* (Philadelphia, 1880); *Excellent Songs for the Church and Sunday School* (Chicago, 1898); *The Gospel Hymnal . . .* (Cincinnati, OH, 1899); ed., *Joy to the World; for the Church and Sunday School* (Chicago, 1915); ed., *The Anti-Saloon League Song-Book* (Westerville, OH, 191-?).

B. SEAP 3, 958; WW 1, 380.

# F

---

**FALLOWS, Samuel** (13 December 1835, Pendleton, Lancashire, England—
5 September 1922, Chicago, IL). *Education*: A.B., Univ. of Wisconsin, 1859;
A.M., Univ. of Wisconsin, 1862; LLD. (honorary), Univ. of Wisconsin, 1894;
D.D. (honorary), Lawrence Univ., 1873, Marietta Coll., 1903. *Career*: vice
president, Galesville Univ., 1859–61; chaplain, 32nd Wisconsin Infantry, Union
army, 1862–63; infantry officer, Union army, 1864–65; minister, Methodist
Episcopal Church, 1859–75; rector, St. Paul's Reformed Episcopal Church,
Chicago, beginning 1875; bishop, Reformed Episcopal church, beginning 1876;
regent, Univ. of Wisconsin, 1866–74; Wisconsin State superintendent of public
instruction, 1871–74; president, Illinois State Reformatory, 1891–1912; active
in various veterans, patriotic, and civic organizations.

Even in the tradition of activist ministry that runs through the Temperance
Movement—and overflows it into all the areas of late nineteenth- and early
twentiety-century reform—the career of Samuel Fallows seems extraordinarily
full of interests, involvements, and impressive attainments. The access of the
ministry to various channels of social and political influence, as well as the strong
capability of individual ministers for exploiting those channels, provides one
important explanation for reformist successes during this period. In the case of
Samuel Fallows, a combination of drive, natural leadership ability, and undeniable intelligence assured that he would exploit such influence to the fullest. A
committed Methodist, young Fallows sought a career in the clergy but instead
took a position as vice president of a small university and then was swept up
into the tragedy of the Civil War. He served first as a chaplain to a Wisconsin
infantry unit; but he considered that the times called for firmer action than prayer,
and he gave up his chaplaincy for a troop command. The reverend proved to be
a tough fighter and was ultimately brevetted to brigadier general for his gallant
war record. Military service brought him considerable regional fame, although
perhaps more importantly it established a pattern for his future conduct in life:
He would rely not only on a burning moral and religious commitment to guide
him but also on a penchant for direct action. For in facing the problems of church
and society after the war, he remained every bit the fighter he was in the army.
Dynamic in the pulpit, he was a popular Methodist minister in the Milwaukee
area, and only a year after switching to the Reformed Episcopal Church he was

elected a bishop in the denomination (1876). At the same time he called for a host of social reforms ranging from temperance and education to prison improvements. Following his activist inclinations, Fallows served willingly on voluntary and governmental bodies concerned with these issues (notably, he was Wisconsin superintendent of public instruction and head of the State Reformatory's Board of Managers). He also served as an intermediary between workers and employers in a number of regional labor disputes. For the busy minister, then, an important part of social leadership involved setting a personal example of commitment and work.

So it was when Bishop Fallows urged his countrymen to temperance. As a leading church figure in the Midwest, he used his considerable influence to denounce the liquor traffic. He emerged, as one temperance source called him, "a firm and uncompromising advocate of the cause of total abstinence and Prohibition." His role in the Temperance Movement, aside from his frequent public pronouncements against drink, lay chiefly in three areas. First, he founded and (for four years) edited a newsletter called *The Appeal* (which became the official organ of the Reformed Episcopalians) and used its pages to champion any number of reform causes. The paper kept up a withering fire against the traffic. Second, the enterprising Fallows launched (in 1907) an experimental "home salon" in Chicago. It was an attempt to demonstrate that a "bar" could forsake liquor and prosper selling soft drinks, coffee, fruit juices, and hot chocolate—while still preserving the social, club-like atmosphere of the rival saloons. The establishment attracted considerable attention, and made money besides, although the idea never caught on as a solid business venture among others. Finally, the bishop financed an unsuccessful but ingenious effort to produce a "beer" with no alcohol content. While he was never able to get an acceptable beverage in this regard, the attempt was indicative of the concern he placed in altering American drinking patterns—and of his belief that the battle against "the demon" was crucial in building a better nation. Indeed, reform in general was an act of patriotism for Fallows. The man was enormously proud of his Civil War service—he was active until his death in many patriotic and veterans groups—and he was equally proud of his service against the social and moral evils he saw as threatening the nation for which he had risked life and limb.

**Bibliography:**

A. *Special Report on Compulsory Education* (Madison, WI, 1873); with Helen M. Fallows, *The Mormon Menace* (Chicago, 1903); with Helen M. Fallows, *Science of Health from the Viewpoint of the Newest Christian Thought* (Chicago, 1903); ed., *Story of the American Flag with Patriotic Selections...* (Boston, 1903, and many other editions); *Health and Happiness: Or, Religious Therapeutics and Right Living* (Chicago, 1908); *Know Thyself...* (Marietta, OH, 1911).

B. DAB 6, 361–62; SEAP 3, 962–63; WW 1, 384.

**FARIS, Herman Preston**    (25 December 1858, Bellefontaine, OH—20 March 1936, Clinton, MO). *Career*: real estate business, Clinton, MO, 1873–77, 1879–1936; acting deputy clerk, District Court, Trinidad, MO, 1878; officer and manager, local bank, Clinton, MO, 1887–1936.

An ardent temperance crusader, Faris was typical of those whose dedication kept the Prohibition Party alive long after it had ceased to be the center of dry political activity. A successful small businessman in Clinton, Missouri, he was active with the local YMCA and took a prominent role in the lay affairs of the Presbyterian Church throughout the late nineteenth and early twentieth centuries. His antiliquor work was also concentrated largely in Missouri. He joined the state Prohibition Party in 1884, and soon gained political visibility as a seemingly perpetual office seeker: Over the years, Faris ran on the dry ticket for positions as diverse as local constable to secretary of state and the governorship (for which he mounted three campaigns). Never successful at the polls, he did manage to keep the temperance issue in the public eye. Aside from electoral politics, Faris was also an energetic organizer—with goals that sometimes bordered on the grandiose. In 1893, for example, he founded the bravely titled ''Anti-Saloon Army,'' which he intended to be a world-wide coalition of all antiliquor forces and styled after benevolent lodges. It failed after two years; but in 1916 he helped launch the Missouri Dry Federation, which effectively aided enforcement officials in closing illegal saloons throughout most of the state. His work in Missouri won him national recognition from the movement, and the Prohibition Party nominated him for president in 1924. For Faris, this last candidacy was a personal honor; but his party was of little political consequence, and such important dry publications as the WCTU's *Union Signal* and the Anti-Saloon League's *American Issue* ignored his campaign.

**Bibliography:**

B. SEAP 3, 964; WW 1, 384; D. Leigh Colvin, *Prohibition in the United States* (New York, 1926).

**FAVILLE, John**    (7 July 1847, Milford, WI—6 September 1927, Lake Mills, WI). *Education*: B.S., Lawrence Coll., 1871; M.S., Lawrence Coll., 1874; B.D., Boston Univ. Sch. of Theology, 1876; A.B., Boston Univ., 1879; D.D. (honorary), Lawrence Coll., 1894; Ph.D (honorary), Boston Univ., 1896. *Career*: ordained in Methodist Church, 1876; minister, pastorates in WI, 1876–86; minister, First Congregational Church, Appleton, WI, 1886–89, 1907–17; minister, First Church, Peoria, IL, 1899–1907; mayor, Appleton, WI, 1917–18; active temperance work, 1880s–1920s.

John Faville was another of those turn-of-the-century ministers, particularly Methodist ministers, who found a comfortable milieu in the increasingly militant and professional field of prohibition organization. Faville, however, was somewhat less common in that he actually found his way into political office. Unlike some of his contemporaries, who occasionally left the pulpit for full-time reform work, the well-educated clergyman continued in pastorates throughout most of his career, mostly at the First Congregational Church in Appleton, Wisconsin (where he had attended Lawrence College). He appears to have retired from active ministry around the age of seventy and soon thereafter became mayor of Appleton (1917), although the office was not the first to which he had aspired. Much earlier, in 1894, a political career had flickered when he received the Prohibition Party nomination for Congress in his district at the Wisconsin State Convention (of which he had been elected chairman). He had earned the nomination. The minister had been an ardent crusader against the liquor traffic and had helped lead the local efforts of the Prohibition Party. With the rise of the Anti-Saloon League, he chose (unlike other members of the Prohibition Party) to cooperate with the new group and even took the initiative in organizing its Wisconsin branch. He served as the first state president of the league (1895–98), and when he moved to a pastorate in Peoria, Illinois, he sat in the same capacity with the Illinois League for a year (1902–3). Once back in Wisconsin, he joined the Board of Directors of the league and served for over twenty years. Faville also worked in church councils (he had become a Congregationalist at age thirty-nine) to assure a strong stand for temperance on the part of local organized religion, and he wrote frequently on the liquor question. His efforts, then, were long and unstinting, and he was a seasoned crusader by the time he took office as mayor. He served only one term but was credited with having started a locally popular "Men's Sunday Evening Club" movement, presumably an activity to divert men from drink and the saloon. His name as a temperance man spread nationally through his several books on the dry crusade as well as on religious topics. Faville's reputation as a reform intellect was such that he was honored with doctorates from two educational institutions (his alma maters of Lawrence College and Boston University), as well as positions on the governing boards of several Midwestern colleges.

## Bibliography:

A. *Christianity and Creed* (Appleton, WI, 1887); *The Interchange of Ministerial Courtesies Across Theological Lines* (Chicago, 1895); *Moral Overstrain: A Sermon* (Peoria, IL, 1906); *I Believe in God the Father* (Boston, 1919).
B. SEAP 3, 970–71; WW 1, 388.

**FELTON, Rebecca Latimer**    (10 June 1835, De Kalb Co., GA—24 January 1930, Atlanta, GA). *Education*: graduated from Madison (GA) Female Coll., 1852; D. Litt. (honorary), Univ. of Georgia, 1922. *Career*: active in political career of husband, Dr. W. H. Felton, 1870s–1890s; newspaper columnist, *Atlanta Semi-Weekly Journal*, 1880s–1920s; active in reform and civic causes, 1870s–1930; member, U.S. Senate, 21–22 November 1922.

Born during Andrew Jackson's second term in office and dying during the presidency of Herbert Hoover, Rebecca Felton's life spanned almost two-thirds of the nation's. For forty of those nearly one hundred years she gave unstintingly of herself in the interests of temperance, prison reform, and the advancement of women's rights. A well-educated young woman (she was a graduate of Madison Female College), in 1853 she married Dr. William H. Felton. Although opposed to secession, they sided loyally with their state during the Civil War and were virtually ruined for their trouble. They were pillaged both by Sherman's invading Union army as well as by Confederate deserters. More tragic, both of her young sons died of measles or malaria before peace was restored. With the coming of Reconstruction, she helped her husband rebuild their home while teaching school at the same time. It was during these hard years that she joined a number of reform groups and became noted as a crusader for temperance and for public aid for Confederate widows and orphans. Dr. Felton subsequently ran for Congress, and for the next several years the Feltons lived in Washington, D.C. Congressman Felton was a well-known liberal and generally sympathetic with a wide variety of reform measures. In his battles with the conservative wing of his party (he was a Democrat), Rebecca was his constant companion. Indeed, she quickly emerged with a reputation for political sophistication (she was also a reformer), and many observers considered her the real power behind her husband's success. Mrs. Felton was also adept in state politics (William was elected to the legislature after losing his congressional seat in 1880), and her prowess in statehouse controversies earned the respect of her contemporaries—and even of her opponents. Moreover, she never shied away from candor, and her book, *My Memoirs of Georgia Politics* (1911), has long been regarded as something of a classic in political exposé. And while Dr. Felton's political career was quite distinguished (it ended in an 1894 bid for Congress as a Populist), there is no doubt that Rebecca came to overshadow him in the popular eye.

Mrs. Felton joined the Woman's Christian Temperance Union in 1886, although she had long advocated total abstinence and prohibition in the column of commentary which she wrote for twenty years for the *Atlanta Semi-Weekly Journal*. She regarded women as the principal victims of male drunkenness, and her vivid portrayals from the lecture platform of suffering wives, neglected children, and broken homes had an undeniable impact on state lawmakers. In 1900 the sale of liquor was banned in Georgia, and there is no doubt that Rebecca Felton deserved considerable credit. She was also an ardent suffragette and an eloquent advocate of equal educational opportunities for women. Matching practice with theory, she founded and for some time was the director of the Georgia Training School for Women, a vocational school for girls. So prominent had Mrs. Felton become in Georgia by the second decade of the twentieth century that she was paid a singular tribute by her native state. In 1922, the death of the fiery Thomas Watson left a vacancy in the U.S. Senate, which was filled by the special election of Walter George. George, however, withheld his credentials for several days, enabling the governor of Georgia to appoint Mrs. Felton to the Senate. She served but two days, November 21 and 22, but she had the distinction of becoming the first woman senator in American history. Late in life Mrs. Felton acquired the reputation of an acerbic and in many ways conservative curmudgeon. While still urging her pet reforms, she also held forth with great forensic skill against those persons and issues she considered benighted or dangerous. Child labor laws, evolution, Woodrow Wilson, the League of Nations, and blacks (she once called for mass lynchings to discourage the rape of white women) were but a few of the targets of her considerable wit and scorn. Nevertheless, Felton's career was remarkable for a woman of her time, and her work on behalf of prohibition and prison reform remained a monument to her devotion and perseverance.

**Bibliography:**

A. *My Memoirs of Georgia Politics* (Atlanta, GA, 1911); *Country Life in Georgia in the Days of My Youth* (Atlanta, GA, 1919); *The Romantic Story of Georgia Women* (Atlanta, GA, 1930).

B. DAB 6, 318; NAW 1, 606–7; SEAP 3, 976–77; WW 1, 390; William P. Roberts, "The Public Career of Dr. William Harrell Felton" (Ph.D. diss., Univ. of North Carolina, 1952); John E. Talmadge, *Rebecca Latimer Felton: Nine Stormy Decades* (Athens, GA, 1960).

**FERGUSON, William Porter Frisbee**    (13 December 1861, Delhi, NY—June 1929, Franklin, PA). *Education*: B.D., Drew Theological Sem., 1887; A.B., Texas Wesleyan Univ., 1889. *Career*: Methodist missionary work, Mexico, 1887–89; minister, various Methodist, Presbyterian, and Universalist pastorates, NY and TN, 1889–1907; principal, Mohawk Inst., Utica, NY, 1891–92; principal, Utica Private Acad., 1892–93; editor, many prohibitionist publications in NY, TN, IL, PA, 1899 to 1920s; archaeological work, MI, 1920s.

Science and temperance reform were the twin passions of William P. T. Ferguson, and he was able to indulge in both with notable success. Graduating from Drew Theological Seminary in New Jersey in 1887, Ferguson left for missionary work in Mexico after marrying Lena Grace Hataway. In Mexico City he was pastor and publishing agent for the Methodist Conference. Subsequently returning to the United States (1889), he served in pastorates in New York State, his last being the Presbyterian Church in Whitehall, New York, Ferguson having withdrawn from the Methodist Church in 1892 (even later, he joined the Universalist Church). Ferguson's contributions to the prohibitionist cause were many and varied. He joined the Prohibition Party in the 1820s and was active in its ranks. He also developed a reputation as a powerful orator, denouncing the liquor traffic from the pulpit and the public podium. However, Fergunson's greatest achievements came as a publicist and editor, in which functions he served on an extraordinary variety of prohibition newspapers, ranging from the Harriman, Tennessee, *Citizen* to the New York *Defender* between the years 1904 and 1919. Ferguson began his attack on alcohol at the age of nineteen, when he had a series of verses published in the Utica, New York, *Living Issue*, and he kept up a steady barrage for the rest of his life. He detested the saloon and went to great lengths to damn it. Indeed, among his targets in this regard was the U.S military.

His pamphlet, *The Canteen in the United States Army, a Study of Uncle Sam as a Grog-Shop Keeper*, was published in 1900. Ferguson was much in demand as a public speaker on the temperance issue and kept up a nonstop series of lectures, ultimately addressing audiences in forty states as well as in Canada. Politics was yet another means of assault on the evils of drink, and in 1914 Ferguson came within a hair's breadth of winning a seat in the U.S. Congress from the Twenty-eighth District in Pennsylvania. In 1918, a change of sixty votes would have elected him to the Pennsylvania legislature. His popularity was such that a hundred delegates were pledged to him at the 1916 Prohibition Party convention. But apparently tiring of politics, Ferguson released them to J. Frank Hanly.*

Ferguson devoted years of intensive effort to the fortunes of the Prohibition Party. It was on its ticket that he made his political races and as one of its most distinguished leaders that he tried to rally the nation for temperance. The active reverend, however, saw his party as the best hope for the dry reform, and he was hesitant to dilute its strength by cooperating with other parties. The rise of the Anti-Saloon League offered a case in point. Ferguson initially welcomed the league (he even did some lecturing for it), seeing promise in its organizing techniques at the local level. But when the new group began to endorse candidates of the two major political parties instead of Prohibitionists, he was outraged and began a long campaign within the party to refuse contact with the league. The resulting conflict between Prohibitionists who favored or opposed the league further weakened the already small party and may have contributed to Ferguson's gradual cooling toward active political participation. At any rate, he did devote more time to his scientific interest, archaeology. His work in this regard had some important results. He conducted several significant excavations in the Lake Superior region of Michigan, and in 1922 he led an expedition that uncovered a prehistoric Stone Age site on Isle Royale, about which he wrote two articles for the *Michigan History Magazine* in 1923 and 1924. As explorer and prohibitionist, Ferguson had no difficulty combining temperance and archaeology in the countless lectures he delivered in the course of an active life, a melding of science and morality that, if not unique, was at least unusual. Of his dedication to the temperance cause there can be little doubt, for he once refused an honorary LLD. when he learned that the granting institution counted a saloon among its property holdings.

**Bibliography:**

B. DAB 6, 334; NYT, June 25, 1926; SEAP 3, 978–79; WW 1, 392; Jack S. Blocker, Jr., *Retreat from Reform: The Prohibition Movement in the United States, 1890–1913* (Westport, CT, 1976).

**FISHER, Irving**    (27 February 1867, Saugerties, NY—29 April 1941, New York, NY). *Education*: A.B., Yale Univ., 1888; Ph.D., Yale Univ., 1891; postdoctoral study, Berlin and Paris, 1893–94; LLD. (honorary), Rollins Coll.,

1932, Univ. of Athens, Univ. of Lausanne, 1937. *Career*: tutor, mathematics, Yale Univ., 1890–93; assistant professor, Yale Univ., 1893–95; assistant professor of political economy, Yale Univ., 1895–98; health leave, NY, CO, CA, 1898–1901; professor of political economy, Yale Univ., 1898–1935; editor, *Yale Review*, 1896–1911; lecturer, Univ. of California, 1917; lecturer, London Sch. of Economics and Political Science, 1921; lecturer, Geneva Sch. of International Studies, 1927; active in writing, consulting, and professional reform organizations, 1890s–1940s.

The Temperance Movement never lacked for friends in academia; it could boast the support of many distinguished scholars over the years. Certainly among the most talented of the campus drys, however, was Professor Irving Fisher of Yale University. The son of a Congregationalist minister, young Fisher grew up with a lively sense of social responsibility, assuring that his interests would always include the state of the world beyond university life and a keen regard for the public welfare. He was a brilliant student, strongly influenced by Josiah Willard Gibbs and William Graham Sumner, and graduated Phi Beta Kappa and valedictorian of his Yale class of 1888. After joining the faculty of his alma mater as a mathematics teacher and completing his Ph.D. (1891), he launched a continuing series of economic studies which, over the course of his career, brought him international recognition and made him the source of major professional debate. (Fisher, after deciding to pursue economics, left the Mathematics Department in 1895 to join the Department of Political Economy.) His academic concerns focused on monetary questions, specifically the issues of capital, interest, and economic statistics. He produced some promising work, but before he could really establish himself he came down with tuberculosis (1898). It took him three years to recover, but he made the most of his time therafter. He wrote prolifically, investigating questions of monetary stability and pioneering the growth of quantitative economics, or "econometrics." Fisher's work never went unchallenged, but he was both persuasive and persistent in presenting his views. Regard for his research grew steadily. He was president of the American Economic Association in 1918, and by the 1920s was one of the nation's leading economists. In 1930 he was elected the first president of the Econometric Society, which indicated a growing acceptance of his quantitative methods.

Given the astonishing level of Fisher's professional activity, it was remarkable that he was able to devote the large amount of time he did to the temperance struggle. The Yale professor, a total abstainer himself, had a deep interest in health-related subjects, perhaps partly as a result of his bout with tuberculosis. At any rate, he saw the liquor traffic as an enemy of the public health and welfare, and he became a vocal advocate of prohibition. In the years before National Prohibition, he used his versatile pen to counter wet arguments, including those of former President William Howard Taft, and to point out the expected economic benefits that would accrue to the nation if it would give up the bottle. After the passage of the Eighteenth Amendment, Fisher set out to defend it, and his efforts in that regard were among the most sophisticated produced during the struggle over the "noble experiment." In espousing the merits of Prohibition, he drew heavily on his skills as an economist. He compiled statistics purporting to demonstrate that the dry amendment had reduced crime, poverty, and alcohol-related health problems, all of which resulted, he claimed, in major savings to the country. Much of what he wrote offered some of the most convincing evidence in favor of Prohibition, and wets could not afford to allow Fisher to go unanswered. Perhaps the strongest counterattack came from no less than attorney Clarence Darrow (with Victor S. Yarros, *The Prohibition Mania*, 1927), who blasted the economist's data in general terms without being able to shake many of his specific arguments. Indeed, Darrow was quite vituperative in places, although Fisher never responded in kind. Fisher himself did not completely endorse the Prohibition enforcement effort, criticizing what he considered government inefficiency and corruption. But while he conceded that Prohibition was not perfect, he adamantly maintained that it was an improvement over the days when liquor was legal. Given time, he believed, the dry experiment would prove itself.

Fisher's reputation at Yale suffered somewhat in his later years. His many reforms and organizational interests frequently kept him off campus and he taught little. Aside from his labors on behalf of the Temperance Movement, the economist was an earnest proponent of public hygiene, labor legislation, world peace (he was a champion of Woodrow Wilson's League of Nations), free trade, health research, and other solutions to American and international ills. Indeed, he was a reformer in the classic Progressive mold. Like all reformers, though, his stands were never universally popular. Also, much of his confidence was shattered by the onset of the Great Depression, in which he lost a considerable sum. More important, however, was a lukewarm professional regard for some of his most significant work. Econometrics was a subject that had not come into its own, and Fisher's efforts in many respects were ahead of their time. Despite his attempts to stimulate interest in other Yale faculty, the university failed to emerge as a center for the study of new economic techniques. In the end, however, his approaches won not only professional acceptance but, in the eyes of one biographer, status for their author as "the leading economic theorist in the United States during the first half of the twentieth century."

## Bibliography:

A. *The Theory of Interest as Determined by Impatience to Spend Income and Opportunity to Invest It* (1907; New York, 1970); *The Attitude of the College Man Toward Alcohol* (New Haven, CT, 1915); *The Case for War-Time Prohibition* (n.p., 1917); *A Clear Answer to Ex-President Taft, the Most Prominent Anti-National Prohibitionist* (Boston, 1918); with Eugene Lyman Fisk, *Alcohol, from How to Live . . .*, 18th ed. (Westerville, OH, 1925); *Prohibition at Its Worst*, rev. ed. (New York, 1927); *Prohibition Still at Its Worst* (New York, 1928).

B. DAB Supp. 4, 272–76; WW 2, 187–88; Paul H. Douglas, "Memorial to Irving Fisher," *American Economic Review* 37 (1947): 661–63; A. D. Gayer, ed., *The Lessons of Monetary Experience: Essays in Honor of Irving Fisher* (New York, 1937); Irving Norton Fisher, comp., *A Bibliography of the Writings of Irving Fisher* (New York, 1961); Irving Norton Fisher, *My Father, Irving Fisher* (New York, 1956).

**FISK, Clinton Bowen**    (8 December 1828, Clapp's Corners, NY—9 July 1890, New York, NY). *Career*: schoolteacher, MI, 1840s to 1846; retail clerk, Manchester, MI, 1846–48; clerk and partner, L. D. Crippen & Son, 1848–59; agent, Aetna Insurance Company, St. Louis, MO, 1859–61; Union soldier, discharged as brevet major general, 1862–65; assistant commissioner, Freedmen's Bureau, TN and KY, beginning 1865; bank officer, New York City, 1860s to 1890; commissioner of Indian affairs, 1874–90.

Fisk's adult life spanned a wide spectrum of activities, in all of which he displayed more than average initiative, self-reliance, dedication, and success. Indeed, one might think that the phrase "self-made man" had been coined to account for the career of this soldier, merchant, educator, and philanthropist. The death of his father, after having moved to Lenawee County, Michigan, from New York State, compelled Fisk, then a teen-aged apprentice farmer, to undertake the sole support of his family in "pinching poverty." In addition, he had to educate himself, since formal schooling was out of the question. By studying in his spare time, Fisk acquired a teacher's certificate and taught school until 1846. Dissatisfied with his prospects, the unhappy teacher became a retail clerk for two years and then entered the employ of L. D. Crippen, a Michigan merchant banker. Within two years he had not only married the boss's daughter, Jeannette Crippen, but had also become a member of the firm, now L. D. Crippen and Son. In 1859 he moved to St. Louis, Missouri, where he was the western agent for the Aetna Insurance Company, although on the eve of the Civil War his business fortunes in fact suffered some reverses. When the war broke out, however, Fisk's economic and social position would have allowed him to escape military service had he chosen that course. But he was an ardent Republican and a friend of President Lincoln (also of Ulysses S. Grant), thus he chose to fight. Characteristically, he scorned the offers of a commission he felt he had not earned and instead enlisted as a private soldier. Yet exceptional valor and leadership qualities quickly carried him from the ranks; he rose to a colonelcy, and by the war's end he wore the stars of a brevet major general of volunteers. The war had carried Fisk a long way.

The still young general was ready to leave the service of his country when Lincoln's assassination caused him to embark on yet another phase of an already full life. In 1865, President Andrew Johnson appointed Fisk to the Freedman's Bureau as assistant commissioner for Kentucky and Tennessee with the typically Johnsonian comment, "Fisk ain't a fool, he won't hang everybody." Fisk's philanthropical and humanitarian impulses found full expression in the Reconstruction era. One of his most notable achievements was the founding of a college to train black teachers, which was chartered in 1867 as Fisk University in

Nashville, Tennessee. Since early manhood Fisk had shown an interest in temperance and while with the Union army had displayed a marked aversion for the profanity and drunkenness that characterized some of military life. His involvement in Prohibition Party politics did not begin until 1884, however, when he supported former Kansas Governor John P. St. John* at the head of the national ticket. Two years later, the New Jersey Prohibition Party persuaded Fisk to run for governor of the Garden State. He did not win, but in 1888 the national party, impressed with his state campaign, nominated him for president. Their confidence was not misplaced, for in 1888 Fisk amassed some 250,000 votes, the most votes for president the Prohibition Party had polled up to that time. Fisk was now through with politics, but not with temperance. Shortly before his death, he helped found Harriman, Tennessee, a factory town premised upon prohibition principles.

**Bibliography:**

B. DAB 6, 413–14; NYT, July 10, 1890; SEAP 3, 997; WW H, 251; Ernest H. Cherrington, *The Evolution of Prohibition in the United States* (Westerville, OH, 1920); Alphonso A. Hopkins, *The Life of Clinton Bowen Fisk* (1888; New York, 1910).

**FISK, Wilbur**    (31 August 1792, Brattleboro, VT—22 February 1839, Middletown, CT). *Education*: attended Univ. of Vermont, 1812–13; B.A., Brown Univ., 1815; studied law, Lyndon, VT, 1815–16. *Career*: family tutor, near Baltimore, MD, 1816–17; Methodist circuit minister, VT and MA, 1818–25; principal, Wesleyan Acad., 1826–30; president, Wesleyan Univ., 1830–39.

Fisk was born in Vermont and spent most of his life in northern New England. A graduate of Brown University, Fisk, like many other prospective lawyers of his generation, was drawn away from his legal studies by a religious call. He became a Methodist Episcopal minister in 1818, making education his special concern, and he was to be a powerful force in moving New England Methodism toward training an educated ministry. (Indeed, he was reputed to be one of the first Methodist preachers in his region to have graduated from college.) Always in frail health, he nevertheless rode a circuit for seven years in Vermont and Massachusetts, becoming noted for his piety and love of study. He gave up the circuit to head Wesleyan Academy in 1826, and then moved on to the presidency of Wesleyan University, which he helped found. His commitment to Wesleyan, plus his health problem, caused him to decline twice when fellow Methodists elected him a bishop. Yet he found the energy to be an effective university administrator, to continue local preaching and lecturing, and to go on a number of fund-raising tours for the school. Fisk never considered that ministers had to attend seminary, arguing instead that practical experience offered better religious training. But there is little doubt that his work and example stimulated major denominational interest in formal education. In 1835, he toured Europe (for health reasons) and surveyed a number of universities on the continent. Back home, he tried to apply what he had learned to running Wesleyan; and although he died (still relatively young at forty-seven) in 1839, before he could institute all of his reforms, Fisk still stood out as a major figure in the history of early American education. He was also an energetic supporter of missionary work among various American Indian tribes.

Fisk, unlike some other ministers of his generation, was not a radical reformer in all respects. While he opposed slavery, for example, he considered the methods of the more extreme abolitionists to be far beyond the bounds of reason. Yet he did take some important stands, and temperance was a particular case in point. The New England minister was strongly opposed to beverage alcohol in all of its forms, and he lost few opportunities to attack it. His denunciations encompassed both those who drank it and those who made and sold it. The traffic, however, drew his special scorn. From the pulpit, he proclaimed that if he had his way, anyone engaged in the traffic would actually be barred from church membership. In this stance he was considered something of a radical (especially in the early 1830s, when not even all other temperance workers were willing to go that far), and some of his colleagues occasionally tried to get him to moderate his position. But over the years he never gave ground on the matter. "Must you, indeed," he once lectured Methodists in the traffic "deal out ruin to your fellow-men, or starve? Then starve!" Such was not the statement of a man of compromise. And he never tired of his temperance work. Although he died before prohibition, even at the state level, had become a major social and political issue, there is little doubt that he helped sow the seeds of dry victories reaped by later reform leaders. As the nineteenth century advanced, Methodism became a spearhead for the dry crusade, and churchmen like Reverend Fisk were owed much of the credit. It was as much a part of his legacy as his work in education or the church.

**Bibliography:**

A. *The Science of Education* (New York, 1832); *Calvinistic Controversy* (New York, 1835); *Travels on the Continent of Europe* (New York, 1838).

B. DAB 6, 415–16; DARB, 161–62; NCAB 3, 177; SEAP 3, 998; Joseph Holdich, *The Life of Wilbur Fisk* (New York, 1842); George Prentice, *Wilbur Fisk* (Boston, 1890).

**FLOURNOY, Josiah**   (17 March 1789, Dinwiddie Co., VA—4 June 1842, Putnam Co., GA). *Career*: planter, GA, circa 1815–42.

The Temperance Movement long considered Josiah Flournoy a Southern martyr in the cause of total abstinence. Immigrating from Virginia as a boy, he was a prosperous Georgia planter by the 1830s. Little is known of the origins of his temperance sentiments, although he had apparently taken the pledge long before he rose to public recognition as a dry leader. He had also become disgruntled with the drinking habits of his state; as in the rest of the nation, imbibing in Georgia was on the increase, with a consequent rise (or so temperance voices alleged) in public drunkenness. There was some popular support for the antiliquor movement, but the 1830s in Georgia lacked a cohesive reform effort. Both moderation and total abstinence groups were virtually moribund; certainly they lacked any political influence. They were even fighting among themselves, extremist teetotalers having no truck with moderationists. Reacting both to this situation and to a substantial number of public complaints over the abuses of the unrestrained liquor traffic, Flournoy launched what became known as the Flournoy Movement. In 1839, he asked the people of the state to support a petition to the legislature demanding the abolition of the drink trade. He organized a committee to circulate the petition and began a tireless speaking campaign across the state on its behalf. The planter-reformer proved an effective organizer, and to the surprise of Georgia liquor interests, his movement started to gather significant support, including some prominent citizens. Joseph Lumpkin,* for example, of the State Supreme Court, stood solidly with Flournoy. The wet opposition, however, quickly rising from its early complacency, mounted a growing counterattack as the year wore on. Events were building to a crucial pass for Flournoy and his adherents.

Flournoy's movement soon ended in bitter defeat. Wets mounted an orchestrated campaign of harassment, disrupting temperance meetings and sabotaging the reformer's wagon. Still, he appeared to be making progress when he made a serious tactical blunder. The Georgia drys decided, with Flournoy's urging, to field a slate of legislative candidates pledged to attack the liquor traffic. The major parties, then locked in a bitter fight between extreme states' rights and Unionist positions, feared both the disruption a third party might cause as well as the loss of wet support if they tried to compromise with Flournoy. Consequently, all factions turned on him, charging that the temperance position was too radical to gain permanent public support. And as the major politicians abandoned Flournoy, so did most of the state's voters: The dry candidates were smashed at the polls—and some of those who won claimed they had done so because their opponents had at one point supported Flournoy's petition. Thus embroiled in the strife-ridden politics of the era, the Georgia Temperance Movement came to grief. Reform morale was shattered and antiliquor work came to a virtual halt. In the recriminations that followed, even some drys charged that Flournoy's decision to send his movement into politics had set the temperance cause back for years. Indeed, it may have. The Georgia dry reform, later hurt as well by the close connections between Northern abolitionists and temperance leaders, never became a potent antebellum political force. Flournoy himself was crushed; during the intense dry struggle he had neglected his estates and his health. Worn out physically and in financial trouble, he died in 1842—a "martyr" in the eyes of the few faithful of his day and honored by temperance advocates of future generations.

**Bibliography:**

B. SEAP 3, 1004–6; H. A. Scomp, *King Alcohol in the Realm of King Cotton* (Chicago? 1888); Alice Felt Tyler, *Freedom's Ferment: Phases of American*

*Social History from the Colonial Period to the Outbreak of the Civil War* (1944; New York, 1962).

**FOLK, Edgar Estes**   (6 September 1856, Haywood Co., TN—27 February 1917, Nashville, TN). *Education*: studied at Brownsville (TN) Acad. and Wake Forest Coll., 1870s; A.M., Wake Forest Coll., 1877; graduated from Baptist Theological Sem., Louisville, KY, 1882; D.D. (honorary), Wake Forest Coll., 1895. *Career*: minister, Murfreesboro (TN) Baptist Church, 1883–85; minister, Millersburg, KY, 1885–86; minister, First Baptist Church, Albany, GA, 1886–88; publisher and editor, *Baptist Reflector* (subsequently merged with other newspapers and moved to Nashville, TN), 1888–1917.

A Baptist clergyman, Edgar Folk was born in Tennessee in 1856, and except for a few years in Kentucky and Georgia, he spent most of his life there, dying at Nashville in 1917. Although he served in a number of different pulpits, Folk's most important work was as an editor and writer. In 1888 he acquired control of the *Baptist Reflector* and assumed the editorship. The next year he consolidated it with the *Baptist*, renaming it the *Baptist and Reflector* (published in Nashville), remaining its owner and editor until his death. He used his editorial position to comment widely on religious and social issues of the day, and like most Baptists, he proclaimed the merits of abstinence and of prohibition. The *Baptist and Reflector* was the most influential religious publication of the region, and thus Folk's views had a considerable popular impact. To further his hold on the local religious press, in 1895 he founded the Southern Baptist Press Association, of which he was president for the remainder of his life. Folk, already a temperance man, came late into the formal Temperance Movement. From 1899 to 1911, he served as president of the Anti-Saloon League of Tennessee and worked along with other local drys to further the interests of state antiliquor fortunes. Mixing his religion with politics, in 1912 he became a member of the Committee on Temperance of the Southern Baptist Convention. Folk remained a prominent temperance figure in Tennessee to the end, and the movement recognized the value not only of his personal leadership but also of his longstanding contributions as a publisher. Nor, it should be noted, were there many better examples of the influence of a committed minister in bringing the faithful of his denomination into the temperance fold.

**Bibliography:**

A. *The Mormon Monster*... (Chicago, 1900); *The Plan of Salvation* (Nashville, TN, 1907); *Baptist Principles*... (Nashville, TN, 1909); *A Southern Pilgrimage in Eastern Lands* (Nashville, TN, 1912).

B. SEAP 3, 1007–8; WW 1, 409; Paul E. Isaac, *Prohibition and Politics: Turbulent Decades in Tennessee, 1885–1920* (Knoxville, TN, 1965).

**FOLK, Joseph Wingate**   (28 October 1869, Brownsville, TN—28 May 1823, New York, NY). *Education*: LLB., Vanderbilt Univ., 1890; LLD. (honorary),

Univ. of Missouri, 1905, William Jewell Coll., 1906, Drury Coll., 1907, West-minster Coll., 1907, Southwestern Baptist Univ., 1908, Baylor Univ., 1919. *Career*: admitted to bar, TN, 1890; legal practice, Brownsville, TN, 1890–94; St. Louis, MO, 1894–1900; circuit attorney, St. Louis, MO, 1900–1904; governor of Missouri, 1905–9; lecturing, 1909–10; solicitor, U.S. Department of State, 1913–14; chief counsel, Interstate Commerce Commission, 1914–18; general counsel, St. Louis (MO) Chamber of Commerce, 1918–23; private legal practice, 1918–23.

Fundamentally a Democratic politician and officeholder, Joseph Wingate Folk served the temperance cause only indirectly—but in ways that endeared him to those in the ranks of the reform. He began his career as a lawyer in Tennessee, moving his practice to St. Louis in 1894. It was in that Missouri city that he began his impressive rise in Democratic politics. Plunging immediately into the public affairs of the city, Folk achieved major public recognition when he successfully mediated a strike of streetcar employees in 1900. That same year he ran for the office of circuit attorney, roughly equivalent to the latter-day district attorney's office, and barely was elected. But he soon established himself as a crusading reformist prosecutor, launching a series of assaults on the crime, graft, and corruption that then bedeviled the cities of America. Not even officials of his own party were immune, and no less than twelve public officials were ultimately convicted, along with scores of lesser culprits. In 1903, Folk won the party's nomination for governor of Missouri, once again on a platform of reform, riding the crest of the Progressive movement in the United States. Folk's popularity was such that he outpolled Theodore Roosevelt in the election of 1904.

It was while he was governor from 1904 to 1908 that Folk made his contribution to the Temperance Movement. Although not a member of any temperance organization, Folk cracked down on illicit grog shops and distillers, and though this was merely part of the reforming spirit of the times, it did serve to advance the temperance cause. Indeed, Folk's strong actions as governor were much in keeping not only with the Progressive conception of the active chief executive but with the contemporary belief that temperance and Progressivism were part of the same political outlook. Certainly drys nationally applauded the Missouri governor. "His fearless and uncompromising attitude toward the liquor interests left its impress on the State," wrote one temperance observer, "and furnished a splendid example worthy of emulation." After leaving office, he received a number of appointments from President Woodrow Wilson and continued as an active foe of special interests in politics. He made one final try at political office when he attempted to secure a senatorial nomination from Missouri; but he lost, as indeed he had in 1912, when he futilely sought the Democratic nomination for the presidency. Folk died in 1923, having a modest but secure place in the history of both American politics and the Temperance Movement.

**Bibliography:**

A. *The Era of Conscience*, Civic Forum Addresses, vol. 1, no. 5. (New York, 1908).

B. DAB 6, 489–90; SEAP 3, 1008–9; WW 1, 409; Louis George Geiger, *Joseph W. Folk of Missouri* (Columbia, MO, 1953).

**FOOTE, Andrew Hull**    (12 September 1806, New Haven, CT—26 June 1863, New York, NY). *Education*: studied at U.S. Military Acad., West Point, 1822. *Career*: midshipman (1822), seeing duty with Commodore David Dixon Porter in West Indies, beginning 1823; naval officer, ship and shore commands in various areas, including Africa, China, Philadelphia, Brooklyn (NY) Naval Yard, 1830–61; promoted to commodore (later rear admiral), commanded Union naval forces on upper Mississippi River, 1862; chief, Bureau of Equipment and Recruiting, 1863; appointed commander, Charleston (SC) Squadron (died en route to assume command), 1863.

Justly remembered as one of the greatest naval commanders of the Civil War, Rear Admiral Andrew Hull Foote was also a man of firm religious beliefs and reform sympathies. Notably, he was a life-long teetotaler and an unrelenting foe of the liquor traffic; and unlike most other Americans enlisted under the temperance banner, Foote ultimately found himself in a position to do something direct and positive about his views. His influence came through his exemplary naval career. He went to sea as a midshipman in 1822 at the age of sixteen and died holding the rank of rear admiral, in his prime as a commander, in 1863. In between he enjoyed a remarkable and successful series of assignments that took him around the globe. In the 1820s, he fought West Indian pirates under Commodore David Porter; in the 1840s the Connecticut sailor tracked down slave traders off the coast of Africa as captain of the brig *Perry* (out of which came a book, *Africa and the American Flag*); and in the 1850s his men stormed a Chinese fortress to avenge an insult to the flag. His most important duty, however, came during the War Between the States. In 1862, commanding a Union river flotilla on the Mississippi and its tributaries, Foote was instrumental in cementing the victories of General Ulysses S. Grant at Fort Henry and Fort Donelson in the Tennessee campaign that helped break the Confederacy in the West. He was in ill health during these crucial operations, however, and he died the following year on the way to a new assignment with the forces blockading the South Carolina port of Charleston. With his passing, the armed forces of the Union lost one of their best.

The Temperance Movement also mourned the admiral's death. Ever since a deep spiritual experience early in his career, Foote had been committed to reform causes, and his views on the liquor question led him to some concrete steps toward drying out the navy. For years, the service had provided its sailors with a rum ration—much to the disgust of Foote. He took the lead in trying to end the spirits ration, and aboard his ships he worked hard to persuade his sailors to take the pledge. He was often successful. Serving on the frigate *Cumberland* before the Civil War, Foote had organized a temperance society and made her the first temperance ship in the navy. He kept in touch with a number of prominent dry leaders during the antebellum years, who cheered his efforts against the rum ration as a sign of general American progress in the battle against drink. When the government finally did eliminate the ration in 1862, Foote, quite rightly, received a good deal of the credit. "Too high a monument," wrote Dr. John Marsh* later, "could not be erected to Rear-Admiral Foote." Foote's temperance sentiments were but one facet of his overall humanitarian and reforming instincts. He was as rigorously opposed to slavery, for example, as he was to the liquor traffic, and it is hard to say which gave him greater satisfaction—the fight against slavery or his victory over "demon rum" in the U.S. navy.

**Bibliography:**

A. *Farewell Temperance Address; Delivered Before the Crew of the U.S. Frigate Cumberland...* (Boston, 1845); *Africa and the American Flag* (New York, 1854).

B. DAB 499–500; SEAP 3, 1009–10; WW H, 255; J. M. Hoppin, *Life of Andrew Hull Foote* (New York, 1874).

**FOSTER, Judith Ellen Horton**    (3 November 1840, Lowell, MA—11 August 1910, Washington, DC). *Education*: studied at Genesee Wesleyan Sem., Lima, NY, 1855–56; studied law with husband, E. C. Foster, Clinton, IA, 1870–72. *Career*: music teacher, Chicago, circa 1865–68; admitted to bar, IA, 1872; legal practice with husband, beginning 1872; superintendent of legislation and petitions, National WCTU, 1880–90; president, Non-Partisan WCTU, 1890–1910; active in Republican Party affairs and governmental commissions, 1888 to 1900s.

One of the most remarkable women to take up the cause of temperance, Judith Foster (born Horton) was born in Massachusetts in 1840. The Hortons were a deeply religious (her father was a blacksmith turned Methodist preacher) and reform-minded family (they were strong abolitionists), and the penchant for commitment was clearly evident in Judith. The death of her parents while she was still a girl compelled her to move in with relatives, and after a marriage to one Addison Avery, she moved first to Montreal and then to Chicago (1865). There, she got her first taste of how the other half lived by working among the poor in the city's slums. She also divorced Avery after their marriage soured and eventually wed a young lawyer named E. C. Foster. The Fosters moved to Clinton, Iowa, in 1869, where Mr. Foster opened a practice, and Judith also expressed an interest in the law. With her husband's help, she read law extensively, and in 1872 was admitted to the Iowa bar—perhaps the first woman to do so in that state's history. Showing a very modern spirit of equality, the shingle outside the office read "Foster and Foster," and it is problematical who had the pride of place. While preparing for the law and tending to her growing family (she finally had four children), Mrs. Foster sought to continue the socially oriented work she had begun in Chicago and thus became involved in the Temperance Movement after the Woman's Crusade spread to Iowa from Ohio in 1873. She founded the Women's Temperance Society of Clinton, which brought her to the attention of Frances Willard* (later the president of the Woman's

Christian Temperance Union). After the WCTU was founded in 1874, Mrs. Foster became an enthusiastic member and in 1880 was named superintendent of legislation for the organization. She was, however, nothing if not an independent spirit, and unlike most in the WCTU, she ultimately developed some major differences with Willard's political views. In the end, things became serious enough to cause a rupture between the two women and to split the temperance group itself.

The chief problem lay in Willard's desire to affiliate the WCTU with the Prohibition Party in order to advance the dry cause. Anticipating the later stance of the Anti-Saloon League, Foster argued instead for a nonpartisan approach, with an emphasis on attempts to work with the major political parties. A loyal Republican herself, she finally led her local chapter of the WCTU out of the parent organization over this issue. With other chapters (including, at one point, most of those in Iowa), Foster established the Non-Partisan Woman's Christian Temperance Union (1890), of which she was president for the rest of her life. The same spirit of independence showed itself when she organized the Woman's National Republican Association; for although women could not vote in national elections, nonetheless, Mrs. Foster believed they could still wield considerable influence in party circles. That this was so is evidenced by the fact that she was called upon to address several national party conventions on the issue of women's rights in which she persuasively argued her position for the political equality of women. Mrs. Foster's personal status eventually became such that she accompanied William Howard Taft to the Philippines, upon his appointment as governor, to investigate the status of women there. During the Spanish-American War she went on a mission for President William McKinley to examine the circumstances under which American volunteers were being trained. Carrying on her tireless campaign on behalf of women, Mrs. Foster ended her long and fruitful devotion to reform by investigating the condition of women in prison and recommending changes and improvements for the benefit of female inmates. Mrs. Foster would have been a remarkable women in any age, but considering the obstacles women faced in the nineteenth century, her career is little short of inspiring and stands as testimony to what one individual dedicated and determined can accomplish.

### Bibliography:

A. *An Argument for the Prohibitory Constitutional Amendment* (New York, 1882); *Constitutional Amendment Manual. . .for Constitutional Prohibition* (New York, 1882); *Scientific Temperance Instruction in the Public Schools* (Boston, 1885); *Constitutional Amendment Catechism* (New York, 1889); *Constitutional Prohibition* (New York, 1889); *The Saloon Must Go* (New York, 1889).

B. NAW 1, 651–52; SEAP 3, 1021–22; 6, 552–53; WW 1, 417.

**FOWLER, Charles Henry**    (11 August 1837, Burford, Ontario, Canada—20 March 1908, Chicago, IL). *Education*: graduated from Genesee Coll., 1859;

studied law, Chicago, 1859; graduated from Garrett Biblical Inst., Evanston, IL, 1861; D.D. (honorary), Garrett Biblical Inst.; LLD. (honorary), Syracuse Univ. and Wesleyan Univ. *Career*: Methodist minister, various Chicago churches, 1861–72; president, Northwestern Univ., 1872–76; editor, *Christian Advocate*, beginning 1876; corresponding secretary, Missionary Society, Methodist Episcopal Church, 1880; bishop, Methodist Episcopal Church, 1884; foreign travel and missionary work, 1880s–1900s.

Fowler's career was characterized by a devotion to the Methodist Church, foreign mission work, and education. He was born a Canadian but was brought to the United States at the age of four and grew up on the family farm in Illinois. After graduating from Genesee College in Lima, New York, Fowler returned to Illinois, where he studied law in Chicago. But he never finished his studies, for he experienced a personal religious conversion and left law school for the Garrett Biblical Institute at Evanston, from which he graduated in 1861. For eleven years he served in pulpits of various Chicago Methodist Episcopal churches, compiling an impressive record as a preacher and commentator on public affairs. Among other subjects, he spoke often on the liquor question and became noted as an advocate of prohibition. During these years, he briefly became engaged to Frances Willard,* future president of the Woman's Christian Temperance Union. The relationship proved unhappy, however, and lingering bitterness remained between the two for years. In 1872, Fowler was chosen as president of Northwestern University and embarked on a major reorganization of the school. Very quickly, he clashed with Willard, who at the time headed an affiliated women's college. Willard became dean of the women's division under Fowler, but in 1874 they fought over who would govern women students. When Fowler made the dean's position all but powerless, she resigned. President Fowler then went on to considerable fame at the head of Northwestern. He continued his interest in temperance and received credit for helping to spread the message of the cause in the ranks of higher education. The Temperance Movement itself counted Fowler as one of its most distinguished allies and lauded his speeches and writings on alcohol problems. In 1876, he became the editor of the New York *Christian Advocate*, the chief publication of the Methodist Episcopal Church. In 1884 Fowler was consecrated a bishop and began a series of overseas mission visits that would take him to South America and Asia, and eventually around the world. He worked with his usual energy while abroad and helped found a number of educational institutions.

### Bibliography:

A. *The Impeachment and Punishment of Alcohol* (New York, 1872); *King Alcohol* (Chicago, 1872); *The Wines of the Bible* (New York, 1878); *Problems of the Twentieth Century* (San Francisco, 1891).

B. SEAP 3, 1024; WW 1, 418; Mary Erheart, *Frances Willard: From Prayers to Politics* (Chicago, 1944).

**FOWLER, Lydia Folger**   (5 May 1822, Nantucket, MA—26 January 1879, London). *Education*: M.D., Central Medical Coll., Syracuse, NY, 1850; studied medicine, Paris and London, 1860–61. *Career*: teacher, Wheaton Sem., Norton, MA, 1842–44; lecturer on women's health topics and author, 1840s; professor, Central Medical Coll., 1851–52; medical practice, New York City, 1852–60; instructor, New York Hygeio-Therapeutic Coll., 1862–63; reform activities and writing, 1863–79.

Lydia Fowler began a career in medicine and reform under rather unusual circumstances. Her husband, Lorenzo Fowler, was one of the leading advocates of the pseudoscience of phrenology in nineteenth-century America. Thus, after a brief teaching career, by the mid-1840s Lydia was involved in the promotion of this fad as a travelling lecturer. She also spoke on health-related issues for women and helped peddle the books published by the firm of Fowler and Wells, some of which she wrote. Bearing such titles as *Familiar Lessons on Phrenology* and *Familiar Lessons on Physiology*, she had some success in reaching the family-oriented book market of the day. Out of this activity Fowler developed an interest in medicine, and in November 1849 she enrolled in the small and struggling Central Medical College in Syracuse, New York. At the time, Central was the only medical school admitting women. When she graduated with a medical degree (1850) she was only the second woman in the United States to have done so. She remained on the faculty at Central Medical as "demonstrator of anatomy to the female students." When the school shut down in 1852, Mrs. Fowler went to New York City, where she practiced medicine until 1860, lectured on the need for women in the medical profession, and published articles in medical journals. She also made a tour of Europe with her husband and used the opportunity to attend medical courses in institutions in Britain and France. They found the Old World pleasant enough, and in 1863 they moved to England to take up permanent residence. Although she continued to write, the relocation meant the end of Fowler's medical career.

She had, however, left her mark on her native United States. While engaged in her medical work, and perhaps because of it, Dr. Fowler became keenly interested in a number of reform movements, especially those involving women. Her greatest concerns were women's rights and temperance, reforms which many contemporaries considered related. Fowler served as an officer of two national women's rights conventions in the early 1850s and devoted a considerable amount of time to the liquor question. She was a delegate to the New York State Daughters of Temperance Convention in 1852 and a year later presided over one of the largest women's temperance gatherings the nation had ever seen (in New York). Her speech was reported favorably in the media, aiding her developing national reputation as a dry worker. The move to Great Britain cut short her temperance career in America but hardly diminished her personal interest in the subject. In fact, before long she was again campaigning against drink, this time as a member of the British Temperance Society, in which she remained active for the rest of her life. She also continued to write and in 1863 produced a temperance novel

(*Nora: The Lost and Redeemed*) depicting the supposed problems of alcohol encountered by young women. It is questionable how original Dr. Fowler's contributions either to practical medicine or to temperance ideas really were; but there is no mistaking the depth of her reform spirit and her willingness to take the lead in advancing the social status of women in her generation.

**Bibliography:**

A. *Familiar Lessons on Physiology and Phrenology*, 2 vols. (New York, 1847); *The Heart and Its Influences* (London, 1863); *Nora: The Lost and Redeemed* (London, 1863); *Familiar Lessons on Astronomy* (Manchester, England, 1877).

B. NAW 1, 654–55.


**FRELINGHUYSEN, Theodore**     (28 March 1787, Franklin Township, NJ— 12 April 1862, New Brunswick, NJ). *Education*: graduated from Coll. of New Jersey (now Princeton Univ.), 1804; studied law with Richard Stockton, 1804– 8. *Career*: admitted to bar, NJ, 1808; legal practice, Newark, NJ, 1808–17; New Jersey attorney general, 1817–27; member, U.S. Senate, 1829–35; mayor, Newark, NJ, 1836–39; chancellor, Univ. of City of New York, 1839–50; president, Rutgers Coll. (now Rutgers Univ.), New Brunswick, NJ, 1850–62.

Son of one of the most distinguished families of early America, Theodore Frelinghuysen was descended from the noted Dutch Reformed divine Theodore Jacobus Frelinghuysen (his grandfather) and Revolutionary General Frederick Frelinghuysen (his father). He was a credit to them both as he combined a number of outstanding careers. As an educator, lawyer, and senator, Frelinghuysen remained always a model for his peers, a "Christian statesman" as abolitionist William Lloyd Garrison* called him. A native of New Jersey, Frelinghuysen graduated from the College of New Jersey at Princeton in 1804, second in his class. He began the practice of law in Newark, and such was his reputation that in 1817 he was appointed attorney general of New Jersey by the state legislature—the majority of whose members did not share Frelinghuysen's political views. He was reelected twice more and then in 1829 elected to the U.S. Senate. He served only one term, but he made his mark as a humanitarian and reformer. Pious and devout, he saw his position in government as a public trust and felt it as his duty to guard national morality and to stand against injustice. He was a foe of slavery, and his principled opposition to President Andrew Jackson's forced removal of the Cherokee Indians from their tribal lands in Georgia attracted national attention; it also won the respect of many of the New Jersey senator's opponents. At the same time, Frelinghuysen exhibited little of the self-righteousness that often accompanied the moral arguments of the period. After leaving the Senate, he returned to Newark, where he was elected mayor in 1837. Politics, however, gradually lost its hold on the devout lawyer, and his interests increasingly turned to education. Indeed, in 1839 he gave up his law practice, resigned as mayor of Newark, and became chancellor of the University of the City of New York. Still later (1850), he accepted the presidency of Rutgers College in New Brunswick, New Jersey, and did much to build that struggling institution. His last foray into politics came in 1844, when the Whig Party prevailed upon him to join its national ticket in a run for vice president. But his friend and running mate, Henry Clay of Kentucky, went down to defeat at the hands of Democrat James K. Polk, ironically on account of the defection of many antislavery New York Whigs to the Liberty Party and its strong abolitionist stand.

As a reformer Frelinghuysen took great interest in many religious and humanitarian causes. In fact, contemporaries noted that few Americans were so active in so many different national reforms. At various times, he played leadership roles on the American Board of Commissioners for Foreign Missions, the American Bible Society, the American Tract Society, the American Sunday School Union (he was president or vice president of all of the foregoing), and the American Colonization Society. He was also a vice president of the American Temperance Union. While he was never strident in arguing his positions on the subject, he was adamant in his belief that liquor was one of the prime evils in American society and ought to be attacked frontally. "He was decided for total abstinence as the only safe principle," noted another dry advocate, long before that position was generally accepted by other reformers, and he urged the legal prohibition of the liquor traffic. Laws protecting liquor sales, he insisted, were contrary to the public good, and elected officials had a duty to resist them. "No man fit to represent a free people," he wrote, "will deny these propositions." Temperance in his view was a cause seeking "the public good" and as such deserved a voice in the highest councils of government. Accordingly, he helped organize the Congressional Temperance Society during his years in the Senate and played an active role in its affairs. The society did not call for immediate prohibition (that was a position too advanced for most of its members), but it did go on record as favoring whatever future legislation might be necessary to protect the morality and well-being of the republic. Frelinghuysen spoke fairly often on the liquor question, and temperance leaders considered him a most effective advocate. At his passing at age seventy-five, antiliquor forces mourned him, noting the loss of "one of the most accomplished Christian gentlemen the world has seen."

## Bibliography:

A. *An Oration...Before the American Colonization Society...* (Princeton, NJ, 1824); *Speech (on the Bill for an Exchange of Lands with the Indians...and for Their Removal West of the Mississippi)...* (Washington, DC, 1830); *Address Before the Merchants' Temperance Society in the City of New York...* (New York, 1842).

B. DAB 7, 16–17; SEAP 3, 1053–54; WW 1, 260; Talbot Wilson Chambers, *Memoir of the Life and Character of the Late Hon. Theo. Frelinghuysen, LL.D* (New York, 1863); Richard P. McCormick, *Rutgers: A Bicentennial History*

(New Brunswick, NJ, 1966); Cortlandt Parker, *A Sketch of the Life and Public Services of Theodore Frelinghuysen* (New York, 1844).

**FUNK, Isaac Kaufman**    (10 September 1839, Clifton, OH—4 April 1912, Montclair, NJ). *Education:* A.B., Wittenberg Coll., 1860; A.M., Wittenberg Coll., ?; D.D., Wittenberg Theological Sem., 1861; LLD. (honorary), Wittenberg Theological Sem., 1896. *Career:* ordained Lutheran minister, 1861; pastorates in OH, IN, and NY, 1861–72; travelled in Europe, Egypt, Palestine, 1872–76; publishing business (president of Funk & Wagnalls Co. after 1890), New York City, 1876–1912.

Known today chiefly as a publisher and lexicographer, Isaac Kaufman Funk began his professional life as a Lutheran minister, having received both his undergraduate and divinity training at Wittenberg College and Theological Seminary in the early 1860s. For over a decade, he served pulpits in the Midwest and New York, during which time he demonstrated an interest in both scholarship and reform. Indeed, he was a decided champion of temperance and vigorously promoted it from the pulpit, even though his Lutheran congregations were not always sympathetic to his message. Resigning from the ministry in 1872 (for reasons not exactly clear), he travelled in Europe and the Holy Land before returning to New York City to enter the publishing business. He started modestly, and his early work was mainly in printing books, pamphlets, and self-help works for ministers. Among these was a journal, the *Metropolitan Pulpit*, which Funk published and edited under various titles until well into the 1880s. In the late 1870s, Funk went into partnership with Adam Willie Wagnalls, an old classmate from Wittenberg, and it was under the rubric of Funk and Wagnalls that the business became a giant in the publishing world. It was also at this point that Isaac Funk's lexicographical reputation was made. This was in the form of *A Standard Dictionary of the English Language*, which Funk worked on between 1890 and 1893 and which was something of a classic of its kind for the period. Funk also published a periodical which was later to gain a certain notoriety, *The Literary Digest*, which he began in 1890. In addition, he brought out the *Voice* in 1880 as a Prohibition Party organ, which proved a quick success. By 1888, the *Voice* had a weekly circulation of some 700,000. Funk kept the dry periodical until 1898, when he sold it to another press (which continued it as the *New Voice*).

Funk remained a zealous Temperance Movement partisan throughout his long and distinguished publishing career. Aside from issuing the *Voice* for some eighteen years, he was active in other dry pursuits. In 1885, he initially accepted the Prohibition Party's nomination for mayor of Brooklyn, New York, although he withdrew in favor of another candidate who promised stringent enforcement of laws against liquor sales to children. He served for a number of years as a vice president of the National Temperance Society and became an early supporter of the Anti-Saloon League when it spread its activities into the New York City region. Funk's dry sympathies gave rise to a number of major investment efforts as well. In 1889, he was a leader in the establishment of Prohibition Park (now the town of Westerleigh on Staten Island), a dry education and conference center. The venture proved successful in its early days, and the enterprising publisher played a major role in its governance. An attempt to found another such venture, this time an entire town run on prohibitionist principles, proved a financial disaster. In 1890, Funk, who had formed the East Tennessee Land Company for the purpose, organized a group of investors to establish the town of Harriman in that state. The town grew, but never on the dry model, and all of its financial backers lost heavily. Funk could absorb his losses, but others could not, and considerable bitterness arose over the incident. Still, he never lost faith in the movement, and until his death (he died working on the letter *s* in a revision of his famous dictionary), he remained a vociferous advocate of personal abstinence and a prohibition amendment to the Constitution.

## Bibliography:

A. "Prohibitory Law and Personal Liberty," *North American Review* 147 (1888): 124; with others, *A Standard Dictionary of the English Language* (New York, 1893, and subsequent editions); *The Psychic Riddle* (New York, 1907); *The Next Step in Evolution: The Present Step* (New York, 1908); *The Widow's Mite, and Other Psychic Phenomena*, 3rd ed. (New York, 1911).

B. DAB 7, 72–73; NYT, Aug. 5, 1912; SEAP 3, 1059–60; WW 1, 432–33.

# G

GAGE, Frances Dana Barker   (12 October 1808, Marietta, OH—10 November 1884, Greenwich, CT). *Career*: reform writing and lecturing, 1840s to 1884; author of children's stories under the pen name of "Aunt Fanny," beginning 1850s; associate editor, *Ohio Cultivator* and *Field Notes*, 1850s to 1861; refugee relief with freedmen, Parris Island, SC, 1862–63; volunteer freedmen and veterans relief work, 1863–65; unsalaried agent, Western Sanitary Commission, 1864.

The social views of Frances Gage (born Barker) were in many ways typical of those of other women reformers of the mid-nineteenth century, as her interest in the Temperance Movement reflected only one side of her varied attachments to the issues of the era. The Barker family was actively involved in the antislavery movement, and young Frances grew up in a heavily reform-conscious atmosphere. As she reached maturity, Gage increasingly addressed herself to women's rights and temperance as well as abolitionism, viewing them as the reforms most likely to eliminate the bulk of the evils she saw as plaguing the nation. In the 1850s, she became a frequent contributor on these themes to magazines (notably the *Ladies Repository of Cincinnati*) and began writing juvenile stories as well under the pseudonym "Aunt Fanny." She also became an effective lecturer, impressing many with the enthusiasm of her style on the podium, and gained wide recognition in the Midwest (and especially her native Ohio) as an avid reformer. She was unable to attend the first Ohio women's rights convention; however, in 1852 she presided over the second such gathering and took part in a national convention in Cleveland, Ohio, in 1853. The same year, the Gages (she had married lawyer James L. Gage in 1829) moved to St. Louis, Missouri, where her antislavery sentiments were not appreciated. She tried to maintain her agitation, but local newspapers eventually refused to print her views, and threats of violence (three mysterious fires struck their home and Mr. Gage's office) finally drove the Gages back to Ohio. They settled in Columbus in 1860, and she quickly took up the pen again as associate editor of the *Ohio Cultivator* and *Farm Notes*. It was soon obvious that the ill-fated sojourn in Missouri had not dimmed her spirits, as she kept up a lively correspondence with suffragettes Susan B. Anthony,* Elizabeth Cady Stanton, and Amelia Bloomer.* In 1861, she also effectively lobbied for an Ohio law granting married women partial property rights. By this time, her reform reputation had made her a national figure.

The coming of the Civil War added an important chapter to Gage's career. The energy she had concentrated on antislavery now went toward relief work with the freedmen of South Carolina, where the local Union army commander placed her in charge of five hundred former slaves on Parris Island in 1862. She returned home in 1863, however, with the death of her husband and then became actively involved in relief work again. She travelled the North and much of the South speaking and raising funds on behalf of freed blacks and wounded Union troops. It was no easy task: Gage set an exhausting pace for herself and was badly hurt in 1864 when her carriage overturned. She was not out of action for long, however. Moving to Lambertsville, New Jersey, in 1865, she poured her energies once more into writing and lecturing. For a time, the Temperance Movement received most of her attention. Her efforts served to awaken many dry reformers from the lethargy that had marked the antiliquor fortunes during the War Between the States, and her publications on the subject enjoyed wide circulation. While playing an active role in reigniting dry sentiments in postwar America, though, Gage never lost contact with the suffrage crusade. She took part in the early activities of the American Equal Rights Association and continued to write on behalf of the female ballot. Later in life she was largely incapacitated by a stroke, although she did manage to do some writing. Gage died on a visit to Greenwich, Connecticut.

**Bibliography:**

A. *The Man in the Well: A Temperance Tale* (London, 185-?); as "Aunt Fanny," *Fanny at School* (Buffalo, NY, 1866); as "Aunt Fanny," *Fanny's Birthday* (Buffalo, NY, 1866); *Elsie Magoon: Or, the Old Still-house in the Hollow* (Philadelphia, 1872); *Poems* (Philadelphia, 1872); *State Upward* (Philadelphia, 1872).

B. DAB 7, 84–85; NAW 2, 2–4; WW H, 264.

**GALLINGER, Jacob H.**    (28 March 1837, Cornwall, Ontario, Canada—17 August 1918, Washington, DC). *Education*: M.D., Medical Inst., Cincinnati, OH, 1858; M.D., New York Homeopathic Medical Coll., 1868; A.M. (honorary), Dartmouth Coll., 1885. *Career*: worked as printer, 1850s; private study and travel in Europe, 1858–60; medical practice, Keene, NH, 1860–62; medical practice, Concord, NH, 1862–85; surgeon general of New Hampshire, 1879–80; member, New Hampshire House of Representatives, 1872–73, 1891; member, New Hampshire Senate, 1878–81; chairman, Republican State Committee, 1882–90, 1898–1907; member, U.S. House of Representatives, 1885–89; member, U.S. Senate, 1891–1918.

While in his political prime in the U.S. Senate, Jacob Gallinger was a veritable paragon of New England conservatism. Yet in certain matters, specifically women's suffrage and temperance, he broke with many of his colleagues and held forth with the zeal of a committed reformer. His early career ambitions had been in medicine, and indeed, after considerable effort he had put himself through medical school and launched a thriving practice (he was one of the most prominent physicians in the Concord, New Hampshire, region for some two decades). But he quickly demonstrated a lively interest in politics and civic affairs, and over the 1870s and 1880s rose steadily to become one of the leading forces in the electoral process in his state. Gallinger first won a seat in the New Hampshire legislature in 1872 as a Republican, and his allegiance to the party never wavered. A thorough and loyal partisan through his years in state office (as he was later in the national government), he also served skillfully as chairman of the Republican State Committee for many years. In office, and at the helm of the party, he usually had little truck with reformers, referring to their issues at one point as "Sunday school politics." He preferred the priveleges of office, the patronage system, and financial issues generally calculated to please conservative business interests. Elected to the national Senate in 1891 (and serving until his death in 1918), he continued in the same vein, clashing bitterly with President Benjamin Harrison over civil service reform (Gallinger was stridently against it). The Granite State politician, however, was also a highly capable champion of the causes he preferred. He fought a constant battle for a strong American merchant marine, devoted much careful effort to the effective administration of the District of Columbia, and received considerable credit for the success in the Senate of the Nineteenth Amendment (women's suffrage). If Gallinger was obstinate in some cases, then, he was also able.

Gallinger's support for National Prohibition showed him at his most effective as a legislator. Though he was at odds with much of the Temperance Movement with respect to broad reform goals, antiliquor workers found him a firm ally on the narrower prohibition effort. He was a temperance man during his years in the House of Representatives, but he reached his full influence in the Senate. He believed beverage alcohol to be at the root of any number of social problems and a prime source of civil disruption. In these positions, he was a worthy successor to his predecessor as senator from New Hampshire, crusading prohibitionist Henry Blair.* Taking an interest in all dry questions, Gallinger made his first major impact on the issue during the 1905 debate over the admission of Oklahoma to the Union. The proposed state constitution was dry, and the senator defended it—successfully—against wet efforts to eliminate its prohibition clauses. In 1915, Gallinger joined Senator Morris Sheppard* of Texas in introducing the legislation that ultimately became the Eighteenth Amendment. He fought consistently for it while also advocating other dry measures. Gallinger took the lead, for example, in framing the laws that dried out the national capital and cast his votes time after time for regulations aimed at curbing or eliminating the liquor traffic. After the final dry victory in 1920—the year the National Prohibition amendment became effective—temperance leaders looked back on Gallinger's contributions to the cause as crucial in bringing about what they termed "an inspiring chapter in our national history."

**Bibliography:**

B. DAB 7, 112–13; SEAP 3, 1065; WW 1, 436; *Washington Post*, Aug. 18, 1918.

**GARRISON, William Lloyd**   (10 December 1805, Newburyport, MA—24 May 1879, New York, NY). *Career*: apprenticed to shoemaker, Lynn, MA, 1814–15; apprenticed to cabinetmaker, Haverill, MA, circa 1816–17; apprenticed to printer, Newburyport, MA, and worked on *Newburyport Herald*, 1818–26; editor, *Newburyport Free Press*, 1826–28; typesetter and editor, *National Philanthropist*, Boston, 1828; editor, *Journal of the Times*, Bennington, VT; editor, *Genius of Universal Emancipation*, Baltimore, MD, 1829–31; editor and publisher, *Liberator*, Boston, beginning 1831; active reform and abolitionist lecturing and organizing, 1820s–1870s.

While best known for his activities in the crusade against slavery, William Lloyd Garrison lent his vigorous support to other social reform efforts as well. Long before he emerged as one of America's leading abolitionists, Garrison advocated laws against imprisonment for debt and profaning the Sabbath, called for an expanded social role for women, urged support for an international peace movement, and came out as a strident and articulate foe of the liquor traffic. In his youth, Garrison was trained as a printer and while still in that role made his first literary contributions to the *Newburyport* (MA) *Herald*. By 1826, he was publisher of the *Free Press* in the same city, and after moving to Boston he became editor of the *Philanthropist* in 1828. The *Philanthropist* was ardently protemperance, one of the nation's first journals to proclaim total abstinence rather than moderation (its motto was "Moderate Drinking Is the Downhill Road to Intemperance and Drunkenness"), and Garrison gave the growing dry cause considerable publicity. He damned church members in the liquor traffic, called upon the town fathers to stop liquor sales on holidays and during militia training, and gladly reported the founding of new temperance societies nationally. Later in 1828, he left the *Philanthropist* to manage a paper in support of the presidential campaign of John Quincy Adams. He maintained his reform interests, however, and went on to edit still other liberal journals over the next few years. In 1831, when he became co-publisher and editor of the famous *Liberator*, he was clearly one of the most accomplished reform journalists in the nation. At its helm, he gave force and form to his already pronounced views against chattel slavery, denouncing it at every turn and helping to organize his countrymen against it (he was a founder of the American Anti-Slavery Society). In 1835, he was brutally beaten and almost lynched by an anti-abolitionist mob in Boston; yet he never lost his zeal and was second to none as a champion of human liberty. Indeed, he was the very epitome of the antebellum reformer.

During his labors on behalf of abolitionism, Garrison never forgot his battle with the "demon rum." Aside from his longstanding reform interests, his specific attachments to the antiliquor cause probably stemmed from an additional and personal motive. His father had been a problem drinker, and his older brother, James, was a confirmed alcoholic whom William watched waste away through the addiction. James died in his younger brother's home in 1842. At any rate, William kept up his attacks on the bottle while he waged his war on slavery. Even during his visits to Great Britain to address antislavery groups, he took the time to speak on temperance as well. In some instances, his bluntness on the issue offended even friendly audiences, but Garrison insisted on total frankness in rebuking what he termed a "criminal indulgence." Indeed, his forceful approach to the liquor question reflected his antislavery style, in which he was equally opposed to compromise with his political and moral opponents. In 1860, however, he did persuade extreme abolitionists to support Abraham Lincoln (who was not for immediate emancipation), thereby helping the new president harness the antislavery movement to the effort against the Confederacy. After the Civil War, with the attendant end of slavery, Garrison, now aging, remained a strident reformer, although at this point he did not emphasize his temperance sympathies. He spoke out widely on behalf of the rights of the newly freed blacks, for women's suffrage, and for the fair conduct of relations with the Indians. He made more trips to Britain (1867 and 1877), where he received considerable recognition as one of the premier veterans of the war against human bondage. His death in 1879 marked the close of a major chapter in the history of American reform.

**Bibliography:**

A. *Thoughts on African Colonization* (Boston, 1832); *Sonnets and Other Poems* (Boston, 1843); *Selections from the Writings and Speeches of William Lloyd Garrison...* (1852; New York, 1968); *The New "Reign of Terror" in the Slave-Holding States* (Boston, 1860); *The Letters of William Lloyd Garrison*, ed. Walter M. Merrill (Cambridge, MA, 1971).

B. SEAP 3, 1072–1073; WW H, 268; George W. Frederickson, ed., *William Lloyd Garrison* (Englewood Cliffs, NJ, 1968); Aileen S. Kraditor, *Means and Ends in American Abolitionism: Garrison and His Critics on Strategy and Tactics, 1834–1850* (New York, 1969); Walter McIntosh Merrill, ed., *Behold Me Once More: The Confessions of James Holley Garrison, Brother of William Lloyd Garrison* (Boston, 1954); John L. Thomas, *The Liberator: William Lloyd Garrison, A Biography* (Boston, 1963).

**GIDDINGS, Joshua Reed**    (6 October 1795, Athens, PA—27 May 1864, Montreal). *Education:* studied law with Elisha Whittlesey, Canfield, OH, 1820–21. *Career:* farmer and schoolteacher, Ashtabula Co, OH, to 1821; admitted to bar, 1821; legal practice, Jefferson, OH, 1821–38; member, Ohio House of Representatives, 1826; member, U.S. House of Representatives, 1838–59; consul general to Canada, 1861–64.

For over two decades, Joshua Reed Giddings held forth in the Congress as one of the leading opponents of slavery. Raised in frontier Ohio (where in the

War of 1812 he served against the Indians), he entered politics in 1826 after establishing a thriving legal practice. That year, he served a single term in the Ohio legislature, but upon election to the national House he made public office his life's work. He fought stubbornly against the "peculiar institution" of the South, frequently at the side of John Quincy Adams and, later, Abraham Lincoln (who held Giddings in particular esteem). His persistent abolitionism once earned him the censure of the House, but his constituents vindicated him with a massive reelection victory. He left office only in 1858, pleading ill health; but he played a prominent role in Republican Party politics and ended his days as President Lincoln's appointee as consul general to Canada. Interested in many other reform causes while in office, he was an early supporter of the Temperance Movement—although he never gained the recognition in its ranks that came to him via the battle against slavery. Still, he was a proud member of the Congressional Temperance Society and voiced his approval when the drinking habits of his colleagues moved toward moderation—all of which garnered him the plaudits of the American Temperance Union. In fact, the dry organization issued a glowing testimonial on his behalf when he retired in 1858. Another aspect of the antislavery warrior's career is worth noting: He serves as a prime illustration of why temperance never took deep root in the antebellum South. The fact that many men like Giddings, such as abolitionist William Lloyd Garrison,* were also protemperance was viewed with alarm below the Mason-Dixon Line. The antislavery and antiliquor causes seemed too closely allied and actually shared some prominent members and leaders, and it simply was too much for proslavery Americans to tolerate. Thus, while there was dry sentiment in the early and midnineteenth century South, the movement never took on mass proportions until after the Civil War. That, too, was part of the legacy of Joshua Giddings.

**Bibliography:**

A. *Speeches in Congress (1841–1852)* (Boston, 1853); *The Exiles of Florida* (1858; New York, 1969); *History of the Rebellion: Its Author and Causes* (New York, 1864).

B. DAB 7, 260–61; SEAP 3, 1105; WW H, 273; George Washington Julian, *The Life of Joshua Giddings* (Chicago, 1892); James Brewer Stewart, *Joshua R. Giddings and the Tactics of Radical Politics* (Cleveland, OH, 1970).

**GLADDEN, Solomon Washington**  (11 February 1836, Pottsgrove, PA—2 July 1918, Columbus, OH). *Education*: studied at Owego (NY) Acad., 1850s; A.B., Williams Coll., 1859; LLD. (honorary), Roanoke Coll., 1882. *Career*: editorial work, *Owego* (NY) *Gazette*, 1850s; schoolteacher, Owego, NY, 1850s to 1859; licensed to preach, Susquehanna Association of Congregational Ministers, 1859; ordained, 1860; minister, First Congregational Methodist Church, Brooklyn, NY, 1860–61; minister, Morrisania, NY, 1861–66; minister, North Adams, MA, 1866–71; editorial work, *The Independent*, 1871–74; minister, North Church, Springfield, MA, 1874–82; editor, *Sunday Afternoon*, 1878–83;

minister, First Congregational Church, Columbus, OH, 1882–1914 (pastor emeritus after 1914); active retirement in writing and speaking, 1914–18.

Through his many pulpits and numerous publications, Washington Gladden waged a long campaign for the spiritual and social betterment of his fellow citizens. He was born Solomon Gladden, but early on dropped his first name. Young Washington, as he was known for the rest of his life, grew up on a New York State farm and worked his way through Williams College as a schoolteacher. At some time during these years he felt a call to religion, and he took his first pastorate (he was a Congregationalist) in 1860 in Brooklyn, New York. Over a succession of other pastorates, and through editorial work in the religious press, he steadily emerged as one of the leading spokesmen of his denomination and as a champion of what he considered a "practical" approach to Christianity. Gladden emphasized the application of Biblical ideas and religious teachings to everyday life, a practice which identified the earnest minister as a major proponent of the "social gospel" of the era. While he never issued a blanket endorsement of reform legislation, he believed firmly that Americans could eliminate most social evils through humane and sincere cooperation. He avowed, for example, that workers should be able to organize on their own behalf and that employers ought to negotiate on such issues as working conditions in good faith. Gladden did more than preach social reform, however; he also became actively involved in the governmental process at times. He served on the City Council of Columbus, Ohio (1900–1902), and urged the creation of any number of civic bodies to address urban needs. He wrote voluminously on reform topics as well. Never a polemicist, he was still an implacable foe of religious and social bigotry. Gladden emphasized no single solution to social ills, and his thinking was hardly systematic. Yet by a pragmatic application of Christian principles to individual circumstances he became noted as one of the most prominent clergymen of his day.

Like many other exponents of the social gospel, Gladden listed intemperance among the evils of the day. His personal commitments to temperance were longstanding: As a youth he had joined the fraternal Independent Order of Good Templars and never was a drinker himself. As he rose to prominence in the pulpit, he denounced the use of distilled liquor as well as the host of problems surrounding the urban saloon. Yet he was not a strident dry and never joined any formal antiliquor organization (other than the Good Templars lodge). Moreover, Gladden specifically eschewed the extremism of more zealous temperance voices, avoiding condemnation of individual drinkers and preferring (as was his wont) what he considered a more practical approach to the saloon issue. He reasoned that since the local drinking establishments—for all of the difficulties they created—were often integral parts of their communities and served as social centers, they could not simply be abolished. Another institution would have to replace them. He was never precise on what form this replacement for the saloon would take, yet he insisted that it offer a social atmosphere imbued with the reform spirit and free from the tainted activities of its predecessor. And while he never saw this rather nebulous alternative to the saloon materialize, Gladden ever remained the reformer. Opposed to violence by nature (although he supported the Spanish-American War), he won a Church Peace Union prize for his writings against international conflict. Self-sacrificing, industrious, and devoted to his fellow man, Washington Gladden's quest for social justice ceased only with his death.

## Bibliography:

A. *Applied Christianity: Moral Aspects of Social Questions* (New York, 1902); *Christianity and Socialism* (New York, 1905); *The Christian Pastor and the Working Church* (New York, 1907); *The Church and Modern Life* (New York, 1908); *Recollections* (Boston, 1909); *Present Day Theology* (Columbus, OH, 1913).

B. DAB 7, 325–27; NCAB 10, 256; NYT, July 3, 1918; SEAP 3, 1109–10; Jacob H. Dorn, *Washington Gladden: Prophet of the Social Gospel* (Columbus, OH, 1966); Richard D. Knudten, *The Systematic Thought of Washington Gladden* (New York, 1968).

**GLEED, James Willis**    (8 March 1859, Morrisville, VT—12 October 1926, Topeka, KS). *Education*: A.B., Univ. of Kansas, 1879; A.M., Univ. of Kansas, 1882; LLB., Columbia Univ., 1884; LLD. (honorary), Columbia Univ., 1904. *Career*: legal practice, Topeka, KS, beginning 1884; instructor, Latin and Greek, Univ. of Kansas, 1879–83; professor of law and real property, Univ. of Kansas, 1887–1900.

A lawyer and educator by profession, James Willis Gleed witnessed and participated in the growth of the prohibition movement in his adopted state of Kansas. Gleed, a characteristic post–Civil War temperance worker, became interested in the antiliquor crusade after the passage of constitutional prohibition in Kansas in 1880. Although the measure had been instituted by popular vote (over the vigorous opposition of the liquor industry and amid the glare of national publicity), the talented young lawyer feared that public complacency would allow the law to become a dead letter. In fact, Gleed anticipated a major wet revival and consequently pledged his personal efforts to keeping the war against drink at full throttle. He joined the Kansas State Temperance Union and quickly became a leading light in the organization. Serving on its executive committee, and for a number of terms as president, he represented the union around the state as a forceful temperance advocate and political campaigner. As Gleed had predicted, wet interests mounted a drive to repeal constitutional prohibition, and he garnered national recognition in his efforts to stop them. Articulate and skillful on the platform, he ranged the state in a highly successful crusade to stay the antitemperance counterattack. In politics, Gleed was a Republican and always preferred to fight in his party's ranks instead of in the Prohibition Party. Thus, while he was never a member of the Anti-Saloon League, he was able to cooperate with the new group when it launched its nonpartisan dry campaign. And although some local Republican leaders were uncomfortable with Gleed's uncompromising stance, the ardent reformer did well enough in shaping party policy. In 1882, for example, he was largely responsible for a local Republican endorsement of a platform advocating prohibition and women's suffrage. Later in life, the demands of Gleed's successful legal practice forced him to devote less time to temperance affairs. But he always remained a loyal member of the Kansas Temperance Union and a staunch supporter of the dry cause.

**Bibliography:**

A. *The Wealth of the Spirit* (St. Louis, MO, 1922).
B. SEAP 3, 1112; WW 1, 461.

**GLENN, Robert Brodnax** (11 August 1854, Rockingham Co., NC—16 May 1920, Winnipeg, Canada). *Education*: studied at Davidson Coll., NC; Univ. of Virginia; Pearson's Law School, NC, 1870s. *Career*: legal practice, 1878–1905; U.S. attorney, Western District, North Carolina, 1893–97; member, North Carolina General Assembly, 1881; North Carolina state solicitor, 1886; officer, North Carolina National Guard, 1890–93; member, North Carolina Senate, 1899; governor of North Carolina, 1905–9; active lecturing and temperance work, 1909–20.

The son of a farmer, Robert Glenn never seriously considered agriculture as his own career. Rather, after academic preparation at a number of Southern institutions, he turned to the law. Practicing first in Danbury, North Carolina (1878–85), and then in Winston-Salem (1885–1905), he established one of the most noted legal reputations in his native state. He numbered among his clients some of the most important economic interests in the region, including the Southern Railway and Western Union. As is so often the case, professional and social prominence soon led to active political participation. Glenn was a loyal and hard-working Democrat, taking a leading role in North Carolina party affairs. He won election to the State Assembly in 1880, was an elector in every presidential election after 1884 until his death, and moved on to the North Carolina Senate in 1898. Aside from party politics and elected office, he also filled a number of other important posts, serving as a U.S. attorney and as an officer in the National Guard. When he won the governorship in 1905, then, Glenn brought· to the office a broad range of public and political service as well as an acknowledged ability to discern the strength of popular opinion on the issues of the day. It was in part this sense of public affairs that saw him quickly emerge as a zealously dry chief executive. Sentiment for prohibition had been building for some years in the Tar Heel State, and Glenn, long privately sympathetic to the antiliquor cause, made the liquor question a central issue of his administration. His unwavering stance against "the demon," as much as anything else, assured the legislative success of legal prohibition in North Carolina in 1908. Indeed, his term as governor alone was enough to mark Glenn as a temperance hero.

Yet Glenn's commitment to the dry crusade extended well beyond politics. He had genuine moral and religious bonds to the issue as well. After leaving

politics in 1909 he devoted his time to Presbyterian missionary work, but reformers sought him out, urging him to renew his efforts on behalf of the battle
against drink. He became a familiar figure on the national lecture circuit, and
he was particularly noted for his denunciation of the liquor traffic. Glenn's
speaking activities were such that he was in no sense in retirement any time
after stepping down as governor. In addition to lecturing, however, he also
assumed an organizational role in the movement. In 1913, the Anti-Saloon
League elected him a vice president, and he kept the post until his death. At no
time did he ever waver in his devotion to the Democratic Party, but he willingly
embraced the league's nonpartisan political techniques, and he had no qualms
over urging the election of individual dry Republicans over wet Democrats.
Glenn's visibility as a temperance leader was quite extensive by the time National
Prohibition became the law of the land. However, his greatest fame lay in his
native South, where other dry stalwarts counted him "among the foremost temperance leaders" of the region. While pursuing his reform activities, the former
governor never completely lost touch with other civic issues. He accepted an
appointment from his old college classmate, Woodrow Wilson, to the International Boundary Commission; and it was while attending one of its meetings in
Canada that he died in 1920.

**Bibliography:**

B. NYT, May 17, 1920; SEAP 3, 1113; WW 1, 461.

**GOODELL, David Harvey**     (6 May 1834, Hillsboro, NH—22 January 1915,
Antrim, NH). *Education*: studied at Brown Univ., 1852–53; A.M. (honorary),
Brown Univ., Dartmouth Coll., 1889. *Career*: schoolteacher and farmer, mid-
1850s; bookkeeper, treasurer, general agent, Antrim (NH) Shovel Co., 1850s
to 1864; founder and owner (with G. R. Carter) of D. H. Goodell & Co., 1864–
1915; member, New Hampshire House of Representatives, 1876–78; member,
New Hampshire Board of Agriculture, 1876–83; member, Governor's Council,
1883–85; governor of New Hampshire, 1889–91.

David Harvey Goodell's contribution to the Temperance Movement was chiefly
an indirect aspect of his involvement in the political life of his native state of
New Hampshire. The son of a prosperous family, the young Goodell had the
advantage of a good primary education as well as the financial means to support
two years of college study at Brown University. After leaving Brown in 1853,
he tried his hand successively at teaching and farming before going to work for
the Antrim, New Hampshire, Shovel Company as a bookkeeper. In this capacity,
Goodell soon revealed a genuine talent for business and rose steadily in the
company. Indeed, his acumen was such that by 1864 he was able (with a partner)
to open his own manufacturing firm, centering first on the production of an apple

parer he had invented. The venture prospered and eventually included seven factories turning out a diversified product line. As so often happens, success in business led to prominence in civil affairs and politics. In 1876, Goodall won election to the lower house of the New Hampshire legislature, and for the next quarter of a century he remained a fixture in the electoral fortunes of the state (as well as a firm Republican). Elected governor in 1889, it was in this office that the noted manufacturer began his public effort on behalf of the antiliquor crusade. He had been a staunch dry since his youth and a member of local temperance societies, but his energies went mostly into his business career and his antiliquor work was not notable. As governor, however, he was able to pursue his latent dry interests. He called prominently for the enforcement of New Hampshire liquor laws and drifted gradually toward an openly militant antiliquor stance. Upon retiring from politics, Goodell became president of the state Law and Order League (1895–1900), which aimed at strict enforcement of liquor statutes, and then worked on behalf of the Anti-Saloon League. The former governor was president of the New Hampshire League from 1902 to 1915, during which time he made numerous public appearances on behalf of the temperance cause. The dry movement credited him with being among the most effective advocates of prohibition in New England. Active in other civic causes as well, he was a trustee of Colby College and the recipient of honorary degrees from both Brown University and Dartmouth College.

**Bibliography:**

B. SEAP 3, 1118; WW 1, 467.

**GOODELL, William**    (25 October 1792, Conventry, NY—14 February 1878, Janesville, WI). *Education*: common schools, Pomfret, CT. *Career*: employed by mercantile firm in Providence, RI, Wilmington, NC, Alexandria, VA, 1817 to circa 1826; director, Mercantile Library Association, New York, 1827; editor, *Investigator and General Intelligencer*, Providence, RI, 1827–28 (merged with *National Philanthropist*, Boston, 1829); editor, *Genius of Temperance*, New York, beginning 1830; editor of various antislavery publications, including the *Emancipator*, beginning 1834; active reform lecturer and author, 1830s–1870s; minister and founder, nondenominational church, Honeoye, NY, 1843–47; co-founder, American Anti-Slavery Society, 1833, Liberty Party, 1840, and Prohibition Party, 1869.

Pious, dedicated, and zealously spirited, William Goodell pursued a career that marked him as an archtypical example of the nineteenth-century reformer. Possessing only a rudimentary education (the Goodells lacked the means to send their son to college), young William formed his early views of the world under the tutelage of his stern-willed and reform-minded grandmother. He also developed a love of libraries and literary pursuits that he held for the rest of his life. At eighteen years old, Goodell entered a mercantile house in Providence, Rhode Island, which led to a two-year voyage to Far Eastern and European ports. He stayed in business until the mid-1820s, when a venture of his own failed in Alexandria, Virginia. The disappointment proved a turning point in his life: It brought him north again (to New York City), where he found work as a bookkeeper and where he helped organize the Mercantile Library Association (which he directed for a time). Goodell also made the contacts he needed to launch himself to national prominence as a reformer, notably as an editor. In 1827, he learned of an opportunity to take over the Providence, Rhode Island, *Investigator and General Intelligencer*, and he soon established it as a successful journal. As editor, he turned the paper into an ardent voice of the fledgling Temperance Movement; indeed, in 1830, when he moved it to New York (after first merging it with the *National Philanthropist* of Boston), Goodell renamed the publication the *Genius of Temperance*. He also took to the lecture circuit. The dry reformer proved an able speaker, stimulating interest not only in the antiliquor movement but in his newspaper as well. As his reputation grew, so did his interests. The reforming publisher became a forceful champion of women's suffrage and antislavery, and over the 1830s his list of journals increased to include the *Female Advocate*, *Youth's Temperance Lecturer*, and the abolitionist papers the *Emancipator* and the *Friend of Man*. Behind this reforming zeal lay a deep spirituality. In fact, in the early 1840s the crusading editor even founded and preached in his own church, the foundation of which was the dignity and inviolability of the individual. Goodell had thus found his place in life: As a reformer, he had not only a political and spiritual commitment but also a substantial business interest in his publications and lecturing.

Goodell's pursuit of reform was tireless, and he proved instrumental in the founding of several important organizations. In 1833, he was a central figure in establishing the American Anti-Slavery Society, and in 1840 he followed his abolitionist bent into the new Liberty Party (which he also helped form). Indeed, he was the party's nominee for the governorship of New York shortly thereafter. Yet Goodell's views, while well in advance of contemporary public opinion, were not actually radical. Unlike William Lloyd Garrison,* for example, Goodell favored reform within existing social and political structures and was never willing to focus his energies upon a single issue. This penchant for diversity eventually led him to abandon the Liberty Party (1847), which he came to believe was too narrowly focused on abolitionism. As an alternative, he founded the Liberty League, which favored a broad spectrum of reforms ranging from peace, antislavery, and tariff revision to land and liquor reform. After the Civil War, he took part in the revival of the dry crusade and worked to make the Prohibition Party a reality in 1869. The following year, he moved to Janesville, Wisconsin, in order to be near his daughters in his later years. All the while, however, he continued to write and to speak on the reform issues of the day. He was honored as a gallant pioneer of the cause in the ranks of temperance crusaders, and reformers generally mourned his passing in 1878. Born only three years after the establishment of the Union under the Constitution, Goodell had lived through the Civil War that preserved it and the centennial of its Independence. And during the greater part of his long life, few Americans were more representative of the great ferment of freedom that so shaped the development of the young republic.

**Bibliography:**

A. *Views Upon American Constitutional Law, in Its Bearing Upon American Slavery* (New York, 1844); *The Democracy of Christianity*, 2 vols. (Honeoye, NY? 1849); *Slavery and Anti-Slavery: A History of the Great Struggle in Both Hemispheres* (1852); *The American Slave Code, in Theory and Practice* (1853).

B. DAB 7, 384–85; SEAP 3, 1118; WW H, 278; Henry Wilson, *History of the Rise and Fall of the Slave Power in America*, vol. 1 (Boston, 1872).

**GORDON, Adoniram Judson**   (19 April 1836, New Hampton, NH—2 February 1895, Boston, MA). *Education*: B.A., Brown Univ., 1860; B.D., Newton Theological Sem., 1863. *Career*: ordained as Baptist minister, 1863; minister, Jamaica Plain, MA, 1863–69; minister, Clarendon Street Baptist Church, Boston, 1869–95.

A Baptist clergyman, the Reverend Adoniram Judson Gordon liked to preface his temperance addresses on the sin of drink by urging his listeners to recognize it for the evil it was and not to "legalize it with the revenue stamp of the state." This view typified Gordon's approach to the liquor question of his generation, preferring to attack it from the pulpit rather than through any of the organized prohibition or temperance groups. The ardent Baptist's interest in the dry debate stemmed primarily from his theological background. Baptists generally lent their denominational strength against "the demon," and Gordon was one of the most prominent Baptist clergy of the day. Well educated and with five years of experience in the pulpit, he took over the well-to-do but theologically sedate Clarendon Street Church in Boston in 1869. He remained there for the rest of his life, building it into a center of evangelical activity and rising to national recognition in the process. Gordon's activities ranged a gamut of social and church concerns. His revival meetings attracted large audiences of the faithful, and he spoke effectively on behalf of aid to Chinese immigrants, women's suffrage, urban relief work among Boston's tenement dwellers, and other philanthropic efforts. This concern for the quality of life, both temporal and spiritual, accounted for many of his statements on the Temperance Movement and closely linked the dry cause to other reforms. Indeed, he became one of the most accomplished reformers in the Boston area.

The church, however, always remained Gordon's first concern. He devoted a major effort to fostering foreign mission work, especially in the Congo and China. He served for years (1871–94) on the executive committee of the American Baptist Missionary Board and in 1889 organized a training center of his own for missionary endeavors (the Boston Missionary Training-School). Gordon also placed great faith in the efficacy of interdenominational revivals. He worked closely with evangelical leaders from other Protestant groups, and openly professed his millennial faith. The Second Coming, he believed, was not far distant. Indeed, as historians of his career have pointed out, he placed little enduring value on theories of social progress, as he insisted that the Bible pointed toward the imminent coming of the end anyway (perhaps explaining his reluctance to join temperance or other social reform organizations with long-term goals). Gordon was, however, a prolific and effective writer on religious matters. He authored a number of books and pamphlets, mostly devoted to mission work or millenial themes, and he edited the *Missionary Review of the World* as well as the *Watchword* (a stridently millennial publication). Within his deliberately limited sphere, then, Gordon was an effective and persistent reform and dry advocate. His major perspective, though, was spiritual, and in his labors on earth he always kept firmly in view the new world soon to come.

### Bibliography:

A. *In Christ, or the Believer's Union with His Lord* (Boston, 1872); *Grace and Glory* (Boston, 1881); *The Twofold Life* (Boston, 1883); *Ecce Venit* (New York, 1889); *Ministry of the Spirit (Philadelphia, 1894); Yet Speaking* (New York, 1897).

B. DARB, 176–77; NCAB 11, 263; SEAP 3, 1119; WW H, 280; Ernest B. Gordon, *Adoniram Judson Gordon: A Biography* (New York, 1896).

**GORDON, Anna Adams**    (21 July 1853, Boston, MA—15 June 1931, Castile, NY). *Education*: studied at Mt. Holyoke Sem., 1871–72; studied at Lasell Sem., MA, 1875; DHL. (honorary), Northwestern Univ., 1924. *Career*: private secretary to Frances E. Willard, 1877–98; full-time temperance work, especially with youth groups, beginning 1877; president, National Woman's Christian Temperance Union, 1914–25; president, World's WCTU, beginning 1922.

Although she was reared a Congregationalist, in her later years Anna Gordon converted to Methodism. Indeed, religion always played a central role in Gordon's life, setting the tone for her work on behalf of the antiliquor crusade. Initially, she had hoped for a musical career as an organist and had in fact spent a year in Europe studying music. But she abandoned these ambitions when, at a revival meeting in Dwight L. Moody's* Boston Tabernacle in 1877, she had a chance meeting with Frances E. Willard.* The young Gordon made an immediate impression on the rising temperance crusader; so spontaneous and reciprocal was the rapport between them that Gordon gave up her musical goals to devote her career to serving as Willard's closest intimate and indispensable aide-de-camp. She was Willard's private secretary until 1898, the year the famous WCTU leader died. Gordon's career in temperance rose with the fortunes of Willard, and when the latter assumed the presidency of the WCTU in 1879, Gordon's star concomitantly brightened. The two were inseparable, not only living together in Evanston, Illinois, but travelling around the United States giving speeches, organizing, inspiring, and in general advancing the cause of temperance. Gordon's special interest was children's work, especially the union's youth organization, the Loyal Temperance Legion. On its behalf she wrote any number of songs and tracts, so that one might say that she had not left her music entirely behind. In recognition of her youth work, in 1891 she was named superintendent of youth activities for the World's WCTU.

As a trusted intimate of Willard, Gordon emerged as something of a power in the National WCTU, invariably supporting the positions and views of her revered leader even when they were unpopular among some of the rank and file. On the death of Willard in 1898, many union members considered it natural that the one who had been so closely associated with her would assume the mantle of the fallen leader. Instead, the presidency went to Lillian M.N.A. Stevens.* If Gordon resented this it did not show, although she was never especially close to Stevens on a personal basis. She continued her work with children, founding the Young Campaigners for Prohibition in 1910. In addition, she labored over a hagiographical life of Willard, *The Beautiful Life of Frances E. Willard*, published in 1898. She also managed to obtain state holidays in honor of Willard's birthday, and it was largely through Gordon's efforts that her beloved mentor joined the nation's illustrious statesmen, writers, and humanitarians by representation in Statuary Hall in Washington, D.C., and the National Hall of Fame in New York City. Anna Gordon became national president of the WCTU in 1914, and she used her office to push vigorously for a National Prohibition amendment by coupling prohibition with patriotism. The achievement of this goal turned her attention to other reforms, notably child welfare, the Americanization of immigrants, and women workers. Her indefatigable energies, even late in life, can be seen in 1923, when she publicly poured three hundred bottles of bootleg whiskey down a sewer in Cleveland, and in 1924, when she successfully completed a million-dollar fund-raising drive for the WCTU. She also took the lead in a campaign that built union membership to over a million women. In 1922 Gordon was elected president of the World's WCTU and travelled to South America and Mexico carrying the message of temperance and prohibition. She retired from active work in 1925 and in 1931 died at the age of seventy-seven.

**Bibliography:**

A. *The Beautiful Life of Frances E. Willard* (Chicago, 1898); ed., *What Frances E. Willard Said* (Evanston, IL, 1905); *What Lillian M. N. Stevens Said* (Evanston, IL, 1914).

B. NAW 2, 63–64; SEAP 3, 1119–20; WW 1, 470; Benjamin F. Austin, ed., *The Prohibition Leaders of America* (n.p., 1895); Julia Freeman Deane, *Anna Adams Gordon: A Story of Her Life* (Evanston, IL, 193?); Helen E. Tyler, *Where Prayer and Purpose Meet: The W.C.T.U. Story* (Evanston, IL, 1949).

**GOUGAR, Helen Mar Jackson**    (18 July 1843, Litchfield, MI—6 June 1907, Lafayette, IN). *Education*: studied at Hillsdale Coll., MI, 1855–58; A.M. (honorary), Hillsdale Coll., 1862; studied law with husband, John D. Gougar, 1870s–

1890s. *Career*: schoolteacher, Lafayette, IN, 1859–63; legal work in husband's office, 1890s; active reform lecturing and writing, 1880s to 1907.

Helen Gougar was one of those figures in the Temperance Movement who began by showing little apparent promise and then, quite without warning, blossomed into a major dry advocate. Mrs. Gougar began life in Litchfield, Michigan, in 1843, and after being compelled to leave Hillsdale College before she could finish her studies, she faced a life of public school teaching in Lafayette, Indiana. But in 1863 she met and married John D. Gougar, a well-known member of the Indiana bar. From this point on Helen Gougar's life took on a new direction and a new dimension. With the help of her husband, Mrs. Gougar began to study law and soon revealed a remarkable legal mind. She combined her outstanding legal ability with a fervent interest in women's suffrage and prohibition. She proved a tireless campaigner. Her efforts in Indiana on behalf of both measures were second to none, and she worked closely with some of the prominent reformers of her region (notably Zarelda Wallace*). By 1881 Gougar was reaching peak form, and she lobbied for both issues to be submitted to a popular referendum. Gougar in the meantime had become one of the most articulate voices of the Indiana Woman's Christian Temperance Union, and under its banner she plunged into the affairs of the 1882 Republican state convention. She was able to win the party's endorsement for both suffrage and temperance, but all for naught as the Democrats won that year's election. It was an especially vicious contest, with the Democrats singling out Gougar (they knew who their most able opponents were) for a smear campaign. She responded by suing successfully for five thousand dollars, although the experience reportedly took a heavy emotional toll on the ardent reformer.

Mrs. Gougar was far from through, however. She embarked on a national lecture tour on behalf of women's suffrage and prohibition. She especially favored the vote for women because she felt that only women could stem the rising tide of the urban masses that seemed bent in the late 1880s and 1890s (in her mind) on revolution. Becoming disenchanted with the Republicans due to their conservatism on what she considered the pressing national issues of the day (the national party would push hard for neither suffrage nor prohibition), she left them for the Prohibition Party in 1888. The broad reform interests of the smaller party appealed to her, but the change of allegiance was the beginning of a political peregrination for Gougar. Ever the reform enthusiast, over the next decade she would wander from the Prohibitionists to the Populists, to Free-Silver, and finally to the Democrats in a vain search for a party that would espouse unreservedly the suffrage and prohibition movements. She was forever doomed to disappointment. Afterward, she would confine herself to writing books and articles for such temperance publications as *Our Herald* and travelling widely around the United States and the world on behalf of her favorite causes. These trips resulted in a wistfully titled book, *Forty Thousand Miles of World Wandering*, in 1905. Like many reformers of her time, her positions tended to be mixed so that she could at one and the same time oppose American imperialism in the Philippines and Oriental immigration into the United States. Mrs. Gougar died of a heart attack in 1907, and her best epitaph would probably have been the description once given her by an admirer, ''a born agitator, leader, and reformer.''

**Bibliography:**

A. *The Constitutional Rights of the Women of Indiana. An Argument in . . . Superior Court . . . , 1895* (Fairfield, IN, 1895); *Forty Thousand Miles of Wandering* (Chicago, 1905; rev. ed., 1913).
B. NAW 2, 69–71; SEAP 3, 1125; WW 1, 473.

**GOUGH, John Bartholomew**    (22 August 1817, Sandgate, Kent, England— 18 February 1886, Frankfort, PA). *Education*: partial elementary schooling in Britain; A.M. (honorary), Amherst Coll. *Career*: bookbinder and itinerant actor, 1830s to 1843; temperance lecturer, from 1843.

Gough was one of the most flamboyant figures in the annals of the temperance reform, and his career as a temperance lecturer was a continuing wonder to thousands in both the wet and dry camps. He immigrated to the United States at age twelve and in his teens began a career as a bookbinder and itinerant actor in New York and New England. A confirmed drunkard, he lived in dire poverty until 1842, when, during the Washingtonian revival in Massachusetts, a temperance worker induced him to take the pledge and reform. In 1843, the newly rehabilitated alcoholic launched a career as a temperance lecturer, bringing to the public rostrum a style marked by an intense delivery enlivened by graphic descriptions of his own battle with the bottle. Like the Washingtonians, Gough saw drunkenness as a disease, and his often lurid discourses on its evils frequently shocked his audiences and excited wide comment among both friends and enemies of temperance. His fame—and his fortune from lecture fees—steadily mounted, even surviving a widely reported binge—the result, he later claimed, of wets tricking him into taking a drink. He took the pledge anew and after major appearances in New York and, in 1844, in Boston on behalf of the Washingtonians, he rose to national stature. In the 1850s he made three successful tours of Britain, while in America his popularity became such that, in his later career, he included nontemperance subjects in his presentations. A tireless speaker to the end, he delivered over 8,600 addresses before collapsing with a stroke in the middle of a speech in 1886.

Over the course of his career, Gough gradually changed his thinking on the best means of eliminating alcohol problems. Although he later claimed to have held prohibitionist views from the beginning, his early lectures emphasized the ''moral suasionist'' approaches of the Washingtonians. That is, rather than relying exclusively on prohibitory legislation—''legal suasion''—as a solution to drunkenness, he urged temperance advocates to work driectly with alcoholics for their social, physical, and spiritual rehabilitation. At one point, he even clashed with other antiliquor crusaders over the effectiveness of the prohibitory Maine Law. But as his reputation spread, he increasingly stressed the importance of legal measures. And despite charges from some moral suasionists that he had abandoned Washingtonianism, Gough insisted that prohibition was a necessary adjunct to individual rehabilitation efforts. He never repudiated the Washingtonian approach, but he argued that only the elimination of the liquor traffic would ensure the safety of reformed drunkards, and he accordingly lent his support to the Prohibition Party after the Civil War. His shift away from full reliance on individual reform to a stress on political action against beverage alcohol was indicative of a national trend in temperance thought during the late nineteenth century.

**Bibliography:**

A. *Autobiography and Personal Recollections of John B. Gough, with Twenty-six Years Experience as a Public Speaker* (1846; Springfield, MA., 1870, and many subsequent editions); *Temperance Address* (New York, 1870); *Sunlight and Shadow: Or, Gleanings from My Life Work ... (Hartford, CT, 1883); Platform Echoes: Or, Leaves from My Notebook of Forty Years*, ed. Lyman Abbott (Hartford, CT, 1885).

B. DAB 7, 445–46; SEAP 3, 1125–27; John Marsh, *Temperance Recollections, Labors, Defeats, Triumphs: An Autobiography* (New York, 1866); Carlos Martyn, *John B. Gough: The Apostle of Gold Water* (New York, 1893); Honore W. Morrow, *Tiger! Tiger!: The Life Story of John B. Gough (New York, 1930).*

**GRADY, Henry Woodfin**    (1 December 1832, Athens, GA—23 December 1889, Atlanta, GA). *Education*: graduated from Univ. of Georgia, 1862; studied law, Univ. of Virginia, 1868–69. *Career*: reporter, *Courier* (Rome, GA), 1871; editor-publisher, *Daily-Commercial*, 1871; co-founder, *Atlanta* (GA) *Herald*, 1872; reporter, *New York Herald*, 1876–77; quarter owner, *Atlanta Constitution*, 1879–89; active lecturing on behalf of the South, 1879–89.

Publicist, journalist, and booster, Henry W. Grady's most persistent devotion was to his native South. Although trained for the law at the University of Virginia, he was never admitted to the bar. Instead, he began an ebullient and successful career as reporter, editor, and publisher, mostly in Georgia, where he was born in 1850. Grady's father was killed in the Civil War, but unlike many Southerners, Grady bore no grudge against the North. Instead, he subscribed to the simple but effective philosophy of joining those you can't lick. And it was this unswerving belief in the capacity of the South to rise again that gave Grady his permanent place in American history. After a brief introduction to journalism as a reporter for a Rome, Georgia, newspaper, Grady embarked on a long search for a paper of his own suitable to his rather considerable talents. First, he bought two papers in Rome and combined them into the *Daily-Commercial*. It quickly failed. He then joined several other like-minded young men and went to Atlanta and founded the *Atlanta Herald*. It met the same fate. Somewhat chastened, Grady returned to reporting for such papers as the *Atlanta Constitution* and the *Augusta Chronicle*, and for a time (1876–77), as special reporter for the *New York Herald*.

Grady's career, it seemed, was destined to run in professionally solid but unexceptional channels.

Yet in 1879 his fortunes took a sudden and dramatic turn. Former Confederate General John B. Gordon introduced the journalist to communications mogul Cyrus W. Field. Field was impressed with the young Southerner and loaned him $20,000 to purchase a quarter interest in the *Atlanta Constitution*. For Grady, it was the opportunity of a lifetime. He emerged as a thoroughly accomplished publisher with a knack for developing stories that gripped the popular imagination. Most particularly, he used his position with the *Constitution* to build the platform for a new Southern political creed—one he never ceased promoting until his untimely death in 1889 at the age of thirty-nine. He christened the idea the "New South." Basically, he argued that the ex-Confederate states ought to abandon the myth of moonlight and magnolias and come into the industrialized modern era. This meant a reexamination of race relations in the South, an end to sentimental doting on the "lost cause," and the strengthening of the regional economy (Grady was especially concerned about the South's overdependence upon cotton production). Instead, he insisted, the new road to prosperity lay in industrialization, modernization, transportation, and diversification of crops. All these themes Grady proclaimed endlessly in speech after speech, editorial after editorial, lecture after lecture, bearing such titles as "The New South," "The South and Her Problems," "The Solid South," "The Farmer and the Cities," "The Race Problem and the South." The appeal of his doctrine was enormous (it made him a national celebrity), and unquestionably, Grady was the prophet and harbinger of a new breed of Southerner, one who looked forward rather than backward. The modern South owes much to the legacy of Henry W. Grady's New South creed.

Grady also considered that temperance would be a part of the New South. He had always been a total abstainer, and he fully embraced prohibition as in the national and Southern well-being. Indeed, Grady's endorsement helped give the Temperance Movement a credence it had lacked in the South. Before the Civil War, Northern temperance affiliations with the abolitionist movement had made the dry crusade highly suspect below the Mason-Dixon Line, and Maine Law and other antiliquor legislation never took hold. Yet in Grady's view, the New South required sobriety as well as capital, and he firmly believed that a dry South would be a progressive and prosperous South. (Many of the same motives were behind the temperance sentiments of some Northern industrial leaders.) As an individual, Grady was an outspoken champion of the dry cause, although the dividend ownership of the *Constitution* never spoke with a single voice on the question. Grady was a powerful force, however, in the contest over local option in Atlanta. When the city outlawed the saloon locally, the journalist defended the measure, as might be expected, on economic grounds. Prohibition, he claimed, had made Atlanta more efficient, freer of crime than ever before, a more profitable place of business and had brought its citizens a higher standard of living. It was an impressive boast but indicative of Grady's penchant for emphasizing the bright side of the South. Eventually, his nonstop efforts on behalf of his native region undermined his health, and in 1889 Grady died of pneumonia, which he had contracted on one of his speaking tours.

**Bibliography:**

A. *The Speeches of Henry W. Grady, with a Short Biographical Sketch of His Life* (Atlanta, GA, 1895); *The Complete Orations and Speeches of Henry W. Grady*, ed. Edwin Du Bois Shafter (Austin, TX, 1910); *The New South: Writings and Speeches of Henry Grady* (Savannah, GA, 1971).

B. DAB 7, 465–66; SEAP 3, 1129–30; WW H, 282; Joel Chandler Harris, *Joel Chandler Harris' Life of Henry Grady, Including His Writings and Speeches* (New York, 1890); Raymond Blalock Nixon, *Henry W. Grady: Spokesman of the South* (New York, 1943); Russell Franklin Terrell, *A Study of the Early Journalistic Writings of Henry W. Grady* (Nashville, TN, 1927).

**GREELEY, Horace**   (3 February 1811, Amherst, NH—29 November 1872, Pleasantville, NY). *Career*: printer's apprentice, VT, 1822–30; printer, New York, 1831–33; publisher, with Francis Story, the *Post* (NY), 1833; founder and publisher, *The New Yorker*, 1834–41; editor, *The Jeffersonian* (NY), 1838; editor, *The Log Cabin* (NY), 1840; founder and publisher, *New York Tribune*, 1841–72; member, U.S. House of Representatives, 1848; president, New York Printers Union, 1850.

Unquestionably one of the giants of American journalism, Horace Greeley began his newspaper career in modest fashion indeed. Born in New Hampshire in 1811, Greeley never mustered more than a common school education, although he early manifested a talent for pithy expression and a facility for spelling. When Greeley was eleven, his father was compelled to flee the state owing to financial difficulties, and young Horace set out to apprentice himself to local printers. But it was not until he was fourteen that he was able to enter the profession in which he was to spend the rest of his life. Greeley began work as an apprentice printer with the East Poultney, Vermont, *Northern Spectator*, where within a few months he was earning all of forty dollars a year, most of which he sent his father. Yet the young Greeley showed an aptitude for newspaper work, and when the *Northern Spectator* folded in 1830, he began to seek his fortune elsewhere. It was in 1831 that he arrived in New York City, the place with which his name is forever associated. At the time he had but ten dollars in his pocket but a burning desire to succeed. Taking on a variety of jobs at a number of New York papers, among them the *Evening Post*, the *Commercial Advertiser*, and the *Spirit of the Times*, he quickly moved into enterpreneurial ranks. With a fellow printer, Francis V. Story, Greeley took over the *Post*, but it soon failed. After Story's death, Greeley joined with Jonas Winchester to publish *The New Yorker*, a weekly which soon became the "best literary weekly in America." As a force in American journalism, Greeley's star was now rising fast.

Greeley had always had a taste for politics, and when in the 1830s a number of New York Whigs headed by William Seward and Thurlow Weed urged him to set up a mouthpiece for the state party, Greeley eagerly undertook the task. The *Jeffersonian* and the *Log Cabin* became the best known and most successful of the party papers, reaching circulations of upwards of ninety thousand. In 1841, Greeley, now a well-known figure in New York, launched the *Tribune*, and it became one of the journalistic wonders of the age. He insisted on greatly improved standards of reporting, reducing the sensationalism that characterized much of the era's press coverage. But perhaps the most noted feature of the *Tribune* was the editorial page, which Greeley used freely to air his views on the issues of the day. And his views were frequently on the unorthodox side. He committed his name, and often his money, to the causes of labor, experimental uptopian communities, antislavery, tariff protection for American industry, vegetarianism, temperance, political reform, and Western settlement (he coined the phrase, "Go West, young man, go West!"), to cite only some of his interests. During the Civil War, his support of Lincoln was always lukewarm at best, and his devotion to the Union was not unalloyed (although once the fighting began, he was a vigorous champion of Northern victory). Greeley thought even less of U. S. Grant, and he allowed himself to be nominated by the Liberal Republicans and Democrats for the presidency against Grant in 1872. Greeley, however, was in ill health. The campaign was a fiasco and Greeley shortly withdrew, and he died within weeks of Grant's smashing electoral triumph.

**Bibliography:**

A. *The American Laborer* (1843; New York, 1974); *Hints Toward Reform* (New York, 1850); with Robert Dale Owen, *Divorce* (New York, 1860); *Alcoholic Liquors: Their Essential Nature and Necessary Effects on the Human Constitution* (New York, 1870); *Essays Designed to Elucidate the Science of Political Economy* (New York, 1870); *Horace Greeley: His First Autobiography with Memoirs of His Late Years and Death* (Brooklyn, NY, 1873).

B. SEAP 3, 1144–46; WW H, 285; William Mason Cornell, *The Life and Public Career of Hon. Horace Greeley* (Boston, 1872); Don Carlos Seitz, *Horace Greeley: Founder of the New York Tribune* (Indianapolis, IN, 1926); Henry Luther Stoddard, *Horace Greeley: Printer, Editor, Crusader* (New York, 1946); Glyndon Garlock Van Deusen, *Horace Greeley: Nineteenth-Century Crusader* (Philadelphia, 1953).

**GREENWOOD, Elizabeth Ward**    (6 February 1850, Brooklyn, NY—?). *Education*: graduated from Brooklyn Heights Sem., 1869; studied at Univ. of Chicago Divinity Sch., 1870s. *Career*: full-time evangelical work for Woman's Christian Temperance Union, 1870s to 1912?

Constancy and devotion were the career hallmarks of Elizabeth Ward Greenwood. Her life centered on but one interest exclusive of all others: evangelism on behalf of the Temperance Movement. Born in 1850 in Brooklyn, New York, we know few details of her early life beyond the fact that she received a comparatively good education. She graduated from the local Brooklyn Heights Seminary in 1869, the nature of her alma mater suggesting an already strong spiritual character in the young woman. Her decision to pursue further studies at the Divinity School of the University of Chicago underscored the trait. Thereafter, Greenwood, who never married, focused her life's work on religious concerns. The vehicle for her activities was the Woman's Christian Temperance Union, which placed a strong emphasis on evangelical work (much of it, when directed at drinkers and alcoholics, was referred to as ''gospel temperance''). Her enthusiasm won her the praise of other temperance advocates, and over the years Greenwood took on a number of prominent WCTU leadership assignments. From 1887 to 1912 she was superintendent of evangelical work for both the National and World's WCTU. In addition, she was president of the Brooklyn chapter of the union for some thirty-four years, as well as serving as superintendent of scientific temperance instruction in the state organization. In this role, she played an important part in the passage of legislation mandating temperance lessons in New York State public schools. Greenwood, however, did not restrict her evangelical work to New York. She took her mission work into jails, asylums, and refuges of the unfortunate all over the United States and in many countries abroad. For over two decades (1887 to 1912) she also was an active summer preacher in Connecticut pulpits. By any measure, she was among the most devout reformers and a true workhorse of the dry movement. She followed the light wherever it led, bringing solace and relief to those most in need. It was, given her work on behalf of others, a somewhat bitter twist of fate that allowed her passing to her final reward to go unrecorded by any notable source, temperance or otherwise.

**Bibliography:**

B. WW 4, 380.

**GRUNDY, Felix**   (11 September 1777, Berkeley Co., VA—19 December 1840, Nashville, TN). *Career*: admitted to bar, KY, 1797; legal practice, beginning 1797; member, Kentucky House of Representatives, 1799–1806; associate justice, Kentucky Supreme Court of Errors and Appeals, 1806–7; member, U.S. House of Representatives (from TN), 1811–15; member, Tennessee House of Representatives, 1819–25; member, U.S. Senate, 1829–38, 1839–40; U.S. attorney general, 1838.

Felix Grundy was part of the ferment of freedom in the presidency of Andrew Jackson that historians have come to call the Age of the Common Man. Grundy himself was almost a paradigm of the rise of this common man in America, for he was born into a frontier family in Virginia and lived most of his life in the frontier states of Kentucky and Tennessee. He was largely self-taught, but his talents were quickly realized. After apprenticing himself to an attorney, Grundy was admitted to the bar of Kentucky at the age of twenty. After that his rise was meteoric. At twenty-two he was chosen to attend the state's constitutional convention in 1799, followed by election to the Kentucky legislature. In 1806 he was an associate justice on the Kentucky Supreme Court, and soon its chief justice. By the time he was thirty, when most men are just embarking on their chosen career, Grundy left the court to set himself up in the lucrative practice of criminal law. He was soon one of the most brilliant trial lawyers in the state of Tennessee, which now became his adopted home. Such was his prowess that only one of his 165 defendants tried in capital cases went to the gallows. But politics called, and as relations between the United States and Great Britain became embittered during the Napoleonic Wars, Grundy left the bar for Congress in 1811 and served two terms. It was a fateful time. Grundy aligned himself with the young Henry Clay, and together with others of similar persuasion, they came to be known as the War Hawks. They played an instrumental role in bringing on the War of 1812 with Great Britain. Grundy was in and out of politics for the next few years. In the legislature of Tennessee he ran afoul of fellow Democrat Andrew Jackson over easy credit for farmers—Grundy was for it, Jackson against it. When Jackson entered the presidency in 1829, Grundy won election to the Senate. Yet the two Tennessee politicians were never close. The two clashed again over Nullification—Jackson against, Grundy in favor. Grundy ended his political career, ironically, as attorney general under Martin Van Buren, a Jackson intimate.

Grundy's activities on behalf of the Temperance Movement were in some respects limited. Aside from the Congressional Temperance Society, of which he was one of the ten vice presidents, he never belonged to any dry organization. Yet his influence as a national leader was such that his antiliquor sentiments, which were indeed public, lent weight to the cause and in fact offered an excellent view of the ideology of a number of early dry enthusiasts. Grundy was a total abstainer, a position which, in his day, was not universally accepted even in temperance ranks. This preference, however, came from convictions deeper than a personal aversion to drink. For the Tennessee lawyer also had a political perspective on the liquor question that placed him in the same reform category as Benjamin Rush* and a number of the Founding Fathers: He believed that drunkenness was a threat to the republic. The "corruption of public morals," he once proclaimed, was the "deadliest foe to the prosperity of our country," and he classed intemperance as one of the surest corruptors. He called for an end to the drinking of toasts on the Fourth of July, praising such public abstinence as "truly republican." Grundy was also acquainted with some of the most prominent temperance leaders of the day and occasionally spoke at their meetings. He helped organize the Congressional Temperance Society in 1833 and applauded the growth of local temperance groups throughout the nation. His death came as the antiliquor crusade was becoming a political force to be reckoned with, and the temperance leaders of a later day looked back with gratitude on the early support rendered by the senator from Tennessee.

**Bibliography:**

B. DAB 8, 32–33; SEAP 3, 1154–55; WW H, 292; Joshua William Caldwell, *Sketches of the Bench and Bar of Tennessee* (Knoxville, TN, 1898); Joseph Howard Parks, *Felix Grundy: Champion of Democracy* (Baton Rouge, LA, 1940).

# H

HAGGARD, Howard Wilcox   (18 July 1891, La Porte, IN—22 April 1959, Fort Lauderdale, FL). *Education*: Ph.B., Yale Univ., 1914; M.D., Yale Univ., 1917. *Career*: physiologist, U.S. Bureau of Mines, 1917, 1919–22; captain, Chemical Warfare Service, U.S. army, 1917–18; instructor in physiology, Yale Univ. Medical Sch., 1919–23; assistant professor, Yale Univ., 1923–26; associate professor of applied physiology, Sheffield Scientific Sch., Yale Univ., 1926–38; director, Laboratory of Applied Physiology, Yale Univ., 1926–56; director, Yale Univ. Office of Development, 1948–51; active consulting and writing activities, 1920s–1950s.

Howard Haggard is one of the truly pivotal figures in the history of America's efforts to deal with its longstanding "liquor question." His career stands as a major benchmark in the evolution of modern thinking on alcohol problems—a path away from prohibitory temperance approaches and toward the research and treatment emphases that came to dominate debate on the subject in the last half of the twentieth century. Haggard's interest in alcohol research stemmed from his training and experience as a physiologist, a discipline in which he had superb credentials. Educated at Yale University, where he earned a bachelor's and a medical degree, he served during World War I as a captain in the army Chemical Warfare Service. He then returned to his alma mater, where he based the rest of his career. The young doctor joined the faculty of the Yale Medical School as an instructor of physiology, rose to associate professor of applied physiology in 1922, and compiled a record distinguished enough to merit appointment as director of the university's Laboratory of Applied Physiology in 1926. He held that post, in addition to other positions, until his death thirty years later. His work at Yale was impressive. In much of it, he was a close associate of Professor Yandell Henderson* in the relatively new field of respiratory physiology, especially as it related to mining. He did pioneer work in mine rescue, the prevention of industrial poisoning, ventilation of vehicular tunnels, decompression in deep sea diving, and resuscitation from drowning, gassing, and electric shock. His accomplishments in research were equalled by his brilliance as a teacher, and several generations of students at Yale recalled him with admiration and affection.

Haggard also maintained a significant interest in the effects of alcohol on the human system, some aspects of which he began to study at the Laboratory of Applied Physiology in 1930. His studies led him to the not surprising conclusion that alcoholism was more than a merely medical or biological phenomenon. But the insight led him to found a Section of Alcohol Studies within his laboratory, a unit which later evolved into the Yale (now Rutgers) Center of Alcohol Studies. Haggard took a number of other critical steps as well: He brought E. M. Jellinek,* the great modern theoretician of alcoholism, to Yale as the section's first director; he established, with Jellinek, the Summer School of Alcohol Studies (now also at Rutgers); he inaugurated the *Journal of Studies on Alcohol* and served as its first editor; and he supervised the opening of the Yale Plan Clinics, which produced some of the best scientific studies of alcoholism in the years following World War II. Haggard, then, stood at the center of events that put the alcohol studies field on its modern scientific footing. It is testimony to his character, though, that he always maintained a wide range of interests, and he was seldom dominated solely by one of them. He loved medical history, for example, and took pains to write it in ways that would enlighten the general public as well as his colleagues in academia. His *Devils, Drugs, and Doctors* (1929) and *Mystery, Magic, and Medicine* (1933) remain two of the more reliable popular histories of medicine. In similar fashion, he was the author or editor of a number of publications aimed at rekindling public thinking on alcohol problems, a subject unpopular since the collapse of National Prohibition. That the topic became an increasingly lively field of popular controversy in his lifetime was in great measure testimony to Haggard's ultimate success.

**Bibliography:**

A. *Are You Intelligent?* (New Haven, CT, 1926); *Devils, Drugs, and Doctors* (1929; New York, 1959); *The Science of Health and Disease: A Textbook of Physiology and Hygiene*, rev. ed. (New York, 1938); with E. M. Jellinek, *Alcohol Explored* (Garden City, NY, 1942); with E. M. Jellinek, eds., *Alcohol, Science, and Society* (New Haven, CT, 1946); *The Physician and the Alcoholic* (n.p., 1946).

B. NYT, April 23, 1959; *Journal of the American Medical Association* 170 (1959): 1439; *Quarterly Journal of Studies on Alcohol* 20 (1959): 211–12; *Time* 73 (1959): 86; *Wilson Library Bulletin* 33 (1959): 726; Max J. Herzberg, *The Reader's Encyclopedia of American Literature* (New York, 1966).

**HAINES, William Thomas**    (7 August 1854, Levant, ME—4 June 1919, Waterville, ME). *Education*: A.B., Univ. of Maine, 1876; LLB., Univ. of Albany, 1878; LLD. (honorary), Univ. of Maine, 1899. *Career*: legal practice, Waterville, ME, beginning 1879; interests in banking, lumber, and manufacturing businesses, beginning 1880s; Kennebec Co. attorney, 1883–87; member, Maine State Senate, 1889–93; member, Maine House of Representatives, 1895; state attorney general, 1897–1901; member, State Governor's Executive Council, 1901–5; governor of Maine, 1913–14.

William Thomas Haines was a Downeaster whose whole career was spent in the state of Maine. A successful lawyer and businessman, Haines saw prohibition as part of the work ethic and a guard against economic waste and social disorder. Like so many other temperance advocates, he used his limited sphere of influence as a local politician and citizen effectively in promoting the dry cause. After graduation from law school in 1878, Haines set up practice in Waterville, Maine, and entered Republican politics as Kennebec County attorney in 1882. The young lawyer subsequently moved through a succession of offices, including state senator, attorney general, and finally governor of the state in 1913. All this time, Haines kept faith with Maine's prohibition laws, even when other politicians were adverse to enforcing them. Indeed, the issue on which Haines won his gubernatorial victory was prohibition. During the campaign, the Democrats had wanted to do away with state-wide prohibition and to replace it with local option. Haines insisted that the issue was long past debate and promised strict enforcement of the existing statutes. Once in office, he read his election as a popular mandate to do just that. His stand was bitterly resented by some local leaders (especially in areas where illegal liquor had previously enjoyed a safe haven), but the governor went ahead with an enforcement effort that had some notable successes. He had no fewer than three county sheriffs and one county attorney whom he considered corrupt or lax (or both) impeached, and there is little doubt that respect for Maine's dry codes gained considerable strength. Haines is not remembered as one of the state's great governors, but he did make his contribution to the national drive for prohibition in the early decades of the twentieth century, and he had the political courage to shape his public policies in accord with his personal moral convictions. For that, he earned the thanks of dry spokesmen nationally.

**Bibliography:**

B. SEAP 3, 1166; WW 1, 501.

**HALE, Edward Everett**    (3 April 1822, Boston, MA—10 June 1909, Boston, MA). *Education*: A.B, Harvard Univ., 1839; private studies for ministry, 1839–42; STD. (honorary), Harvard Univ., 1879; LLD. (honorary), Williams Coll., 1904. *Career*: minister, Church of the Unity, Worcester, MA, 1846–56; active writing on reform subjects, religion, fiction, beginning 1850s; minister, South Congregational (Unitarian) Church, Boston, 1856–99; active retirement, beginning 1899, including election as chaplain of U.S. Senate, 1903.

Author of whimsical stories, romantic tales, historical romances, autobiographies, and scholarly works, Edward Everett Hale managed somehow between his literary outpourings and religious activities to lend important help to the Temperance Movement in the second half of the nineteenth century. Hale was born into a well-to-do Boston family in 1822 and early on displayed the interest in writing and journalism that played such a large role in his later career (he published his first article—a translation from French—in his father's newspaper at age eleven). Entering Harvard at thirteen years old, he graduated Phi Beta Kappa and, fully in character, as class poet. Rather than pursue his literary bent professionally, however, Hale studied for the Unitarian ministry and took his first pastorate in 1846 at Worcester, Massachusetts. Ten years later he took the prestigious pulpit at Boston's South Church, where he remained for the rest of his ministerial career. Over the years, he garnered great acclaim as a pastor, winning a number of public honors, including election as chaplain of the U.S. Senate (1903). By all accounts, he was an eloquent speaker and devoted to the service of his congregation. Yet Hale's interests flowed in many channels, some of which took expression in his talents as an author. He was a prolific writer, and his articles and stories dealt variously with relief for the needy, the antislavery struggle, temperance, church affairs, and other concerns. But easily his most famous work was the short story for which he is probably best known. "The Man Without a Country" first appeared in the *Atlantic Monthly* in December 1863 and was an instantaneous success. Hale, the grand-nephew of Revolutionary War hero Nathan Hale, came by his own patriotism naturally, and his tale of Philip Nolan's fifty-five years of wandering at sea without a country to call home served to make the Union seem dearer to a people engaged in a bitter Civil War.

Hale's reform activities, however, were also noteworthy. He had a particular compassion for the poor and urged efforts to help them, to "lend a hand." This was the theme of two of his most popular inspirational volumes, *Ten Times One Is Ten* (1871) and *In His Name* (1873), and they addded considerable stimulus to the growth of the "Lend-a-Hand Clubs" across the nation, pledged to assist the unfortunate back on their feet. It was in this spirit that Hale lent his support to the Temperance Movement. To Hale, it seemed a natural reform cause: As a Harvard student, he had been a firm and articulate believer in total abstinence on a personal basis; and as a matter of public policy, he saw the liquor traffic as a chief contributor to the social misery that so distressed him. As a young minister, he felt strongly enough on the issue to protest the abuses of the traffic even if the interests of his family were involved. At one point he wrote his father, an officer of a local railroad, urging the closing of a hotel owned by the railroad because of the pernicious influence of its bar. Never a strident man, Hale nevertheless spoke consistently against alcohol and, with the founding of the Unitarian Temperance Society in 1886, became one of the more prominent participants in its activities. He also promoted the medical and institutional treatment of alcoholics. With the proper attention, he hoped they could be healed and reformed, and with the right assistance, once more become productive members of society. Hale was certainly one of the most versatile and humane temperance advocates and, with his fame as an author, one of the most prestigious.

**Bibliography:**

A. *If, Yes, and Perhaps* (1868; New York, 1969); *The Man Without a Country and Other Tales* (1868; Freeport, NY, 1971); *His Level Best, and Other Stories* (1872; New York, 1969); *Philip Nolan's Friend's* (1877; Upper Saddle River,

NJ, 1970); *A New England Boyhood* (Boston, 1893); *Memories of a Hundred Years*, 2 vols. (Boston, 1902).

B. DAB 8, 99–100; SEAP 3, 1167–68; John R. Adams, *Edward Everett Hale* (Boston, 1977); Edward E. Hale, Jr., *The Life and Letters of Edward Everett Hale*, 2 vols. (Boston, 1917); Jean Holloway, *Edward Everett Hale: A Biography* (Austin, TX, 1956).

**HANLY, James Franklin**     (4 April 1863, St. Joseph, IL—1 August 1920, near Kilgore, OH). *Education*: studied at Eastern Illinois Normal Sch., late 1870s; private study of law, 1880s. *Career*: schoolteacher, IN, 1881–89; admitted to bar, IN, 1889; legal practice, Williamsport and Lafayette, IN, beginning 1889; member, Indiana Senate, 1891–94; member, U.S. House of Representatives, 1895–97; governor of Indiana, 1905–9; publisher, *National Enquirer* and *National Commercial*, beginning 1915; active public lecturer and temperance organizer, 1910–20.

James Hanly's career offered one of the best examples of how successful a politician could be if he understood the national mood on the prohibition question. Ambitious and politically astute, Hanly grew up in the strongly protemperance Midwest. While teaching in the public schools of Indiana, young Hanly studied law in his spare time and passed the bar in 1889. His legal practice, however, soon took second place to his chief interests—politics and the antiliquor crusade. He wasted no time in entering the political ring (as a Republican), running successfully for the Indiana Senate in 1890. Hanly used that office as a springboard for a leap to greater heights: In 1894 he won a seat in Congress, and after an unsuccessful campaign for the Senate in 1899, he was elected governor in 1904. The race for the governorship allowed Hanly to give free reign to his dry sentiments. He called for a county-option program in order to assist local prohibitionists in drying out the state. He portrayed his Democratic opponent, Thomas R. Marshall, as a pronounced wet and beat him by the widest plurality ever won by an Indiana governor. (It is worth noting, however, that Marshall's career was hardly ruined: He went on to make a modest name for himself later as Woodrow Wilson's vice president and as the father of that imperishable observation, "All this country needs is a good five-cent cigar.") As governor, Hanly actively supported the Temperance Movement in his state and did yeoman service in moving Indiana toward eventual state-wide prohibition. Had his career ended upon leaving office in 1909, his reputation as an antiliquor champion would have been secure.

In fact, however, Hanly's temperance activities hit their full stride only after he left the statehouse. By this time, the war against liquor had become his consuming interest; he believed without question that the liquor traffic lay at the root of most American social and political ills, and the former governor devoted the rest of his life to its abolition. Over the next five years, he garnered national recognition as a nation-travelling lecturer at the head of the Flying Squadron of America. The Flying Squadron was a touring dry speakers' group composed of such antiliquor stalwarts as Daniel A. Poling,* Clinton N. Howard,* and Dr. Wilbur Fletcher Sheridan. They expounded before large and enthusiastic audiences on the evils of drink and urged the passage of a national prohibitory amendment to the Constitution. "A Saloonless Land, a Stainless Flag, a Sober People" was its motto, and Hanly, chairman of the group's executive committee and later its president, was one of the most popular speakers. His favorite address was a veritable tirade against the traffic entitled, "I Hate It," in which he bitterly castigated all aspects of beverage alcohol use. His passion for the cause carried him out of the Republican Party in 1916, when he ran for president on the Prohibition ticket. It was, of course, a losing bid, but he characteristically threw all of his energy into the campaign. With the passage of National Prohibition, Hanly remained in the vanguard of the struggle. He defended the new Volstead Act against challenges in Ohio courts, maintained his active lecture schedule, and in conjunction with the Flying Squadron mapped an extensive campaign to elect congressmen favorable to strict enforcement of the Volstead Act. The plans went forward, however, without the avid reformer: Hanly was killed in an automobile accident in August 1920 near Kilgore, Ohio, while en route to a speaking engagement.

**Bibliography:**

A. *Messages and Documents, January 9, 1905–January 11, 1909* (Indianapolis, IN, 1909); *The Conqueror of the World* (Indianapolis, IN, 1918).
B. SEAP 3, 1174; WW 1, 515.

**HARDMAN, Lamartine Griffin**   (14 April 1856, Commerce, GA—18 February 1937, Atlanta, GA). *Education*: M.D., Univ. of Georgia, 1877; postdoctoral medical studies, Bellevue Hosp., New York; Polytechnic Hosp., Univ. of Pennsylvania; Guy's Hosp., London; Birmingham, England; Paris; B.S. (honorary), Univ. of Georgia, 1922. *Career*: medical practice, Commerce, GA, beginning 1876; interests in Georgia banking, real estate, cotton mills, drugs, telephone, and power businesses, beginning 1880s; member, Georgia House of Representatives, 1902–7; member, Georgia Senate, 1908–10; member, State Fuel Administration, 1917–18; governor of Georgia, 1927–31.

Lamartine Hardman combined most of the attributes of the so-called New South in his distinguished and active Georgia career. Born as the secession crisis loomed over the nation, he made his mark in life in a Georgia forever changed from the slave-holding region of his boyhood. Hardman seized the opportunities available to the skilled and talented as the South industrialized: Well trained as a medical doctor, he devoted much of his time to making a fortune in a variety of business enterprises. Even in agriculture he looked to the future, as he put his scientific training to work in soil improvement experiments and developing methods of crop diversification. By the turn of the century he was one of the leading citizens of his native region, and it was no surprise to find this prominence soon translated into political participation. He served nearly a decade in the state legislature (1902–10), where he became a spokesman for reform measures encompassing agricultural education and the public school curriculum. Hardman was also a champion of prohibition, which he saw as essential to an orderly and economically prosperous South. While in the legislature, he stood solidly for statutory state prohibition, and he played a leading role in securing passage of the measure. He was also a leading dry speaker, travelling the state on behalf of the Temperance Movement. For some years, Hardman was a member of the Georgia branch of the Anti-Saloon League and sat as that group's representative on the board of the National League. Antiliquor crusaders were therefore pleased when he won election as governor in 1927. In the statehouse, Hardman remained firmly in the dry camp, although popular support for the Eighteenth Amendment was on the wane. Hardman's influence, despite the support he enjoyed as governor, was hardly enough to stem the tide, and he never put his political career on the line to mount a major defense of the measure.

**Bibliography:**

B. NYT, Feb. 19, 1937; SEAP 3, 1181; WW 1, 519.

**HARPER, Frances Ellen Watkins**    (24 September 1825, Baltimore, MD—22 February 1911, Philadelphia, PA). *Education*: studied in Baltimore, MD, school for free blacks run by Reverend William Watkins, 1830s. *Career*: author, beginning circa 1845; sewing teacher, Union Sem., Columbus, OH, 1850–52; schoolteacher, Little York, PA, 1852–54; antislavery lecturer for abolitionist groups, 1854–65; reform lecturer and organizer in temperance, black rights, peace, and suffrage groups, beginning 1860s.

One of the few black women in the Temperance Movement to leave a clear record of her career, Frances Harper was born of free black parents in Baltimore, Maryland, in 1825. Her mother and father died, however, when she was three years old, and young Harper grew up in the care of her uncle, the Reverend William Watkins. Watkins proved a powerful influence, as he was no ordinary preacher. He was a forthright abolitionist who numbered among his friends such firebrands as William Lloyd Garrison* and Benjamin Lundy. In a state where slavery was legal, Watkins still worked on behalf of his race, establishing a school for free blacks when they were barred from Baltimore public schools. Self-taught in medicine and languages, he offered an excellent model for his niece, who grew to match him in talents and determination to make the most of life. Harper left his household in 1839 (to work variously as a seamstress and teacher of sewing in Ohio and Pennsylvania) but took with her important lessons in self-reliance and discipline that enabled her to carve an important place for herself in both the abolitionist and the Temperance movements. She became caught up in the antislavery struggle as the abolitionist fervor increased throughout the North in the early 1850s, and especially in response to a Maryland law of 1853 which made free blacks entering the state liable to enslavement. Living in Philadelphia, she became active in the Underground Railroad, which provided escape routes for Southern slaves fleeing North, and was on close terms with both black and white abolitionists. In 1854, she began a successful career as an abolitionist lecturer, which took her on speaking tours across the North and earned her considerable public recognition. Her reform views also found an outlet in poetry, which she had begun writing in the 1840s (her first book, *Poems on Miscellaneous Subjects*, appeared in 1845). Although critics have never lauded her technical style, her antislavery verse had strong emotional appeal. It was published widely in the reform press, and Harper became the most popular black writer since Phyllis Wheatley. Harper's career, then, had assumed national significance.

In the late 1860s, however, her path took new direction. With the slavery issue decided by the Civil War, and following the death of her husband, Fenton Harper, in 1864, she took an an active interest in the growing Temperance Movement. Her motives, moreover, evidently stemmed from her continuing concerns over the welfare of her fellow blacks. Drink, she believed, would hinder their ability to enter the mainstream of American life. During the Reconstruction years, she never gave up writing and speaking on black rights (she also met the issue of white racism head on, denouncing it in front of racially mixed audiences), but her reform activities increasingly involved the antiliquor crusade, peace, and women's suffrage. Her chief temperance work came in the 1880s and 1890s, when she campaigned extensively among blacks, warning them away from alcohol. During these years she was superintendent of "work among the colored people" for the Woman's Christian Temperance Union, and she made a number of antiliquor speaking tours in the South (an area previously less than pleased—at least among its white citizenry—with her reputation as a public figure). She maintained her impressive record as a reform organizer, and in 1896 she founded the National Association of Colored Women. Two years earlier she had become the director of the American Association of Education of Colored Youth, and later served as an officer of the Association for the Advancement of Women and of the Universal Peace Society. Her work for women's rights twice led her to take part in conventions of the American Woman Suffrage Association (in 1875 and 1887), although in the 1890s she placed a greater stress on working for black suffrage. Throughout, Harper continued to write, and one of her novels, *Iola Leroy: or Shadows Uplifted* (1892), was popular enough to go through three editions. Her passing in 1911 brought to an end a reform career that had made its mark in both the nineteenth and early twentieth centuries.

### Bibliography:

A. *Poems on Miscellaneous Subjects* (1845; Boston, 1854); *Sketches of Southern Life* (1872; Philadelphia, 1891); *Iola Leroy: or Shadows Uplifted* (Philadelphia, 1892); *Atlanta Offering: Poems* (1895; New York, 1969); *Idylls of the Bible* (1901; New York, 1975).

B. NAW 2, 137–39; SEAP 3, 1184; Theodora Williams Daniel, "The Poems of Frances E. W. Harper'' (Master's thesis, Howard Univ., 1937); William Still, *The Underground Rail Road* (1872).

**HASTINGS, Samuel Dexter**    (24 July 1816, Leicester, MA—26 March 1903, Evanston, IL). *Career*: merchant, Philadelphia, 1837–45; farmer, banker, real estate agent, merchant, WI, 1846 to 1870s; member, Wisconsin legislature, 1849, 1857; state treasurer of Wisconsin, 1858–66; officer and organizer, Independent Order of Good Templars, 1840s–1900s; active in antislavery and temperance reform groups, 1840s–1900s.

Samuel Dexter Hastings was one of a large number of reformers whose interests spanned humanitarian causes from antislavery to temperance. Born in Leicester, Massachusetts, in 1816, Hastings lived close to a full century and during that time labored to emancipate mankind from what he conceived to be the two great scourges of his day: involuntary servitude and alcohol. At the age of nineteen he became actively involved in the antislavery crusade, and he was ultimately to be an associate of the leading abolitionists of the pre–Civil War era. The young reformer numbered such radicals as William Lloyd Garrison,* Wendell Phillips,* and John Greenleaf Whittier among his friends. In the late 1830s he was one of the founders of the Liberty Party in Pennsylvania, which was dedicated to the freeing of the slaves; although he himself did not seek public office under its banner, he played a major role in the party's internal affairs. But in 1848, without his knowledge, he was nominated for the state legislature of Wisconsin, to which he had moved in 1846, and was elected overwhelmingly. As a member of the state's first legislature, Hastings took the lead in antislavery agitation and was instrumental in placing Wisconsin firmly against the extension of the internal slave trade. Indeed, Hastings was recognized as one of the most prominent antislavery men in the Midwest. Very popular politically, he ran successfully for state treasurer in 1857 and held the post through the Civil War, when he won high praise for his capable management of Wisconsin's finances in a difficult period.

In addition to his antislavery stand, Hastings was also an implacable foe of alcohol. Enslavement to liquor, he believed, was as bitter an enemy of humanity as chattel slavery. (He was no less opposed, we should note, to the use of tobacco.) From his youth, the zealous reformer stood firmly in the total abstinence camp, and he easily translated his personal views on the liquor question into political action. When he took his first seat in the Wisconsin legislature, he moved quickly against the state's liquor traffic. He served on a committee dealing with licenses to sell alcoholic beverages and drafted a bill that would have repealed the licenses of all dealers in such drinks. But it was defeated narrowly in the State Senate by a margin of only two votes. This setback, however, hardly discouraged the bill's author, as he took up the battle again outside of the local government. Hastings was an active and influential member of the Sons of Temperance and of the Independent Order of Good Templars (of which he ultimately became grand worthy patriarch), and he used these groups as forums to expound on the merits of prohibition. With the end of the Civil War, he felt free to devote all of his reform efforts to the temperance struggle. In 1882 he joined the Prohibition Party, and until 1901 he was one of its most stalwart members. For years, he served on its executive committee and as its national treasurer. He was also one of the founders of the National Temperance Society and served on the boards of many other temperance-related organizations. Throughout his antiliquor career, Hastings gave much of his time to travel for the cause as well. As a brother in the Good Templars, he journeyed to Australia and New Zealand on missionary duty as early as 1847, and he crossed the Atlantic no fewer than six times—once to Scotland on Templar business when he was seventy-seven. Always a firm member of the Congregational Church, Hastings took as his personal text the Biblical admonition, "Whatever you do, do all to the glory of God." On this basis he waged a lifetime campaign against sin and evil as he saw them; and upon his death in 1903, after some seventy years of reform effort, few could deny that he had labored mightily for the benefit of his fellow man.

### Bibliography:

A. *Address Before the Hastings Invincibles...Wisconsin Volunteers...1862* (Madison, WI, 1862); *Remarks of Hon. S. D. Hastings, Chairman of the Committee Appointed to Investigate the Affairs of the State Hospital for the Insane...* (Madison, WI, 1868); "The Present Condition of the Common Jails of the County," Wisconsin Academy of Sciences, Arts and Letters, *Transactions* 1 (1872): 90–97; *Some Grand Tributes to a Sublime Character: Eloquent Eulogy on the Life and Work of the Late Frances E. Willard...* (Green Bay, WI, 1898).

B. DAB 8, 386–87; SEAP 3, 1191–92; L.N.H. Buckminster, *The Hastings Memorial* (n.p., 1866); *International Good Templar* (Oct. 1889).

**HAWKINS, John Henry Willis**    (23 October 1799, Baltimore, MD—26 August 1858, Parkersburg, WV). *Career*: hatter, to 1840; temperance lecturer and organizer, 1840–58.

In 1840, the Washington Temperance Society was born in Baltimore, Maryland. The creation of six heavy drinkers who elected to take the pledge and carry the dry message to others, the Washingtonian movement quickly emerged as a full-blown revival, the most dramatic explosion of temperance sentiment in national history. Before the enthusiasm cooled several years later, Washingtonian groups, displaying many of the self-help characteristics of modern Alcoholics Anonymous, sprang up in cities across the nation, often in the wake of movement speakers sent out to spread the dry gospel. One of the most successful of these proselytizers was John Hawkins. A hatter by trade, we know little of the man's early years other than that he apparently had some elementary education and that he certainly was a hard drinker. He also had a daughter, Hannah, who figured largely in his story. Worried about her father's drinking, Hannah persuaded him to join the Washingtonian movement soon after its founding, and he quickly discovered latent talents as an orator. Speaking on behalf of the group before the Maryland legislature, he came to the attention of temperance leaders in a number of Eastern cities, notably in New York, and they invited the Washingtonians to send Hawkins and other delegates to spark the crusade there. The mission (conducted later in 1840) was a major success as Hawkins and his colleagues spoke before thousands of New Yorkers at a series of mass meetings. Some 2,500 people took the pledge as a result. As the fame of the Washingtonians spread, Hawkins went on to lead equally successful rallies in Boston and later, except for California, in each of the states until his death in 1858. In all, he travelled some 200,000 miles and gave about 5,000 lectures.

Aside from his services in the Washingtonian reform, the career of John Hawkins was important in other respects. Although dry speakers were in the field before the Washingtonians, Hawkins proved one of the first of a new type. He appealed successfully to mass audiences and to actual drinkers. He also led the field as an independent career lecturer and organizer—perhaps the first American reformer to make his living in such a fashion. His success in this regard opened the way for others, although Hawkins (and his fellow Washingtonian John B. Gough*) always remained among the most popular dry speakers of the day. His appeal lay in his ability to keep his message alive even after the Washingtonian movement itself ebbed by the mid-1840s. His personal story of fighting the bottle allowed him to reach other drinkers with effect over the years; and while some Washingtonians ultimately differed bitterly over tactics with the organized temperance societies of the period (the Washingtonians were seldom prohibitionists and usually concentrated solely on the salvation of the alcoholic), Hawkins made his peace with them. Thus he readily found sponsorship for his lectures even after most itinerant Washingtonians had long since left the field. Temperance workers were loud in his praise over the years and mourned his passing for what it was—the loss of a sincere and able reform champion who never lost sight of his goal to rescue the drinker from his drink. Even his daughter was later immortalized by the dry press. Soon after the great lecturer's death, the Reverend John Marsh* penned *Hannah Hawkins: or, the Reformed Drunkard's Daughter*. Placed in schools and private hands throughout the nation (more than 100,000 copies were distributed), it sought to inspire families to similar dedication against the "demon rum."

### Bibliography:

B. SEAP 3, 1202–3; Daniel Dorchester, *The Liquor Problem in All Ages* (New York, 1888); W. G. Hawkins, *Life of John H. W. Hawkins* (New York? 1859); Alice Felt Tyler, *Freedom's Ferment: Phases of American Social History from the Colonial Period to the Outbreak of the Civil War* (1944; New York, 1962).

**HAY, Charles Martin**    (10 November 1879, Wayne Co., MO—16 January 1945, St. Louis, MO). *Education*: A.B., Central Coll., MO, 1901; LLB., Washington Univ., 1904; LLD. (honorary), Washington Univ., 1926. *Career*: legal practice, various locations in MO, beginning 1904; member, Missouri House of Representatives, 1913–14; active in Democratic Party affairs, 1900s to 1945; counselor, City of St. Louis, 1932–35; legal specialist in railroad labor affairs, 1930s to 1945; general counsel, War Manpower Commission, 1943–45.

Democrats were not rare among the ranks of temperance leaders, but in the late nineteenth and early twentieth centuries, the liberal (or Progressive) wing of the party shared a greater enthusiasm for the dry cause than did party conservatives. The career of Charles Martin Hay was an ample demonstration of this fact, as well as of the connections between temperance and American liberalism in general. After establishing a successful legal practice, Hay became actively involved with the Democrats, serving repeatedly over the years on party committees, working on campaigns, and sitting as a convention delegate. His own term as an elected official, however, was brief. He won a seat in the Missouri legislature (1913–14) but thereafter failed in a bid for his party's nomination for the national Senate (1920). Throughout, he was identified as a Progressive, and he loyally served the administrations of both Woodrow Wilson and Franklin Roosevelt. During World War I, Hay was one of Wilson's so-called four-minute speakers, a task force of prominent men and women who traversed the nation giving brief talks in support of the allied war effort against Germany. After the conflict, he was an enthusiastic supporter of Wilson's League of Nations, and he took a major part in the effort to rally popular support for the organization. Largely out of public life (at least on the national level) during the Republican ascendancy of the 1920s, the Missouri Democrat became civically active again with the election of Roosevelt. During the New Deal, Hay served in the Justice Department as special assistant to the attorney general, mostly involved in defending the Railroad Retirement Act and other railroad labor legislation in the courts. During World War II, Hay served on the War Labor Board and was General Counsel of the War Manpower Commission when he died in 1945.

During his years of public life, Hay was a firm believer in the values of temperance, and he took part enthusiastically in the activities of the antiliquor crusade. Indeed, the scope of his contributions to the dry cause was impressive. As a college student, he was noted for his oratorical skills, and he won at least one prize in a speaking competition sponsored by the Temperance Movement: the Interstate Prohibition Contest, held in Buffalo, New York, in 1901. For the next two years, he served as a prohibitionist lecturer, appearing at educational institutions across the state of Missouri. His reputation as a local dry was considerable, and when the Anti-Saloon League established a chapter in the state, it was no surprise to find Hay not only involved but moving quickly to a leadership position. For years he sat on the Missouri League's Board of Trustees, and then added to his busy schedule similar responsibilities with the National League. As a Progressive, he saw prohibition as part and parcel of the reforms needed to set right American social and political problems, and much of his effort in politics was based on this sentiment. As early as 1905 he was spearheading local-option campaigns throughout the state; in fact, he chose local option as the key issue of his single campaign for a seat in the legislature. In office, he successfully introduced a county-level local-option measure, and led the fight which finally made it a law. In the fight for National Prohibition, Hay was a leader in the drive for the ratification of the Eighteenth Amendment in Missouri. Yet as deep as his antiliquor commitment was, Hay was also possessed of a great degree of common sense: When the nation, and especially the Democratic Party, turned against the dry cause, the Missouri reformer saw no sense in defending it to the last ditch. Like other Americans of similar outlook, he considered the problems inherent in the Great Depression, and in launching the New Deal, of more importance than keeping Prohibition alive. Thus Hay made his peace with his wet brethren, and he served loyally the national administration that had brought about the final repeal of the "noble experiment" for which he had worked so long.

**Bibliography:**

B. SEAP 3, 1203–4; WW 2, 242.

**HAY, Mary Garrett**    (29 August 1857, Charlestown, IN—29 August 1928, New Rochelle, NY). *Education*: studied at Western Coll. for Women, Oxford, OH, 1873–74. *Career*: temperance and women's suffrage reform activities, 1870–1928.

Mary Garrett Hay was one of those persons who spend much of their lives as self-effacing righthand aids to famous personages and only emerge later in life as significant individuals in their own right. Hay was born in Indiana in 1857, the daughter of a well-to-do doctor who had an interest in local politics. He imparted to young Mary his enthusiastic partisanship for the Republican Party, although she quickly developed political interests of her own. After a brief sojourn at Western College for Women in Oxford, Ohio, she launched a long and active reform career. A deeply religious woman (she was a Presbyterian), she was attracted to the newly organized Woman's Christian Temperance Union, which evinced a highly spiritual tone in many of its activities. Hay quickly became an officer in her local chapter of the union and for seven years was treasurer of the Indiana state branch. By 1885, she had risen to a national position, heading one of the WCTU's smaller departments. Influenced by the broad range of the union's reform pursuits, Hay grew increasingly interested in the women's suffrage movement—a course in which other WCTU leaders encouraged her. She became active in Indiana suffrage affairs, during which she met Carrie Chapman Catt, the noted suffragette, who was in the Midwest on an organizing campaign. They quickly developed a life-long association. In 1895, Hay left Indiana, following Catt to New York City and work with the Organization Committee of the National Woman Suffrage Association. She and Ms. Catt made a dynamic combination, and they soon were travelling the nation organizing, fund raising, and generally proselytizing for the suffrage movement. After 1905, the relationship had become so close that they lived together upon the death of Catt's husband.

The common effort with Catt brought an important degree of power and influence to Hay within suffrage ranks. She held a succession of important posts, including president of the Federation of Women's Clubs (1910–12); director of the General Federation of Women's Clubs (1914–18); and president of both the New York Equal Suffrage League (1910–18) and the New York City Woman Suffrage Party (1912–18). In the last group, she did yeoman work organizing parades, local rallies, and getting out literature, ultimately swinging New York into the suffragist camp. After the victory, Hay went to Washington to lobby among Republican congressmen in support of the women's vote. In 1918, she masterminded an impressive victory over Nicholas Murray Butler to win the chairmanship of the platform committee at the Republican National Convention— the first woman to do so. She used her extraordinary position to push through a plank supporting a national suffrage amendment. She was also a member of the Republican Women's National Executive Committee in 1918. But in 1920 her opposition to the reelection of Republican Senator James W. Wadsworth, a bitter enemy of the female ballot, led to her withdrawal from politics. She then began to take a more active part in the prohibition movement and worked through the Women's Committee for Law Enforcement to support the Eighteenth Amendment. In this effort she supported Robert F. Wagner for the Senate, although he was a Democrat, and was a factor in his defeat of her longtime foe, Senator Wadsworth (who was as opposed to prohibition as he was to suffrage). Hay died in 1928 at the age of seventy-one (in fact, on her birthday), having achieved recognition as one of her generation's most formidable advocates of women's rights and temperance. As a champion of the suffrage movement, she was second only to the redoubtable Carrie Chapman Catt, whose able second in command she was.

**Bibliography:**

B. DAB 8, 436; NAW 2, 163–65; NYT, Aug. 31, 1928; WW 1, 538; Mary Gray Peck, *Carrie Chapman Catt* (New York, 1944).

**HAYES, Lucy Ware Webb**  (28 August 1831, Chillicothe, OH—25 June 1889, Fremont, OH). *Education*: studied at Ohio Wesleyan Univ., 1840s; graduated from Wesleyan Female Coll., 1850. *Career*: volunteer work with Union army wounded and veterans, 1861 to 1870s; White House hostess as First Lady to President Rutherford B. Hayes, 1877–81; active in community and church philanthropic work, 1870s–1880s.

Descended from a line of Revolutionary and War of 1812 veterans, Lucy Ware Webb Hayes grew up with a strong sense of civic duty and pride. Raised in Ohio, her parents provided a comfortable (her father was a successful doctor) but highly moral home life: The Webbs were strict Methodists, and from her earliest days young Lucy was pledged, like the rest of the Webbs, to total abstinence; she was also taught to share her father's abhorrence of slavery. (In fact, Dr. Webb died on a trip to Lexington, Kentucky, where he had gone to free some slaves he had inherited.) Upon the death of Dr. Webb, his widow saw to the education of Lucy and her two brothers, and in 1850 the future Mrs. Hayes entered the relatively thin ranks of American women college graduates. She married Rutherford B. Hayes, then a young Ohio lawyer, in 1852. The couple generally shared the same moral and social outlook: Both were Methodists and antislavery, both looked favorably on the Temperance Movement (although Mr. Hayes was a moderationist and not a teetotaler), and both were prime examples of what one historian has called the "wholesome, religious, family-oriented respectability" that marked the values of America's middle class. They also believed in public service: Rutherford compiled a distinguished military record as a Union officer during the Civil War, while Lucy devoted long hours to working with Union wounded. Serving as a volunteer nurse and writing letters home for the troops, she became known as Mother Lucy. After the conflict, and as her husband's political star rose (he served variously in Congress and as governor of Ohio from 1865 to 1877), she maintained her devotion to the veterans. She spoke on behalf of veterans relief measures and in 1869 played a leading role in the founding of the Ohio Soldiers' and Sailors' Orphans' Home. While she was not a major reformer, then, nor, evidently, did she seek an independent career, there was no question of her intelligence, moral certainty, and good intentions.

In 1877, these were the qualities that Lucy Hayes brought to the White House after her husband was declared the winner of the disputed presidential election of 1876. She quickly put her stamp on Washington society as she emerged as perhaps the most influential (and certainly one of the best-educated) First Ladies since Dolly Madison. Although her critics probably overestimated her influence on President Hayes, there was no doubt that she had some definite notions about what social life at the White House should be. And none of them included alcohol. Adopting a role analagous to the then reigning monarch of Great Britain, Mrs. Hayes assumed, in some respects, the moral outlook of an American Queen Victoria. She firmly eschewed dances, lawn parties, balls, card parties, and other frivolities. Family gatherings replaced the usual Washington social whirl, and a typical evening was likely to include sedate readings of improving literature, hymn singing, and prayers. The White House wine cellar was padlocked and nonalcoholic beverages became standard, earning Mrs. Hayes the sobriquet of "Lemonade Lucy." In this she had the firm and principled support of President Hayes, who was only slightly less an adherent of temperance than his wife. In response to detractors, she answered that her children had "never tasted liquor," that they never would from her hands, and that she would never sanction a habit that might prove the ruin of "the sons of other mothers." The Temperance Movement was thrilled, with one spokesman proclaiming that her stand would rank next to the Emancipation Proclamation in the annals of history. When President Hayes left the White House in 1881, a grateful Woman's Christian

Temperance Union donated a portrait of the dry First Lady to the collection of the Executive Mansion. On her part, Lucy Hayes showed little remorse over leaving the capital. She returned with her husband to Ohio, where she spent the rest of her life in church work, principally with the Woman's Home Missionary Society of the Methodist Church.

**Bibliography:**

B. NAW 2, 166–67; SEAP 3, 1204–6; WW H, 311; Mrs. John Davis, *Lucy Webb Hayes: A Memorial Sketch* (Cincinnati, OH, 1890); Emily Apt Geer, "Lucy Webb Hayes: An Unexceptionable Woman" (Ph.D. diss., Western Reserve Univ., 1962).

**HECTOR, John Henry**   (17 March 1847, Windsor, Ontario, Canada—8 April 1914, York, PA). *Career*: cowboy, IL, late 1850s to 1862?; soldier, Union army, circa 1862–65; locomotive engineer, PA, 1860s–1870s; temperance lecturer, beginning 1870s.

Historians have paid relatively little attention to the careers of black temperance workers, whose activities and contributions on behalf of the dry cause (particularly among other blacks) were nevertheless significant. Occasionally, however, a black voice was able to command the attention of the entire crusade, and such was the case of the antiliquor "Black Knight" (as his contemporaries called him), John Henry Hector. He was the son of slaves who escaped their bondage in Virginia and fled to freedom in Canada, where Hector was born. Young Hector lacked any formal schooling and made only a precarious living as a cowpuncher on the plains of Illinois. During the Civil War he enlisted in the Union army and fought with splendid gallantry. In all, he was wounded no less than five times. Hector came into his own during these hard years, emerging with what one source described as an "indomitable will" to make something of his life. Upon his discharge he taught himself to read and write, found skilled work as a locomotive engineer, and began a steady climb to public prominence. Settling in York, Pennsylvania, Hector was elected commander of the local post of the Grand Army of the Republic, and he became a pillar of his community's African Methodist Episcopal Church. In these capacities, he developed his latent talents for leadership and public speaking, which led directly to the launching of his career as a full-time temperance lecturer. It was in this calling that the son of former slaves would make his greatest public mark.

Temperance was a central tenet of both the black and white divisions of the Methodist Church. Hector was convinced of the dry message, and as a church member he carried the gospel to the community with genuine zeal. Indeed, he was so effective that the African Methodist Episcopal Church asked him to accept an appointment as a travelling temperance missionary, taking the antiliquor cruasade to blacks throughout the nation. Hector seemingly was perfect for the job: He had the emotional commitment of a true believer; and his impressive physique and speaking eloquence made him a dominating presence on the podium. He travelled widely in his lecturing role and received much credit in the drive to close the saloons in Atlanta, Georgia. While Hector's primary audience was black, his reputation was such that white reformers sought him for their programs as well. He spoke in front of interracial audiences in both the United States and his native Canada, garnering the praise of listeners wherever he went. He was the first speaker employed with a year-long contract by the National Committee of the Prohibition Party, ample testimony to the regard Hector's abilities commanded. It is clear, then, that the Temperance Movement saw itself in the black reformer's debt. Further study, however, has yet to determine how his efforts reflected old temperance sympathies for the antislavery movement (if at all) or general black attitudes toward the dry crusade. In any event, as an individual Hector could lay claim to one of his day's most noted reputations as a dry lecturer, which was perhaps enough for any one man.

**Bibiography:**

B. SEAP 3, 1210–11.

**HENDERSON, Yandell**   (23 April 1873, Louisville, KY—19 February 1944, La Jolla, CA). *Education*: A.B., Yale Univ., 1895; Ph.D., Yale Univ., 1898; postgraduate study, Univ. of Marburg and Univ. of Munich, 1899–1900; M.D. (honorary), Connecticut State Medical Society, 1942. *Career*: instructor in physiology, Yale Univ., 1900–1903; assistant professor, Yale Univ., 1903–11; professor, Yale Univ., 1911–21; professor of applied physiology, Yale Univ., 1921–38 (professor emeritus after 1938); ensign, U.S. navy, 1898; consulting physiologist, U.S. Bureau of Mines, 1913–25; chairman, Medical Research Board, Aviation Section, Signal Corps, U.S. army, 1917–18; active consulting work, 1900s–1940s.

Yandell Henderson's career was another that figured prominently in the shifting of American thinking about alcohol problems away from temperance activities and toward scientific research and medical treatment. His family background inclined the young Henderson toward scientific interests: His maternal grandfather was dean of the Medical School of Transylvania University, while his uncle was a surgeon of considerable reputation. Henderson's personal interests lay in physiology, in which he took his Ph.D. at Yale in 1898 (he was also an undergraduate alumnus of 1895), to which he added postdoctoral studies in Germany. An active man, however, he did not confine himself to academia. During the Spanish-American War he took time off from his studies to serve in the navy, seeing duty aboard the U.S.S. *Yale* when the fleet supported the American invasion of Puerto Rico. He was back at his alma mater in 1900, beginning a faculty career that lasted until 1938 (after which he was professor emeritus). A full professor of physiology by 1911, Henderson's work emphasized the practical application of scientific knowledge rather than basic research, and he specialized in human respiration. The Yale professor was an authority in his field, consulting broadly with industry and government while he pursued his teaching and research career. Notably, he headed the Medical Section of the Army War Gas Investigation during World War I, which perfected a serviceable gas mask for American troops. In addition, he chaired the Medical Board of the Aviation Section of the Army Signal Corps and administered the devising of medical tests to determine flight ceilings for pilots. Back at Yale after the war, he worked closely with Professor Howard Haggard* in various lines of research. Among their many joint efforts, they pioneered resuscitation in cases of carbon monoxide poisoning, developed the Henderson-Haggard technique for stimulating breathing in newborn babies, and devised the ventilation safety standards used in many larger tunnels throughout the world. Not all of Henderson's projects were successful, and some of his ideas provoked heated professional controversy, but there is no denying that his contributions were many and valuable.

Henderson's interests in alcohol problems stemmed from his career in physiology and his concern for civic affairs. He had not been a temperance worker, but he was no stranger to reform causes. Before World War I he had been an ardent member of the Progressive Party and, with Theodore Roosevelt at the head of the ticket, the Yale researcher ran unsuccessfully for Congress in 1912. (Undaunted, he tried again two years later.) Like other Progressives who held no particular brief for the Eighteenth Amendment, he nevertheless supported the coming of National Prohibition as a worthwhile reform and the law of the land. However, as the "noble experiment" encountered popular resistance, Henderson reconsidered his position, coming to believe that Prohibition was fostering a dangerous public taste for high-proof distilled liquor. (Subsequent historical research, at least to a limited extent, has supported Henderson in this conclusion, even though demonstrating that overall American consumption of beverage alcohol was at its lowest ebb in history during most of the Prohibition years.) He argued that a safer course for public policy was to shift popular tastes to weaker beverages such as wine and beer. When he adopted this view, Henderson drew on his knowledge of the history of drinking in America: It was the same course that Benjamin Rush* had advocated in the late eighteenth century. In reviving the idea, Henderson hoped to discourage the use of the strongest drinks through taxation—heavier levies on high-proof beverages, he hoped, would turn the public away from them. The proposal was nothing if not controversial. Henderson presented it in some detail before the House Ways and Means Committee in 1932, and his testimony created something of a stir. He claimed that a beer, for example, with a 4 percent alcohol content, was virtually nonintoxicating—less intoxicating, in fact, than a cigar. Little came of his proposals until 1933, when the government voted to modify the Volstead Act and made beers of up to 3.2 percent alcohol legal. With the coming of Repeal, however, Henderson's arguments for a broad national policy of encouraging the use of weaker beverages went nowhere, although he presented his case compactly in a book, *A New Deal in Liquor: A Plea for Dilution* (1934). Yet the alcohol-related research begun in his Yale laboratory did carry on and was an important element in the rise of the Yale Center of Alcohol Studies. In that sense, Henderson's career was a direct link between the debate over National Prohibition and the modern alcoholism research effort.

**Bibliography:**

A. *Fatal Apnoea and the Shock Problem* (Baltimore, MD, 1910); *The Physiology of the Aviator*, the Harvey Lectures (New York, 1917–19); with co-workers, series of twelve articles entitled "Hemato-respiratory Functions," *Journal of Biological Chemistry* (1919–21); with Howard W. Haggard, *Noxious Gases and the Principles of Respiration Influencing Their Action* (New York, 1927); *Modification of the National Prohibition Act...[Report to accompany H.R. 13742]*, U.S., Congress, Senate, Committee on the Judiciary (Washington, DC, 1933); *A New Deal in Liquor: A Plea for Dilution* (Garden City, NY, 1934).

B. NCAB 36, 25–26; NYT, Feb. 20, 1944; WW 2, 247–48; Cecil Drinker, [obituary notice], *Journal of Industrial Hygiene and Toxicology* 26 (1944): 179–80; Howard W. Haggard, "Current Notes: Yandell Henderson, 1973–1944," *Quarterly Journal of Studies on Alcohol* 4 (1944): 658–59; Howard W. Haggard, [obituary notice], *Year Book: American Philosophical Society* (1944): 369–74.

**HENRY, Sarepta M.**    (4 November 1839, Albion, PA—17 January 1900, Graysville, SD). *Education*: studied at Rock River Sem., Mount Morris, IL, late 1850s. *Career*: temperance lecturer and author, 1873–1900.

Sarepta Henry was another of those indefatigable dry Methodists who provided the marrow of so much of the nineteenth-century Temperance Movement. Born the daughter of a Methodist parson (her maiden name was Irish), she moved with her family to Illinois as a child and grew up drinking deeply of the tenets of her father's denomination. Such was the depth of her belief that for a time she attended seminary in Mount Morris, Illinois. In the month of Abraham Lincoln's first inauguration, with the storm clouds of the Civil War gathering, Miss Irish married James W. Henry. It was a difficult marriage, as he was shortly to march off to battle and a serious wound in action. He never fully recovered his health and finally died in 1871 of his war-related disability. Sarepta Henry, left a widow with three children, showed considerable pluck after her loss and chose not to remain idle. Always temperance-minded, she quickly devoted her time and energy to the steadily building dry crusade. She was one of the first women of Illinois to become involved in the newly founded Woman's Christian Temperance Union in 1873 and 1874. It was the start of a vigorous and distinguished reform career. For long years Henry served as a WCTU evangelist, denouncing the drink traffic and laboring in gospel temperance campaigns (she received credit for persuading impressive numbers to swear off alcohol). Much of this activity was concentrated in Rockford, Illinois, then regarded as one of the state's chief centers of the liquor trade. Forceful and convincing as a speaker, Henry directed her fire at the purveyors of drink—the saloons and the bartenders—and consequently orchestrated the closing of a number of drinking establishments in that city and in several surrounding communities. Later in life,

Henry moved to Evanston, Illinois, home of the National WCTU, where she turned to writing and produced a number of temperance volumes. While she never had the stature of some of her colleagues in reform, Sarepta Henry was nevertheless a staunch soldier in the crusade; her efforts typified the devotion that carried the Temperance Movement to national moral and political influence.

**Bibliography:**

A. *One More Chance* (Evanston, IL, n.d.); *Pledge and Cross* (Evanston, IL, n.d.).
B. SEAP 3, 1215–16.

**HEWIT, Nathaniel**    (28 August 1788, New London, CT—3 February 1867, Bridgeport, CT). *Education*: graduated from Yale Coll., 1808; studied law with Lyman Law, New London, CT, 1808; graduated from Andover Theological Sem., 1815. *Career*: minister, Presbyterian Church, Plattsburg, NY, 1815–18; minister, First Congregational Church, Fairfield, CT, 1818–27; agent, American Temperance Society, 1827–30; minister, Second Congregational Church, Bridgeport, CT, 1830–62; retired, 1862.

In the late 1820s and early 1830s, drinking in America was reaching unprecedented levels. Some historians have estimated that during these years annual per capita consumption of beverage alcohol (that is, only the ethel alcohol, not including water or other substances in the liquor) had topped seven gallons per year, or considerably more than twice the per capita consumption levels of Americans in the 1980s. In great measure, the social complications inherent in this "national binge" gave rise to the early Temperance Movement and helped account for the zeal of many of the first antiliquor reformers. So it was with Nathaniel Hewit, a New England pastor who became one of the first, and one of the most effective, full-time proselytizers in the service of the dry crusade. Hewit's first inclination was for the law, but he left it quickly after feeling the pull of a religious calling. After finishing seminary he served churches in New York State and Connecticut and established himself as a tireless advocate of moral reform. Society, in the ardent pastor's view, suffered under a multitude of sins, most of which, he claimed, stemmed from drink. When, around the time he began his ministerial career, the major Protestant denominations called for attention to the temperance question, Reverend Hewit was already a leader in the growing reform. Consequently, his pulpit regularly castigated the liquor traffic, and even his private conversations with parishioners and fellow clergymen often turned to the subject. Such was his reputation for zealousness that the newly organized American Society for the Promotion of Temperance (later the American Temperance Society), upon deciding to hire a full-time agent to spread the dry gospel, could think of no one better for the job. Hewitt accepted the post (although apparently with considerable soul-searching) and between 1827 and 1830 demonstrated just how effective a professional reformer could be. He toured New England and the Middle and Southern states, speaking before church groups, public gatherings, medical societies—almost anywhere he could find a forum—urging on his listeners the dangers of drink and asking their support for the movement. He returned to the ministry in late 1830, but almost immediately agreed to yet another mission on the society's behalf, this time in Great Britain, where he helped organize still more dry efforts. His work brought thousands into the antiliquor fold, and Hewit was justly dubbed the "Luther of the early temperance reform."

Hewit's position on drink was consistent throughout his reform career. From the beginning he was a total abstinence man, and he had little patience with the moderationist position. In the early days of the crusade, his strident advocacy of teetotalism identified the New England reformer as a radical, and later Temperance Movement leaders were generous in crediting him with the final victory of the abstinence view. Yet there were some clear limits to Hewit's reform vision. While other temperance workers had no difficulty linking their battle against the "demon rum" to other reform efforts, such as antislavery and women's suffrage, Hewit balked at going beyond the war on booze. Indeed, he developed a profound dislike for the women's rights movement generally, and he was implacably opposed to women taking leadership roles in the temperance struggle. It was an aspect of the crusader that troubled many of his friends and that ultimately caused an open break with some of them. The most serious incident came in May of 1853, when a large temperance group met at the Brick Church in New York City, with the intention of laying plans for a massive World's Temperance Convention. Most of those in attendance had assumed that women would be seated as delegates, but Hewit violently objected and the meeting was thrown into turmoil. The planning session broke up over the issue, as many women, including Susan B. Anthony* and Lucy Stone, and male insurgents such as Thomas Wentworth Higginson, William Lloyd Garrison*, and Wendell Phillips* all walked out. Meeting in another building, they organized their own *Whole* World's Temperance Convention. The affair left Hewit bitter, and even some of his admirers later admitted that the aging crusader was "out of step with the times" and lacked "the breadth of vision which should have enhanced the value of his work." Yet if he stood still as his colleagues in reform broadened the scope of their horizons, Hewit still received due credit as one of the most important temperance pioneers. He could even be magnanimous in his chosen areas: Later in life he helped found Hartford Theological Seminary, and he was one of its most generous benefactors.

**Bibliography:**

A. *A Discourse Delivered Before the General Association of Connecticut . . .* (Hartford, CT, 1840).

B. SEAP 1220–21; Samuel F. Cary, ed., *American Temperance Magazine, and Sons of Temperance Offering* (New York, 1853); Daniel Dorchester, *The Liquor Problem in All Ages* (New York, 1884); *Proceedings of the Whole World's Temperance Convention, 1853* (New York, 1853).

**HINSHAW, Virgil Goodman** (15 January 1876, Woolson, IA—3 August 1952, Pasadena, CA). *Education*: A.B., Penn Coll., IA, 1900; LLB., Univ. of Minnesota, 1908. *Career*: officer, National Intercollegiate Prohibition Assoc., 1900–1906, 1908–10; legal practice, Portland, OR, 1910–12; chairman, National Committee, Prohibition Party, 1912–24; superintendent and various offices, International Reform Federation, beginning 1923; active in wide variety of temperance groups nationally, 1900s–1940s.

Hinshaw's was a life devoted to the temperance crusade. Indeed, except for two years (1910–12) when he opened a law office, his entire professional career centered on various aspects of the antiliquor movement. The precise roots of his enthusiasm for the dry reform are obscure; but he was born (and remained) a Quaker and perhaps drew some of his motivation for following what he saw as the good fight from his intense religious faith. At any rate, Hinshaw grew up dry, and his formal association with the Temperance Movement began when he was still an undergraduate at Penn College, in Oskaloosa, Iowa. He was an ardent member of the Intercollegiate Prohibition Association, one of the leading student reform groups of the era, and after graduation the association offered him his first job. For most of the next decade he made his living as a professional reformer, travelling the country as a secretary of the organization. Hinshaw visited over two hundred colleges around the United States, lecturing students on the evils of drink and recruiting members into the association. His work showed results, and he rose progressively in the group, becoming successively treasurer, vice president, and finally president. Hinshaw had displayed a genuine talent for reform organization and leadership and clearly demonstrated the benefits that accrued to the cause when it could keep such devoted servants in the field full time. Personally, the Quaker reformer found the work satisfying: He labored in a cause that he felt just and one that also seemed to be winning in the first decade of the twentieth century. And as the possibilities for the crusade brightened, Hinshaw determined to remain at the cutting edge of the drive toward a final prohibitionist victory.

In fact, Hinshaw became one of the nation's leading dry organizers in the early 1900s. After 1910 he left the management of daily operations in the association to to others (he remained on the board of the organization, however) and became intimately involved in other dry groups. Politically, he was a staunch member of the Prohibition Party, sitting on its National Committee for some twelve years (and looking askance, at times, at the nonpartisan politics of the Anti-Saloon League). He founded and led the Prohibition Foundation, a philanthropic group designed to educate the public on Prohibitionist issues, and he served long periods as an officer in such groups as the International Reform Federation, the National Temperance Council, the Committee of Sixty, and the Council of One Hundred. (These last two groups were organized during World War I in order to advance the fortunes of the Temperance Movement during the waging of the war.) Hinshaw took his temperance work abroad as well. After the war, he spoke and organized dry groups in Austria, Czechoslovakia, Australia, and Mexico. Even the Repeal of National Prohibition failed to slow the old crusader, and he maintained his quest for a dry nation well into his seventies. He fought the Repeal movement stubbornly, and over the 1930s and 1940s, Hinshaw remained a driving force (indeed, *the* driving force by this time) in California antiliquor activity (he had taken up residence in the state in the 1930s). He ran for state office as late as 1950, polling the largest tally of any Prohibition Party candidate in the country, and even travelled to Kansas in 1948 on behalf of a campaign to save state prohibition there. Tenacious and capable throughout his career, the life's work of Virgil Hinshaw was ample testimony not only to the zeal but also to the administrative skills that drove the Temperance Movement in its years of national social and political leadership.

**Bibliography:**

B. SEAP 3, 1226–27; WW 3, 404.

**HOBSON, Richmond Pearson**    (17 August 1870, Greensboro, AL—16 March 1937, New York, NY). *Education*: studied at Southern Univ., 1882–85; graduated from U.S. Naval Acad., Annapolis, MD, 1889; postgraduate study at Ecole National Supérieure des Mines, France, circa 1891; graduated from Ecole d'Application du Génie Maritime, Paris, 1893; M.S., Washington and Jefferson Coll., 1898; LLD. (honorary), Southern Univ., 1906. *Career*: various naval construction projects, 1894–97; instructor in naval construction, U.S. Naval Acad., 1897–98; fleet duty during Spanish-American War, combat in Santiago Harbor, Cuba, 1898; ship salvage duty and construction supervision, 1899–1903; member, U.S. House of Representatives, 1907–15; active reform lecturer and writer (especially on alcohol and drug problems), 1900s–1930s.

Richmond Hobson pursued his dream of a sober and drug-free America with the single-minded dedication of a true zealot. An incident from his student days at the Naval Academy reveals something of his character: Of a highly moral and deeply religious background (he was a strict Baptist), he was notorious for reporting the disciplinary infractions of his fellow midshipmen. For a semester, no one spoke a word to him in retaliation. When a classmate suggested a rapprochement, however, Hobson refused, saying that he had done well enough without their comradeship. It was Hobson's way: If he thought he was in the right, he would press on no matter what others thought of him, and this was the outlook that governed his approach to reform. Typical of other Progressives of his day, he advocated changes not only to improve the quality of life but also to make the nation more efficient and productive. This was true even of his military career. His specialty was naval construction, and he pioneered efforts to improve navy repair services and training for officers. He never had a regular ship command, and his fame as a sailor came only under unusual circumstances. While at sea off of Cuba during the war against Spain, he volunteered to sink the old collier *Merrimac* in the channel of Santiago Harbor, thus bottling up the Spanish fleet. The attempt failed as intense enemy fire drove *Merrimac* off course and sunk her outside of the channel, but Hobson's undeniable gallantry made him a national hero over night. He came home to a tumultuous welcome, his feat commonly compared with Theodore Roosevelt's charge up San Juan Hill. (In a somewhat curious lapse of time, Congress honored his bravery by awarding him the Congressional Medal of Honor and naming him a rear admiral on the retired list—all in 1933!). Bored by his postwar assignments, however, he resigned from the service in 1903, at which point his fame allowed him to begin a new career as a reformer and politician.

Returning to his native Alabama, Hobson ran successfully for the House of Representatives in 1906 and served for four consecutive terms. He proved a tireless legislator who made no secret that he considered his nation's greatness divinely ordained. To project America's majesty abroad he labored endlessly to expand and reform the navy, and he deserved much of the credit for establishing the post of chief of naval operations. The internal salvation of the country also captured his attention, and in this cause he waged what he saw as a veritable holy war against drug and alcohol addiction. He spoke repeatedly against the liquor traffic and emerged as a vociferous proponent of National Prohibition. Indeed, in 1913 he introduced into Congress a prohibition amendment to the Constitution. It failed to obtain the necessary two-thirds majority, but it was a sign of things to come. He also spoke and wrote heatedly against alcohol use (he considered booze a "protoplasm poison"), and one of his books, *The Great Destroyer* (1911), stood as one of the most effective polemics produced by any dry author. His persistence on behalf of his chosen reforms won him low marks with some of his legislative colleagues, a few of whom termed the Alabamian a "national nuisance." But his stock with drys and with much of the public, which remembered his wartime heroism, remained high. The Temperance Movement considered him nothing less than a national resource. After leaving Congress in 1915, he pursued his war on addiction uninterrupted. Until 1922 he was a touring lecturer for the Anti-Saloon League, speaking in front of large and enthusiastic audiences. He also organized the American Alcohol Educational Association, as well as the International Narcotic Educational Association. He was an officer in both groups until his death. Hobson was a difficult man to characterize. He was unquestionably talented and dedicated, not to mention courageous. But he was also erratic and prone to see issues in extremes of good and evil. Still, his outspoken opinions at least let everyone—friend or foe—know exactly where he stood.

**Bibliography:**

A. "America Mistress of the Seas," *North American Review* (Oct. 1899); *The Great Destroyer* (New York, 1911); *Destroying the Great Destroyer* (New York, 1915); *Alcohol and the Human Race* (New York, 1919); *Milestones in the War Against the Narcotic Peril* (New York, 1925); *The Modern Pirates— Exterminate Them* (New York, 1931).

B. DAB Supp. 2, 308–9; NYT, March 17, 1937; SEAP 3, 1230–31; WW 1, 572.

**HODGES, George Hartshorn**    (6 February 1866, Orion, WI—7 October 1947, Olathe, KS). *Education*: private study of law. *Career*: laborer, Olathe, KS, 1886–89; senior partner, Hodges Brothers (lumber and hardware), beginning 1889; owner, *Johnson County Democrat*, beginning 1890s; president, Olathe Building & Loan Co., beginning 1890s; member, Kansas Senate, 1904–12; governor of Kansas, 1913–15; civilian staff member with Major General Leonard Wood, circa 1917–18; active reform lecturing and writing, beginning circa 1912.

A classic self-made man of the American West, George Hodges grew up with the state of Kansas as it left the frontier stage and entered the Progressive Era. His parents were of moderate means and could not afford to send him beyond the level of an elementary public education. Consequently, he went to work early in life, starting as a day laborer in a lumberyard in the mid-1860s. Hodges, however, proved not only ambitious but able; three years later, at only twenty-three years old, he opened his own lumber business, and he made it pay. He was a partner in that original venture—Hodges Brothers—until he died, although over the years his holdings expanded considerably; he ultimately owned twelve lumberyards and as many hardware stores in various parts of Kansas, as well as a newspaper, the *Johnson County Democrat*. Wealthy and sucessful, Hodges tried his hand at politics, and he did it the hard way. In a largely Republican state, the active businessman was a loyal Democrat. He served in the Kansas State Senate from 1904 to 1912, compiling a record that identified him with the Progressive wing of his party. He strongly endorsed the streamlining of government, humanitarian reforms, prohibition, women's suffrage, and the interests of Western agriculture. His personal popularity was considerable; indeed, it was probably greater than that of the Democratic Party generally. When he ran successfully for the governorship he was the only member of his party to win a state-wide electoral contest. The new governor gained a measure of recognition during World War I when he spearheaded a Kansas relief drive for Belgium. As a result of his efforts, the state raised tons of supplies for the war-torn nation, and later a grateful King Albert decorated Hodges with one of Belgium's highest awards. Out of office when the United States entered the conflict, the former governor served as a civilian volunteer on the staff of Major General Leonard Wood. Raised on the frontier, then, Hodges played an active role as his country shifted its attention from westward internal expansion to international participation.

Hodges's career also exemplified the relationship between prohibition and Progressivism. The antiliquor crusade was at the heart of his reform thinking. It was the firm belief of the businessman-governor that with the drink trade eliminated, a host of other evils of modern society, from poverty to political corruption, would disappear. He was an articulate champion of prohibition during his years in the State Senate and met the issue head-on when opponents tried to use his position against him in his run for the governorship. Hodges never relented on the liquor question, however, and he assigned the protection of the Kansas dry laws a high priority while he sat as the state's chief executtive. To his credit, he never tried to gain partisan advantage from his stand, always insisting that the fight against "the demon" should be above party politics. Hodges acquired considerable national renown as a result of a speech he delivered to the national convention of the Anti-Saloon League of America in Columbus, Ohio, in 1913. Ironically titled, "How Prohibition Ruined Kansas," the address soon became a minor temperance classic, being reprinted many times in booklet form and distributed to thousands across the country. It purported to show that the abolition of legal liquor in the state had brought an impressive range of benefits to Kansas. Thirty years of prohibition, Hodges claimed, had led to sharp declines in the general death rate, while at the same time producing dramatic increases in literacy, taxable ratables, and general social and economic prosperity. Hodges was well pleased with the startling popularity of his talk, genuinely happy to have advanced national dry sentiments. After leaving office, he continued in the crusade. The former governor was acclaimed as a public speaker, and he became a wide-ranging figure on the podium on behalf of prohibition. Years later, however, as the national mood swung away from temperance under the impact of the Great Depression, Hodges chose to remain with his party, even as the Democrats turned avowedly wet. Yet in his day, George Hodges had amply demonstrated the reform faith in freeing Americans from the curse of the liquor traffic as a means of bringing about a general reformation of the nation.

### Bibliography:

A. "Distrust of State Legislatures: The Cause, the Remedy," *Governors' Conference Proceedings*, No. 6 (Madison, WI, 1913); *How Prohibition Ruined Kansas* (Topeka, KS, 1914).

B. SEAP 3, 1232; WW 2, 256.

**HOHENTHAL, Emil Louis George**   (15 October 1864, New York, NY—8 December 1928, South Manchester, CT). *Career*: carpenter, 1882–97; construction contractor, South Manchester, CT, 1897–1913; full-time temperance organizing, 1913 to 1920s.

George Hohenthal's life exhibited a Horatio Alger pattern of poverty and lack of education overcome by hard work and right living. When he was only thirteen, the death of his father forced young Hohenthal to leave school and go to work. He earned a meager wage in a tailor shop for five years, the sole support of a family of seven. At eighteen years old, he became a carpenter's apprentice, and he worked at the trade for more than twenty years. Hohenthal had a good head for business and after 1897 worked for himself as the head of his own contracting firm in South Manchester, Connecticut, where he had lived since 1886 (and remained for the rest of his life). During his formative years (in fact, at the time he became a carpenter), Hohenthal strictly abstained from drink and tobacco. His motives are unknown, but there was never any question of his dedication, as he devoted most of his nonworking hours to temperance activities. He joined the Prohibition Party in 1886, his first political affiliation, and remained a committed member until his death. The following year, he entered the local lodge of the Sons of Temperance. In both organizations, Hohenthal displayed remarkable enthusiasm, and he began a steady rise to leadership. He managed the affairs of the Prohibition Party in his community with genuine skill and by 1901 had risen to the post of chairman of the party's state committee. The story was similar in the fraternal lodge: After holding a succession of local offices, he was head of the state organization by the 1890s. Reform, then, had offered the hardworking carpenter a considerable degree of social mobility. Certainly he had become Connecticut's premier antiliquor crusader.

Hohenthal's temperance activities finally became so time-consuming, and his reputation as a champion of the cause so noted, that he decided to focus his career solely on reform work. In 1913, then, after more than two decades in carpentry, and at the request of his comrades in the Prohibition Party, he closed his business and took on even greater antiliquor responsibilities. At the head of his party, he ran for Congress, the Senate, and the governorship; and while unsuccessful, the tireless dry always ran a spirited campaign and did manage to win several local elections (something of a novelty for Prohibition Party candidates). In the Sons of Temperance, he served three terms as most worthy patriarch (1916–22), the highest national office in the organization. In that capacity, he travelled the country extensively and made two visits to Britain and Ireland to meet with lodges there. A frequent participant in the International Congresses Against Alcoholism, Hohenthal went to the 1921 Congress in Lausanne, Switzerland, as President Warren G. Harding's officially appointed delegate. He also visited Central Europe a number of times in the early 1920s as a lecturer for the International Reform Bureau. Hohenthal's work demonstrated how thoroughly the temperance cause had penetrated many American communities. His activities brought him considerable respect in Connecticut (despite the fact that wet strength was always great in the region), and he was a welcome and influential member of his church (he was a Congregationalist), various governmental agencies, and the Chamber of Commerce. Of German heritage, Hohenthal was also living proof that the antiliquor cause could appeal to members of traditionally wet ethnic groups.

**Bibliography:**

B. SEAP 3, 1236–37; WW 1, 576.

**HOOFSTITLER, Jacob Hostetter**  (9 January 1846, Salunga, PA—?). *Education*: private study of law, 1860s. *Career*: soldier, Union army (mustered out as second lieutenant), 1861–65; legal practice, Sterling, IL, 1865–66; army scout, Fort Omaha, NB, 1866–67; clerk, U.S. District Court, Julesberg, CO, 1867–70; temperance lecturer, 1870 to 1920s.

There were many routes by which individuals entered the ranks of the Temperance Movement, but it is doubtful that any was as varied, circuitous, and exciting as the one travelled by Jacob Hoofstitler. Of German heritage, young Jacob grew up in the quiet Pennsylvania-Dutch area of Lancaster County, where he received an elementary education. At fifteen years old, however, the relative tranquility of his early life ended abruptly. With the coming of the Civil War, he enlisted in the Union army as a drummer and served until the end of the conflict. He saw some tough soldiering before the last shots were fired, and when he mustered out Hoofstitler wore the rank of a second lieutenant, won in a battlefield commission. Somehow during the war he had also found enough spare time to study law and in 1865 was licensed to practice in Pennsylvania. Apparently, legal advocacy was too tame for Hoofstitler, because he shortly took himself off to the West, where he became a government scout at Fort Omaha, Nebraska. There, he hunted down outlaws in the socially unstable period after the War Between the States. He faced some rather nasty situations, once staring down a hostile crowd, a revolver in each hand, while making an arrest. During part of his experience, he served as clerk of the regional federal district court, where he worked closely with a judge who carried a pistol himself—and also knew how to use it. The former drummer boy stayed in Nebraska until 1870, establishing a reputation that struck terror into the local outlaws, whom he stalked with such effect that his years on the job marked the beginning of law and order in the area. By any measure, then, Jacob Hostetter Hoofstitler was a tough customer.

Although Hoofstitler's career up to this point would seem poor preparation for a temperance advocate, it was actually the turning point in his life. For he became convinced that at the root of much of the lawlessness he combatted on the frontier was the drinking habit. So, in 1870, Hoofstitler began yet another career, battling the evils of drink as he had battled the evils of outlawry. He moved back to his native Pennsylvania-Dutch country, married, and launched one of the more memorable temperance careers of his day. He joined the Prohibition Party and immediately plunged into politics, running repeatedly for state, national, and local office. The ex-lawman never won an election, but his political efforts certainly enhanced his popular notoriety. This was fortunate, for his source of income came almost exclusively from the lecture platform for the next forty-seven years. Moving to Illinois in 1873, he spent little time in his new home as his hectic speaking schedule kept him on the road throughout the United States and Canada. He held forth to large audiences on the evils of drink, the promise of women's suffrage, and the need for a range of other reforms; his listeners found apealing his combination of law and order and moralizing rhetorical style. With the entry of the United States into World War I, Hoofstitler's lecture tours shifted to patriotic themes and support for the war effort. His German ethnic background made him especially valuable in countering pro-German sentiment, although his comments evidently evoked the hostility of some German-Americans. After 1918, however, he returned to his favorite theme, once more denouncing the ''demon rum'' and, during the 1920s, urging the strict enforcement of National Prohibition. While the busy orator belonged to a number of dry organizations and remained active in the Prohibition Party, his greatest call on temperance gratitude was as a speaker. He was one of the most colorful—and there is a certain sad irony in the fact that his passing (which came as popular opinion was losing interest in the dry crusade) escaped major public notice.

**Bibliography:**

B. SEAP 3, 1246–47.

**HOPKINS, Alphonso Alva**    (27 March 1843, Burlington Flats, NY—25 September 1918, Cliffside, NJ). *Education*: Ph.D., American Temperance Univ., TN, 1895. *Career*: schoolteacher, NY, 1860s; editor, *Moore's Rural New Yorker*, *American Rural Home*, *American Reformer*, 1867–85; vice chancellor and professor of political economy; American Temperance Univ., Harriman, TN, beginning 1868; editor, *National Advocate*, beginning 1913; editorial staff, Funk & Wagnalls Co., NY, 1918.

Alphonso Hopkins made his mark in the Temperance Movement chiefly through his literary activities, although his contributions to the reform ranged over a number of fields. Growing up in rural New York State, he secured a sound elementary education as well as proficiency in Latin and Greek under private tutors. After several years of teaching and part-time writing, his interest in languages led him to an editorial career, beginning with the Rochester-based *Moore's Rural New Yorker* in 1867. Soon after this, he founded and edited his own rural journal. The young editor's interests, however, lay beyond the confines of stories on country living. He was deeply drawn to the reform sentiments then at large in the nation, and in 1882 he established a publication reflecting his feelings, the *American Reformer*. In its pages he emerged as a crusading editor, voicing concern over any number of issues then current in the public mind. The Temperance Movement, though, received most of his attention. In Hopkins's hands, the *Reformer* blistered the liquor traffic while singing the praises of the dry cause generally and the Prohibition Party in particular. During these years, Hopkins also tried his hand at politics, joining the Prohibition Party in 1872. Under its aegis he ran at various times for governor and secretary of state of New York, as well as for Congress. He was never elected to any office, however, and he never let his political ventures interfere with his editorial work. Indeed, after the *American Reformer* merged with another temperance journal in 1884, he increased his own writing considerably. As the turn of the century neared, the New York editor wielded one of the most active pens the dry movement could boast.

Yet editing and writing expressed only part of Hopkins's zeal for the dry crusade. He was also a public speaker of some note. He was frequently on the Chautauqua circuit, and his lecture tours on behalf of temperance took him to most sections of the country. While on the stump, he appeared on the platform with such antiliquor luminaries as John B. Finch, John P. St. John,* and General

Clinton Fisk.* He also believed that education offered an effective means of dealing with the liquor question, and in this area he had grand hopes indeed. He took an important role in the founding of the American Temperance University in Harriman, Tennessee. For several years in the 1890s he served on the faculty of the institution as professor of political economy, while at the same time sitting as the school's first vice chancellor. In 1895, the university awarded him the doctor of philosophy degree. In addition to his teaching at American, he also taught courses off campus for various community groups, a practice he continued upon returning to his native East a few years later. His academic work led to the writing of still more titles, which he used in the classroom. These included prohibitionist works such as *Wealth and Waste* (1896), *Profit and Loss in Man* (1909), and *The Bugle of Right* (1913). (In addition, Hopkins wrote several biographies and one verse novel.) After resettling in New Jersey in the early 1900s, he edited the *National Advocate* for the National Temperance Society and Publication House, and went to work on the editorial staff of Funk and Wagnalls in New York City. He died at home in 1918 at age seventy-five, remembered by his colleagues in reform as one of the most active of their number.

**Bibliography:**

A. *Prohibition from the Front Porch. . .* (n.p., 1897); *His Prison Bars: A Temperance Story* (Chicago, 1901); *Sinner and Saint: A Story of the Woman's Crusade* (Chicago, 1902); *Geraldine: A Souvenir of the St. Lawrence* (Boston, 1909); *Profit and Loss in Man* (New York, 1909).

B. SEAP 3, 1247–48; WW 1, 586.

**HOPKINS, Mark**   (4 February 1802, Stockbridge, MA—17 June 1887, Williamstown, MA). *Education*: A.B., Williams Coll., 1824; M.D., Berkshire Medical Coll., 1829. *Career*: tutor, Williams Coll., 1825–27; medical practice, New York City and Binghamton, NY, 1829–30; faculty member, Williams Coll., 1830–87; president, Williams Coll., 1836–72; ordained Congregational minister, 1836; president, American Board of Commissioners for Foreign Missions, 1857–87; president, National Temperance Society and Publication House, 1883.

One of the most celebrated educators of his time, Mark Hopkins, the son of a poor farmer and the nephew of renowned minister Samuel Hopkins, based his long career at Williams College in Williamstown, Massachusetts. In a sense, he was connected with the college before he enrolled, as one of his ancestors, Colonel Ephriam Hopkins, had helped to found it. After completing his undergraduate studies (he graduated in 1824), he went on to acquire an M.D. and to a brief medical practice; but his heart was never in medicine. He gave it up gladly when his alma mater called him back in 1830 to a position as professor of moral philosophy and rhetoric. Hopkins remained at Williams, teaching without major interruption until his death over five decades later, serving as president of the school a good deal of the time (1836–72). To his commitment to Williams, the professor added a deep religious faith (like his famous uncle, he was a

Congregationalist). Although he lacked formal theological training, the Berkshire Association of Congregational Ministers licensed him to preach in 1833, and ordination followed in 1836. Hopkins delivered many sermons, and by all accounts he was a popular speaker on religious and moral subjects. Many of his addresses were collected and published in book form, and all sold well. But Hopkins achieved his greatest fame as a teacher. He was not especially widely read himself, nor was he a particularly original scholar. Even in his teaching he had little use for formal aspects of education and he scorned modern methods. Yet he drew the best from students. It was necessary, he believed, only to appeal "directly to the consciousness of the hearer. No learning is needed; no science, no apparatus, no information from distant countries." His method was basically Socratic, a dialogue between teacher and pupil. So effective was this approach that those who had been exposed to it never forgot it. His influence can clearly be seen in the familiar comment made by President James A. Garfield (a Hopkins student) in an address to Williams alumni in 1871. No better education could be imagined, he said, than a log in the woods with a student at one end of it and Mark Hopkins at the other.

If Williams was the center of Hopkins's universe, however, he still had important interests off campus. The famous educator developed a considerable reputation as a moral reformer. For thirty years he was president of the Board of Commissioners for Foreign Missions, and he consistently lent his name and prestige to the efforts of the Temperance Movement. He often spoke on the subject, and he authored at least one tract for the National Temperance Society in which he deplored the impact of social drinking on education. He became actively involved in the dry cause during the Civil War, when a number of Northern states began to repeal or modify their prohibitory statutes. In response to this wet offensive, a number of reformers, Hopkins among them, organized the National Temperance Society and Publication House. The New York–based group was intended to educate the public in temperance values and to provide a literary outlet to be used in maintaining the prohibitionist crusade. Hopkins's association with the new group lent it considerable credence, and he followed its affairs with keen interest. Upon the death of its first president, William E. Dodge,* in 1883, the Williams professor stepped into the vacancy and led the society personally. When Hopkins himself died in 1887 (at age eighty-five, and still teaching), the society was a healthy and important part of the postwar onslaught against drink, and temperance workers, as well as educators and former students, mourned the passing of an inspirational leader.

## Bibliography:

A. *The Connexion Between Taste and Morals . . .* (Boston, 1842); *Lectures on the Evidences of Christianity . . .* (Boston, 1861); *Lectures on Moral Science . . .* (Boston, 1871); *An Outline Study of Man . . .* (1873; New York, 1903); *Temperance and Education: Or, the Relation of the Social Drinking Customs to the Educational Interests of the Nation* (New York, 1876); *The Scriptural Idea of Man* (Boston, 1883).

B. DAB 9, 215–17; SEAP 3, 1248–49; Franklin Carter, *Mark Hopkins* (New York, 1892); John Hopkins Denison, *Mark Hopkins: A Biography* (New York, 1935); Frederick Rudolph, *Mark Hopkins and the Log: Williams College, 1836– 1872* (New Haven, CT, 1956); Leverett Wilson Spring, *Mark Hopkins, Teacher* (New York, 1888).

**HOSS, Elijah Embree**    (14 April 1849, Washington Co., TN—23 April 1919, Muskogee, OK). *Education*: A.B., Emory and Henry Coll., VA, 1869; D.D., Emory and Henry Coll., 1885; LLD., Emory and Henry Coll., 1890; LLD. (honorary), Emory Coll., GA, 1898, Ohio Wesleyan Univ., 1906. *Career*: ordained, Methodist Episcopal Church, South, 1870; minister, Knoxville, TN, 1870–72; minister, San Francisco, 1872–74; minister, Asheville, NC, 1875; president, Martha Washington Coll., Abington, VA, 1876–81; vice president (later president), Emory and Henry Coll., 1881–85; professor of ecclesiastical history, Vanderbilt Univ., 1885–90; editor, *Nashville Christian Advocate*, 1890– 1902; bishop, Methodist Episcopal Church, South, beginning 1902.

A noted academician and temperance advocate, Elijah Hoss centered his life's work on his devotion to the Methodist Church. Educated in the law and theology, he served in pulpits from Tennesee to California throughout the 1870s, his sermons carrying much of the dry message inherent in Methodist social and moral tenets of the day. A forceful and eloquent speaker, as well as a good organizer, Hoss established a considerable reputation among his fellow churchmen. In 1878, he put his leadership talents to work in academia, serving as president of two colleges for the next seven years: Martha Washington College in Abington, Virginia, from 1878 to 1881, and his alma mater, Emory and Henry College in Virginia, from 1881 to 1885. Leaving college administration in 1885, he taught ecclesiastical history at Vanderbilt University in Nashville, Tennessee, for the next half decade, when he gave up the academic life to become editor of the *Nashville Christian Advocate* (1890). In the meantime, Hoss was busy establishing himself as one of the most active temperance reformers in the state. He played a central role in founding the Tennessee chapter of the Anti-Saloon League (which always had close ties to Methodism), and he served for a number of years as its president and treasurer. As an editor and speaker, he labored diligently to sway popular opinion in favor of the league's policies, to influence legislation, and to fight off counterattacks by the state's considerable wet forces. He argued consistently that his fellow citizens must follow a path of abstinence and prohibition as a prerequisite to the Christian life. In all of this he enjoyed a major degree of success, and he proved able to organize and finance an enduring dry structure that did yeoman service in building a popular base of support for prohibition of the region. After his denomination named him a bishop in 1902, Hoss continued zealous in the crusade until his death on a trip to Muskogee,

Oklahoma, in 1919. In Bishop Hoss, the Temperance Movement had found, as one dry commentator put it, "a leading spirit and a perpetual source of inspiration."

**Bibliography:**

A. *Elihu Embree: Abolitionist* (Nashville, TN, 1897); *Sunday School Studies...* (Nashville, TN, 1903); *Methodist Fraternity and Federation* (Nashville, TN, 1913); *The Call and Equipment of the Christian Minister* (n.p., 1915); *David Morton: A Biography* (Louisville, KY, 1916); *William McKenovee: A Biographical Study* (Nashville, TN, 1916).

B. SEAP 3, 1252–53; WW 1, 590; Paul E. Isaac, *Prohibition and Politics: Turbulent Decades in Tennessee, 1885–1920* (Knoxville, TN, 1965).

**HOWARD, Clinton Norman**    (28 July 1868, Pottsville, PA—25 April 1955, Washington, DC). *Education*: privately educated. *Career*: reform lecturer and organizer, beginning 1889.

Reform was almost second nature to Clinton N. Howard. His ancestry boasted a long line of preachers and reformers of all types, and though he himself had been trained for the ministry, he never took a pastorate; rather, he preferred to devote his life to the causes he held so dear, world peace and temperance. Originally from Pennsylvania, Howard moved to Rochester, New York, in 1889, and he did most of his work there. After an education at the hands of private tutors, he began a long career of public service, chiefly as a lyceum and Chautauqua lecturer. He spent ten years conducting a Sunday afternoon forum, addressing large crowds on topics heavily concerned with "civic righteousness" and "public rectitude." The Rochester orator was dynamic in front of audiences, and he soon established a reputation as the "Little Giant" of reform. Temperance was one of his favorite topics. Indeed, during his climb to notoriety, the subject led to some of his most memorable speeches. Howard also devoted his formidable energies to antiliquor organizing. In 1890 he founded the Prohibition Union of Christian Men, of which he was president, and in time the group enrolled over three thousand members. Over the next twenty-five years, Howard made more than 1,500 speeches on behalf of prohibition and became so identified with the cause that the public thought of him almost solely in connection with the dry crusade. (Indeed, he went so far as to name two of his sons after dry heroes: John Gough Howard, in honor of the great Washingtonian temperance lecturer, and Neal Dow Howard, after the Maine Law crusader.) With the ratification of the Eighteenth Amendment, he gave perhaps his greatest address, a funeral oration for "John Barleycorn" entitled "A Joy Ride to the Grave." Thousands listened as Howard delivered it in cities from Boston to San Francisco. With the coming of National Prohibition, however, the Rochester orator considered the dry battle won (a fatally shortsighted view for a temperance worker, as things turned out). While he never lost touch with antiliquor work, beginning in the early 1920s he turned most of his attention to the issue of world peace. He spoke fervently on the issue, planned a speaking tour with William Jennings Bryan (although Bryan's death brought the scheme to nought), and sat for a time as president of the World Peace Commission. In his old age, little was heard of Howard, and upon his death in 1955 few Americans knew his reputation as one of the great public speakers of his generation.

**Bibliography:**

A. *The Handwriting on the Wall...* (Chicago? 1912); *The World on Fire* (Rochester, NY, 1918); *A Joy Ride to the Grave* (Rochester, NY, 1919, and subsequent printings).

B. SEAP 3, 1254–55; WW 3, 420.

**HOWARD, Oliver Otis**   (8 November 1830, Leeds, ME—26 October 1909, Burlington, VT). *Education*: graduated from Bowdoin Coll., 1850; graduated from West Point, 1854; LLD. (honorary), Waterville Coll., 1865, Shurtleff Coll., 1865, Gettysburg Theological Sem., 1866, and Bowdoin Coll., 1866. *Career*: army officer, 1854–94 (included major Civil War commands in Union army; major commands in Indian Wars; superintendent, U.S. Military Acad., 1881–82; retired as major general); commissioner, Freedmen's Bureau, 1865–74; philanthropic activities, 1860s to 1909.

A graduate of Bowdoin College and the U.S. Military Academy, O. O. Howard, the son of a well-to-do farm family, spent almost all of his adult life in the military. After serving briefly in the Seminole Wars in Florida in 1857, Howard taught mathematics at West Point and then, with the outbreak of the Civil War, was appointed a colonel of the Third Regiment, Maine Volunteer Infantry. Beginning with First Bull Run, Howard served throughout the entire war, often with great bravery, from the Peninsular Campaign to Sherman's "March to the Sea." In the course of these campaigns Howard was several times wounded, losing his right arm at the Battle of Fair Oaks in June 1862. The following year, his division bore the brunt of Stonewall Jackson's devastating flank assault at Chancellorsville; but his men were back in fighting trim in time to take a prominent part in the crucial engagement at Gettysburg shortly afterward. Although some historians have questioned Howard's judgement on the field (as did some contemporaries), there was never any doubt about his personal bravery. He received many honors and decorations for heroism under fire, including the thanks of the Congress and the Congressional Medal of Honor. By the close of the Civil War, Howard had been elevated to the rank of brigadier general in the regular army, with brevet rank of major general. In the postwar years, his more interesting assignments took him to the West, where he campaigned against the Indians and negotiated a number of important treaties (notably with Cochise, the Apache chief, in 1872).

Although Howard's claim to public notice had come chiefly through his military activities, his longstanding humanitarian proclivities added another aspect to the general's call on popular gratitude. Howard had been a firm antislavery man during the Civil War, and he did not shirk what he saw as his duty when called upon to help the newly freed slaves after the defeat of the Confederacy. In 1865, President Andrew Johnson appointed him commissioner of the Bureau of Refugees, Freedmen and Abandoned Land (popularly known as the Freedmen's Bureau), which the federal government had established in order to provide for the needs of the emancipated slaves. Howard showed great sympathy, interest, and concern for the freedmen and as head of the bureau provided much-needed protection and assistance for them in the uncertain period during Reconstruction. He left much to be desired, however, administratively, and his ardent defense of black rights outraged many Southern whites; but his conduct of the bureau was such as to leave it free from the taint of corruption that so besmirched the Grant administration. While Howard's critics raised serious charges of mismanagement, congressional investigation completely cleared him, and he left the agency in 1874 with his reputation intact. The reform-minded soldier's concern for the freed black population did not end when he left the bureau, however. He was a central figure in the founding of the Washington, D.C., school that was named in his honor, Howard University, an institution dedicated to the education of black youth. Later he was instrumental in establishing Lincoln Memorial University in Cumberland Gap, Tennessee, which offered educational opportunities to poor whites. Until his death, Howard never lost interest in these ventures or in the welfare of the groups these schools were intended to help.

Howard's reform concerns encompassed other causes as well. In fact, he was a notable temperance advocate throughout his military career. As a commanding officer, he was stern in his condemnation of drunkenness in the ranks (an all too frequent occurrence), an attitude fully in keeping with his reputation for personal probity and morality. At the head of the Freedmen's Bureau, he was appalled at what he saw as the drinking excesses of the black population he dealt with, and he took a direct role in sponsoring dry organizations to counter the situation. Howard advocated the founding of Lincoln Temperance Societies and encouraged the former slaves to join. On occasion, the general also took to the stump himself, delivering antiliquor speeches throughout the Southern states. As a direct proponent of total abstinence, he tried to point out that the demands of citizenship and the requirements of making a living were incompatible with drink. He also offered temperance groups considerable help in spreading this message. Returning to duty after his tour with the bureau, he was no happier about the drinking he saw among his troops. In 1888, for example, when placed in command of the army's Department of the East, he lodged a strong protest with the secretary of war, objecting heatedly to the practice of selling liquor in army canteens. Howard remained active upon his retirement in 1894. He wrote extensively on reform and military subjects, raised money for charitable causes, and continued a staunch Republican until his death at seventy-nine in 1909.

### Bibliography:

A. *Nez Perce Joseph...* (1881; New York, 1972); *Fighting for Humanity; or, Camp and Quarter-Deck* (New York, 1898); *Henry in the War; or, the Model*

*Volunteer* (Boston, 1899); *My Life and Experiences Among Our Hostile Indians...* (1907; New York, 1972); *Autobiography of Oliver Otis Howard, Major General, United States Army*, 2 vols. (New York, 1908); *General Taylor* (New York, 1912).

B. DAB 9, 279–81; SEAP 1255–56; WW 1, 594; John Alcott Carpenter, *Sword and Olive Branch: Oliver Otis Howard* (Pittsburgh, PA, 1964); William S. McFeely, *Yankee Stepfather: General O. O. Howard and the Freedmen* (New Haven, CT, 1968); Harriet Beecher Stowe, *Men of Our Times, or Leading Patriots of the Day...*, 8 vols. (New York, 1869).

**HUDSON, Grant Martin**    (23 July 1868, Eaton Township, OH—26 October 1955, Lansing, MI). *Education*: B.A., Kalamazoo Coll., MI, 1894. *Career*: retail business, 1896–1909; member, Michigan House of Representatives, 1905–8; state superintendent, Michign Anti-Saloon League, 1910–20; state manager, Occidental Life Insurance Co., 1916; member, State Industrial Accident Compensation Commission, 1920–21; member, U.S. House of Representatives, 1923–27; field representative, State Tax Commission, 1939–42.

Born in Ohio in 1868, but spending almost all his adult life in Michigan, Grant M. Hudson made his chief contribution to the prohibition movement in the first decade of the twentieth century. It was after more than a decade in the retail business that Hudson entered state politics by being elected to the Michigan House of Representatives in 1905. There he found the opportunity to put to practical use his longtime hatred of the liquor traffic and his commitment to prohibition. His views were typical of many in his situation: He was a successful merchant, active in civic and business groups (he was a Mason and a Rotary International member, for example), a pillar of his church (he was a devout Baptist), and prominent in his community; in short, Hudson was the kind of solid citizen to whom the political influence and social disorder attributed to the drink trade was anathema. Rallying the Republican forces in the legislature, he sponsored a statute that became known as the Hudson Bill. The legislation aimed at making it easier for temperance forces to dry out Michigan through local option—a favorite technique of the Anti-Saloon League, of which Hudson was an ardent member. The proposed law would have replaced county local-option districts with smaller municipal units, thus giving greater opportunities to township-level dry forces. A second part of the bill called for more stringent enforcement provisions against liquor law violations. Although wet groups strongly opposed the law, Hudson mounted a dynamic campaign for it with his fellow legislators and the general public; it carried and was rightly seen as a major prohibitionist victory. It was also a personal victory for Hudson, who became even more involved with the politics of temperance. He took on a number of assignments with the Michigan League, serving as financial secretary in 1910, superintendent of the Detroit district in 1911, and superintendent of the full Michigan League in 1914, which office he held until 1920. In 1916, Hudson, at the head of the league, led the drive that resulted in a popular majority of some 68,000 votes for state-wide prohibition. Making the most of his popularity, Hudson then ran successfully for the U.S. House of Representatives, and was reelected in 1924. Not surprisingly, he was among the firmest supporters of the Volstead Act and other National Prohibition laws during his four years in Washington, D.C. Returning home after his second term, Hudson capped his temperance career by election to the National Board of Directors of the Anti-Saloon League.

**Bibliography:**

B. SEAP 3, 1260; WW 3, 425.

**HUGHES, Harold Everett**    (10 February 1922, Ida Grove, IA— ). *Education*: studied at Univ. of Iowa, 1940–41; D.Sc. (honorary), Government Coll. of Osteopathic Medicine and Surgery, 1965; LLD. (honorary), Cornell Coll., 1966, Buena Vista Coll., 1967, Graceland Coll., 1967, Loras Coll., 1968, Lehigh Univ., 1969, Grinnell Coll., 1969; DHL. (honorary), Marycrest Coll., 1967; DCL. (honorary), Simpson Coll., 1969. *Career*: private, U.S. army, 1942–45; trucking business, 1946–53; field agent, Iowa Motor Truck Association, 1953–55; manager, Iowa Better Trucking Bureau, 1955–58; member, Iowa State Commerce Commission, 1959–63; member, Interstate Commerce Joint Board, 1959–62; governor of Iowa, 1963–69; member, U.S. Senate, 1969–75; brief campaign for Democratic presidential nomination, 1971; missionary work with various groups, beginning 1975.

The career of Harold Hughes served to demonstrate much of the continuing impact of alcohol-related issues on American political life. A deeply religious man (and a licensed Methodist preacher), his years in public office were marked by a conscious effort to apply the tenets of his faith to his responsibilities as an elected official. After service during World War II, he emerged as a leader—both in business and as a commerce commissioner—in the reform of the Iowa trucking industry, a task in which he was especially sensitive to the interests of small truckers. Later, as a Democratic governor, he displayed the same concern for the disadvantaged, fighting consistently for civil rights, improved social services for the needy, and freer access to the political system. Throughout his years in pursuit of these goals, however, Hughes also fought a more personal battle—with alcoholism. A hard drinker for years, he finally managed to quit drinking over the early 1950s through the aid of a personal religious experience and a continuing affiliation with Alcoholics Anonymous. Although he had won his struggle with the bottle, though, alcohol and alcoholism still became major issues in his political career in Iowa. In his initial campaign for governor, for example, in 1962, one of the most heated controversies raged over permitting the sale of liquor by the drink, which the state only allowed in private clubs. Although a total abstainer himself by this time, candidate Hughes urged the legality of by-the-drink sales in order to better regulate the liquor business in the state, and his forthright stand contributed to his victory over a popular incumbent Republican. In a later campaign, Hughes easily overcame a vicious attempt to use his alcoholism as a political issue. Indeed, by candidly discussing his former drinking, the Iowa governor probably contributed to a growing national effort to lessen the social stigma attached to the condition. At any rate, when he left the statehouse in 1969, Hughes took with him a record of solid legislative accomplishment, major credit for stimulating vital economic growth for his state, and a reputation for honesty and compassion in office.

In the Senate, Hughes continued his affiliation with the liberal wing of the Democratic Party. He was an outspoken critic of the Vietnam War, active in framing labor and veterans legislation, and generally an advocate of expanding the federal role in the provision of human and social services. One of his chief interests in this regard was forging national policies and programs to deal with drinking problems. During his single term in the Senate (as assistant majority whip) he chaired the first congressional subcommittee on alcoholism and narcotics, procured funding and legislative approval for alcoholism and narcotics treatment and education programs in the armed forces and Office of Economic Opportunity, sponsored efforts to bar job discrimination against recovered drug addicts and alcoholics, and was the driving force behind the passage of the Comprehensive Alcohol Abuse and Alcoholism Prevention, Treatment, and Rehabilitation Act (1970). The act (sometimes called the Hughes Act), a far-reaching piece of legislation, firmly established the national government in alcohol-related issues while avoiding the prohibitionist policies of previous generations. It created the National Institute on Alcohol Abuse and Alcoholism (which in turn initiated a variety of research, treatment, and education projects), put the government on record as viewing alcoholism as a medical and public health concern, and encouraged the states to increase their efforts in the field as well. Amended since originally passed, the Hughes Act remains the basis of federal involvement with alcohol-related questions. Taken as a whole, the work Hughes devoted to alcohol problems was probably more substantial than that of any other federal legislator since the legal efforts of the Prohibition era.

Despite his popularity in Iowa and the high regard of much of the Senate (including many conservatives), Hughes did not seek reelection in 1974. Thereafter, he committed most of his time to religious or social outreach work with various groups, often in conjunction with acquaintances from his years in government. He took a special interest in the problems of the American Indian, remained active in prison Bible fellowships and other religious circles, and worked closely with a number of organizations addressing alcoholism and its related problems. Already named president of the World Council on Alcoholism in 1972, he continued in that capacity while being named to the board of the National Council on Alcoholism in 1974. Remaining active with Alcoholics Anonymous, Hughes also worked in a consultant capacity with alcoholism treatment facilities and philanthropic groups, notably the Christopher D. Smithers Foundation in New York. To some extent, he maintained ties to national politics as well. In 1975 and 1976 he served as a consultant to the Senate Judiciary

Committee, advising members on negotiations over the Panama Canal Zone, as well as chairing a commission on Senate operations. Yet his ultimate political goals also centered on his faith. In the late 1970s, Hughes and his wife, Eva, established what they hoped would become, in effect, a spiritual retreat for national leaders in Cedar Point, Maryland. Beyond that, however, it also became home to a local chapter of Alcoholics Anonymous.

**Bibliography:**

A. with Dick Schneider, *The Man from Ida Grove: A Senator's Personal Story* (Lincoln, VA, 1979).

B. Christopher D. Smithers Foundation, *Pioneers We Have Known in the Field of Alcoholism* (Mill Neck, NY, 1979); Carolyn L. Wiener, *The Politics of Alcoholism: Building an Arena Around a Social Problem* (New Brunswick, NJ, 1981).

**HUGHES, Matthew Simpson**    (2 February 1863, Doddridge Co., VA—4 April 1920, Portland, OR). *Education*: studied at Univ. of West Virginia, 1880s; D.D., Hamline Univ., 1909. *Career*: ordained Methodist Episcopal Minister, 1887; minister, Chestnut Street Church, Portland, ME, 1890–95; minister, Wesley Church, Minneapolis, MN, 1895–98; minister, Independence Avenue Church, Kansas City, MO, 1898–1908; minister, First Church, Pasadena, CA, 1908–16; professor of practical theology, Maclay Coll. of Theology, Univ. of Southern California, 1908–11; bishop, Methodist Episcopal Church, beginning 1916.

The son of a Methodist preacher and brother of a bishop in the Methodist Episcopal Church, it seemed only natural when Matthew Hughes turned to religion as his chosen profession. After schooling in West Virginia, where he was born in 1863 (it was then Virginia), Hughes went on to study theology, first at the University of West Virginia and then at Hamline. Before earning his doctor of divinity in 1896, however, he was able to launch his long and distinguished ministerial career. He was ordained in 1890 by the Methodist Episcopal Church and then began service to a succession of pastorates in Maine, Minnesota, Missouri, and California. Hughes proved an able and dynamic church leader in his various assignments, and his views were typical of those of his fellow churchmen on the pressing social issues of the day—especially the question of prohibition. His sermons and writings thundered against the liquor traffic and urged the public to rally behind the dry standard. While pastor to a Methodist congregation in Pasadena, California (1908–16), the fiery preacher became active in organized antiliquor activities. He ultimately became president of the California Dry Federation and later a member of the Executive Committee of the Anti-Saloon League of America. In 1916, the Temperance Movement lauded the appearance of his only major book, *The Logic of Prohibition*, a less-than-original summary of standard temperance arguments, which further contributed to his public recognition as a dry champion. Hughes's untiring performance as a church leader and reformer also brought denominational recognition: In 1916 the Methodist Church elected him a bishop. The decision was in fact more than a means of honoring Hughes's service to the church. It was an era of close ties between Methodism and the Temperance Movement, especially the Anti-Saloon League, and the elevation of Hughes served to underscore the fact. He had done well not only by his denomination but by the antiliquor crusade as well. His ideas had never been original, nor his contributions especially novel, but he had proven staunch in the cause, devout, and unquestionably a good administrator— a combination of value to any large organization seeking to get the most from its personnel. The new bishop promptly moved to Portland, Oregon, where he died (1920) before he could really make his mark on local affairs.

**Bibliography:**

A. *The Higher Ritualism: Sermons...* (Cincinnati, OH, 1904); *Fraternal Address to the General Conference of the Methodist Episcopal Church, South...* (Oklahoma City, OK? 1914); *The Logic of Prohibition* (Pasadena, CA, 1916); *Dancing and the Public Schools* (New York, 1917).

B. SEAP 3, 1263–64; WW 1, 603.

**HUMPHREY, Heman**    (26 March 1779, West Simsbury, CT—3 April 1861, Pittsfield, MA). *Education*: graduated from Yale Coll., 1805. *Career*: minister, Fairfield, CT, 1807–17; minister, Pittsfield, MA, 1817–23; president, Charitable Collegiate Inst. (Amherst Coll.), 1823–45; active retirement, 1845–61.

Born while the War of Independence still raged, Heman Humphrey, clergyman and educator, was to make his mark as a devoted and effective soldier in the war against drink in the first half of the nineteenth century. Humphrey enjoyed some excellent schooling in his youth. Yet he was of a serious frame of mind and never took his future success in life for granted; thus he prepared himself through strict self-discipline and dogged study for entrance into Yale College as a junior in 1803. The fact that by then he was already in his twenty-fifth year indicates some measure of his determination. After graduation in 1805, Humphrey began his theological studies, over the course of which he developed the appreciation of Congregational orthodoxy that guided the rest of his career. In 1806 he was licensed to preach by the Litchfield (Connecticut) North Association of the Congregational Church, and the following year the new minister assumed the pulpit in Fairfield, Connecticut. His firm convictions, however, made his first pastorate anything but tranquil. Humphrey's sense of orthodoxy led to his rejection of the liberal Half-Way Covenant, and he had to use all of his powers of persuasion to convince his congregation of the correctness of his refusal to baptize children whose parents were not church members. Humphrey quickly emerged as equally strict on other questions. What his original motives were is obscure, but as early as 1810 the Fairfield preacher declared for total abstinence on religious grounds. He was one of the first ministers in his area to do so— and in an age when most of his neigbors, including most of the clergy, saw little or nothing wrong with moderate drinking. It was a radical position, but Humphrey proclaimed it with a passion, and his message helped prepare the way for the organized Temperance Movement that arose to spread the dry gospel a decade later. Indeed, his protest against drink led to authorship of two of the earliest and most forceful temperance tracts by any New England minister. In 1813, in conjunction with two other clergy, he wrote *Intemperance: An Address to the Churches and Congregations of the Western District of Fairfield*, in which he castigated the liquor traffic as the root of immorality and civic ruin. Later (1828), he wrote a more compelling pamphlet, *Parallel Between Intemperance and the Slave Trade*. Clearly, he had become established as a champion of moral reform in all of its guises and as one of the most sophisticated opponents of the "demon rum."

Humphrey's prominence took him on to progressively more important assignments over the years. In 1817 he took the pulpit of Pittsfield, where he healed a major rift in the congregation. Indeed, his reputation for strong and consistent moral leadership spread widely, as did notice of his firm insistence on linking religious orthodoxy with moral reform. Along with Lyman Beecher* and a few others, Humphrey was also acknowledged as one of the most influential temperance leaders of the day. All of this brought him to the attention of the trustees of the Charitable Collegiate Institution—soon to be renamed Amherst College—when they pressed their search for a president of the school in 1823. The crusading minister accepted the call and began a tenure of leadership that lasted twenty-two years. At Amherst, he maintained his acclaimed probity and dedication in guiding the educational fortunes of some 765 young men and was doubtless a major factor in persuading over 400 of them to enter the clergy. His convictions regarding drink and sin formed an important part of this preparation, and his beliefs found characteristic expression in 1830, when he founded the college Antivenenean Society. The new organization's members were sworn to abstain from alcohol, tobacco, and drugs. Significantly, while Humphrey was president of Amherst, fully 80 percent of the student body subscribed to this self-denying ordinance. Education, according to the college leader, had as its main goal the training of the "habits of industry, temperance, and benevolence," and none could gainsay that he failed to instill these principles in his students. After his stewardship at Amherst, the old reformer retired to write hortatory books on morality, travel, and his memoirs.

## Bibliography:

A. *Intemperance...* (Ballston Spa, NY, 1814); *The Good Pastor...* (Amherst, MA, 1826); *Parallel Between Intemperance and the Slave Trade* (New York, 1826); *Miscellaneous Discourses and Reviews* (Amherst, MA, 1834); *Great Britain, France, and Belgium: A Short Tour in 1835* (New York, 1838); *Debates of Conscience, with a Distiller, Wholesale Dealer, and a Retailer* (New York, 18—?).

B. DAB 9, 369–70; WW H, 336; Z. M. Humphrey and Henry Neill, *Memorial Sketches: Heman Humphrey and Sophia Porter Humphrey* (Philadelphia, 1869).

**HUNT, Mary Hannah Hanchett**    (4 June 1830, Canaan, CT—24 April 1906, Boston, MA). *Education*: studied at Amenia Sem., Amenia, NY, 1840s; studied at Patapsco Female Inst., near Baltimore, MD, 1848–50. *Career*: chemistry and physiology teacher, 1851–52; family governess, plantation in VA, 1850; superintendent, Department of Scientific Temperance Instruction, Woman's Christian Temperance Union, 1880–1906; editor, *School Physiology Journal*, 1892–1906.

Modern alcohol education in the public schools is in part a continuing legacy of the efforts of Mary Hunt. She became active in temperance work only in the late 1870s, when her training as a science teacher convinced her that misinformation on the physiological effects of alcohol had prevented decisive public action against the liquor traffic. As a solution, she urged the teaching of ''scientific temperance'' in the public schools. Properly taught, she believed, students not only would learn the dangers of drink, and consequently grow up dry, but also would carry a school-bred bias toward prohibition to the ballot box when they reached voting age. In temperance eyes, Hunt's educational approach therefore offered the nation both health and political benefits. She argued her position vigorously before local audiences in Massachusetts and then, at the urging of Frances Willard,* explained her ideas to the National WCTU in 1879. The following year the union appointed Mrs. Hunt superintendent of its new Department of Scientific Temperance Instruction in Schools and Colleges; her mission was to assist in the creation of suitable instructional materials and to advocate their inclusion in public school curricula. The pursuit of these goals became her life's work and earned her international recognition.

Hunt concentrated her department's efforts jointly on politics and educational policy. She led a sophisticated effort at the state level to induce passage of laws mandating temperance education, including curriculum content. The first success came in Vermont in 1882, and by 1902 every state and territory had adopted similar legislation. In 1886 her efforts resulted in a federal law for such instruction in all nationally owned schools, including the military academies. While waging her political battles Mrs. Hunt also moved to assure both the supply and quality of teaching materials. Under her direction, the WCTU endorsed texts it considered adequate and actively recruited authors and publishers to maintain the flow of new books. (Indeed, the rapid spread of mandated temperance education made the field lucrative for many publishers.) In order to keep teachers abreast of health education issues, she founded the *School Physiology Journal* in 1894, which she edited until her death. A tireless exponent of her cause, she explained her methods before a number of international conferences and assisted groups in Canada and Europe in attempts to institute similar educational programs. She also proved an able defender of scientific temperance instruction. Her efforts helped fend off attacks on its methods and content from a variety of quarters; and in 1903 her testimony before a Senate committee successfully blunted the criticisms of the Committee of Fifty, which had charged temperance education with distortion, bias, and inaccuracy. And while they have been radically altered in the years since Repeal, the laws sponsored by Mary Hunt remain the genesis of modern alcohol education statutes.

**Bibliography:**

A. *A History of the First Decade of the Department of Scientific Temperance Instruction in Schools and Colleges* (Boston, 1891); *An Epoch of the Nineteenth Century* (Boston, 1897); "Reply to the Committee of Fifty," *Sen. Doc.* 171, 58 Cong., 2d sess., 1904.

B. DAB 9, 388–89; NAW 2, 237–39; SEAP 3, 1268–70; David Leigh Colvin, *Prohibition in the United States* (New York, 1926); Norton Mezvinsky, "Scientific Temperance Instruction in the Schools," *History of Education Quarterly* 1 (1961): 48–56; Frances E. Willard and Mary A. Livermore, eds., *American Women* (New York, 1897).

**I**

---

**IGLEHART, Ferdinand Cowle** (8 December 1845, Warrick Co., IN—21 July 1922, Dobbs Ferry, NY). *Education*: A.B., DePauw Univ., 1867; A.M., DePauw Univ., 1869; D.D., DePauw Univ., 1892. *Career*: minister, various pastorates in IN, IL, NY, NJ, 1870–1905; district superintendent, Anti-Saloon League of New York, 1906–15; editorial staff, *Christian Herald*, beginning 1908; lecturer in sociology and temperance, Syracuse Univ., 1900s.

Ordained as a Methodist Episcopal minister in 1870, Ferdinand Iglehart was an earnest advocate of temperance throughout his career. Something of an itinerant in his early years, he held pulpits in six Indiana cities and one in Illinois before moving to New York in 1882, where he spent the following twenty-three years serving as pastor. For varying time periods Iglehart ministered to eight churches in the New York metropolitan area, including one in New Jersey. During these years he was generally active in local temperance affairs—which was typical of many of the Methodist clergy of the period—and his interests gradually shifted from pastoral to full-time work on behalf of prohibition. In 1906, Iglehart accepted the position of district superintendent with the New York Anti-Saloon League, and he dedicated himself entirely to the work of the league for the next decade. Tireless and devoted, he saw the league's efforts as an extension of the Progressive "social gospel," and under his leadership the organization grew in numbers and prestige. While superintendent, with the cooperation of his close friend Theodore Roosevelt, then police commissioner of New York City, the reforming minister saw to it that the city's Sunday-closing law was strictly enforced and obeyed by the regional saloons. His efforts in the state's urban areas helped to demonstrate that the message of the Temperance Movement could find receptive ears in the cities of the nation—that the antiliquor crusade was not simply a rural assault on the metropolis. Iglehart's tenure with the league made it a force to be reckoned with in New York State politics, and when he retired from the superintendency in 1916 (at age seventy-one), he could look back on his years at the helm with satisfaction. Yet his retirement from the league hardly ended his contributions to the movement as a whole. He remained active in the cause, devoting himself to writing and occasional teaching. He also submitted works to various magazines and served on the editorial staff of the *Christian Herald*, a position he had held since 1908. In 1917 his most important book, *King Alcohol Dethroned*, was published and quickly gained fame in dry circles as one of the most eloquent and penetrating analyses of the liquor question in the contemporary literature. Temperance advocates retained a high regard for it years afterward. He also lectured briefly at Syracuse University on sociology and temperance issues.

**Bibliography:**

A. *The Spreading Oak* (n.p., 1903); "The Liquor Problem," pp. 400–402, in *American Yearbook* (Westerville, OH, 1913); *King Alcohol Dethroned* (New York, 1917); *Theodore Roosevelt: The Man as I Knew Him* (New York, 1919).
B. SEAP 3, 1282; WW 1, 617.

**INGALLS, Eliza Buckley**    (24 August 1848, St. Louis, MO—9 February 1918, St. Louis, MO). *Education*: brief college study in Philadelphia, early 1860s. *Career*: secretary, St. Louis Woman's Christian Temperance Union, beginning 1879; vice president-at-large, Missouri WCTU,1880–91; president, St. Louis WCTU, 1891–1918.

In common with many temperance advocates, Eliza Ingalls took an interest in almost every species of reform that promised to free humankind from dependence on drugs of any type. In a major respect, as Frances Willard* was frequently to remind the dry crusade, the reform struggle was "a fight for the clear mind." And one of the chief stalwarts in that fight was Ingalls, the wife of a temperance-minded St. Louis businessman who encouraged her in her antiliquor career. Her interest in temperance preceded her marriage, however. As a girl of fourteen, she received special permission to enroll in the Independent Order of Good Templars, and she kept her total abstinence pledge until she died. While still a young woman, she achieved local recognition for her efforts on behalf of the dry cause. In 1879, when Frances Willard* organized the St. Louis branch of the Woman's Christian Temperance Union, Ingalls became the new groups's first secretary and then shortly afterward took an at-large vice presidency in the state organization. She held that post for eleven years and in 1891 moved up to the presidency, where she oversaw the affairs of the Missouri WCTU for the next twenty-seven years. Indeed, aside from her home and a few other charitable activities, the WCTU became the chief focus of her life. Her interest in drug problems brought her a leadership post with the National Union, which she served for over twenty years as superintendent of anti-narcotics. From this position, she worked to educate the public on the dangers of drug addiction and in the process emerged as a fairly able pamphleteer and illustrator. She was one of the pioneers in pointing out the adverse impact of cigarette smoking on health, and she campaigned vigorously against the habit. Another side of Eliza Ingalls was revealed by her service of many years on the Missouri State Board of Charities (a succession of governors reappointed her periodically). She worked voluntarily and gave of her time freely. Ingalls was thus a superb example of Willard's "Do Everything" reform policy; she typified the commitment and range of activities that temperance workers undertook, and her long service says much on how the dry movement was able to muster the leadership talent that brought it to national prominence.

**Bibliography:**

B. SEAP 3, 1324.

**IRELAND, John**    (1838, Burnchurch, Ireland—25 September 1918, St. Paul, MN). *Education*: graduated from college, Meximieux, France, 1857; graduated from sem., Montbel, France, 1861. *Career*: chaplain, Union army, 1861–62; curate, St. Paul, MN, 1861–67; rector, St. Paul, MN, 1867–75; bishop, Diocese of St. Paul, 1875–88; archbishop of St. Paul, 1888–1918.

Irish born, French educated, and American by citizenry, John Ireland was one of the most prominent Catholic churchmen in the nation during the late nineteenth and early twentieth centuries. He was the first archbishop of St. Paul, and he demonstrated considerable administrative capacity as he steadily improved the affairs of his diocese. His concerns, however, went beyond the church, as Ireland was also an energetic and forthright proponent of the "social gospel." Indeed, he set his hand to a number of Progressive era reform causes, advocating them with a frankness that surprised even some of his friends. While always maintaining the worth of parochial education, for example, the archbishop also insisted on strong state-supported school systems, and for years he attempted to find grounds on which the Catholic and public schools could cooperate. He did his best to combat racial prejudice and segregation in his church, called for improved working conditions and wages for Americn labor, and advocated public support for many social services. Ireland also struck out bluntly at the liquor traffic, accusing drink and intemperance of impeding reform in other areas—not to mention their roles in bringing about innumerable social ills in the first place. He was thus a vocal and active member of the Temperance Movement, in which he assumed an important leadership role. The St. Paul priest encouraged the growth of the Catholic Total Abstinence Union and along with Protestant clergy took the initiative in calling the dry convention that resulted in the founding of the Anti-Saloon League of America in 1895. He then agreed to serve as a league vice president, a post which clearly established his reputation nationally as a champion of the antiliquor cause.

Much of Ireland's outlook on church governance seemingly reflected his liberal attitude toward reform. He sought to demonstrate that modern Catholicism was compatible with republican ideals and that Catholics could work actively and democratically for social change. At least in part, he saw this stance as a means of reducing the "foreign" image that many American Protestants still attached to the Roman church. This concern was clearly evident in some of Ireland's temperance work. He noted, for instance, that many Catholic immigrants to the United States had indeed brought their traditional drinking habits with them, but that American Catholic leaders were trying to change things. He pointed out that thousands of Catholics were working hard on behalf of temperance and that some church organizations had barred members of the liquor traffic from membership. Old charges that Catholics were tolerant of intemperance and the saloon, he claimed, were untrue. "The American saloon," the archbishop wrote, was "a personification of the vilest elements in our modern civilization." It was a danger to "virtue, to piety of soul, to peace of family, to the material, moral, and intellectual welfare of the people, to the free institutions of the republic." No native-born Protestant could have put the temperance position better, and some dry reformers saw in such statements a sign that an "Americanization" of the immigrant population was underway. Ireland probably hoped so, as long as the process left attachments to church hierarchy intact. But apart from his dry sympathies, other Catholics, usually of a more conservative persuasion, began to fear that the archbishop was going too far in his liberal stances—that he had opened the path to a schism in the church. Ireland and his closest associates protested their innocence of any such intentions; but the controversy ultimately led to a papal warning against any tampering with church teachings or doctrine. Some historians have suggested that the controversy prevented Ireland's selection as cardinal.

**Bibliography:**

A. "The Catholic Church and the Saloon," *North American Review* 159 (1894): 498–505; *L'Eglise et le siècle* (Paris, 1894); *The Church and Modern Society: Lectures and Addresses* (Chicago, 1896).

B. DAB 9, 494–97; DARB, 225–27; NCAB 9, 226; NYT, Sept. 26, 1918; Joan Bland, *Hibernian Crusade: The Story of the Catholic Total Abstinence Union of America* (Washington, DC, 1951); James H. Moynihan, *The Life of Archbishop John Ireland* (New York, 1953); Cuthbert Soukus, *The Public Speaking of Archbishop John Ireland* (St. Cloud, MN, 1948); J. V. Tracy, "Prohibition and Catholics," *Catholic World* 51 (1890): 669–74.

**IRVINE, Stella Blanchard**    (21 July 1859, Beaver Dam, WI—?). *Career*: schoolteacher, La Crosse, WI, early 1880s; active in Woman's Christian Temperance Union, especially with Sunday School Department, 1884 to 1920s; Prohibition Party organizer and candidate, CA, 1902 to 1920s.

Stella Blanchard Irvine was yet another member of the Woman's Christian Temperance Union who saw compatability between temperance work and the campaign for women's rights. Beginning her adult life as a schoolteacher in her native Wisconsin, she took up efforts with the dry crusade in a serious way after her marriage to husband Lew Irvine in 1882 and their subsequent move to Minnesota. It was in her adopted state that she joined the WCTU in 1884, having watched the rise of the woman's group for the previous several years. From the beginning, Irvine's religious sentiments influenced her relationship with the temperance organization. From girlhood, she had been involved with Sunday school work, and over the years she came to believe that a strong national network of

Sunday schools would prove an essential boon to American morality and well-being. Consequently, she put these interests to use by focusing her temperance work on the WCTU's Sunday School Department—a division established not only to foster Sunday schools in churches but to provide them with dry instructional materials. Her energy soon carried her to the position of department superintendent, and she eventually became national director. As such, Irvine was responsible for organizing the Bureau of Sunday School Temperance Literature, which was ultimately to put out over five hundred publications on temperance topics for distribution to Sunday schools in Europe as well as the United States. Mrs. Irvine capped this phase of her work in 1922, when she was elected world superintendent of the bureau. For the former schoolteacher from Wisconsin, then, work with the WCTU had offered a career ladder, which she climbed to successively more responsible levels.

Irvine's most notable work, however, came later when her attention shifted from Sunday schools to women's rights. The cause of this new emphasis in her activities is not precisely known, although as her own leadership talents emerged, Irvine may have become more aware of (and angry with) the social limits put on women of her generation. At any rate, following a move with her husband to California in 1902, she increasingly coupled her temperance arguments with agitation on behalf of the female vote. Her base of operations was the Prohibition Party, a small and politically uninfluential group in California—but willing to allow a woman to assert herself in the electoral arena. In 1914, Irvine ran as a Prohibitionist for the state legislature and lost, and then came right back to run for Congress. Even in defeat she surprised the public with the vigor of her campaigns, her abilities as a speaker, and the relatively impressive number of votes she tallied. And even though her own races ended in losses, Irvine had the satisfaction of seeing her bids open up politics (at least to a limited extent) for other women: Soon after, four women did win seats in the State Assembly. Irvine also broke other frontiers for her sex. Following her religious calling, she pursued a career in another area long dominated by men—the ministry. Applying for the right to preach in the Southern California Conference of the Methodist Episcopal Church, she became the second women to be licensed to preach in the denomination in the region. Throughout these years, she maintained a leadership role in the state WCTU, helping to build it to unprecedented levels of membership and local influence. During the battle for the ratification of the Eighteenth Amendment, Irvine was instrumental in marshalling state support for the measure, and she received due credit when California finally voted to ratify.

**Bibliography:**

B. SEAP 3, 1359–60.

# J

**JELLINEK, Elvin Morton** (15 August 1890, New York, NY—22 October 1963, Palo Alto, CA). *Education*: studied at Univ. of Berlin, 1908–11; studied at Univ. of Grenoble, 1911; M.Ed., Univ. of Leipzig, 1914; Sc.D. (honorary), Univ. of Leipzig, 1935. *Career*: biometric consultant, 1914–19; biometrician, plant research, Sierra Leone, 1920–25; biometrician, United Fruit Co., Honduras, 1925–30; chief biometrician (later associate director of research), neuroendocrine research, Worcester State Hosp., MA, 1931–39; alcohol research, Research Council on Problems of Alcohol, NY, 1939–40; alcohol research, Laboratory of Applied Physiology, Yale Univ., 1940–50; associate editor, *Quarterly Journal of Studies on Alcohol*, 1940–50; associate professor of applied physiology, Yale Univ., 1940–50; director, Yale Summer Sch. of Alcohol Studies, 1943–50; lecturing, consulting, writing, and teaching, including the World Health Organization, Texas Addiction Research Foundation, Toronto, and Stanford Univ., 1950s to 1963.

Modern conceptions of alcoholism as a disease have evolved from a variety of sources. But of all of these, the ideas pioneered by E. M. Jellinek and his co-workers probably have been the most influential. In the years since Repeal, Jellinek did as much as anyone to advance the notion that alcoholism is a treatable disease, and he offered the post-prohibition era its most plausible explanation of the condition's etiology. Jellinek did most of his best work on alcoholism at the Yale University Labroratory of Applied Physiology, where he came in 1940 after a distinguished career in biometrics (he was of sufficient stature to have shared a platform once with Sigmund Freud). He had come to the laboratory at the request of its director, Professor Howard W. Haggard,* who asked him to conduct a series of scientific investigations of the nature of alcoholism. To begin, Jellinek produced a number of classic reviews of alcohol-related phenomena in psychiatry and psychology. He then followed with publication on the drinking habits of various societies, the "Jellinek estimation formula" (still used by some researchers to estimate the number of alcoholics in a given population), and efforts to link the study of drinking and alcohol to the established academic disciplines. Although he did not cast himself in an administrative role, his organizational contributions were also of the first magnitude. With Haggard, he founded the Yale Center of Alcohol Studies (serving for years as its director), worked on the *Quarterly Journal of Studies on Alcohol* (of which he was associate editor), and directed the Summer School of Alcohol Studies and the first alcoholism treatment clinics launched by the Yale Center. Jellinek also helped establish the World Health Organization Committee on Alcoholism and the National Council on Alcoholism. By the late 1950s, his mark on the field was indelible.

Jellinek was best known, however, for his efforts to define the nature of alcoholism itself. He identified five varieties of alcoholism (he called them "species"), although he always noted that there could be more. Of these, however, only two fit the disease model: "Gamma" and "delta" alcoholism, he noted, involved increasing adaptation to alcohol, changes in cell metabolism, withdrawal symptoms, a physical or psychological "craving" for alcohol, and a "loss of control" over drinking. That is, these were states of physical addiction. Gamma alcoholics, Jellinek believed, could frequently abstain for periods without going into withdrawal, while deltas quickly suffered withdrawal symptoms after abstinence and therefore drank almost continuously. In addition, he saw a symptomatic progression of "phases" leading from psychological to physical addiction. "Alpha" and "beta" alcoholics, who were only psychologically dependent (betas having more severe physical complications), and "epsilon" alcoholics, characterized by unpredictable periodic episodes of uncontrolled drinking, lacked the "progressive process" and did not fall clearly under the disease rubric. Thus for Jellinek, the term *alcoholism* per se was confined to gammas and deltas and lacked the wider meaning it often carried later. The thoughtful researcher contended at the outset that his theory was only a hypothesis: It would do "for the time being" he wrote in 1960, "but not indefinitely." Despite warnings, however, much of the emerging alcohol studies field adopted his ideas as virtual gospel, and over the years even dissenting voices have acknowledged the wide appeal of Jellinek's formulations. In fact, it is not too much to say that in the almost half century following Repeal, the work of this extraordinary individual framed most aspects of the modern debate over the nature of alcoholism and its treatment.

In addition to this typology of alcoholism, though, Jellinek also took a number of other steps which, if less heralded, were equally important in fostering continuing scholarship. The significance of the *Quarterly Journal of Studies on Alcohol* should not be underrated: For years, it was one of the only reliable forums for reporting on scholarship in the field. He also initiated (and for a time directed) the compiling of the *Classified Abstract Archive of the Alcohol Literature*, which for more than a generation stood as the world's definitive literature collection on all aspects of drinking and alcohol. Jellinek's influence was also intensely personal. He captured the ardent loyalty of his colleagues, and his work inspired other scholars to pursue paths of inquiry that otherwise would have gone unexamined. Notably, he was one of the first researchers to see the value of Alcoholics Anonymous, and his interest in the group helped spark continuing scientific attention to the dynamics and methods of the self-help fellowship. (Jellinek used data gathered from AA members as the basis of his famous study on the "phases" of alcoholism.) After he left the Yale Center, he moved through a succession of university appointments and work with the World Health Organization, teaching, writing, and encouraging the further study of alcohol-related phenomena (he was concerned with more than just alcohol problems) by other researchers. When he died at seventy-three years old, he was, fittingly, in his office—still at work.

**Bibliography:**

A. with Ross A. McFarland, *Analysis of Psychological Experiments on the Effects of Alcohol* (New Haven, CT, 1940); with Howard W. Haggard, *Alcohol Explored* (Garden City, NY, 1942); *The Problems of Alcohol* (New Haven, CT, 1945); *Phases in the Drinking History of Alcoholics: Analysis of a Survey Conducted by the Grapevine...* (New Haven, CT, 1946); *Recent Trends in Alcoholism and in Alcohol Consumption* (New Haven, CT, 1947); with Mark Keller and Vera Efron, *CAAAL Manual: A Guide to the Use of the Classified Abstract Archive of the Alcohol Literature* (New Brunswick, NJ, 1953); *The Disease Concept of Alcoholism* (New Haven, CT, 1960).

B. NYT, Oct. 23, 1963; WW 4, 492; Selden D. Bacon, "E. M. Jellinek, 1890–1963," *Quarterly Journal of Studies on Alcohol* 24 (1963): 587–90; Mark Edward Lender, "Jellinek's Typology of Alcoholism: Some Historical Antecedents," *Journal of Studies on Alcohol* 40 (1979): 361–75; Harry Milt, *Revised Basic Handbook on Alcoholism* (Maplewood, NJ, 1977); Robert E. Popham, ed., *Alcohol and Alcoholism: Papers at the International Symposium in Memory of E. M. Jellinek* (Toronto, 1966); A. E. Wilkerson, "A History of the Concept of Alcoholism as a Disease" (DSW diss., University of Pennsylvania, 1967).

**JEWETT, Charles** (5 September 1807, Lisbon, CT—3 April 1879, Norwichtown, CT). *Education*: study of medicine in physician's office, CT, 1820–30. *Career*: medical practice, East Greenwich, RI, 1830–40; agent, Massachusetts Temperance Union, 1840–54; editor, *Temperance Journal*, 1840 to 1850s; farmer, Batavia, IL, 1854; farmer, Faribault, MN, beginning 1855; member, Minnesota legislature, late 1850s; temperance lecturer and author, 1850s to 1870s.

Charles Jewett grew up on a relatively poor Connecticut farm, with few opportunities for formal education. Yet he had an intense desire to learn, saved enough for limited study at a local academy, and found a doctor willing to let him study medicine in his office. Opening his own practice in 1830 in East Greenwich, Rhode Island, he quickly built a large clientele and became a prosperous member of the community. In addition to treating the more common maladies of his patients, Jewett also added a preventive aspect to his practice. A total abstainer himself for many years, he would, as he recalled later, mix "a little temperance" with his medicine. Over the years, his constant attention to the antiliquor gospel made him as widely known as his medical practice, and he began to appear regularly before public groups as a temperance lecturer. For the Temperance Movement, Jewett was quite a find: Physicians of the period often used alcohol freely as a treatment for a wide variety of complaints, and to have an established doctor publicly denounce the practice (which Jewett did at length), and drink in general, was a major boon to the growing reform effort. Much of his speaking was on behalf of the Rhode Island Temperance Society, which he had joined in the 1830s, although occasionally he spoke out of state. The reform-minded doctor proved especially effective in inducing listeners to sign abstinence pledges. Finally, in 1840, his reputation as a temperance campaigner led to an employment offer that took him out of medicine (to which he had been devoting less and less time anyway) and into full-time reform work. The Massachusetts Temperance Union hired him as its agent, and for the next fourteen years he toured much of the nation in a concerted effort to carry the fight to the liquor traffic. His travels took him repeatedly through the Eastern and Midwestern states, where temperance forces considered him one of their most potent allies and wets developed a particular dislike for him. Throughout, he had the able and tireless support of his wife, Lucy Adams Tracey Jewett, who was an ardent reformer in her own right. By 1854, however, Jewett's rigorous schedule had helped to break his health, and he was compelled to leave the field. After an unsuccessful attempt to homestead acreage in Illinois, he and his sons began a prosperous farm in Minnesota—seemingly closing a brief but productive chapter in temperance history.

But it was not to be, for as his health improved on the farm, so did his enthusiasm for the reform wars. Jewett returned to the lecture circuit, still as cutting an enemy of the traffic as ever. Moreover, he became enmeshed in local politics, running successfully for the state legislature. He was not an especially successful lawmaker, but his presence in the halls of government gave his reform pleas additional credence in the public eye. To the end of his career, he gave particular emphasis to his warnings against the medicinal use of alcohol. Jewett saw his own ideas (which were not really novel) as flowing from the addiction theories of Benjamin Rush.* While Rush was not an advocate of total abstinence, however, Jewett insisted that even light alcoholic beverages could set a drinker on the path to addiction. Eventually, he explained, the drink would control the individual, with addiction demanding ever increasing amounts of alcohol, leading to the alcoholic's spiritual and physical demise. The evidence for this, he proclaimed, was clear for all to see, and he repeatedly castigated physicians who chose to ignore it and continued to send patients to their dooms. In his efforts to spread the alarm, Jewett authored a number of titles on various aspects of the liquor question, but his best-known work dealt with the issue of medicinal alcohol. Colleagues of the old campaigner considered him one of the best of their number: "No advocate of temperance," wrote Theodore Cuyler*, "has ever compressed more sound common sense into his speeches than Charles Jewett." And as a final legacy to the cause, Jewett left his son, Professor F. F. Jewett of Oberlin College in Ohio, who in the 1880s and early 1890s assisted the Reverend Howard Hyde Russell* in the work that led to the founding of the Anti-Saloon League.

## Bibliography:

A. *Speeches, Poems, and Miscellaneous Writings, on...Temperance and the Liquor Traffic* (Boston, 1849); *The Temperance Cause: Past, Present, and Future* (Hartford, CT, 1865); *Bound, and How: Or, Alcohol as a Narcotic* (New York, 1873); "The Medical Uses of Alcohol," 258–79, in *Centennial Temperance Volume...* (New York, 1877); *A Forty Years' Fight with the Drink Demon: Or, a History of the Temperance Reform...and of My Labor Therewith* (New York, 1882); *The Medical Use of Alcohol* (New York, 1885).

B. SEAP 4, 1399–1400; W. H. Daniels, *The Temperance Reform and Its Great Reformers* (Cincinnati, OH, 1878).

**JOHNSON, William Eugene ("Pussyfoot")**    (25 March 1862, Coventry, NY— 2 February 1945, McDonough, NY). *Education*: studied at Western Reserve Normal Sch., OH, 1880s, and at Univ. of Nebraska, 1880s. *Career*: school-teacher, NY and NB, early 1880s; reporter, *Lincoln* (NB) *Daily News*, 1884–86; manager, Nebraska News Bureau, 1886–87; feature news writer, mostly on prohibition, 1887–95; associate editor, *New York Voice* (later *New Voice*), 1899–1905; lobbyist for antiliquor legislation, Washington, DC, 1905–6; special agent, Department of the Interior (later with the Indian Service), 1906–11; active temperance lecturing, organizing, and editing, beginning 1911.

Perhaps the most glamorous of all temperance advocates, Johnson's life was the stuff out of which movie serials were made. Born in New York State of sternly temperance parents, Johnson began his career calmly enough as a teacher, a vocation he continued upon moving to Nebraska as a young man. But he wanted a position in journalism, a goal perhaps born of his happy experience editing his college newspaper, and he finally landed a job with the *Lincoln Daily News* in 1884. He subsequently became manager of the Nebraska News Bureau and, combining his love of journalism with his dedication to the Temperance Movement, a special correspondent for the dry *New York Voice*. He also briefly brought out his own antiliquor sheet, the *Daily Bumblebee*, and he revealed something of his combative nature when he beat up some hooligans who had been paid to harass his newsboys. In the 1890s, Johnson moved to Kansas City and continued his newspaper work, concentrating on exposing the corruption in the liquor traffic, and in 1896 he moved on to New York City, where he joined the staff of the *Voice*. By this time, Johnson had established a major reputation as an investigative reporter, a line in which he was to continue. In fact, his repeated success in uncovering illegal liquor operations made him internationally famous as the scourge of the beverage industry. His list of "credits" was amazing. For example, in Nebraska he posed as a liquor dealer purveying "Johnson's Pale Ale" in order to trap liquor dealers into revealing their plans to defeat pending prohibition legislation. In addition, Johnson exposed electoral frauds by which proliquor forces attempted to pad the voter rolls. In New York City, the journalist-detective continued his muckraking by producing evidence that the Raines Law was working contrary to its intended purpose by increasing drinking rather than reducing it. Similarly, Johnson later investigated college campus drinking and the South Carolina dispensary system. He also visited a number of U.S. army installations abroad and found extensive corruption in the canteens. He reported all of this in a sensationalist style that captivated readers.

All of these activities brought Johnson to the attention of President Theodore Roosevelt, who admired the temperance man's direct approach to matters. In 1906, the president appointed Johnson to enforce federal liquor laws in the Indian Territory, soon to become the state of Oklahoma. In the region what was left of the American frontier was still raw, and Johnson's technique for dealing with lawbreakers was well suited to the situation. He believed in taking on outlaws in rough-and-tumble fashion. Relying on a handpicked crew of deputies, Johnson would swoop down on illegal saloons, literally smashing them, destroying illegal hooch, furniture, and fixtures, in the process cracking a few skulls. Naturally, Johnson made plenty of enemies during these irregular proceedings, and for some time he was a marked man. He was assaulted, shot at, and generally made the target of the wrath of the liquor interests. This caused him to alter his tactics somewhat, preferring to attack by stealth rather than by direct assault, thus earning for himself the sobriquet "Pussyfoot." But Pussyfoot was a tough customer and he often gave as good as he got, although he took casualties: Eight of his deputies were killed and others were wounded. In the end, Johnson was credited with closing down some four hundred saloons and getting over 4,400 convictions during his five years of operations—statistics impressive by any standard. Through all of this Johnson enjoyed the unqualified support of President Roosevelt, who perhaps viewed it as another aspect of the Strenuous Life, or a domestic version of the diplomacy he had displayed in taking the Panama Canal. Once, when reproached for tolerating Johnson's dubious methods, Roosevelt replied, "Let Johnson alone: more power to his elbow." But Roosevelt's successor, William Howard Taft, a man of a more constitutional frame of mind, took a dim view of Johnson's private war on liquor. Having lost official support, Johnson resigned as special agent for the Department of the Interior in 1911. But "Pussyfoot" he remained for the rest of his days.

Retirement from public office did not mean that Johnson would rest on his laurels. Instead, he committed all of his considerable energy to the Temperance Movement, joining the Anti-Saloon League of America in 1912. In his new capacity, Johnson performed chiefly as publicist, travelling about the United States, and indeed the world, promoting prohibition. His itinerary was as impressive as it was diverse. To cite only a few of his efforts: He travelled widely in Europe, toured Russia extensively, conducted dry organizing efforts in India, and founded a chapter of the Anti-Saloon League in the Philippines. It was while he was in London on just such a mission that, during a debate, someone in an anti-temperance mob threw an object that hit the dry crusader in the face, costing him the sight of one eye. The Temperance Movement considered him something of a martyr ever afterward. The incident hardly slowed Johnson, however, as he continued his speaking engagements with his accustomed vigor. In 1918, he joined the editorial staff of the *Standard Encyclopedia of the Alcohol Problem*, first as managing editor and then as associate editor. Johnson also wrote extensively on the liquor question, as well as on his own experiences in law enforcement. He died in 1945 at the age of ninety-three and still awaits the full biography that his fascinating life so richly deserves.

**Bibliography:**

A. *The Basis for Total Abstinence Life Insurance* (New York, 1899); *The Gothenburg System of Liquor Selling* (Chicago, 1903); *The Federal Government and the Liquor Traffic* (Westerville, OH, 1917); *The Liquor Problem in Russia* (Westerville, OH, 1917); *Prohibition in Kansas* (Westerville, OH, 1919); *The South Carolina Liquor Dispensary* (Westerville, OH, 1919).

B. SEAP 3, 1408–13; WW 2, 285; Frederick Arthur McKenzie, *"Pussyfoot" Johnson: Crusader, a Reformer, a Man Among Men* (New York, 1920); G. V. Krishna Roo, *"Pussyfoot" Johnson: The Man and His Work* (Madras, India, 1921); Tarini Prasas Sinha, *"Pussyfoot" Johnson and His Campaign in Hindustan* (Madras, India, 1922).

**JOLLIFFE, Norman Hayhurst**    (18 August 1901, Knob Fork, WV—1 August 1961, New York, NY). *Education*: B.Sc., Univ. of West Virginia, 1923; M.D., New York Univ., Bellevue Medical Sch., 1926. *Career*: intern and resident, Bellevue Hosp., NY, 1927–30; chief, Medical Service of Psychiatric Division, Bellevue Hosp., 1932–45; faculty member, physiology, New York Univ., 1930–46; faculty member, Sch. of Public Health, Columbia Univ. Coll. of Physicians and Surgeons, 1946–61; active research and writing, mostly in nutrition, 1930s to 1961; service with international and national governmental, professional, and philanthropic groups dealing with nutrition issues, 1930s to 1961.

In the years immediately following the demise of National Prohibition, when most of the country wanted little to do with further discussion of alcohol problems, Norman Hayhurst Jolliffe was instrumental in reviving scientific interest in the subject. He approached alcoholism from the perspective of nutrition and diet, areas in which he was superbly trained and experienced. His medical background was extensive: Upon completing medical school and his internship and residency at New York's Bellevue Hospital, he joined the faculty of the New York University College of Medicine in 1932, and taught there until 1946. That year, he joined the faculty of the School of Public Health of the Columbia University College of Physicians and Surgeons, and he remained there until his death in 1961 (although during the last two years he was confined to a wheelchair). In addition, Jolliffe served as chief of the Nutrition Clinic of the New York City Department of Health from 1932 to 1946, and was director of the Bureau of Nutrition from 1949 until 1961. His chief interest was diet, and it was largely through his influence that the deleterious consequences of the vitamin-poor and high-fat foods of Americans came to be seen as the hazard they were to the nation's health. He coined the word *appestat* to describe what he thought was an appetite-controlling mechanism in the human brain. And he all but singlehandedly made Americans cholesterol conscious, pointing out its relationship to coronary attacks. Such was the professional foundation Jolliffe brought to the study of alcoholism. He was particularly interested in the role of vitamin deficiency as a factor in alcoholic diseases, and in the 1930s he proposed a seven-year study to determine the origins of alcoholism, including the effects of family and social environments. He envisaged a broad interdisciplinary approach to the problem that would mobilize the resources of physicians, psychiatrists, sociologists, social workers, and others. But the project, which would have been the most ambitious of its kind, failed to get the funding needed, and the great study never materialized. In 1937, however, Jolliffe did much in organizing the Research Council on Problems of Alcohol, along with Karl M. Bowman.* In 1939, he enlisted E. M. Jellinek* to direct a review of the biological literature on alcohol for the Research Council. The reports of that review prompted Dr. Howard W. Haggard* to found the *Quarterly Journal of Studies on Alcohol* in 1940, which figured importantly in placing the study of alcoholism on a firm professional and scholarly basis.

**Bibliography:**

A. ed., *Clinical Nutrition* (New York, 1950); *Reduce and Stay Reduced on the Prudent Diet* (New York, 1952).

B. NCAB 45, 44–45; NYT, Aug. 2, 1961; WW 4, 502; Mark Keller, "Norman Jolliffe, 1901–1961," *Quarterly Journal of Studies on Alcohol* 22 (1961): 531–34; Robert R. Williams, "Norman H. Jolliffe: A Biographical Sketch," *Journal of Nutrition* 80 (1963): 3–5.

**JONES, Charles Reading**    (9 November 1862, near Philadelphia, PA—26 March 1944, Evanston, IL). *Career*: family saddlery and hardware business, 1880–90; partner in saddlery business, 1890–93; publisher, horse and prohibition publications, 1885 to 1900s; treasurer, National Lincoln Chautauqua, 1914–19.

Born on a farm near Philadelphia, young Charles Jones turned from agriculture to a career as a small businessman—and came to exemplify the type of citizen who saw the antiliquor reform as a prime means of maintaining social order and prosperity. He began his adult life in the hardware and saddlery business as a member of the firm of Charles Jones and Sons, his father's enterprise. In 1890, Jones joined the partnership and for three years, until 1890, was secretary and manager of the Frink, Barcus and Jones Manufacturing Company (also saddlery makers), and became a well-known member of the local commercial community. Jones also had become involved in what was to be his true interest, publishing and editing. Between 1885 and 1890 he published the *Horesman's Guide*, and between 1891 and 1896, the *Harness Journal*. In addition to these special interest publications, he also put out a more general periodical, *The People* (1900–1905).

From the start of his career, Jones was also deeply interested in the prohibition question, and as his prominence in business grew, so did his belief that a favorable economic climate depended on national sobriety. Beginning in the early 1890s, he became increasingly involved in the struggle against booze, electing to work on behalf of the Prohibition Party. He was Philadelphia county chairman of the party for five years (1892–97) and then served as state chairman from 1897 to 1905. His administrative talents proved adequate to running the small reform organization, and in 1905 the party selected Jones as its national chairman (a post he held until 1912). Jones never brought his party close to real political influence, but he was deeply devoted to it. From 1892 until his death he never failed to attend its conventions. In keeping with his publishing interests, Jones was for a time the president of the Associated Prohibition Press and briefly an associate editor of the *American Prohibition Yearbook* (1910–11). He also helped to found a number of other dry groups, including the International Prohibition Confederation, and he served as an officer in many more. Perhaps his most important contribution to the history of the Temperance Movement was his leadership role in the Business Men's Research Foundation, a national group of small businessmen (like Jones) who argued that prohibition was essential to sound business and economic activity. The foundation has long survived Jones and the old crusade that gave it birth, and it remains (as of the 1980s) a legacy of an age when community leaders saw in temperance a key ingredient in the social order.

**Bibliography:**

B. SEAP 3, 1415; WW 2, 286.

**JONES, Samuel Porter**    (16 October 1847, Chambers Co., AL—15 October 1906, near Perry, AR). *Career*: legal practice, Cartersville, GA, 1868–71; laborer, 1871–72; travelling minister, Methodist Church, GA, 1872–80; agent, North Georgia Conference Orphan's Home, 1880–92; evangelist, 1892–1906.

The career of Samuel Porter Jones was the stuff of which Temperance Movement dreams were made. The movement never had a more potent ally; for when the fiery and flamboyant, yet utterly sincere evangelical preacher attacked the evils of drink, he knew whereof he spoke. Jones had started his professional life as a lawyer in 1868, and prospects for his practice in Cartersville, Georgia, seemed bright. Yet he had long been a heavy drinker, and his habit soon degenerated into alcoholism. His promising legal career went down the drain in a sea of booze, and Jones dragged his young wife and infant child into poverty with him. He was unable to stop drinking and was reduced to a bare existence as a day laborer. Then, as Jones hit bottom, his fortunes rebounded in the midst of another family crisis. As his father lay near death, Jones promised the dying man that he would reform; with that vow, Jones began his climb from the depths of alcoholism to national fame. He stopped drinking, found religion, and started preaching as a travelling Methodist minister in Georgia. He made only a modest living for the first eight years of his new career, but he stayed sober and his reputation as a speaker grew. In 1884 and 1885 he answered calls, based on his success in Georgia, to do evangelical work in Tennessee and in Brooklyn, which launched him into the national speaking circuit. He was an electrifying orator who was able to blend fundamentalist religion, direct and simple language, humor, and reform subjects in a single delivery. Audiences, North and South, loved him, and one historian has suggested that by 1900 he was perhaps "the foremost American public speaker of his generation." While his emotional style and fundamentalism lent themselves to easy caricature in some of the press, Jones was no charlatan and was popular with most sectors of the public.

One of Jones's favorite themes was the liquor question. His personal battle with the bottle had made him a convinced prohibitionist, and he spoke and wrote widely on behalf of the temperance cause. On the podium, he could move audiences deepy with the telling of the story of his own descent into alcoholism and his eventual recovery. He was a mortal enemy of the liquor traffic, and especially in his early preaching in Georgia, he made a particular effort to attack the purveyors of drink. "He probably would not regard a sermon as finished," recalled one account of the Georgia dry crusade, "until liquordom had received a drubbing." In some areas, notably Atlanta, Rome, and in other larger towns of the state, speeches by Jones were probably telling in finally swaying popular opinion against the traffic. Although he never joined the Prohibition Party, the hard-working evangelist was known to be kindly disposed toward it, a sentiment proudly touted on occasion by party members. In his later years, Jones reduced his public appearances, restricting his travel mostly to his native South. His death in 1906 was cause for widespread mourning in the region.

**Bibliography:**

A. *Quit Your Meanness* (Cincinnati, OH, 1886); *Sermons*, 2 vols. (Chicago, 1886); *Sam Jones' Sermons*, 2 vols. (Chicago, 1896); *Popular Lectures* (New York, 1909); *Revival Sermons* (New York, 1912); *Lightning Flashes and Thunderbolts* (Louisville, KY, 1912).

B. DAB 10, 199; NYT, Oct. 16, 1906; SEAP 3, 1417–18; WW 1, 650; Walt Holcomb, *Sam Jones* (Nashville, TN, 1947); Laura M. Jones, *The Life and Sayings of Sam P. Jones* (Atlanta, GA, 1906).

**JONES, Wesley Livsey**   (9 October 1863, Bethany, IL—19 November 1932, Seattle, WA). *Education*: A.B., Southern Illinois Coll., 1886. *Career*: legal practice, WA, beginning 1890; member, U.S. House of Representatives, 1899–1909; member, U.S. Senate, 1909–33.

A holder of national political office for close to thirty-three years, Wesley Livsey Jones grew up in Illinois. After completing his law studies in 1886, Jones moved to the Washington Territory just as it was on the verge of achieving statehood. The ambitious young lawyer had arrived on the scene just in time to get in on the ground floor of state politics, and he moved ahead quickly. Devoting as much time to Republican Party affairs as he did to the law, Jones was soon a prominent member of the party in Washington. (Indeed, he was already a firm member of the GOP back in Illinois, where he had worked hard on behalf of the unsuccessful presidential bid of James G. Blaine and the winning effort of Benjamin Harrison four years later.) In 1898 he made his move for national office and handily won a seat in Congress as an at-large representative. He served five full terms before he ran for the Senate in 1908. Victorious again, Jones was reelected in 1914, as he was over and over until his death in 1932. His record in the national legislature was never especially distinguished, but he had a knack for keeping his constituents happy, and he seldom faced major political opposition at home until late in his career. He was generally middle-of-the-road on most issues of his generation, although he did come out decidedly for a number of reforms (including women's suffrage)—the most prominent of which was prohibition, where Jones was anything but hesitant in his support.

In fact, Jones proved one of the staunchest drys ever to sit in Congress, and the Temperance Movement considered him one of its particular champions. The Anti-Saloon League found Jones usually ready to sponsor league-endorsed bills and in turn marshalled it support on the senator's behalf at election time. Jones was active in the fight to legislate prohibition in the District of Columbia and took the lead during World War I to urge restrictions on the liquor traffic as a food conservation measure. At one point, he tried to attach a rider to one conservation bill that would have barred the conversion of any grain or foodstuffs into alcohol. President Woodrow Wilson scuttled the attempt with a veto, insisting that any prohibition measure would have to face consideration on its own merits. Disappointed in this rebuff, Jones tried again and in 1917 was able to get the Congress to adopt the Jones-Randall Antiliquor Advertising Law. It was an important dry victory, which barred the use of the mails and public prints to lobby against prohibition efforts. With the advent of National Prohibition, the Washington senator emerged as a strident proponent of the Volstead Act, and when public support for the measure began to wane in the mid-1920s, the Anti-Saloon League turned to him to shore up enforcement efforts. In 1929, he secured passage of a Draconian law—the Jones Act—which called for a jail term of five years *and* a ten thousand dollar fine for a first offender who violated the Volstead statutes. Opponents sarcastically called the measure the "Jones 5 & 10 law," but it was really the handiwork of Bishop James Cannon* and the league. Jones, however, as the law's chief legislative sponsor, also reaped the political repercussions. The harshness of the law produced widespread dismay and probably cost National Prohibition further popularity. Jones himself came under intense political fire, which never abated until his death in late 1932. Prohibition, which Jones had supported for most of his political life to such advantage, thus had brought his electoral career to a close under a dark cloud indeed. His death at least spared him the added pain of fighting the losing battle against the repeal of the Eighteenth Amendment.

**Bibliography:**

A. *Woman-Suffrage* (Washington, DC, 1913); *Results of National Prohibition. Speech...in the Senate...* (Washington, DC, 1921); *The Problem and Policy of Prohibition* (Washington, DC, 1929).

B. SEAP 3, 1418–19; WW 1, 651; Mark Edward Lender and James Kirby Martin, *Drinking in America: A History* (New York, 1982); *Memorial Services Held in the House of Representatives...in Eulogy to Wesley L. Jones...* (Washington, DC, 1933).

# K

**KEARNEY, Belle** (6 March 1863, Vernon, MI—27 February 1939, Jackson, MI). *Career*: schoolteacher, 1880s; state superintendent, Youth Department, Mississippi WCTU, 1889–91; lecturer and organizer, National WCTU, 1891–1912; president, Mississippi WCTU, beginning 1895; president, Mississippi Woman Suffrage Association, 1906–8; lecturer, War Work Council, YMCA, 1917–18; field secretary, World's Purity Federation, 1920s; member, Mississippi Senate, 1924–28.

Belle Kearney grew up the daughter of a slaveholding Mississippi family whose fortunes suffered badly during the Civil War. Her father was a successful planter before the conflict (during which he was a Confederate officer), and although he eventually got his family back on its feet afterward, for a time the Kearneys were desperately poor. Young Belle therefore had little formal education. She proved to be a self-reliant young woman, however, and, self-taught, she opened a school in her own bedroom to raise extra money for the family. She then made her way in life for six years as a schoolteacher. Yet Kearney was apparently not happy: She was clearly a talented and ambitious individual, but career opportunities for women in the archconservative Mississippi of the 1880s were few and far between. It was in this social context that Kearney fortuitously met Frances E. Willard* in 1889. Willard was in the state on an organizing mission for the Woman's Christian Temperance Union, and although Kearney had had no prior knowledge of the union (nor much interest in the Temperance Movement), Willard pursuaded the Mississippi schoolteacher to enlist under the dry banner. There is no doubt that Kearney was a sincere convert to the temperance cause—her later record was ample testimony in that regard—but it was just as true that she saw working with the WCTU as an opportunity for fuller social participation. Indeed, she wasted no time in establishing herself as a force in the movement. The Mississippi Union selected her as a departmental superintendent (of youth work) in 1889, and two years later the National WCTU made her a national lecturer. It was an illuminating experience for a woman who had known only Mississippi. Until she gave up temperance lecturing in 1912, she toured both the United States (repeatedly) and Europe on behalf of the antiliquor crusade, garnering applause as one of the most popular WCTU speakers in the field. Back home, Kearney's work won quick recognition as the state union elected her president in 1895.

Kearney's reform career rose in meteoric fashion after her affiliation with the WCTU. While maintaining her work on behalf of temperance over the years, she became an active suffragette and crusader for moral reform. By the early twentieth century, Kearney was perhaps the leading advocate of the woman's vote in Mississippi (from 1906 to 1908 she was president of the state Woman Suffrage Association), and she spoke widely on the subject in other regions as well. Her suffrage attitudes, however, reflected the racial outlook of the day: she regarded the vote as "the medium through which to retain the supremacy of the white race over the African." The "sexual purity" of the young also attracted her attention. For years, Kearney worked with the World's Purity Federation, urging the strict monitoring of the sexual mores of American youth. Her novel, *Conqueror or Conquered* (1921), inveighed against the dangers of sexual permissiveness and the threat of venereal disease. With the passage of woman's suffrage in 1920, Kearney became the first Mississippi woman to pursue high political office. She challenged incumbent John Sharp Williams for the Democratic nomination for the U.S. Senate, and although she lost, polled a remarkable 18,285 votes. Four years later, though, she was a winner, taking a contest for the State Senate (and later winning reelection). She was the first woman in the South elected to such an office. Her record won her considerable regard as a careful and meticulous legislator, and she took a conscientious part in the national affairs of the Democratic Party as well. Still a committed dry, Kearney fought the nomination of Alfred E. Smith for the presidency in 1928.

**Bibliography:**

A. *A Slaveholder's Daughter* (1900; New York, 1969); *Conqueror or Conquered; or, the Sex Challenge Answered; A Revelation of Scientific Facts from Highest Medical Authorities* . . . (Cincinnati, OH, 1921).

B. NAW 2, 309–10; SEAP 4, 1444–45.

**KEELEY, Leslie Enraught**   (1832, Kings Co., Ireland—21 February 1900, Los Angeles, CA). *Education*: M.D., Rush Medical Coll., 1864; LLD. (honorary), Univ. of St. Louis, 1891. *Career*: medical cadet, Union army, 1861–64; major, Union army, 1864–65; medical practice, Chenoa, IL, 1865–67; medical practice, Dwight, IL, 1867–80; ran alcoholism and addictions treatment business, Dwight, IL (and subsequent other locations), 1880–1900.

The late nineteenth century saw considerable interest in the disease conception of alcoholism and in alcoholism treatment. Both the Temperance Movement and important elements of the medical profession engaged in various treatment efforts and scientific study of the issue. Perhaps the most controversial such effort of the period, however, was the so-called Gold Cure or Keeley Cure allegedly discovered by Dr. Leslie Enraught Keeley in the early 1880s. Brought from Ireland to the United States by his parents while a young child, Keeley grew up in Buffalo, New York. He obtained a medical degree while on leave from the Union army in 1864, and after being commissioned a major he served with distinction for the rest of the war (he was on Sherman's March to the Sea and was captured by the Confederates). After the war, the veteran doctor settled eventually in Dwight, Illinois; there, he proclaimed (based on what research, if any, is unknown) the discovery of a specific remedy for alcoholism and drug addictions. Soon he opened a "Keeley Institute" and began treating patients. His activities received no special notice until 1891, when the *Chicago Tribune* published a number of laudatory articles on Keeley and his cure, launching a wave of popularity for the treatment. Thousands of alcoholics flocked to Dwight and then to branch institutes which proliferated during the 1890s. By the turn of the century, each state had a Keeley Institute, and some had as many as three; by the second decade of the twentieth century, some estimates put the number of individuals taking the Gold Cure at about 400,000.

Keeley's secret was "bichloride" or "double chloride of gold" (whence "Gold Cure"). Pharmacology has recognized no such substance, and Keeley never revealed the formula; but bichloride of gold was evidently a gold salt mixed with vegetable compounds and traces of other drugs (including strychnine). It was not a unique approach, as other Gold Cure promoters were active around the turn of the century as well. Keeley's gigantic success stemmed from his business acumen in promoting his institutes. He argued that addiction (inebriety) came from the alcoholic or narcotic poisoning of the nerve cells, which came to require repeated doses of alcohol or drugs in order to function. In many respects, the idea was not much different from those advanced by others in the medical community who branded Keeley a quack. In retort, Keeley pointed to thousands of satisfied customers and insisted that precisely scheduled doses of his secret compound could break addiction in most people (although he carefully never claimed universal success). The best method, he claimed, was through intravenous injection under institute care, although he did a large mail order business in oral doses of the formula. (In fact, patients probably did receive some benefits, although in many cases only briefly, through a placebo effect. The Gold Cure formula itself has no known pharmacological impact on alcoholism.) To keep new patients coming, Keeley and his institute managers were adept at organizing former patients as virtual missionaries for the cure. In the early 1890s, they flocked to join the "Keeley League," which held annual conventions and hired lecturers to spread the Gold Cure gospel. The league even staged a "Keeley Day" at the Columbian Exposition in Chicago in 1893. Wives of patients organized as auxiliaries of the league in "Ladies' Bichloride of Gold Clubs." It was all good for business, a fact which even Keeley's sternest critics acknowledged.

Enthusiasm for the Keeley Cure, however, did not long survive Keeley's death in 1900. The last Keeley League convention was held in 1897, even before his passing; and as time went on, relapses of former patients (often highly publicized by Keeley's detractors) made it increasingly difficult to maintain business at old levels. Medical charges that Keeley's methods were ridiculous also began to tell, and by the 1920s there were only eleven institutes left. Eventually, these survivors either closed or ended their affiliation with the cure, although the original facility in Dwight—no longer offering the Keeley Cure—has remained open as an alcoholism treatment center. The Gold Cure, then, ended as only a curiosity of the period. In an age when relatively little was known about alcoholism treatment, thousands had turned to Leslie Keeley because he promised a miracle that few others dared offer.

**Bibliography:**

A. *Double Chloride of Gold: Cure for Drunkenness* (Dwight, IL, 1892); *The Keeley Institutes of the United States, Canada, and Other Countries* (Dwight, IL? 1895); *One Hundred Cases, (with testimonials) of Opium and Other Drug Patients, Successfully Treated...by the Leslie E. Keeley Double Chloride of Gold Remedies* (Dwight, IL, 1895?); *Opium: Its Use, Abuse and Cure; or, from Bondage to Freedom* (Chicago, 1897); *A Treatise on Drunkenness* (Dwight, IL, 18—?); *The Non-Heredity of Inebriety* (Chicago, 1902).

B. DAB 10, 280; SEAP 4, 1445; WW 1, 659; *Dr. Haines' Golden Specific for the Cure of Drunkenness* (Cincinnati, OH, 1887?); C. S. Clark, *The Perfect Keeley Cure: Incidents at Dwight...* (Milwaukee, WI, 1893); Mark Edward Lender and James K. Martin, *Drinking in America: A History* (New York, 1982).

**KELLER, Lewis Henry**    (24 February 1858, Upper Sandusky, OH—5 August 1938, Penney Farms, FL). *Education*: studied at Valparaiso Univ., 1879–80; studied at Adrian Coll., 1881–85; B.D., Yale Univ. Divinity Sch., 1889; D.D., Ripon Coll., 1909; postgraduate study, Univ. of Chicago, 1910. *Career*: ordained in Congregational Church, 1886; minister, WI and MN, 1886–1912; general superintendent, Wisconsin Congregational Conference, 1912–18; superintendent, Congregational Extension Boards of the Southeast, 1918–25; president, Atlanta Theological Sem., 1925–29.

The histories of American Protestantism and temperance were inextricably bound during the late nineteenth and early twentieth centuries. The Anti-Saloon League in particular was a classic demonstration of the relationship, the league originally being the brainchild—and then the actual creation—of the clergy. Indeed, even when league membership spread beyond church congregations and built support among secular groups, church leaders of various denominations retained prominent roles on all levels of the antiliquor organization's administration. Their efforts were often unheralded, but they provided the backbone of the league's grassroots activities and were thus critical in marshalling popular support in the final drive for National Prohibition. Lewis Henry Keller was just such an unsung temperance stalwart. A Congregationalist minister with a Yale degree in divinity, he came by his dry sentiments early. As a child in Ohio, he had watched his mother take part in the famous Woman's Crusade in the 1870s. The sight of her praying in the streets in front of saloons galvanized his hatred of the liquor traffic, and as an adult his pulpits rang with the temperance convictions he had adopted as a boy. Keller served four pastorates in Wisconsin and Minnesota over the course of his career and took an active hand in regional church governance; but he served the Anti-Saloon League with the same dedication. He helped run the headquarters of the Wisconsin League for some eight years (1900-1908), spent five more years as president of its Board of Trustees, and for two years edited the Wisconsin edition of the *American Issue*. His untiring efforts won Keller considerable recognition in regional temperance circles, and from 1912 to 1918 he was chosen to represent the Wisconsin, Iowa, and Minnesota leagues in the deliberations of National League headquarters. All the while, the dedicated minister saw his work for the league as a natural part of his religious calling. In laboring for the league and for temperance, he was laboring for the Lord. Keller rejoiced with the passage of the Eighteenth Amendment, fought the movement for Repeal bitterly, and devoted his life after the defeat of Prohibition to his church and to his duties as president of Atlanta Theological Seminary. Never in the first rank of dry leadership, Keller's career still offered a clear lesson in the value of skilled and dedicated "middle management" in the Temperance Movement—and in the ability of the Anti-Saloon League to marshal the loyalty of so much of the American clergy.

**Bibliography:**

B. SEAP 3, 1446–47; WW 1, 661.

**KELLER, Mark**   (21 February 1907, Austria— ). *Education*: privately educated. *Career*: various editing positions, to 1941; lecturer in applied physiology, Yale Univ. Center of Alcohol Studies, 1941–61; editor, *Quarterly Journal of Studies on Alcohol* (later *Journal of Studies on Alcohol*), 1941–77, editor emeritus, beginning 1977; acting editor, 1981–84; research specialist, Rutgers Univ. Center of Alcohol Studies, 1962–77; visiting scientist, National Institute on Alcohol Abuse and Alcoholism, 1974–75; professor emeritus, Rutgers Univ., beginning 1977; adjunct professor, Brandeis Univ., beginning 1980.

The alcoholism treatment and research field long identified the career of Mark Keller with the *Quarterly Journal of Studies on Alcohol* (later the *Journal of Studies on Alcohol*, when it became a monthly publication). There was every reason: Keller edited the *Journal* for the better part of four decades before his retirement in 1977, and for two years more upon his recall to active duty by the *Journal's* publisher in 1981. Over that period, both Keller and the *Journal* did good service. The *Journal* was established at the Yale University Center of Alcohol Studies in 1941 and moved with it to Rutgers in 1962. Its founders, Howard W. Haggard* and E. M. Jellinek,* intended the publication to offer a forum for scientific reports in the nascent post-Prohibition field of alcohol research. It was Keller, however, who brought the *Journal* to maturity. Over the years, he firmly eschewed the old wet–dry controversy and concentrated on publishing papers conforming to the established canons of science; the policy not only served a needed academic function (the *Journal* was the only international scientific publication devoted to the subject for years) but also tacitly moved alcohol studies well beyond the realm of the Temperance Movement. The concern for alcohol problems remained, but the *Journal* did not deal with them in the traditional contexts of political or moral reform. In the early years of its existence, the publication effort of the Yale Center did come under some (although never unanimous or even serious) temperance fire for its posture; but, to the benefit of the field, the *Journal* prospered.

Keller's work with the *Journal* and its related publications (the center also issued a large number of books and pamphlets) had a marked influence on the growth of the modern alcohol studies effort. He was one of the first to insist, for example, that alcohol-related experiments include adequate control groups as part of the research design. He also assumed a much-needed critical stance, demanding that scholars ground their work on firm theoretical foundations. He was critical, in this regard, of those in the field ready to discard the disease conception of alcoholism without offering any scientifically persuasive grounds. Perhaps less recognized, his bibliographic and reference contributions have been equally important to progress in alcohol studies. Over his many years at the Center of Alcohol Studies, Keller fostered the growth of the world's most complete alcohol-related library, the Classified Abstract Archive of the Alcohol Literature, as well as the collection's data retrieval system. It remains one of the most widely used research archives on alcohol-related subjects in the world (at its inception, it was the only such collection of its kind). He was also editor of the *International Bibliography of Studies on Alcohol*, the most complete reference series in the field. In addition, Keller took charge of editing many special publications and monographs, introducing some of the most significant research findings of the post-Prohibition era. Keller's own writings have been extensive, and he has lectured and taught before groups in many parts of the world. While far apart in their techniques and goals, then, both the Temperance Movement and the modern alcohol research effort have placed major emphasis on an adequate literature; in making that literature available and in assuring its quality, no one's contributions surpassed Keller's. The Mark Keller Award, for the best article of the year in the *Journal of Studies on Alcohol*, has been established in his honor.

### Bibliography:

A. *What Do People Do About Alcohol Problems?* (New Haven, CT, 1955); with Vera Efron and E. M. Jellinek, *CAAAL Manual: A Guide to the Use of the Classified Abstract Archive of the Alcohol Literature* (New Brunswick, NJ, 1963); with Mairi McCormick, *A Dictionary of Words About Alcohol* (New Brunswick, NJ, 1968; rev. ed., 1982); "The Oddities of Alcoholics," *Quarterly Journal of Studies on Alcohol* 33 (1972): 1147–48; "Alcohol Consumption," *Encyclopedia Britannica*, vol. 1 (Chicago, 1974), 437–50; ed., *Alcohol and Health: Second Special Report to the U.S. Congress* (Rockville, MD, 1975);

"The Disease Concept of Alcoholism Revisited," *Journal of Studies on Alcohol* 37 (1976): 1694–1717.

B. Christopher D. Smithers Foundation, *Pioneers We Have Known in the Field of Alcoholism* (Mill Neck, NY, 1979).

**KELLEY, David Campbell**   (25 December 1833, Wilson Co., TN—1909, Lebanon, TN). *Education*: A.M., Cumberland Univ., 1851; M.D., Univ. of Nashville, 1853; D.D., Cumberland Univ., 1868; LLD. (honorary), Univ. of Nashville, 1896. *Career*: medical missionary, China, 1853–57; cavalry officer, Confederate army, 1861–65; minister, various Methodist churches near Nashville, TN, beginning 1860s; trustee, Vanderbilt Univ., 1872–85; secretary and treasurer, Board of Missions, Methodist Episcopal Church, South, 1875–84; presiding elder, Nashville District, Methodist Church, 1898–1909.

Clergyman, soldier, educator, David C. Kelley's life was as varied as one could wish for, and in each of its three major phases it was a highly successful one. A devout Methodist, Kelley grew up in the countryside of pre–Civil War Tennessee. After his education, which included an M.D. from the University of Nashville, he went on to combine his medical training and his penchant for religion as a medical missionary to China in 1853. Kelley served in China for four years, although details of his activities there are sketchy. He returned to Tennessee in 1857, and little more is known of him until the coming of the Civil War, when the former missionary emerged as a cavalry colonel under Confederate General Nathan Bedfort Forrest (which suggests that Kelley had a reasonably prominent social standing on the eve of the war). He served with distinction under the hard-hitting Forrest and fought throughout the grueling western campaigns of the conflict. Even in defeat, the memories of the war stayed alive, as Kelley later won election (seven times) as a lieutenant general among Forrest's old troopers in the United Confederate Veterans. From war, the cavalry officer finally turned full time to religion. He earned a doctor of divinity from Cumberland University and began his ministry in the Methodist Church, serving as pastor in various churches in the Nashville area. Always interested in education, Kelley devised the project out of which there came the Central University of the Methodist Episcopal Church, South, which later changed its name to Vanderbilt University in honor of its principal benefactor. As a companion institution the Nashville College for Young Ladies emerged at the same time. Kelley's career, then, was hard to match for diversity and accomplishment.

Like so many other Methodists of his generation, Kelley also placed great value on work with the Temperance Movement. He had been a total abstainer since his youth, when he first became involved with the dry crusade as a member of the Cadets of Temperance (a youth arm of the fraternal temperance lodges of the era). As a Cadet, he helped with prohibitionist campaign efforts in his home area of Wilson County, Tennessee. After his ordination, he resumed his antiliquor bent and became a leading advocate of constitutional prohibition in the Volunteer State. His labors on behalf of local option contributed greatly to the piecemeal drying out of a good deal of Tennessee, and Kelley won widespread recognition as one of the most effective dry organizers in the region. Ironically, all of this got him into considerable trouble with his church (overwhelmingly dry itself). His conference charged that the ardent reformer was devoting too much time to prohibition at the expense of his pastoral duties, an issue that came to a head in 1890. That year, Kelley received an unsolicited nomination for governor of Tennessee from the Prohibition Party. He was then pastor of a church in Gallatin, and he had not wanted the nomination. Nevertheless, the Methodist conference then suspended him, although on appeal it restored him to the ministry in good standing. In his later years, Kelley worked closely with the Anti-Saloon League and, while taking care not to further antagonize his fellow churchmen, ended his life as one of the state's most accomplished anti-liquor crusaders.

**Bibliography:**

A. *A Short Method with Modern Doubt* (Nashville, TN, 1882); *Address on Female Education...* (Jackson, TN, 1884); "General Sam Houston: The Washington of Texas," 145–74, in *The Scotch-Irish Society of America, Second Congress* (1890); *Bishop or Conference?* (Nashville, TN, 1893); *Life of Mrs. M. L. Kelley* (n.p., 1900).

B. WW 1, 661; SEAP 4, 1447.

**KELLOGG, John Harvey**    (26 February 1852, Tyrone, MI—16 January 1943, Battle Creek, MI). *Education*: studied at State Normal Sch., MI, 1870s; M.D., Bellevue Hosp. Medical Coll., NY, 1875; postdoctoral study in Europe, 1883, 1889, 1899, 1902, 1907, 1911; LLD. (honorary), Olivet Coll., and Lincoln Memorial Univ.; Dr. Pub. Service (honorary), Oglethorpe Univ., 1937. *Career*: editor, *Good Health*, beginning 1873; medical practice, Battle Creek, MI, beginning 1875; superintendent, Battle Creek Sanitarium, beginning 1876; member, Michigan State Board of Health, 1878–90, 1912–16; inventor of surgical instruments and various medical and dietary treatment techniques, beginning 1870s; breakfast food business with brother, Will Keith Kellogg, 1890s; founder and president, Battle Creek Coll., 1923–38; founder and president, Race Betterment Foundation, beginning 1914.

The man who revolutionized America's breakfast habits was one of the more interesting and talented—if not eccentric—medical men of his era. Reformer, surgeon, businessman, and medical researcher, John Harvey Kellogg grew up in Tyrone, Michigan, earned his medical degree in New York, and returned to Michigan (Battle Creek) to open his first practice. From the start, however, Kellogg set his sights on considerably more than the life of a small-town doctor. Only a year after settling in Battle Creek, he put into practice certain theories of diet and health that he had been maturing for some years. Raised in the Seventh Day Adventist faith, Kellogg had come under the influence of the teaching of Ellen G. White and her notions of health reform, including vegetarianism. As early as 1873, he had become editor of *Health Reformer*, an Adventist publication; and upon his return to Michigan he changed the name to *Good Health* and began a lifetime dedicated to improving the health of America through a variety of dietary and other reforms. Kellogg developed what he called the Battle Creek Idea, a regimen that included the elimination from the diet of all meat, the reduction of milk, cheese, and eggs, and total abstinence from tea, coffee, chocolate, tobacco, and alcohol (whence came a great deal of his vociferous support for the Temperance Movement). The Battle Creek Sanitarium, which Kellogg had founded to put these notions into practice, became a haven for many of the great and near-great social and political figures of the era who sought to improve their health through Kellogg's diet and therapy, which included such exotic items as an electric light bath. In his search for the perfect health food, Kellogg, in collaboration with his brother, experimented with various grains and cereals. Ultimately, they produced a flaked cereal later christened "corn flakes." At first, this new food was to be eaten dry just as it came in the box. It was not a success, and it languished on grocers' shelves until someone got the idea of serving it in milk. In this form, corn flakes swept the nation, changed the eating habits of countless Americans, and survived challenges from imitators, including "grape nuts," a similar cereal food developed by one of Kellogg's patients, C. W. Post.

While Kellogg's dietary beliefs labeled him, at least in part, as something of a genial eccentric, he was also enormously talented. He was in fact a busy and outstanding surgeon (who performed some 22,000 operations over the course of his career) who employed novel antishock methods and postoperative excercises successfully on some of the most trying surgical problems of the period. He turned all of his fees over to the Battle Creek Sanitarium. Aside from his dietary and medical interest, Kellogg was also an ardent social reformer, especially when his pet reforms touched on medicine. He was a deadly foe of the liquor traffic, for example, and a firm prohibitionist. For years (1885–1902), he headed the Medical Temperance Society, a group of abstaining doctors, and helped bring out their publication, the *Medical Temperance Quarterly*. Later, he was a major source of financial aid to the Association for the Study and Cure of Inebriety, which sought to put the treatment of alcoholism and addiction research on a scientific footing. In his own writings, Kellogg frequently emphasized the value of personal abstinence, and he was a major supporter of the activities of the Woman's Christian Temperance Union. Later in life, the reformer-doctor developed a keen interest in eugenics, which prompted him to found and promote the Race Betterment Foundation (1906); while still later he launched Battle Creek College, which he supported mostly out of his earnings from food sales for the fifteen years the college remained open. In addition, Kellogg was a prolific writer, turning out reams of articles, pamphlets, and books, as well as technical papers. His *Plain Facts About Sexual Life* (1877) was one of the first straightforward books on its subject to be written, and it sold over half a million copies. *Rational Hydrotherapy* (1901) was also a pathbreaker in its field. In the 1930s, the aging doctor suffered some serious financial reverses. As a result of overexpansion and the Great Depression, Battle Creek Sanitarium went into receivership and never regained its former popularity. Yet Kellogg refused to be discouraged. He was in the midst of launching new projects when he died of an attack of acute bronchitis at age ninety-one.

**Bibliogaphy:**

A. *The Physical, Moral and Social Effects of Alcoholic Poison as a Beverage and as a Medicine* (Battle Creek, MI, 1876); *Temperance Charts, Showing in a Series of 10 Plates, the Physical Effects of Alcohol and Tobacco* (Battle Creek, MI, 1882); *The Home Handbook of Domestic Hygiene and Rational Medicine*, rev. ed. (Battle Creek, MI, 1900); *Plain Facts for Young and Old...* (Battle Creek, MI, 1903); *The Truth About Alcohol as a Medicine* (Battle Creek, MI, 1906); *Tobaccoism*, rev. ed. (Battle Creek, MI, 1946).

B. DAB Supp. 3, 409–11; SEAP 4, 1447–48; WW 2, 292; Gerald Carson, *Cornflake Crusade* (London, 1957); Ronald M. Deutsch, *The Nuts Among the Berries* (New York, 1961); Richard M. Schwarz, *John Harvey Kellogg, M.D.* (1970).

**KENT, Edward**    (8 January 1802, Concord, NH—19 May 1877, Bangor, ME). *Education*: A.B., Harvard Univ. (Phi Beta Kappa), 1821; study of law under Benjamin Orr and Chancellor Kent, ME, early 1820s; LLD. (honorary), Colby Coll., 1827. *Career*: legal practice, Bangor, ME, beginning 1825; member, Maine state legislature, 1828–29; mayor, Bangor, ME, 1836–38; chief justice, Court of Sessions, Penobscot Co., ME, 1827–29; governor of Maine, 1838, 1841; party to Maine boundary negotiations, 1842; U.S. consul, Rio de Janeiro, 1849–53; associate justice, Maine Supreme Court, 1859–73; member, Maine Constitutional Amendment Commission, 1875.

The late 1830s saw the first serious rumblings of political prohibitionist sentiment in the United States. It found its most fertile ground in New England, which had given birth to some of the earliest organized dry groups, and where enthusiasm for moral and social reform was steadily becoming enmeshed in the politics of the era. In the eyes of many New Englanders, reform held the promise of shaping the nation's future in accordance with their perceptions of the good society and of preserving existing institutions from social disorder. Into this mold fit Edward Kent, successful lawyer, Whig politician, and one of the first legislative leaders in his native state of Maine to advocate the coercion of law to control the evils of drink. Kent was fully convinced that the liquor traffic was a wellspring of poverty, profligate behavior, and political corruption—that familiar litany of dry complaints against the trade—and that it was therefore a mortal danger to individuals and to society itself. The abolition of beverage alcohol, he concluded, was the only safe answer if society was to defend itself, and to that end he worked hard on behalf of the Maine Temperance Union. He also used political office as a platform to belabor wets. A frequent and successful office seeker, he openly made prohibition an issue in his campaigns. Kent won the governorship twice (both in hotly contested elections) and upon entering the statehouse surprised some of his colleagues by trying to get a prohibitory bill through the legislature. He failed in the attempt in 1838, but the vote was close, revealing unexpected dry strength and demonstrating the importance of temperance as an electoral issue in the public mind. During his second term, the governor chose not to press the matter, but he never gave up his hope for an eventual victory. When it came a decade later under Neal Dow's* leadership, the "Maine Law," the first state-wide prohibition act in the nation, owed much to the foundation previously laid by Kent. In other areas aside from temperance, the former governor proved a useful citizen, playing distinguished roles in a number of state and national diplomatic missions and in the history of Maine jurisprudence.

**Bibliography:**

B. DAB 10, 343–44; SEAP 4, 1451; WW H, 361; L. V. Briggs, *Genealogies of the Different Families Bearing the Name of Kent* (n.p., 1898); John E. Godfrey, "Memoir of Edward Kent," *Maine Historical Society Collections*, vol. 8 (Portland, 1881).

**KENYON, William Squire**    (10 June 1869, Elyria, OH—9 September 1933, vacationing in ME). *Education*: studied at Iowa Coll., 1880s; law courses at Iowa State Univ., 1890. *Career*: admitted to bar, IA, 1891; legal practice, Fort Dodge, IA, beginning 1891; prosecutor, Webster Co., IA, 1893–97; district judge, IA, 1897–99; special assistant U.S. attorney general, 1910–11; member, U.S. Senate, 1911–22; judge, U.S. Circuit Court, 1922–33.

The ratification of the Eighteenth Amendment to the Constitution came only after a long train of prohibitionist legislative victories. Some of these earlier triumphs had done a great deal to dry out the nation even before the advent of National Prohibition, and one of the most important of these was the Webb-Kenyon Act of 1913, the principal architect of which was Senator William Squire Kenyon of Iowa. The law made it a federal crime (with stiff penalties) to transport intoxicating beverages from a wet state into a state where they were legally prohibited. It closed a major loophole in many state dry statutes, whereby local enforcement officials, having no power over interstate commerce, were largely powerless to stop shipments of alcohol legally manufactured in neighboring states into their own, making its illegal distribution at a later date a relatively simple affair. Federal enforcement of the Webb-Kenyon law also constituted the most significant national intervention to that point in the war against the traffic. In the light of the times, it was a drastic step, bitterly resented and fought by wets. Kenyon himself, however, was anything but a radical. A generally moderate man, and personally dry, he had been a highly distinguished lawyer, prosecutor, and judge before going to the Senate in 1911. He backed temperance legislation because he honestly believed it would "do something for human rights and moral laws and decency in politics." Much of the nation shared this view, and the

Iowa senator had many supporters in the fight for the Webb-Kenyon Act, although President William Howard Taft was not among them. The president vetoed the measure, and it became law only when Congress overrode him. Despite the president's opposition, however, the law's success was a clear sign that the Temperance Movement was gathering political momentum.

Kenyon's career was also a demonstration of the close bonds between temperance and Progressivism. From the beginning of his tenure in the Senate, he played a prominent role in the liberal wing of the Republican Party. (Indeed, even earlier, while briefly a federal prosecutor, he had pursued antitrust cases with the applause of Progressive opinion.) He fought hard for labor reform legislation and industrial regulation, opposed the entry of the United States into World War I (he was on President Woodrow Wilson's list of a "little group of willful men"), and advocated a benign foreign policy after the conflict. Kenyon was also a prominent spokesman for agricultural interests. In his mind, National Prohibition fit easily into this overall context of reform—it was part and parcel of a broader effort to make America's industrial and urban economy, which was rapidly emerging fullblown, beneficial to all citizens. Kenyon, however, was never completely happy as a politician. Rather, he preferred a judicial career, and he resigned from the Senate in 1922 (at the height of his influence) when President Warren G. Harding offered him a seat on the federal bench. He was an able jurist and garnered considerable recognition when he rendered a strong decision voiding the Teapot Dome oil leases. As a circuit judge, though, he was still to play a part in the Prohibition controversy. With the Eighteenth Amendment under fire by the mid-1920s, Kenyon agreed to serve on the Wickersham Committee, charged with investigating the effectiveness of the Volstead Act and recommending changes in the dry laws. His subsequent criticisms of Prohibition enforcement, given his prior advocacy of temperance issues, generated major public comment. But the judge was not about to become embroiled in partisan politics again and refused to become further involved with the debate on the liquor question. Such was his preference for the relative tranquility of the bench that he turned down offers of cabinet positions under President Calvin Coolidge and declined to pursue encouragement from some Republicans for a presidential bid in 1928.

**Bibliography:**

A. DAB Supp. 1, 465–66; NYT, Sept. 10, 1933; SEAP 3, 1456–57; WW 1, 669; H. E. Kershner, *William Squire Kenyon and the Kenyon-Duncombe-Williams-Squire Family Histories* (New York, 1935).

**KIRK, Edward Norris**   (14 August 1802, New York—27 March 1874, Boston, MA). *Education*: B.A., Coll. of New Jersey (now Princeton Univ.), 1820; legal study in private law office, NY, 1820–22; studied at Princeton Theological Sem., 1822–26; D.D. (honorary), Amherst Coll. *Career*: agent, American Board of Commissioners for Foreign Missions, 1826–28; minister, Second Presbyterian

Church, Albany, NY, 1829; minister, Fourth Presbyterian Church, Albany, NY, 1829–37; founder, Troy and Albany Theological Sch., 1833; travelling preacher, Europe, 1837–39; secretary, Foreign Evangelical Society, 1839–42; minister, Mt. Vernon Congregational Church, Boston, 1842–71; president, American Missionary Association, 1865.

Born the son of a not very successful Scotch immigrant storekeeper in New York City, Edward Kirk was raised by his mother's more prosperous relatives in Princeton, New Jersey. Intellectually precocious, he entered the College of New Jersey as a sophomore at age fifteen and after graduation went back to New York to study for a legal career. By 1822, however, Kirk found that he was indifferent to the law, and a religious conversion turned him to a pastoral calling. Following seminary and two years of missionary preaching in the Southern states, he was ordained in 1828 and called to his first pastorate by the affluent congregation of the Second Presbyterian Church in Albany, New York. Kirk's theology, however, which emphasized revivalism and the saving of souls, did not sit well with his parishioners—who summarily dismissed him. Yet those who relished his uncompromising emphasis on salvation and his evangelical preaching style (a style at which he became quite accomplished) founded a new church for him, and his fame as a proponent of the Second Great Awakening steadily spread. He attracted large and enthusiastic audiences as he doggedly pursued the conversion of sinners and holding the faithful to the fold. In this cause he opened his pulpit to the evangelizing mission of the great revivalist Charles G. Finney, even when other pastors had shied away from Finney's radical theology. Later, in the 1840s and 1850s, Kirk launched his own crusade, preaching throughout the urban centers of the East and taking part in the evangelical organizing efforts in Europe. His reputation finally brought him to Boston, where a group of believers had established a Congregational church especially for him. To the end of his days, Kirk maintained his revivalist zeal and was one of the most noted preachers in a city famed for the distinction of its clergy.

Kirk's enthusiasm for personal salvation was matched only by his commitment to social reform. His efforts in this vein were quite similar to those of other revivalists of the era, and his labors began early and seldom stopped. As a young minister, his preaching lashed out at slavery and intemperance as fonts of godlessness and sin, and as time went on he lent his support to an entire range of other reforms as well. Sunday schools, public education, tract societies, and missionary groups all won his endorsement. As the Civil War approached, Kirk was vociferous in his abolitionism and his hatred of secession. During the conflict, which he welcomed as a final means to deal with slavery and rebellion, he was, as one historian put it, "a fiery supporter of the Union." He staunchly believed that the Northern armies were engaged in doing God's bidding, and he lent his hand to relief efforts for the newly freed slaves. The Boston minister was equally fiery in his denunciations of drink. Intemperance was a source of all manner of social misery, he proclaimed, while the individual drunkard was not only a poor example to others but at risk of sacrificing his soul to alcohol. Unless he heard the call of the Word and repented, Kirk warned, the drunkard was doomed. Doomed too were those who for personal profit would sell the drunkard his drink. It was stern stuff but fully in accord with the zealous refomer's general outlook on personal and social conduct. At the same time, Kirk was fully prepared to welcome the repentance and salvation of the worst sot or rum seller. A life-long bachelor, Kirk's later years were slowed by eye and throat problems, although he continued to write (he wrote or edited eight major books and many pamphlets and articles) until his death in 1874.

### Bibliography:

A. *Sermons Delivered in England and America* (New York, 1840); *The Drunkard's Character and Destiny: A Discourse* (Boston, 1846); *Results of the Temperance Reformation* (Boston, 1851?); *Lectures on the Parables of Our Savior* (New York, 1856); *Discourses Doctrinal and Practical* (Boston, 1860); *Children Taught About God*, 3rd ed. (New York, 1892).

B. DAB 10, 427–28; DARB, 246–47; NCAB 6, 194; NYT, March 28, 1874; WW H, 366; David Otis Mears, *Life of Edward Norris Kirk, D.D.* (Boston, 1877).

**KRESGE, Sabastian Spering**    (31 July 1867, Bald Mount, PA—18 October 1966, East Stroudsburg, PA). *Education*: studied at Polytechnic Inst., Gilbert, PA, 1880s; graduated from Eastman Business Coll., 1889; DBA. (honorary), Albion Coll., 1941; LHD. (honorary), Dickinson Coll., 1950; LLD. (honorary), Wayne Univ., 1950, Michigan State Univ., 1963. *Career*: salesman, PA, 1892–97; partner in store, Memphis, TN, 1897–99; principal, Kresge & Wilson (later sole owner as S. S. Kresge), Detroit, MI, beginning 1900 (incorporated as S. S. Kresge Co. in 1912); philanthropic and reform pursuits, beginning 1920s.

In 1916, a bitterly contested and nationally watched campaign for state prohibition in Michigan succeeded at the polls by some 68,000 votes. The Anti-Saloon League, which had done much to orchestrate the winning political effort, was exultant while temperance enthusiasts all over the country rejoiced. And among those who celebrated the dry victory, few were happier than five-and-dime-store magnate Sabastian Spering Kresge. Kresge had made considerable donations of time and money to make that campaign work, and the triumph made his many years of antiliquor efforts seem worthwhile. One of the most successful retailers in American history, he had been involved with organized temperance work since his early days as a salesman in Pennsylvania, where he had joined the Central Prohibition League in Scranton in the 1890s. From that time on, as his various business dealings took him to different locations, he made it a point to look at the temperance record of any candidate before casting his vote. With the headquarters of his company in Detroit, Michigan, after 1900, Kresge became a major force in the antiliquor battles of the state. He not only donated to Anti-Saloon League coffers but served as well on the Michigan League's headquarters committee and on the Executive Committee of the National League. After the battle to dry out Michigan had been won, the energetic corporate leader turned immediately to the struggle for the Eighteenth Amendment, the passage of which he applauded and then worked to enforce. Realizing that wet opposition would make National Prohibition a dead letter unless popular support for the measure remained high, Kresge organized and financed the National Vigilance Committee for Prohibition Enforcement. The intention was to assist enforcement officals in upholding the dry laws and to combat political efforts to weaken them. Rarely did the Temperance Movement enjoy a patron so willing to commit not only his labor but also his financial resources to the cause.

Kresge came by his prohibitionist enthusiasm early in life. His parents neither drank nor smoked, and young Sabastian grew up a teetotaler. He detested both alcohol and tobacco and had a dim view of those who took part in either, remarking once that he "made it a practice never to give a dollar to a church the pastor of which used tobacco" (churches with drinking pastors, we may suppose, also went without). Later, however, the established business executive took a more hard-nosed economic view of the matter. Drink, he concluded—as did a great many other business and industrial leaders of the era—was productive only of waste and inefficiency. It was anathema to men who depended on clear thinking themselves and on the effective performance of their employees. Kresge was convinced that mankind's abilities would be appreciably better without alcohol—and certainly he did well enough without it. Starting his business life as a struggling salesman with virtually no capital to invest, he rose to wealth and fame pioneering chain retail stores (which, for a time, actually were "five and tens"—with no item costing more than a dime). He ended his career with a retail empire of 930 stores which employed over 42,000 people. Personally frugal—a product of spare beginnings—over the years he often proved a kind and generous benefactor to others. He offered good pay and benefits (at least in his view) to his employees, endowed the Kresge Foundation (and then managed its assets to make it one of the wealthiest charitable foundations in the nation), and contributed liberally to causes he favored. The Temperance Movement was a case in point. In all, he gave over a million dollars to the Anti-Saloon League, some half a million of it coming in a single pledge in 1927 to help finance a Prohibition enforcement campaign. Repeal was a bitter disappointment to Kresge, for he had never lost his faith in the dry experiment. But he remained active in other charitable work and with his company. Although he was rarely in the public eye after 1940, when he died at age ninety-nine he was still deeply involved with the management of the enterprise he had built so well.

**Bibliography:**

B. NYT, Oct. 19, 1966; SEAP 4, 1483; WW 4, 544.

**KYNETT, Alpha Jefferson**   (12 August 1829, Adams Co., PA—23 February 1899, Harrisburg, PA). *Education*: D.D., Cornell Coll., IA, circa late 1840s;

LLD., Allegheny Coll., early 1850s? *Career*: Methodist minister and presiding elder, IA, 1851–67; staff of governor of Iowa, 1861–65; active in Methodist General Conference and Church Extension Society, IA, 1867–99; editor, *Christianity in Earnest*, 1889–99; co-founder, Anti-Saloon League of America, 1895.

Reformer and Methodist Clergyman, Alpha Jefferson Kynett had as deft an administrative and organizational touch as anyone who worked under the temperance banner. Able to plan effectively on a large scale, the Iowa minister was one of the prime movers in launching the Anti-Saloon League to national prominence. For that labor alone drys would have accorded him an honored place in Temperance Movement history; Kynett's record, however, was considerably more extensive. He assumed fairly important administrative responsibilities early in his career, being chosen a presiding elder of a large church district in Iowa while in his late twenties. Shortly afterward, the Civil War having erupted, the hard-working minister agreed to serve on the staff of the state governor. Kynett was deeply involved in recruiting and equipping Iowa troops, becoming adept at organizational routine. Even while the war still raged, he was able to use what he had learned on behalf of his church. Working with the Methodist General Conference, he was instrumental in regional church governance and in the founding of the Church Extension Society (an organization to assist in the founding of new churches). Kynett was an officer in the society for the next thirty-two years, leading it with such efficiency that it was able to help fund the establishment of hundreds of other churches, mainly on the Western frontier. In addition to his administrative skills, Kynett was also a reformer and took the lead in advocating lay and women's representation in the General Conference. He fought for temperance as well. While still a new minister, he thought of linking Methodist congregations into a single social and political bloc to attack the liquor traffic, and he had achieved some local success. As his stature in the church hierarchy grew, however, his plans for a league of churches united against alcohol grew with him. By the 1890s, he was ready to help reshape the nature of the Temperance Movement.

With the last decade of the nineteenth century, Kynett's church responsibility saw him working in Ohio and Pennsylvania, as well as in his native Iowa, and in Methodism's national affairs. He established the Board of Temperance (later renamed the Board of Temperance, Prohibition and Public Morals) to coordinate Methodist antiliquor activity throughout the nation and took part in major dry conventions. In Pennsylvania, he was instrumental in putting a Union Prohibitory League into the field, and the group successfully marshalled the vote that made the state dry. Encouraged by the result, Kynett organized (1893) the Interdenominational Christian Temperance Alliance in Ohio, which sought to link congregations across the state together in the prohibitionist cause. At the same time, he wrote to the Reverend Howard Hyde Russell,* who was already pursuing the same kind of goal, calling his organization the Anti-Saloon League. Kynett offered to merge his group with Russell's, and after both leaders conferred with colleagues an organizational convention took place in December 1895. The result was the Anti-Saloon League of America, which, over the next decade, steadily consolidated its position as the single most powerful political voice in the Temperance Movement. When National Prohibition finally came in 1920, it was correctly identified as having provided the political muscle and leadership for getting the job done. Kynett, though, never saw the final victory. He died in 1899, but he went down fighting: The old reformer collapsed in the middle of a speech before the Anti-Saloon League of Pennsylvania. In retrospect, it seems a fitting place to have ended his career. (Several years later, Kynett's son, Alpha G. Kynett, followed his father's path into the Methodist clergy and the ranks of temperance leadership.)

### Bibliography:

A. *Laws and Forms Relating to Churches and Other Religious Societies...* (New York, 1887); *The Union Prohibitory League...* (Asbury Park, NJ, 1889); "Citizen's Prohibitory Leagues," 177–82, in *Essays Written for the National Temperance Convention...* (n.p., 1891?); *The Church and the Saloon at War...* (Philadelphia, 1892); *The Religion of the Republic and Laws of Religious Corporations...* (Cincinnati, OH, 1895); *Christian Temperance Leagues and Alliances* (n.p., 189-?).

B. DAB 10, 516–17; SEAP 3, 1487–88; WW H, 370; Ernest Cherrington, *History of the Anti-Saloon League* (Westerville, OH, 1913).

# L

**LANDRITH, Ira**  (23 March 1865, Milford, TX—11 October 1941, Pasadena, CA). *Education*: B.S., Cumberland Univ., TN, 1888; LLB., Cumberland Univ., 1889; studied theology, Cumberland Univ., 1889–90; LLD., Cumberland Univ., 1903; D.D. (honorary), Trinity Univ., TN, 1906. *Career*: editor (assistant and chief), *Cumberland Presbyterian*, 1890–1903; president, Belmont Coll., Nashville, TN, 1904–12; president, Ward Sem., 1912–13; president, Ward-Belmont Coll., 1913–15; national lecturer, Anti-Saloon League of America and World League Against Alcoholism, 1915–25; president, Intercollegiate Prohibition Association, 1920–27; president, National Temperance Council, 1928–31; membership in editorial, temperance, and YMCA groups, beginning early 1900s.

A clergyman by profession, Ira Landrith probably had greater impact in his role as a prohibition advocate than he did as a man of the cloth. In fact, he never had a congregation, and his religious work, when not inextricably bound to his temperance activities, came in other than ministerial capacities. For thirteen years he helped to bring out the *Cumberland Presbyterian* (Nashville, Tennessee), serving as editor-in-chief from 1896 to 1903, and then took the presidencies of three religiously-affiliated Nashville colleges between 1904 and 1915. Landrith was also a joiner, taking part in the affairs of the Religious Education Association, the Presbyterian Brotherhood of America, the General Assembly of the Cumberland Presbyterian Church, and the Young Men's Christian Association. At one time or another he was an officer in all of these groups, and he generally took a reform outlook toward their activities. He was instrumental, for example, in reuniting the Cumberland church with the parent national Presbyterian body, and he saw work with the YMCA as a prime means to ensure the moral standards of the nation's youth and future. Indeed, his commitment to the reform of American morality and society—he was desperately concerned to ensure a Christian (read *Protestant*) social order and to cleanse the country of what he considered disruptive and alien ideologies—was such that he ultimately went full time into reform work. A convinced dry, he saw the Temperance Movement as the vehicle most capable of forging the homogeneous and orderly society of his ideals, and to it he devoted the bulk of his considerable energy.

Landrith's first effort on behalf of organized temperance came just before World War I. He joined the celebrated prohibitionist Flying Squadron of America and as a paid lecturer travelled the nation proselytizing for the dry cause. He proved a real asset to the movement. Possessed of a good bearing on the podium, the clergyman-reformer was popular with audiences and emerged as something of a sloganeer: "The saloon is an unmixed evil and unmixed evils are never necessary evils" was one of his favorites. Indeed, the man had a positive flare for alliteration. Thus he summed up his views on the political parties of the era: "Democracy Must Be Decent or Die! Republicanism Must Be Respectable or Ruined! Progressivism Must Be Pure or It Is Pre-ordained to Perish." Landrith was one of the organizers of the Tennessee Anti-Saloon League, and at one of the national conventions he coined the slogan, "A saloonless nation by 1920, the three hundredth anniversary of the landing of the Pilgrims." It proved to be one of his most popular, and probably no one had greater claim to the title of phrasemaker to the movement. But he was in deadly earnest about his work. He saw the war against booze as a struggle against the forces of darkness and openly branded opponents of National Prohibition traitors and Bolsheviks. The enemy, in his view, deserved no mercy; the stakes were too high. Although he urged the election of drys, Landrith himself was not much attracted to political office. He did consent to run as the vice presidential candidate of the Prohibition Party in 1916, but he had no expectations of victory. Instead, when not lecturing full time, he was involved with the Anti-Saloon League and the Intercollegiate Prohibition Association, in which he served as president. Landrith fought hard to defend National prohibition in the 1920s and 1930s, and even with the coming of Repeal, he maintained his old faith in the dry cause. He died at seventy-six years old, still dreaming of a prohibitionist resurgence.

**Bibliography:**

A. *Some Extracts from the Bill of Complaint...by Dr. Landrith and His Associates, and the Presbyterian Church in the United States of America...* (Louisville, KY, 1906); "Opposition to Prohibition Bolshevistic," *Union Signal* 49, No. 37 (1923): 6.

B. SEAP 3, 1502; WW 1, 701–2.

**LAWSON, Albert Gallatin**    (5 June 1842, Poughkeepsie, NY—8 March 1929, Danbury, NH). *Education*: studied at Coll. of City of New York, 1870s; studied at Madison Univ. (now Colgate Univ.), 1870s; A.M. (honorary), Madison Univ., 1876; D.D. (honorary), Madison Univ., 1883. *Career*: ordained Baptist minister, 1862; pastorates in NY, CT, NJ, 1862 to 1920s; secretary, American Baptist Union, 1884–86; general secretary, Colgate Univ., 1906–9; instructor, Italian Dept., Colgate Sem., 1917.

Educator and Baptist clergyman, Albert Gallatin Lawson combined a long and distinguished career in the ministry with an abiding commitment to the Temperance Movement. He grew up dry and as a young man apparently considered involvement in temperance activities quite natural. Before his twentieth birthday, and before launching his ministerial career, Lawson joined the fraternal Sons of Temperance and became one of the organization's leading members. The Sons of Temperance served not only as a means to hold their own rank and file to the pledge but as a vehicle for prohibitionist agitation as well. And as Lawson worked in various pulpits later in life across New England, New York, and New Jersey, he always affiliated with the local fraternal lodge in order to continue his part of the struggle against the traffic. Indeed, the existence of the lodge made it possible for Lawson to keep some continuity in his dry activities, as his career kept him on the move. Ordained in 1862, he took a succession of pastorates in Brooklyn, New York; Newark, New Jersey; his native Poughkeepsie; Waterbury, Connecticut; Woodside and Meredith, New York; and Camden, New Jersey. In addition, he lived in Boston as secretary of the American Baptist Union (1884–86) and Hamilton, New York, as general secretary of Colgate University (1906–9) and instructor of Italian (1917). Credited with hard work and competence in all of these positions, Lawson was one of the best-known clergy of his denomination in the East and one of the most influential Baptist spokesmen for temperance.

Lawson's reputation as a temperance worker was probably as widely recognized as his role as a clergyman (if not more so). Through his efforts on behalf of the dry crusade, beginning with his involvement with the Sons of Temperance, he worked closely with other denominations and secular leaders from many parts of the nation. His climb to prominence within temperance circles was fairly steady. In 1867, he was elected grand worthy patriarch of the New Jersey division of the order and the same year was initiated into the National Division, where he became active in directing the national affairs of the group. In 1898, after more than three decades of service, the order selected him as its leader, putting Lawson at the head of the largest fraternal temperance organization in the country. Throughout this long tenure of leadership with the Sons of Temperance, the Baptist reformer also did good service in other sectors of the dry movement. With the founding of the National Temperance Society and Publication House in 1865, he became a life member; later he joined its executive committee. Lawson always devoted time to keeping the church in the fore of the crusade, and with that end in view he sat as chairman of the Temperance Commission of the Federal Council of Churches. In all of these capacities, he regularly attended national and international prohibitionist conventions, usually in some official position. His reform career was indicative of a pattern in temperance leadership which, in the long run, assisted the movement in coordinating its political efforts: Sitting on a number of different social and religious bodies concerned with the liquor question, Lawson, and dry leaders like him all across the nation, were able to keep their activities in concert. In effect, it gave the dry crusade the same advantages of control that business leaders gained through serving on interlocking boards and directorates.

**Bibliography:**

A. *Methods of Church Temperance Work* (New York, 1882); *The High License Method of Dealing with the Liquor Traffic* (n.p., 1891); *A Short Method with Christian Science* (Philadelphia, 1902); *The Religion of Jesus* (Philadelphia, 1920); *The Duty of the Christian Church with Reference to the Temperance Question* (New York, n.d.).

B. SEAP 3, 1520–21; WW 1, 711.

**LEAVITT, Mary Greenleaf Clement**    (22 September 1830, Hopkinton, NH—5 February 1912, Boston, MA). *Education*: graduated from State Normal Sch., MA (as valedictorian), 1851. *Career*: schoolteacher, VT, NH, MA, 1846–57; founded and taught in private sch. for girls, Boston, 1867–81; temperance work with Boston and National WCTU, beginning 1882; named honorary life president, World's WCTU, 1891.

Mary Leavitt was another of those women in the Temperance Movement who was singled out early by Frances Willard* for a major role in the antiliquor crusade and who in fact came to occupy a place of preference and responsibility in the Woman's Christian Temperance Union. But unlike most other WCTU reformers, Leavitt came to a falling out with the organization's president, and their once close relationship ended in bitterness and animosity. Leavitt (born Clement) grew up in New Hampshire, the daughter of a Baptist minister who had been an active social reformer in his day. He was a staunch antislavery and temperance man who supposedly bore a strong likeness to George Washington, and the elder Clement passed on to his daughter not only his penchant for reform but reportedly also his resemblance to the first president. As a young woman, Mary Clement was well educated, having graduated first in her class from the Massachusetts State Normal School in 1851, and she embarked on a career as a teacher. She worked in schools for odd terms in Vermont, New Hampshire, and Massachusetts, finally quitting to marry Thomas Hooker Leavitt, a real estate broker, in 1857. Thomas Leavitt, however, proved a spendthrift and a poor provider, and after ten years of unhappy marriage his wife had to open and run a private school for girls in Boston in order to help pay the family bills. Thomas subsequently left home (for Nebraska) and divorced Mary. It was after the collapse of her marriage that Mary Leavitt became actively involved with the Temperance Movement, and specifically the WCTU. As a mother left to raise a family alone, she was perhaps attracted by the union's credo of "Home Protection." At any rate, she worked skillfully in organizing the Boston chapter of the group, and in 1877, while visiting evangelist Dwight L. Moody,* she met Frances E. Willard (soon to be president of the WCTU). Leavitt impressed Willard as a woman who "would do good service for any cause to which she was committed." In 1881, she gave up her private school and went to work full time for the union, travelling about New England on behalf of temperance and the woman's vote (she also represented the New England Woman Suffrage Association). It was the start of a notable temperance career.

Leavitt in fact developed a considerable reputation as a speaker, and the WCTU leadership pushed her to take on bigger assignments. After the death of her father in 1883, she agreed, albeit reluctantly, to accept Frances Willard's suggestion that she travel abroad as a temperance missionary. In 1884, she left for the Pacific and the Orient on a journey that was to last for seven years. Travelling through New Zealand, Australia, the Far East, and Europe, Leavitt performed prodigies of lecturing. Often speaking three times a day, using a total of 229 interpreters in forty-seven different languages, she claimed to have established eighty-six branches of the WCTU. Her travels stimulated interest in the founding of a World's WCTU, which changed the motto of the National WCTU, "For God and Home and Native Land," to "For God and Home and Every Land." Leavitt was named honorary president for life of the new organization in 1891. Circulating the WCTU "Polyglot Petition," she got 7.5 million signatures by 1895 supporting international prohibition. But the famous lecturer had her detractors. A number of critics claimed that, like other missionaries, her work was ephemeral and that little survived of it after she had passed through an area. Nonetheless, Leavitt was undaunted and soon after her return left on a similar mission to Latin America. But there came a gradually disintegrating relationship with Frances Willard after the latter's assumption of the presidency of the World's WCTU in 1891. The reasons are not precisely known, although Leavitt was highly critical of Willard's long residence in Great Britian in the 1890s. Whatever their origins, Leavitt's attacks grew in vehemence, and many reformers were mystified and repelled by their virulence. Leavitt died in 1912, alienated from most of her old friends in the WCTU, but the record of her international lecturing achievements would never be surpassed.

### Bibliography:

A. *John Bidwell, Josiah Royce: A Letter of Mary Clement Leavitt to Bidwell on Behalf of Royce* (San Francisco, 1943); *Report Made to the First Convention of the World's Christian Temperance Union...* (Boston, 1891).

B. DAB 11, 85–86; NAW 2, 383–85; SEAP 3, 1525; WW 1, 714; Mary Earhart, *Frances Willard: From Prayers to Politics* (Chicago, 1944); Elizabeth Putnam Gordon, *Women Torch Bearers* (Evanston, IL, 1924).

**LENNON, John Brown**   (12 October 1850, Lafayette Co., WI—18 January 1923, Bloomington, IL). *Career*: tailor's apprentice, MO, 1865–69; tailor, CO, 1869–84; secretary, Tailor's Union, Denver, CO, 1883; president, Tailor's Union, 1884; vice president, Journeyman Tailor's Union of America, NY (later IN), 1885–87; general secretary, Journeyman Tailor's Union of America, 1887–1910; editor, *The Tailor*, 1887–1910; treasurer, American Federation of Labor, 1889–1917; member, Commission on Industrial Relations, Washington, DC, 1912; member, Board of Mediators, U.S. Department of Labor, 1917–23.

One of the relatively few prominent labor leaders in the ranks of the Temperance Movement, John Lennon was born in Wisconsin but grew up in Hannibal, Missouri, where his family moved when he was only two. Young Lennon early learned to deal with adult responsibilities, for in 1861 his father enlisted in the Union army and left John the sole support of his family. After the Civil War, Lennon apprenticed himself to his father's newly opened tailor shop, and after four years learning the trade he left for Colorado, where he settled in Denver in 1869. There he opened his own tailor shop and the following year sent for his family, whereupon his father took over the shop while John Lennon became a journeyman tailor. He learned quickly that working for wages was something different from working for yourself, and Lennon developed an active interest in the rights of labor. He became an enthusiastic trade unionist and was one of the pioneer organizers of the Denver Tailor's Union (of which he served as secretary). In 1883, the Denver union became affiliated with the new Journeyman Tailor's Union of America, a national organization, and the way was opened for Lennon to become a full-time union leader. He won election two years later to a vice presidency in the national union and thereafter held a succession of important labor posts for the rest of his life. After becoming general secretary of the Journeyman Tailors in 1887, he moved to New York, the location of national headquarters. There, he also edited *The Tailor*, the official union publication, and became a key figure in labor politics. Throughout his climb to leadership, he maintained a firm belief in the basic value of the American social and economic system. He had no use for labor radicals who sought the overthrow of the old order; rather, Lennon sought to improve the lot of the workingman within the established American system and to reform the system where necessary. His orthodoxy won him high marks with many other labor leaders of similar outlook, and in 1890 he was rewarded with election as treasurer of the American Federation of Labor.

Lennon's views on social reform fit the general Progressive mold of the era. He sought not only humane changes in society but also the elimination of sources of disorder, poverty, political corruption, and similar ills—and he believed firmly that the elimination of the saloon and the liquor traffic would do wonders toward these ends. The fact that the liquor industry was an important employer nationally and that many other labor leaders consequently looked askance at the Temperance Movement (or were outright hostile to it), did not bother Lennon; he felt that the dangers posed by the traffic overrode all other considerations and that, in fact, the saloon on the whole lowered the quality of life for the vast majority of working Americans. "To the trade-unionist," he said, "there is no redeeming feature in the saloon." The union leader campaigned hard for prohibition and even joined the Anti-Saloon League of Illinois as one of its vice presidents, a post he held proudly for more than ten years. He welcomed the coming of the Eighteenth Amendment, considering the dry triumph a victory for "social well-being, civic benefits, and moral uplift." While working for temperance, however, Lennon stayed active on other fronts. A Democrat in politics, he was one of the three labor members appointed to the Commission of Industrial Relations by President Woodrow Wilson in 1913, and in 1917 he agreed to serve on the Board of Mediators of the U.S. Department of Labor. Lennon died in 1923 at the age of seventy-three, having taken a significant part in the progress of organized labor in America and, perhaps thankfully, before seeing the failure of the "noble experiment" for which he had worked so hard.

**Bibliography:**

B. *American Federationist*, March 1923; DAB 11, 170–71; NYT, Jan. 19, 1923; SEAP 3, 1532; *The Tailor*, Jan. 23, Feb. 5, 1923; WW 1, 721.

**LEONARD, Adna Wright**    (2 November 1874, Cincinnati, OH—3 May 1943, Iceland). *Education*: A.B., New York Univ., 1899; B.D., Drew Theological Sem., 1901; postgraduate study, American Sch. of Archaeology, Rome, 1901–3; D.D. (honorary), Ohio Northern Univ., 1909; LLD. (honorary), Coll. of Puget Sound, 1916, Univ. of Southern California, 1916, Syracuse Univ., 1930, Allegheny Coll., 1932, American Univ., 1941; STD. (honorary), Syracuse Univ., 1926; LHD. (honorary), West Virginia Wesleyan Coll., 1938. *Career*: ordained Methodist minister, 1899; minister, NJ, Puerto Rico, Rome, OH, IL, WA, 1898–1916; bishop, Methodist Church, beginning 1916; active on various national committees of the Methodist Church, beginning 1900s.

Adna Wright Leonard grew up a prohibitionist. His father, Adna Bradway Leonard, also a Methodist clergyman, was an active and deeply committed temperance man who once ran for governor of Ohio as a member of the Prohibition Party. Thus in entering the church and the ranks of the dry crusade, young Adna Wright followed closely in the steps of Adna Bradway. After his ordination in 1889, Leonard travelled widely as he served pastorates in the East, Midwest, Pacific Coast, Puerto Rico, and Rome, Italy. Wherever his ministerial duties took him, he never failed to speak on behalf of the Temperance Movement. Quite regularly, he also took part in dry political and organizational activities. In Ohio, he campaigned for local-option laws, while in Washington a call from his pulpit launched the movement for state-wide prohibition. With Leonard maintaining a leadership role, the effort was victorious in 1914—a significant dry triumph—and the crusading pastor was elected a member of the Washington Anti-Saloon League Central Headquarters Committee the following year. Leonard's elevation to bishop enabled him to increase his contributions to the cause. In 1922 he marshalled public support in California for that state's "Little Volstead Act" (its local enforcement statute for National Prohibition); and the next year, having moved to New York State, he was elected president of the New York Anti-Saloon League. Throughout his years as a temperance worker, Leonard also did good service in other church causes, wrote extensively on a variety of topics, and established a highly respected record for church leadership (he was the recipient of no fewer than eight honorary degrees). He remained an active churchman after the collapse of the Eighteenth Amendment, notably in a Methodist effort to assist army and navy chaplains during World War II. He was on such a mission, heading to an army position in Iceland, when he died in an aircraft crash in 1943.

**Bibliography:**

B. SEAP 3, 1532–33; WW 2, 319.

**LEVERING, Joshua**    (12 September 1845, Baltimore, MD—5 October 1935, Baltimore, MD). *Career*: worked in family coffee importing business, E. Levering & Co., Baltimore, MD (co-owner after 1870), 1860s–1880s; various official positions in Prohibition Party, beginning 1884.

As a successful importer of coffee, it may have appeared that Joshua Levering was waging a battle in his own self-interest by attacking a rival beverage— alcohol. Yet Levering, in addition to his business acumen, was a sincerely committed philanthropist and reformer throughout his adult life. A deeply religious Baptist, he devoted most of his initial concerns to affairs of the denomination. Over the years, he helped found a new church, served as an officer in a number of Baptist organizations, and later in life sat as president of the trustees of the Southern Baptist Theological Seminary in Louisville, Kentucky. His importing business proved lucrative enough to allow him to retire from the active direction of the company while still a relatively young man in the early 1880s. From then on, the scope of his reform and civic activities broadened considerably. Levering donated funds to and worked on behalf of a variety of charities and reform groups in the Baltimore area—he was especially fond of the Young Men's Christian Association. Yet he quickly singled out the Temperance Movement as his chief interest. As a Baptist, he had long been a total abstainer and favorably disposed toward the dry cause, and given the opportunity, he threw himself into the fray with a passion. Formerly a Democrat, he quit the party when it did not take a strong prohibitionist stance. Instead, he joined the Prohibition Party, in which he earned a national reputation as a scourge of the "demon rum."

Levering's rise in the party was quick, a fact owing much to his ability to give its affairs a great deal of his time. He frequently attended Prohibitionist conventions and served a term as president of the Maryland State Prohibition Committee (1892–93). Not content simply to manage campaigns and conduct lobbying efforts, he also ran for office himself, beginning at the state level. In 1891, he made a bid for Maryland state comptroller, and in 1895 he headed the state Prohibition Party ticket in a run for governor. Levering's electoral efforts, however, reached the national scene in 1896, when the party's nominating convention broke up in an acrimonious ideological dispute. Two factions emerged: "broad-gaugers," who wanted to couple prohibition with work on behalf of other reforms; and "narrow-gaugers," who insisted that the party concentrate solely on the liquor question. The sides would not be reconciled, and the "broad-gaugers" finally walked out, held a rump caucus, founded a new National Party, and nominated Charles E. Bentley,* of Nebraska, for president. The "narrow-gaugers,'' who remained with what was left of the party, then put Levering forward as their candidate. Neither man did well at the polls, Levering having the dubious distinction of bringing in one of the lowest Prohibition Party votes in some time. Still, the Baltimore reformer had never expected to win, only to show the party flag as evidence of the vitality of the cause. The cause was indeed quite alive, but by 1896 it had become clear that the Prohibition Party would never be its chief political vehicle.

**Bibliography:**

B. SEAP 3, 1534–35; WW 1, 724; Jack S. Blocker, Jr., *Retreat from Reform: The Prohibition Movement in the United States, 1890–1913* (Westport, CT, 1976).

**LEWIS, Dioclesian ("Dio")**    (3 March 1823, Auburn, NY—21 May 1886, Yonkers, NY). *Education*: studied at Harvard Medical Sch., 1845–46; M.D. (honorary), Homoeopathic Hosp. Coll., OH, 1851. *Career*: founder and teacher, private school, OH, early 1840s; medical practice, Port Byron, NY, beginning 1846; publisher, *Homoeopathist*, Buffalo, NY, 1840s; lecturer and women's gymnastics instructor, 1852–63; founded Boston Normal Physical-training Sch., 1863 (and a similar school in Lexington, MA, 1864); reform lecturer, 1860s to 1881; active writing on reform subjects, 1881–86.

Dioclesian Lewis (or "Dio" Lewis, as he was usually called) holds a special and generally misunderstood part in the annals of the temperance reform. He was a reformer-entrepreneur who made a comfortable living from his various private schools, writings, and extensive lecturing and who, whatever his personal motives, was able to move his listeners to action. He aspired originally to a medical career, although he never finished his medical education (his M.D. was an honorary degree). Nevertheless, he established a practice in homoeopathic medicine near Buffalo, New York, in the 1840s. Eventually, however, his interest turned chiefly to the efficacy of physical exercise, which he believed of greater value than drugs in preventing illness. To put into practice his idea, he founded two schools in the mid-1860s, one in Boston and the other in Lexington, Massachusetts, in which he offered instruction in his exercise system—"free gymnastics." Many of his students were women, and Lewis became a vocal proponent of physical education for females. He added the subject to his stock of lectures, which usually attracted enthusiastic audiences. Indeed, Lewis had been an accomplished public lecturer since the late 1840s, when he had spoken on temperance themes throughout the Midwest, the South, and Canada. His theories on physical education constituted, in his mind, yet another reform which, like temperance, would contribute to the national welfare and therefore merited dedicated advocacy. Despite his successes in popularizing his medical views, however, his greatest fame would come from a renewal of his interest in the Temperance Movement.

Given Lewis's views of the harmful effects of even the most benign of medical drugs, it is little wonder that he saw alcohol as an evil. His commitment to temperance was no doubt sincere—but there was also no question that he made his antiliquor work pay. He had done well with his dry lectures before the Civil War but had concentrated on his other interests when popular attention waned on the liquor question. Yet by the early 1870s the issue had come alive once more, and Lewis again took to the podium. His delivery was as effective as ever, and, quite unwittingly, one of his speeches provided the spark for the so-called Woman's Crusade of 1873 and 1874. After a lecture in Hillsboro, Ohio, in 1873, the women of the town asked what they should do to protect their families from the illegal liquor business that flourished in the locale. Lewis replied with a story about his mother's response years before to a similar situation: She knelt by the saloon and prayed, which act melted the heart of the barkeep—who closed up shop! (Or so went the story.) Soon afterward, "praying bands" descended on the liquor sellers of Hillsboro and then on their brethren in the trade all across the country. By late 1874 the crusade had coalesced into the Woman's Christian Temperance Union, and temperance partisans looked back with gratitude on the inspiration originally provided by Lewis (not to mention the heroic Delecta Barbour Lewis, his pious mother). Overlooked, however, was the fact that Lewis simply did not subscribe to the most significant element in the women's program: He was not a prohibitionist. The reformer insisted that prohibitory laws were useless, that true temperance could not come through the force of legislation. Instead, he advocated "moral suasion," the appeal for voluntary abstinence first used on a mass basis by the Washingtonian Movement in the 1840s. Over the years until Lewis's death in 1886, the WCTU was thus in the curious position of having one of its honored heroes actively denouncing legal prohibition as folly.

### Bibliography:

A. *The New Gymnastics* (New York, 1862, and many subsequent editions); *In a Nutshell: Suggestions to American College Students* (New York, 1883); *Prohibition: For and Against. Containing the Correspondence Between, and Speeches of Dr. Dio Lewis . . . and Hon. John B. Finch . . . on This Great Question* (New York, 1884); *Our Digestion . . .* (New York, 1886); *Chastity; or, Our Secret Sins* (New York, 1890); *Prohibition a Failure; or, the True Solution of the Temperance Question* (New York, 1892).

B. DAB 11, 209; *New York Tribune*, May 22, 1886; SEAP 3, 1536; WW H, 383; Mary F. Eastman, *Biography of Dio Lewis* (n.p., 1891); W. C. Steel, *The Woman's Temperance Movement* (New York, 1874).

**LITTLEFIELD, Charles Edgar**    (21 June 1851, Lebanon, ME—2 May 1915, Rockland, ME). *Education*: private study of law, 1870s. *Career*: admitted to bar, ME, 1876; legal practice, Rockland, ME, beginning 1876; member, Maine House of Representatives, 1885–89; Maine attorney general, 1889–93; member, U.S. House of Representatives, 1899–1909.

Charles Edgar Littlefield spent most of his adult life in state and national politics and was typical of the kind of legislator the Temperance Movement could count on to carry the dry message to the halls of government. A lawyer by training, Littlefield had a penchant for politics and was soon one of the most active members of the Republican Party in Maine. He won his first political contest in 1885, taking a seat in the state House of Representatives, and he served half of his four-year term as speaker. The following four years (1889–1893) saw him in office as Maine's attorney general; and after further work within GOP ranks as a convention delegate and party organizer, he was elected in 1899 to the national House of Representatives to fill the unexpired term of his recently deceased predecessor, Nelson Dingley.* Littlefield was elected in his own right to the next four Congresses, serving until 1909, when he voluntarily retired. While in Congress, Littlefield not unexpectedly devoted much of his time to temperance issues. In this, he fully reflected the concerns of his constituents—the legacy of Neal Dow* and the Maine Law still being powerful forces back home. He joined the Congressional Temperance Society and played an instrumental role in framing legislation to bar the sales of alcoholic beverages in army post exchanges—the so-called anticanteen law—in 1901. The Maine congressman was also a central figure in getting a prohibition clause inserted in the Oklahoma statehood bill. In addition, in the absence of a constitutional amendment, Littlefield sought the passage of national laws to prohibit the shipment of intoxicating beverages across state lines. The proposed Littlefield-Dolliver Bill, Littlefield-Carmack Bill, and Littlefield-Hansborough Bill all sought this end, though none succeeded in passage. These setbacks, however, never discouraged him, and until he left Congress he continued to campaign, on the floor of the House and in print, for his chosen cause. His record as a legislator was never major, but his dedication to temperance was sincere, and his persistence aided the accumulation of piecemeal dry victories that pointed the way toward the Eighteenth Amendment. Upon stepping down from his House seat, Littlefield returned to the practice of law.

**Bibliography:**

A. *Puerto Rico: The Pearl of the Antilles, the Everfaithful Isle. Speech...* (Washington, DC, 1900); *The Insular Cases...Address by Charles E. Littlefield...* (n.p., 1901); "Sherman Anti-Trust Law...Address," Illinois State Bar Association *Proceedings* (1908); *Class Legislation* (New York, 1911?).

B. SEAP 3, 1575; WW 1, 721.

**LITTLEFIELD, Nathan Whitman**   (21 May 1846, Bridgewater, MA—5 December 1929, Pawtucket, RI). *Education*: A.B., Dartmouth Coll. (valedictorian), 1869; LLB., Boston Univ., 1876; A.M. (honorary), Dartmouth Coll., 1909. *Career*: principal, Newport, RI, high school, 1871–73; high school principal and superintendent of schools, Westerly, RI, 1873–74; admitted to bar, MA, 1876, RI, 1877; legal practice, Providence, RI, beginning 1877; member, Rhode

Island Senate, 1897–98; extensive memberships on civic and governmental commissions and bodies, beginning 1870s.

Nathan Whitman Littlefield came early to his recognition of the evils of the liquor traffic. His family was firmly under the temperance banner, so he was raised without tasting "the demon rum." In addition, his father took the dry cause with particular seriousness—to the point of taking the offensive against booze. One of young Nathan's earliest memories was his liquor-hating father taking him on a trip through the countryside around Plymouth, Massachusetts, in an effort to gather evidence against illegal beverage sales. Without probing the local geography in similar fashion, Nathan, in his day, followed closely his father's lead in pushing the attack against drink. And he did so with solid social and legal credentials. He was well educated, completing studies at prestigious Philips Academy, Dartmouth College, and Boston University. Deciding on a career in law, he set up practice in Providence, Rhode Island, and steadily built a lucrative business. His legal skills attracted influential clients, and Littlefield became active politically (he was a Democrat), serving in a number of capacities on public administrative and judicial panels. To cite only several examples: He was variously a referee in bankruptcy for the District of Rhode Island from 1898 to 1918, a member of the commission to revise the judicial system of Rhode Island (1904–5), as well as a leading force on the commission to redistrict the state and to write the statutes implementing the new Rhode Island Constitution in 1910. Littlefield also briefly tried his hand at elective politics, serving as a member of the Rhode Island State Senate (1897–98) and running for governor without success in 1900. His interests in other civic, church (he was a Congregationalist), and historical groups were wide. In short, Nathan Littlefield was a man of considerable talent and public standing—precisely the kind of indivudual the Temperance Movement prized as a dry leader.

Littlefield did not disappoint the cause. Indeed, his youthful hatred of the liquor traffic remained at white heat as he matured in his legal and public careers. He spoke frequently on temperance issues, and his popular stature was such that he commanded a hearing. He also used his legal talents in support of prohibitionist measures, and he won some important victories in the courts. In the face of fierce wet opposition, he played a critical role in securing a decision from the Massachusetts Supreme Court allowing voters to consider the question of liquor licensing at every general election without gathering petitions requesting such a vote each time. In cooperation with other attorneys, he successfully aided in the prosecution of illegal beverage dealers and Rhode Island gamblers. The crusading attorney became a major force in the state chapter of the Anti-Saloon League. He served as its legal adviser and in 1908 was elected one of its trustees. Four years later he advanced to the presidency, a position he held until 1925. From 1912 on he represented the Rhode Island League on the national board of directors of the Anti-Saloon League of America, rising to vice president of the national organization in 1918. Littlefield was also active in supporting the drive for the enactment of the Eighteenth Amendment to the Constitution. The dry reform could hardly have asked more of any one man, and temperance leaders were properly appreciative. Yet public support for many of his activities was never unanimous. Rhode Island had a large Roman Catholic population, much of it composed of recent immigrants, and wet sentiments were strong. The state was in fact one of the bitterest foes of National Prohibition. Littlefield, however, never hesitated to follow the right as he saw it, and he never failed to proclaim temperance as an American virtue necessary to the national welfare and social order.

**Bibliography:**

A. "Governor Marcus Morton . . .," *Old Colony Historical Society* 7 (1909): 75–93; *James C. Hunter vs. Mabel B. Conrad, et al. Brief . . .* (Providence, RI, n.d.).

B. SEAP 3, 1575–76; WW 1, 721.

**LITTLE TURTLE**    (circa 1752, Eel River area, near Fort Wayne, IN—14 July 1812, Fort Wayne, IN). *Career*: led Indian forces against American expansion in Northwest Territory, 1790s; signed Treaty of Greenville, 1795; frequent negotiations on behalf of Indians, 1795–1812.

The son of a Miami chief and (probably) a Mohican mother, Little Turtle (Michikiniqua) became one of the most prominent Indian leaders of the old Northwest Territory in the late eighteenth and early nineteenth centuries. His youth is obscure, but he came to white attention as an ally of the British during and after the American Revolution. Determined to halt the expansion of the United States into the traditional homeland of his people, the Miami leader counseled a determined opposition to the Americans over the 1780s and led an effective military defense in the early 1790s. Indeed, he proved one of the most able Indian commanders the United States ever faced in battle. In 1790, Little Turtle helped plan and lead the assault that smashed the forces of Josiah Harmar; a year later he repeated the success against Arthur St. Clair's army. Again, in 1792, he clashed with Kentucky militia and in 1794 was a central figure in the opening stages of the campaign against the invading American columns under Anthony Wayne. Always brave and determined, Little Turtle was also a realist. Concluding finally that battle would prove catastrophic to the tribes in the end, he urged peace talks while the Indians were still strong enough to negotiate. This advice cost him his prestige with his people, and he did not lead them in the disastrous engagement against Wayne at Fallen Timbers. Thereafter, however, he once more became spokesman for his tribe, signing the Treaty of Greenville and conducting a series of negotiations with the Americans into the 1800s.

Little Turtle's arguments for peace instead of war made him more popular with many Americans than with substantial numbers of Indians. Nevertheless, he retained enough influence with the Miami to prevent their joining Tecumsa and the British during the War of 1812. And he devoted many of his later days to campaigning against social problems besetting the tribes. In particular, Little Turtle denounced the spread of intemperance and actively sought to restrain the flow of alcohol to the Indians. White traders and settlers encouraged the Miami in their drinking over the late 1790s and early 1800s, helping to weaken tribal society and spread demoralization. Angered at the deleterious impact of drinking on Indian culture, as early as 1801 Little Turtle travelled to Baltimore to address a Quaker gathering, asking their help in halting beverage shipments to the Miami. A year or so later he made a similar plea to the Kentucky legislature, and shortly after that he spoke on the subject to Ohio authorities. He painted a villainous picture of white traders, accusing them of plying the Indians with liquor and then leaving them destitute. "My people barter away their best treasures," he supposedly complained, "for the white man's miserable firewater." Such objections brought little relief, as white officials were generally unwilling or unable to control the lucrative trade with the Indians. But Little Turtle's efforts were a further demonstration that many Indian leaders were fully aware of the damage intemperance spread in its wake and that they saw liquor control as an important element in the preservation of Indian society. The Miami chief, much as he deplored Indian sufferings at the hands of whites, spent his final years in a house the American government built for him, frequently visited Eastern cities, and died while receiving medical treatment at Fort Wayne.

**Bibliography:**

B. DAB 11, 300; WW H, 387; Charles H. L. Johnston, *Famous Indian Chiefs: Their Battles. . .for the Possession of America* (Boston, 1909); Alvin M. Josephy, *The Patriot Chiefs* (New York, 1961); Norman B. Wood, *Lives of Famous Indian Chiefs* (Aurora, IL, 1906).

**LIVERMORE, Mary Ashton**   (19 December 1821, Boston, MA—23 May 1905, Boston, MA). *Career*: teacher (including several years while a student), Charleston Female Sem., 1836–38; teacher, plantation in VA, 1839–42; founder and principal of private sch., Duxbury, MA, 1842–45; associate editor, *New Covenant*; work with the Northwestern Branch, U.S. Sanitary Commission, 1861–65; editor, *The Agitator*, which merged with the *Woman's Journal*, 1869–72; reform author and lecturer, 1872–95.

Mary Livermore's career epitomized the broad reform interests of the early Temperance Movement. Raised a strict Baptist, her personal ethical standards were reflected publicly in a passion for social justice and service to others. She formed early commitments to antislavery, women's education, and, through work with the Washingtonians, temperance. In 1845 she married a Massachusetts temperance man and Universalist minister, Daniel P. Livermore, in whom she found a life-long reform partner. While working on charitable projects with Daniel's congregations, she began writing on religious, moral, and reform subjects and continued in this vein when, in 1857, the Livermores moved to Chicago to edit the Universalist *New Covenant*. During these years her reputation as a reform author grew considerably, and she added to it by being the only woman reporter to cover the Republican presidential nomination in 1860. Mary worked with the Sanitary Commission during the Civil War, and her efforts on behalf of Union wounded and army health standards also gained national attention. After the war, she entered the woman's rights movement with equal determination, convinced that involving women in politics would expedite the causes for which she had labored before and during the war. She became the first president of the Illinois Woman's Suffrage Association and then began editing the feminist *Agitator* in 1869; she merged this publication with the Boston-based *Woman's Journal* when the Livermores moved back to Massachusetts. Giving up editing in 1872, she became a full-time reform author and lecturer, speaking on a variety of issues throughout the United States and Britain. While suffrage and temperance remained two of her favorite themes, she ultimately became involved with such other causes as industrial, educational, and prison reform, Indian relief, and local charities. Livermore was clearly one of the premier reformers of her generation.

Livermore's approach to reform was well suited to the postwar Temperance Movement, particularly the "Do Everything" policy of Frances Willard* and the WCTU. While maintaining her other reform interests, she assumed a decisive leadership role in antiliquor work in the 1870s. When the Massachusetts WCTU arose in the wake of the Woman's Crusade in 1875, she assumed the presidency and held it for ten years. Linking temperance with woman's rights, she lobbied effectively with Massachusetts Republicans to obtain endorsements for both prohibition and suffrage. She also proved highly successful in organizing youth temperance groups and as an advocate for temperance issues on the national lecture circuit. Willard considered her the WCTU's foremost orator, and co-edited with her a popular temperance volume, *A Woman of the Century* (1893). Livermore retired from active reform work in 1895, and, deeply hurt by the death of her husband in 1899, she was lost as a major force in temperance work. During her years of service, however, she was perhaps the only other major leader of the WCTU with organizational abilities and intellectual talents equal to Willard's.

### Bibliography:

A. *The Children's Army* (Boston, 1844); *Pen-Pictures* (Chicago, 1863); *What Shall We Do with Our Daughters? and Other Lectures* (Boston, 1883); *My Story of the War: A Woman's Narrative of Four Years of Personal Experience...* (Hartford, CT, 1888); with Frances E. Willard, eds., *A Woman of the Century* (New York, 1893, and many subsequent editions under various titles); *The Story of My Life: Or, the Sunshine and Shadow of Seventy Years* (Hartford, CT, 1897).

B. DAB 11, 306–7; NAW 3, 410–13; NCAB 3, 82; SEAP 4, 1576–77; WW 1, 736; William M. Thayer, *Women Who Win: Or, Making Things Happen* (New York, 1896).

**LOCKE, David Ross**    (20 September 1833, Vestal, NY—15 February 1888, Toledo, OH). *Career*: trained as a printer, Cortland, OH, circa late 1840s; local reporter, various newspapers, Western states; publisher, *Plymouth* (OH) *Advertiser*, 1852; reporter, *Mansfield* (OH) *Herald* and *Bucyrus Journal*, 1850s; editor, *Jeffersonian* (Findlay, OH), 1861–65; editor and partner, *Toledo* (OH) *Blade*, 1865–88; managing editor, *Evening Mail* (New York City), 1871.

David Ross Locke has been called "the most powerful political satirist of his day and country." After reporting and editing jobs of no great promise with various Midwestern and Western journals, Locke, who was an ardent Unionist, hit his professional stride during the Civil War. The vehicle of his influence was his literary creation, "Petroleum V. Nasby," an itinerant Kentucky preacher whose ignorance, horrid speech, and general dissoluteness served as a stinging caricature of Copperhead Democrats. By allowing Nasby to drawl stupidity on behalf of slavery and drink, Locke achieved the satirical purpose of ridiculing the entire Southern cause. The "Nasby Letters," as Locke's columns quickly became known, appeared first in 1861 in the Findlay, Ohio, *Jeffersonian*, of which he was editor at the time. They came out regularly after that over the course of the war and Reconstruction. As wretched an individual as Petroleum V. Nasby was, the fictive character brought his creator wealth and fame as he delighted Northern readers and infuriated partisans of the Confederacy. President Abraham Lincoln was known at times to read the Nasby letters to official guests, and both he and President Grant offered Locke government positions. Grant's secretary of war, George Boutwell, once observed that the Union victory in the war was attributable to "the army, the navy, and the Nasby letters." In addition to their efforts against the Confederacy, the letters also added a new dimension to the war against drink. It was a novel vein in the temperance literature for liquor to be linked with disloyalty; through Nasby, however, Locke presented liquor as the motivating force behind not only crime and poverty but slavery and secession as well. For the antiliquor cause, it was an important contribution, as Locke's sort of temperance propaganda helped to maintain the continuity of the Temperance Movement while preoccupation with the war largely supplanted interest in other issues. After the war, especially in his later years, Locke persistently attacked the liquor trade from the editor's desk at the *Toledo Blade*. Writing under his own name, he denounced the liquor traffic at length, heading articles and punctuating paragraph after paragraph with the slogan, "Pulverize the Rum Power." Shortly before his death the American Temperance Society published a number of his tracts. But he was always best recalled for Petroleum B. Nasby, who was eventually given pictorial representation by cartoonist Thomas Nast.

**Bibliography:**

A. *Prohibition* (New York, 1886); *High License Does not Diminish the Evil!* (New York, 1887); *"Swingin Round the Circle": His Ideas of Men, Politics, and Things as Set Forth in His Letters to the Public Press*, illus. Thomas Nast

(Boston, 1888); *Civil War Letters of Petroleum V. Nasby*, ed. Harvey S. Ford (Columbus, OH, 1962); *The Struggles of Petroleum V. Nasby*, ed. Joseph Jones, notes by Gunther Barth (Boston, 1963).

B. DAB 11, 336; *New York Herald*, Feb. 16, 1888; SEAP 4, 1587–88; WW H, 338; James C. Austin, *Petroleum V. Nasby (David Ross Locke)* (New York, 1965); Robert Ford, *American Humourists, Recent and Living* (London, 1897); John M. Harrison, *The Man Who Made Nasby: David Ross Locke* (Chapel Hill, NC, 1969).

**LONG, John Davis**   (27 October 1838, Buckfield, ME—28 August 1915, Hingham, MA). *Education*: A.B., Harvard Univ., 1857; studied law in Harvard Law Sch. and with a private law office, 1861; LLD. (honorary), Harvard Univ., 1880, Tufts Univ., 1902. *Career*: principal, Westford Acad., MA, 1857–59; admitted to bar, 1851; legal practice, ME, 1861–62, legal practice, MA, beginning 1862; member, Massachusetts House of Representatives, 1875–78; lieutenant governor of Massachusetts, 1879; governor of Massachusetts, 1880–83; member, U.S. House of Representatives, 1883–89; secretary of the navy, 1897–1902.

John Davis Long's major contribution to the Temperance Movement was made as secretary of the navy. In 1899 he ordered a prohibition against the sale of all alcoholic beverages to enlisted men aboard ships and in naval stations. (In 1914, under one of his successors, Josephus Daniels,* this prohibition was extended to officers as well.) The motivating current of thought behind this measure was a concept of efficiency and safety which had already found expression in similar regulations throughout business and industry during the late nineteenth century. It was clear enough that the availability of alcohol to servicemen and workers threatened the sure functioning of the systems within which they worked; the fact had long been a major point in the rhetoric of temperance argument. Long's action, however, went further. He also saw prohibition as a patriotic measure. In the case of the navy, which owed something of its splendid performance during the Spanish-American War to Long's efforts as secretary, military efficiency was arguably bound to the national destiny. And any measure furthering the national interest, in Long's mind, had to be pursued as an obligation of civic duty. Indeed, that was his view of the prohibition question in general throughout his long and distinguished public career.

The values which informed this antiliquor concept of the national good may be seen, in Long's case, as a function of a larger cultural ethic. "I was brought up with a wholesome abhorrence of liquor drinking," Long recalled. He drank after college, he noted, but he returned to the dry fold, becoming a strong advocate of total abstinence. For many years, he served as president of the Massachusetts Total Abstinence Society. In his description of how he became a proponent and adherent of the antiliquor cause, Long cited first the influence of his upbringing, which was in the tradition of upper-class New England social and moral stewardship. It was not, however, until what Long referred to as "a sense of responsibility'' as a father, husband, and citizen set in that he actually recognized abstinence as a personal and communal duty. With marriage, and an appreciation of the securities of domestic society, he began to attach a religious value to the maintaining of established institutions and of a nationwide standard of personal and public behavior and values. Long came to see alcohol as a direct threat to this normative ideal. It led to crime, poverty, waste, and disorder—all deviations from his vision of the good society—and thus it had to be eradicated. Long expressed this view consistently as a public servant, from his first election to the Massachusetts legislature in 1875 (as a Republican) through his years as governor, a member of Congress, and ultimately, secretary of the navy. He wasted no sympathy on the liquor industry, believing that government had every right to intervene in its affairs or even abolish it in the name of the public good. When he issued his prohibitory order to the navy, Long also expressed the hope that it would serve as an example to the fleets of other nations and that America's friends would issue similar orders to their sailors. It would be a step, he believed, toward securing world order under the banner of international sobriety.

### Bibliography:

A. *After Dinner and Other Speeches* (Boston, 1897); *The Republican Party: Its History, Principles, and Policies* (New York, 1900); *The New American Navy*, 2 vols. (Boston, 1903); with others, eds., *The American Business Encyclopedia and Legal Advisor*, 5 vols. (Boston, 1913); *At the Fireside* (Boston, 1914); *Papers of John Davis Long, 1897–1904*, ed. Gardner Weld Allen (Boston, 1939).

B. *Boston Transcript*, Aug. 30, 1915; DAB 11, 377–78; SEAP 3, 1595; WW 1, 743; Lawrence Shay Mayo, *America of Yesterday, as Reflected in the Journal of John Davis Long* (Boston, 1923).

**LUMPKIN, Joseph Henry**    (23 December 1799, Oglethorpe Co., GA—4 June 1867, Athens, GA). *Education*: studied at Franklin Coll. (now Univ. of Georgia), circa 1814–15; A.B., Coll. of New Jersey (now Princeton Univ.), 1819; LLD. (honorary), Princeton Univ., 1851. *Career*: admitted to bar, GA, 1820; legal practice, GA, beginning 1820; member, Georgia legislature, 1824–26; justice, Georgia Supreme Court, 1845–67.

Joseph Henry Lumpkin is one of the most famous names in the annals of Southern jurisprudence and in the history of early temperance sentiment in the American South. He was a member of one of the more prominent families in the state, the seventh son of parents who moved to Georgia from Virginia shortly after the American Revolution. One of his brothers became governor, while Joseph became a justice on the State Supreme Court, as did two of his grandsons after him. Lumpkin was eminently successful as a lawyer and was highly esteemed for his eloquence in the courtroom. His fellow citizens also prized his sense of fair play, a faith he kept when he played a major role in the framing of the Georgia Penal Code in 1833. Appointed (without his knowledge) to the state's first Supreme Court in 1845, he did yeoman service establishing the authority and reputation of the bench. He sat until his death, adding teaching duties soon after his appointment at a new law school at the University of Georgia (named the Lumpkin School of Law in his honor). He was devoted to his profession and to the court, generally eschewing politics (although he somewhat reluctantly served two terms in the legislature) and turning down offers of appointment to other prestigious posts. Notably, he refused a seat on the federal bench when President Franklin Pierce asked him to serve, just as he refused to take the job when he was actually elected chancellor of the University of Georgia in 1860. Few Georgians, then, could claim the public regard accorded Lumpkin.

Lumpkin's sense of public duty also made him something of a reformer, although never of the radical stripe. He favored the industrialization of the South, primarily to uplift poor whites, and he saw temperance as a means of maintaining personal health and social order. He became a teetotaler himself in 1828, the same year that he joined the new Georgia Temperance Society. In 1833, he served as a Georgia delegate to the convention of the American Temperance Union and several years later became an ardent supporter of the antiliquor movement initiated by Josiah Flournoy.* Flournoy aimed at the enactment of prohibitory legislation, and in getting involved with this effort Lumpkin made one of the few mistakes of his career in reading popular opinion on an important issue. With Flournoy, Lumpkin challenged the state liquor interests to a petition-signing contest, the legality of the liquor traffic to hang on the issue of which side garnered the most signatures. While some petitions actually did circulate, the effort never led to a resolution of the issue. It did, however, do much to politicize the temperance debate. The antiliquor cause had generated promising early strength, relying solely on moral suasion; but the shift to a drive for legislative prohibition—Flournoy's goal—generated a concerted opposition. Flournoy's radicalism, despite the support of Lumpkin and other prominent Georgians, ultimately cost the local temperance forces much of their popular support, and by the mid 1840s they were no longer a serious political pressure group. Nor was the cause able to rebuild its strength quickly: Too many Northern dry leaders were allied to the abolitionist movement, and as the antislavery controversy deepened, most Southerners wanted little to do with temperance men. Thus, despite the personal abstinence and public sympathies of Georgians like Lumpkin, the dry crusade did not resume a major presence in the Peach State until after the Civil War.

**Bibliography:**

A. *An Address to the Religious Community of Georgia, in Six Essays* (Washington, GA, 1828); *An Address on Natural History...* (Washington, GA, 1836); *An Address Delivered Before the South Carolina Institute...* (Charleston, SC, 1850); *The Industrial Regeneration of the South* (1852).

B. DAB 11, 502–3; SEAP 3, 1612–13; WW H, 395; L. L. Cody, *The Lumpkin Family of Georgia* (Macon, GA, 1912); W. J. Northen, ed., *Men of Mark in Georgia*, vol.2 (Atlanta, 1910); H. A. Scomp, *King Alcohol in the Realm of King Cotton* (Chicago, 1888).

# M

**McAULEY, Jeremiah ("Jerry")**  (1839? Ireland—18 September 1884, New York, NY). *Career*: founder and manager, Water Street Mission, NY, beginning 1872; editor, *Jerry McAuley's Newspaper*, beginning 1882.

Jeremiah McAuley's biography has been transmitted in all the colors of a certain kind of romance that became an essential part of temperance propaganda around the turn of the century. Yet in "Jerry" McAuley's case, almost every dramatic word was the truth. The son of an Irish counterfeiter, he grew up a thief upon immigrating to America. At nineteen years old he was sentenced to fifteen years in Sing Sing penitentiary in New York State for a crime he did not commit. There he claimed to have reformed and was pardoned after seven years, only to fall back to his old ways and then to reform again and again. Finally, he gained his footing once and for all, found honest work, had a religious conversion, and in 1872 opened the Water Street Mission in New York City. In its early stages, the mission ran mostly on McAuley's faith and the tireless and devoted efforts of his wife, Maria; financially, it was a dubious proposition at best. Yet the McAuleys carried on, ministering and bringing help to the city's poor and needy, often braving attacks from the criminal element from whose ranks Jerry had emerged. He became "apostle to the drunkard and outcast," recalled one of his converts, a Samuel H. Hadley; at Water Street "the drunkard was more welcome than the sober man, the thief than the honest man, the harlot than the beautiful pure woman." He published a regular journal of mission meetings and testimonies and a biography which was widely circulated. He continued to depend for assistance in all this work on his wife, also a convert from "a life of degradation," who continued the mission after he died. The McAuley missions, at Water Street and later at a second location on West Thirty-second Street, became havens of rest for people from throughout the world who had heard of them by word of mouth among the diffuse legions of the itinerant and dispossessed.

The imagery of Christianity obviously played a large part in McAuley's sense of his role, as to be sure, the agencies and imagery of religion figured largely in his own salvation. And as McAuley tried to offer both spiritual and material comfort through his rescue missions, his work was of a type in many respects with the "gospel temperance" efforts already in the field. In fact, his labors helped to further this special branch of the dry crusade, which earlier had taken the downfallen as the objects of its ministry and whose effective feature was the public testimony by those who, like McAuley, were once lost but now redeemed. Indeed, McAuley attributed the difficulty of his own reformation to drink. Having once been saved from alcohol at Sing Sing with the help of a reformed felon, and having been pardoned after developing his own program of religious revivalism at the prison, back on the streets it was booze, as he told it, that again took him astray. Introduced to a drink that had only come into wide use in New York during his imprisonment, läger beer, and with whose properties and effects he was thus unfamiliar, the future mission worker fell into drunkenness. McAuley's report is in the popular tradition of those who described firsthand the insidious workings of even minimal quantities of alcohol in awakening lascivious and criminal impulses. Thus McAuley's own exposure to mission workers on Water Street helped to make total abstinence the cornerstone of his own rebuilding and that of his effort to rescue others. The reformer's hard life caught up with him eventually, however. His difficult years had undermined his health, and he died, probably of tuberculosis, only twelve years after his religious conversion at some forty-five years old.

**Bibliography:**

A. *Transformed, or the History of a River Thief* (New York, 1876); *Jerry McAuley: His Life and Work*, ed. R. M. Offord, intro. S. Irenaeus Prine (New York, 1907, and subsequent editions).

B. DAB 11, 553–54; NYT, Sept. 19, 1884; *New York Tribune*, Sept. 22 1884; SEAP 4, 1619–20; Helen Campbell, *The Problem of the Poor* (New York, 1882); W. H. Daniels, *The Temperance Reform and Its Great Reformers* (Cincinnati, OH, 1878); Samuel H. Hadley, *Down in Water Street* (New York, 1902).

**McBRIDE, Francis Scott**    (29 July 1872, Carroll Co., OH—23 April 1955, St. Petersburg, FL). *Education*: B.S., Muskingum Coll., 1898; graduated from Allegheny Theological Sem., 1901; D.D. (honorary), Muskingum Coll., 1915. *Career*: ordained in Presbyterian ministry, 1901; minister, Kittanning, PA, 1901–9; minister, Monmouth, IL, 1909–11; state superintendent, Anti-Saloon League of Illinois, 1912–24; general superintendent, Anti-Saloon League of America, 1924–36; state superintendent, Anti-Saloon League of Pennsylvania, 1936–43.

F. Scott McBride figured importantly in one of the most crucial historical tensions within the ranks of the Temperance Movement. There was a longstanding debate within the movement about the degree of militancy and coercion that ought to inform crusade strategies. In the earlier stages of this debate, there were on one side those who regarded constitutional prohibition as the logical and necessary end of the movement; on the other side were those who opposed coercion and felt that public education was the better approach to solving the alcohol problem. The argument was often subdued (although by no means always), and temperance workers generally managed to keep it from interfering with the movement's larger objectives. But once National Prohibition had been legislated into existence, the old polarity set itself up between those who supported the most rigorous measures of enforcement and those who preferred a gentler appeal to the public mind in order to maintain support for the Eighteenth Amendment. McBride had established himself as an effective partisan of militancy during the struggle to ratify the Eighteenth Amendment in Illinois. As a Presbyterian cleric, he had participated in the great interdenominational unification of churches initiated by the Anti-Saloon League, which marshalled the most powerful array of forces against the liquor industry the nation had ever seen. As superintendent of the Illinois Anti-Saloon League, McBride was operating in one of the real strongholds of the industry, where the liquor forces waged one of their most desperate and violent battles for survival. And while McBride had come out on the winning side of the struggle, he had seen nothing to make him believe that a moderate approach would enhance Prohibition enforcement. His hard-line stance soon played a critical role in the internal politics of the league, and thus in the entire attempt to dry up America under the Volstead Act.

During the early years of National Prohibition, a note of ambivalence toward enforcement approaches threatened to divide the Anti-Saloon League into two factions: the militant, so-called evangelical wing, and a more persuasion-oriented "social gospel" wing. The evangelicals controlled the league in the persons of national superintendent Purley Baker,* legislative committee chairman Bishop James Cannon,* and legislative superintendent Wayne B. Wheeler.* When Baker died in 1924, McBride somehow mediated a personal rivalry between Cannon and Wheeler and became their compromise choice for the national superintendency. He took to his role with a passion, committing himself and the league to a relentless fighting posture he felt was enjoined by the essential spirit of the Temperance Movement—indeed, by God himself. He met strong opposition at the 1928 convention from Ernest Cherrington,* director of the league's publishing activities, who opposed the magnitude of the law-and-order doctrine; Cherrington favored a better balance with a public information approach. It was a close election and McBride won, though as a gesture of appeasement Cherrington was installed as head of a new department of education and publicity. When Wayne Wheeler died in 1927, McBride extended his own duties and influence by taking over Wheeler's high-pressure legislative politics, which Cherrington so opposed. With the reins thus firmly in hand, McBride gathered the dry forces to the side of Herbert Hoover in the 1928 presidential campaign against Alfred E. Smith; but the effort was one of the last in which the league could claim any success. During the Great Depression the league found its resources so depleted that its activism in legislation and enforcement became too great a burden to maintain. In fact, the zeal with which Prohibition enforcement was pursued evoked a widespread public antipathy, ironically reversing the mood of support that had determined the league's legislative power in the first place.

**Bibliography:**

B. DAB Supp. 5, 442–43; NYT, April 24, 1955; SEAP 4, 1621; WW 3, 567; Ernest Cherrington, *History of the Anti-Saloon League* (Westerville, OH, 1913).

**McCABE, Harriet Calista Clark**    (19 January 1827, Sidney Plains, NY—25 September 1919, Delaware, OH). *Education*: studied at Elmira (NY) Acad., circa late 1830s. *Career*: preceptor, Dickinson Sem., PA, 1851–57; temperance organizer and reformer, OH, 1873–79; president, Ohio WCTU, 1874–79; editor, *Woman's Home Missions*, 1884–1902.

The dramatic Woman's Crusade, which began as a local protest against illegal liquor sales in Hillsboro, Ohio, in 1873 and became a national phenomenon by 1874, was the start of an impressive number of reform careers. Many women who had never been involved with organized temperance work, or who had never taken leadership roles, were tested campaigners at the end of 1874, when the initial crusade coalesced into the more formally structured Woman's Christian Temperance Union. Indeed, the WCTU would never have emerged unless a talented and dedicated cadre of women reformers had moved to continue the work of the crusade on an organized basis. One of these was Harriet McCabe, wife of a distinguished Ohio Wesleyan University professor. After settling in Delaware, Ohio, with her husband, McCabe became active in the missionary work of the Methodist Church, particularly the Woman's Home Missionary Society. Thus when the Woman's Crusade broke out she already had some reform and leadership experience behind her. She used it to good advantage against the liquor traffic, playing a central role in organizing Ohio women in their protests against drink and then taking the lead in moving to consolidate the gains of the crusade in 1874. McCabe took part in a woman's temperance meeting in February 1874, which elected her head of an information office to assist other reformers around the state. From there, she was a key planner in calling a much larger state temperance convention in June, which proceeded to found the Ohio Woman's Christian Temperance Union. McCabe drafted the new group's constitution, suggested its name, and won election as its first president. It was the first such organization in the field. As leader of the Ohio WCTU, McCabe next hosted the national antiliquor convention in November in Cincinnati, at which the idea for a national WCTU was discussed. It had been a hectic but satisfying year, and Harriet McCabe had accomplished much—not the least of which was giving the largest woman's organization in the country its name. By 1879, however, her temperance leadership days were over, although she always remained a firm antiliquor partisan. The Ohio Union was stable, and she gave up its presidency to return to her Home Missionary Society, serving for years as editor of its journal and an officer in its Indian Bureau. Her years of service as a captain in formal dry ranks were thus relatively short, but none could say that they were not productive.

**Bibliography:**

B. SEAP 4, 1621; WW 1, 797.

**McCARTHY, Raymond Gerald**    (30 April 1901, Brockton, MA—25 June 1964, New Brunswick, NJ). *Education*: studied at Boston Coll., 1920s; M.A., Harvard Univ., 1939. *Career*: teacher and superintendent, Kingston, MA, public schools, 1930s–1940s; research, teaching, administration, Yale (later Rutgers) Univ. Center of Alcohol Studies, 1944–64; assistant director, Summer Sch. of Alcohol Studies, Yale Univ., 1948–61; associate professor of health education, Yale Univ., 1954–61; director, State Program on Alcoholism, MA, 1961; director, State Program on Alcoholism, NY, 1962; professor of education, Rutgers Univ. Center of Alcohol Studies, 1962–64; director, Rutgers Univ. Summer Sch. of Alcohol Studies, 1962–64.

Professor, clinician, and alcohol studies researcher, Raymond G. McCarthy, as his colleague Selden Bacon* put it, was "a leader among those attacking the problems of alcohol and alcoholism in the twentieth century," and was one of the first to rise to prominence from within the post-Prohibition alcohol studies field itself. Beginning his career as a teacher and administrator in the public schools of Kingston, Massachusetts, McCarthy became interested in alcohol problems in part through his familiarity with the writings on the subject by Richard Peabody. His direct involvement began in 1943, with his enrollment in the first session of the Summer School of Alcohol Studies sponsored by the Section of Alcohol Studies (later the Yale Center of Alcohol Studies) of the Yale Laboratory of Applied Physiology. The director of the summer school was then the noted alcohol researcher E. M. Jellinek,* who was impressed with Mc-Carthy's talents and interest in the field. With Jellinek's endorsement, McCarthy was enlisted as the first staff member of the Yale Plan Clinics, established in 1944 to investigate alcoholism (and its treatment) in a clinical setting. He devoted the next several years to the clinics, becoming their executive director and authoring a number of important papers on clinic operations and the nature of alcoholism itself. He pioneered the group therapy literature in alcoholism, and was co-author of one report on differentiating types of alcoholics that some students of the field considered a classic study. McCarthy's rise to distinction as an alcoholism researcher, then, was steady and built upon a solid scholarly foundation.

Yet research was only one dimension of his work. McCarthy became equally if not better known as an educator. Four years after joining the center, he became assistant director of the summer school, and he remained a major force in its operations and growth for the rest of his life. He was an active teacher at the school, where a number of his students founded the Association of the Advancement of Instruction on Alcohol and Narcotics (he rose ultimately to associate director and then director of the group in 1962). The school was then at Rutgers University, where the Center of Alcohol Studies had moved in 1962, and McCarthy conducted a sweeping revision of its function, stressing graduate-level instruction and training. As a professor of education at Rutgers, he also took an active role in the efforts of the rest of the center: He designed major studies of alcohol use in student populations, formulated an ambitious fifteen-year investigation of alcohol problems at the community level, and launched other educational and public health proposals. In many respects, McCarthy emerged as the father of modern alcohol education, authoring a number of important titles on how to teach the young about alcohol. As regard for his talents as an instructor and the breadth of his knowledge of alcohol problems assumed national proportions, the Yale (later Rutgers) professor became one of the most sought after consultants and speakers in the field. And he always tried to shoulder what to his colleagues seemed more than his share of professional responsibilities. To cite only two examples: He devoted long hours of work to the American Public Health Association and to the leadership of the North American Association of Alcoholism Programs. Thus McCarthy was highly respected not only as a professional but also for his qualities as a person. The McCarthy Memorial Collection, housed at the Rutgers University Center of Alcohol Studies, and the finest single collection of the alcohol literature in the world, was named in his honor.

**Bibliography:**

A. with Edgar M. Douglass, *Alcohol and Social Responsibility: A New Educational Approach* (New York, 1949); *Clinical Practice and Community Education on Alcoholism: A Research Report on the Program of the Connecticut Commission on Alcohol* (New Haven, CT, 1959); ed., *Drinking and Intoxication: Selected Readings in Social Attitudes and Controls* (New Haven, CT, 1959); *Teenagers and Alcohol: A Handbook for the Educator* (New Brunswick, NJ, 1962); ed., *Alcohol Education for Classroom and Community: A Source Book for Educators* (New York, 1964).

B. NYT, June 26, 1964; Selden D. Bacon, "Raymond G. McCarthy, 1901–1964," *Quarterly Journal of Studies on Alcohol* 25 (1964): 413–16.

**MacCLEOD, Donald Campbell**    (13 November 1869, Nova Scotia, Canada—27 October 1942, Wilmington, DE). *Education*: A.B., Franklin Coll., OH, 1895; A.M., Franklin Coll., 1898; studied at Western Theological Sem., PA, 1898; D.D. (honorary), Franklin Coll., 1912. *Career*: ordained in Presbyterian Church, 1898; minister, Meadville, PA, 1898–99; minister, Washington, DC, 1899–1913; minister, Springfield, IL, 1913–18; minister, St. Louis, MO, 1918–23; minister, Dundee Presbyterian Church, Omaha, NB, 1923–29; secretary, Presbytery of St. Louis, 1929; minister, Lower Brandywine Presbyterian Church, Wilmington, DE, 1933–42.

Donald MacCleod's was a life dedicated in equal parts to prohibition and to the Presbyterian Church. By the time he was ordained in 1898, he had already been a member of the Anti-Saloon League for five years. Indeed, MacCleod had been a member of the league since it was first organized. Not unexpectedly, he made temperance a central part of his preaching and involved himself as fully as possible in the affairs of local antiliquor groups. His years as a reformer, however, were most notable for his work on behalf of the Anti-Saloon League. He took his first important leadership role in Washington, D.C., where he assumed the pulpit of the First (Presbyterian) Church in 1899. As president of the Anti-Saloon League of the District of Columbia, his performance as a dry organizer was in the national spotlight—the league being concerned that its activities in the capital city receive maximum impact on public opinion. MacCleod lived up to temperance expectations as he chaired the effort to coordinate a drive by several reform groups to restrict liquor licenses in the district. And it was no ordinary local-option battle: The law had to be passed by Congress, which finally acquiesced only in 1913. The long-awaited victory was symbolic, indicating the increasing willingness of the national legislature to move against the liquor traffic. For the liquor industry, the publicity surrounding the affair was a body blow— it appeared to many Americans that the traffic had been told that it was no longer welcome in the capital.

Upon his move to Illinois, MacCleod remained a league officer. He sat on the Board of Trustees of the league for years (as well as on its Executive Committee), and took a hand in the political effort that dried out the Illinois capital of Springfield. (The reforming Presbyterian seemed to specialize in capitals.) In recognition of his work, the National Anti-Saloon League also named him to its Board of Directors. MacCleod's commitment to the Temperance Movement was always unquestioned, the thought of compromise with the liquor industry playing no part in his thinking. He had entered the cause with a missionary zeal which he never lost. In fact, over time his fervor for spreading the antiliquor message seemed to grow more intense. For years, he worked with the International Reform Bureau, based in Washington, D.C., with an eye to carrying the prohibition gospel abroad. It was, of course, a task doomed to failure in light of the eventual collapse of the "noble experiment" in America; but there is little question that to the end the Reverend MacCleod was convinced that he was fighting the good fight.

**Bibliography:**

B. SEAP 4, 1638; WW 2, 338.

**McCULLOCH, Catherine Gouger Waugh**    (4 June 1862, Ransomville, NY— 20 April 1945, Evanston, IL). *Education*: studied at Rockford Sem., 1882; LLB., Union Coll. of Law, 1886; simultaneous B.A. and M.A., Rockford Sem., 1888; LLD. (honorary), Rockford Coll., 1936. *Career*: admitted to bar, 1886; legal practice, Rockford, IL, 1886–90; partner (with husband), McCulloch & Mc-Culloch, Chicago, beginning 1890; justice of the peace, Evanston, IL, 1907–9,

1909–13; master in chancery, Cook Co. Superior Court, 1917–25; author, reform and legal subjects, beginning 1890s; active memberships in reform, civic, and professional organizations, beginning 1880s.

The ferment of Progressivism that shaped so much of American social and political thinking in the late nineteenth century involved any number of individual reform movements and causes. Frequently they shared memberships and goals and not uncommonly leaders. Catherine McCulloch was a prime example of this interlocking pattern of reform activity. A distinguished jurist, suffragette, temperance worker, world peace advocate, and author, McCulloch began her professional life with a determined effort to succeed in the male-dominated world of the law. Her early frustrations helped make her an ardent suffrage worker, although her prospects flourished in 1890 when she and her husband joined forces to form their own legal firm. As a lawyer, she proved highly skilled in her private practice. She helped break new ground for women in the profession by being admitted to the bar of the U.S. Supreme Court in 1898 and by serving ably in local judicial posts. Throughout her legal career, however, she maintained her interests in reform, especially women's rights. Indeed, McCulloch was tenacious in pursuit of the female ballot. As legislative superintendent of the Illinois Equal Suffrage Association, for example, she tried for twenty years to get the state legislature to approve women's suffrage in presidential elections (it passed in 1913). She was also a leading proponent of wives' rights to equal guardianship of their children, of raising the legal age of consent in women from fourteen to nineteen, and of women's access to professional opportunities and civic participation. In this regard, McCulloch was a classic role model: She was the first woman trustee of the University of Illinois, an officer of the League of Women Voters, and an active leader in church (she was a Congregationalist) and professional society affairs. She managed all of this, we should add, while raising four children—three of whom also became lawyers, while the fourth married one.

McCulloch's views on the Temperance Movement were typical of many other women whose primary reform interest was in suffrage. The rise of the Woman's Christian Temperance Union provided new opportunities for women to influence social and political events, which won McCulloch's quick applause. The fact that the WCTU also worked strongly for suffrage made it even more attractive, and the reform-minded lawyer joined the organization soon after beginning her legal career. None of this is to say that she did not favor temperance as a goal in and of itself. She did: Reformers of the Progressive era frequently endorsed prohibition as a means of attacking an entire range of social and political ills. For years, McCulloch used her legal talents on behalf of WCTU activities, advising the group on local and national legislative matters and helping with its routine legal affairs. She also joined the Illinois branch of the Anti-Saloon League, viewing with satisfaction the growth of its successful drive for National Prohibition. When the Eighteenth Amendment finally proved unworkable, however, McCulloch did not join in last-ditch efforts to save it. She was not a zealot by nature, and at any rate other activities had greater claims on her time by the

1930s. During these years, she and her husband spent considerable time in travel and undertook a private study of social legislation in Europe (she was particularly impressed with the rights accorded women under the Soviet legal system). Her death in 1945, at eighty-two years old, closed a distinguished chapter in the history of American reform and in the use of one's talents for the benefit of others.

**Bibliography:**

A. *Mr. Lex: On the Legal Status of Mother and Child* (Chicago, 1899); *Before the Chicago Charter Convention: In the Matter of the Power of the Illinois Legislature to Grant Municipal Suffrage to the Women of Chicago . . .* (Chicago, 1906); *Mayors of Five States Recommend Municipal Suffrage for Women* (Evanston, IL, 1909?); *Northwestern University and Woman Suffrage* (Evanston, IL, 1909); *Guardianship of Children* (Chicago, 1912); with Frank A. McCulloch, *A Manual of the Law of Will Contests in Illinois* (Chicago, 1929).

B. NAW 2, 459–60; NYT, April 21, 1945; WW 2, 358; Frances E. Willard and Mary A. Livermore, eds., *A Woman of the Century* (New York, 1893).

**McGINNIS, George**   (28 July 1858, Mendota, IL—?). *Education*: studied law in legal office, NB, 1870s; studied at Union Coll. of Law., IL, 1878–79; B.Th., Univ. of Chicago Divinity Sch., 1893; LLB., Gale Coll., WI, 1902. *Career*: coal, salt, and grain business, Utica, IL, 1884–88; feed and flour business, El Paso, TX, 1888–89; Baptist minister, various pastorates in IL, 1890–1914; secretary and treasurer, Chicago Ministers' Association, 1896–97; district superintendent, Northern District, Illinois Anti-Saloon League, beginning 1914; reform lecturer on various subjects, beginning circa 1914.

An American Baptist clergyman, George McGinnis reflected the temperance sentiments shared by so many other members of his denomination. His first inclination was for the law, and he pursued legal studies both in a law firm and at law school, but for reasons unknown he finally chose not to launch a career at the bar. Instead, he followed business opportunities in Illinois and Texas and then turned to the ministry. He took his first pastorate in Earlville, Illinois, in 1890, some three years before he was formally ordained. From the beginning, Reverend McGinnis made temperance a central tenet of his pastoral message. For him, it was nothing new. He had been a total abstainer since his youth and recalled having made his first temperance speech at age sixteen. Ever since, he had been an ardent reformer. His initial public acclaim as a dry came during his years in business in Utica, Illinois, where he led the victorious forces opposed to issuing any local liquor licenses. Although the triumph was only in one municipality, drys across the state took heart, seeing McGinnis' efforts as a sign of better things to come. The prohibitionist minister did his best to keep the cause moving, lending a hand to dry initiatives in each of the six Illinois towns in which he held pulpits over the years. Finally, in 1914, he left the ministry for full-time temperance work. Assuming duties as a district superintendent in the Illinois Anti-Saloon League, he became a key figure in the dry campaigns then shaping the politics of the state. When necessary, he took on special organizing assignments from the league and emerged with a reputation as one of the most effective temperance leaders in the state. McGinnis also wrote and lectured widely on antiliquor and reform subjects, becoming a regular speaker on the Chautauqua circuit. He developed a special interest in the preservation of the "Anglo-Saxon race"—a cause, he argued, that prohibition would advance—and this was one of his favorite platform themes in the 1920s. (In this regard, he also served as head of an "American Saxon Federation.") McGinnis continued with the Anti-Saloon League under National Prohibition, although he faded abruptly from public view with Repeal and the relatively quick demise of the league.

**Bibliography:**

B. SEAP 4, 1629–30; WW 4, 638.

**McINTYRE, Robert**    (20 November 1851, Selkirk, Scotland—30 August 1914, Chicago, IL). *Education*: studied at Vanderbilt Univ., 1877. *Career*: bricklayer, circa 1868–77; ordained, Methodist Episcopal Church, 1878; minister, various churches, IL, Denver, CO, and Los Angeles, 1879–1908; bishop, Methodist Episcopal Church, 1908–14.

In the story of Robert McIntyre lay something of the experience of Paul of Tarsus—the sinner suddenly converted and joined to the ranks of those most ardent in doing the work of the Lord. To those who knew McIntyre as a young man, his conversion must have seemed a miracle indeed. Born of Scottish parents who brought him to America as a child, his early years were marked with tragedy and hardship. Robert's mother died shortly after the family immigrated to Philadelphia, and his father passed on when he was seventeen, leaving him the sole support of his younger brothers. Unable to afford an education, he was lucky to find training as a bricklayer, a trade he followed in an effort to pay the family bills. The bricklayer's trade was a rough one, and McIntyre, wandering from town to town in search of seasonal employment, found little time for the finer things in life. He had as little time for religion and was in fact hostile to the church. One day, however, at the age of twenty-six, to escape the cold he walked into the First Methodist Church in St. Louis, Missouri. He heard his first sermon and was converted on the spot. Resolving to dedicate his life to the ministry, he gathered all of his resources to attend a year at Vanderbilt University, following which he entered the Illinois Conference of the Methodist Episcopal Church. In 1879, he took his first pastorate at Easton, Illinois, where he was able to combine a gift for his new vocation with the skills of the old: McIntyre not only preached effective sermons but helped to build a new church with his own hands. As his reputation as an inspirational minister increased, he answered calls to carry his message farther afield. The former bricklayer preached in Chicago, Denver, and Los Angeles and finally was elected bishop at the Methodist General Conference at Baltimore, Maryland, in 1908. The young man of little faith had come a long way.

As McIntyre's stature as a clergyman grew, he used his influence to damn the liquor traffic and to bolster the fortunes of the dry crusade. The evils of the saloon were frequent topics in his pulpit, and he allowed no defense for what he considered an institution with no redeeming values. In all of this, he was quite moving. "Men came out from his church and from the auditorium where he lectured," reported one temperance source, "amazed at their own and society's long toleration of this enormous evil." After his appointment as bishop, McIntyre maintained his assault on the traffic and was chosen as president of the Temperance Society of the Methodist Episcopal Church. He also wrote extensively on the subject, including poetry, as part of his dedicated effort to sway the country against drink. His reform vision always had a touch of the millenial. He "contemplated," one account of his life noted, "the creation of a new earth in a single generation." Prohibition, he hoped, would help realize that vision. He died in 1914, before the passage of National Prohibition but after he had seen the Temperance Movement hit the organizational and political stride that would make the Eighteenth Amendment a reality only six years later. Perhaps he at least thought he saw the "new earth" coming.

**Bibliography:**

A. *A Modern Apollos (A Story)* (Cincinnati, OH 1901); *At Early Candle Light and Other Poems* (Cincinnati, OH 190–?); *The Boy, the Booze, and the Bishop* (n.p., 19—?); *From the Trowel to the Pulpit: How an Infidel Workingman Became a Christian and a Preacher* (n.p., 19—?).

B. SEAP 4, 1630; WW 1, 814.


**MALINS, Joseph** (21 October 1844, Worcester, England—5 January 1926, Birmingham, England). *Career*: bookbinder, printer, pursemaker, England, 1854–58; grainer's and decorative painter's apprentice, England, 1858–66; decorative painter, England, 1866; grainer, Pennsylvania Railroad, Philadelphia, 1866–68; decorative painter, Birmingham, England, beginning 1869; county councillor, Worcester Co., England, 1888–1909; county magistrate and alderman, beginning 1907; active work internationally with Independent Order of Good Templars, beginning 1867.

The Temperance Movement was never an exclusively American phenomenon. Europe in particular also witnessed considerable antiliquor activity in the nineteenth century, and there were some prominent examples of reformers in the Old and New Worlds working in cooperation. This transatlantic aspect of temperance was clearly evident in the career of British-born Joseph Malins, whose prodigious efforts in the struggle against the liquor traffic saw him cross the Atlantic no fewer than nineteen times. Malins confronted the problems of drink at an early age, when his father's intemperance dragged his family into poverty, forcing young Joseph out of school. He eventually learned to make a living as a skilled and prosperous decorative painter, but the road was not easy for him and he never stopped hating the alcohol that had so damaged his family. Indeed, at sixteen years old, soon after his father had gone to a drunkard's grave, Malins took a pledge of total abstinence and joined the local Temperance Society of the Church of St. Thomas in Birmingham (England). For the rest of his life, he was never without an affiliation with an organized temperance group. Shortly after his marriage in 1866, Malins moved to America for two years, working as a wood grainer for the Pennsylvania Railroad. Looking for an antiliquor group, he joined the Independent Order of Good Templars, a fraternal brotherhood organized on temperance principles. Once initiated, he became an enthusiast, and when he returned home to Great Britain he set about organizing Templar lodges there. Over the years, Malins prospered in his trade and rose to civil prominence in his home locality, but he gained international recognition for his work with the Templars. In 1870, he was elected the first grand chief templar in England, a post he would hold for the next forty-four years. And when, in 1920, the order created the post of patriarch templar, Malins was the logical choice to fill it. By then he was renowned as an enemy of the liquor interests in America and Europe and as an influential friend of an array of social reform legislation.

Not content with achievements that would have been enough for most men, Malins devoted his years to organizing efforts on behalf of the Templars, extending the order worldwide. He introduced Templar lodges throughout the British Isles in the 1870s, and for the remainder of the nineteenth century he saw to the planting of the organization in most of Europe, the Mediterranean, Southern Asia, and Latin America. As international chief templar, he supervised a good deal of this work personally, preferring not to act through agents unless absolutely necessary. Annual travels of 20,000 miles were not uncommon as he labored to build new foundations for temperance, and one biographical account has claimed that in the course of his lifetime he logged as many as 700,000 miles, a staggering total for an age that did not know the airplane. The chief templar also carried the temperance battle into the complex world of British politics, where, during the early twentieth century, his massive propaganda activities were able to influence parliamentary legislation that might otherwise have been favorable to the liquor interests. He also worked in support of old-age pension laws, the Local Government Act, and other reform efforts. To his many other pursuits, Malins added talents as an extraordinarily prolific writer. Over the years, he authored scores of temperance pamphlets of every conceivable variety, historical, moral, hortatory, and inspirational, plus a number of temperance songs. In addition to all of this, the stalwart campaigner hardly ever missed a temperance convention or meeting of importance anywhere in the world. It was characteristic of Malins that on the day of his death he was making preparations, at the age of eighty-two, for his twentieth visit to the United States to attend yet another temperance convention.

**Bibliography:**

A. *Professor Alcoholico* (London, 1876); *The Unlawful Exclusion of the African Race* (London? 1877); *British Restrictive and Local Option Legislation Throughout the Present Century* (n.p., 1889); *The Russian Government Liquor Monopoly* (London? 1905); *The Temperance Movement: Its Origin and Development* (London, 19—?).

B. *Alliance News and Temperance Reformer* (Feb. 1926); SEAP 4, 1667–71.

**MANN, Eugenia Florence St. John**    (1847, Kane Co., IL—? Long Beach, CA?). *Education*: theological courses, WCTU, 1885, and Methodist Protestant Church, 1887. *Career*: schoolteacher, IL, circa 1862–69; minister's assistant, IL, 1878; temperance lecturer, Colorado WCTU and Independent Order of Good Templars, circa 1881–85; national lecturer, National WCTU, beginning 1885; ordained, Methodist Protestant Church, 1887; minister, various pastorates, KS, 1880s–1890s; homestead farmer, CO, beginning 1907.

A tireless worker in the temperance cause and a woman of talents ranging from preaching to homesteading a farm by herself, Eugenia Mann left more of her career on the public record than she did of her private life. We do not know exactly when she was born, and even her date of death (probably in the 1920s) is osbscure. We do know, however, that during her long lifetime she compiled a formidable record of personal and civic accomplishment. Born Eugenia Florence Schultz, she taught school in her native Illinois for most of the 1860s, until she married the Reverend Charles Henry St. John, a Methodist minister, in 1869. After almost nine years of relatively tranquil marriage, however, her life took an eventful turn: In 1878, the Reverend St. John was taken seriously ill and was forced to suspend his work with his congregation in Bloomington, Illinois. At the invitation of the church members, Eugenia St. John stepped into the breach, and for several years she preached three times every Sunday as well as continuing with her husband's pastoral duties. In addition, she served for a number of years as an officer in the state chapter of the Methodist Woman's Home Missionary Society. In 1879, a year after she assumed the Bloomington pulpit, she joined the Prohibition Party, having already become affiliated with the Woman's Christian Temperance Union and the Independent Order of Good Templars. Her busy schedule then made room for temperance activities on a major scale. WCTU president Frances Willard* arranged her appointment as president of the Illinois Union, and she did good service in the struggle for local option in the state. By the time she and the Reverend St. John moved to Colorado in the early 1880s, she had established a reputation as one of the most active temperance workers in the Midwest.

The move to Colorado did nothing to dampen her reform and religious enthusiasm. She was active in the temperance organizations of the Denver area, where she once more lectured on behalf of the WCTU and the Good Templars.

Elected a delegate to the Right Worthy Good Templar's Lodge of the World in 1883 (an international convention of the order), she subsequently went on a speaking tour that took her through New York, Pennsylvania, and Canada for five consecutive years. Not to go without the services of such an effective speaker, the WCTU also named her to the post of national lecturer. In 1887, however, she and her husband moved to Kansas, where she was ordained in the Methodist Protestant Church. Taking various pulpits in the state, the new Reverend St. John was credited with converting over four thousand of the unchurched and founding almost ninety children's temperance organizations and ten adult groups. Sunday schools also captured her attention, and she attended at least one international conference on the subject in London. Temperance, though, remained her special reform passion. She spoke on behalf of prohibition all over the West, giving more than sixty-three speeches during the campaign for Nebraska state prohibition alone. At sixty years old, over a decade after the death of Charles St. John, she finally gave up the lecture circuit, although "taking it easy" never seems to have occurred to her (or perhaps it was financially impossible). At any rate, she homesteaded a 320-acre farm in Colorado by herself, and in 1920—at age seventy-three—married Francis W. Mann, who had been an old childhood friend back in Illinois. Reportedly, the new couple moved on to Long Beach, California, at which point this extraordinary woman dropped from public view.

**Bibliography:**

B. SEAP 4, 1684–85.

**MANN, Horace**    (4 May 1796, Franklin, MA—2 August 1859, Yellow Springs, OH). *Education*: graduated from Brown Univ., 1819; studied at Litchfield (CT) Law Sch., 1821–23. *Career*: tutor in Latin and Greek, Brown Univ., 1820–21; admitted to bar, MA, 1823; legal practice, Dedham, MA, 1823–33; member, Massachusetts House of Representatives, 1827–32; legal practice, Boston, 1833–37; member, Massachusetts Senate, 1835–37; secretary, Massachusetts Board of Education, 1837–48; editor, *Common School Journal*, 1838–48; member, U.S. House of Representatives, 1848–53; president, Antioch Coll., OH, 1852–59.

Horace Mann, the educational reformer who did so much to create the modern American public school system, began life with few prospects for schooling himself. His parents were poor farmers, and until his late teens Mann had almost no formal education. Yet he had a persistent will to better himself, and his quest for knowledge reads like something out of a Horatio Alger novel. To get what schooling he could, he braided straw to earn money for his own books, and at twenty years old he satisfied the entrance requirements for Brown University, graduating in 1819. After teaching for two years at his alma mater, he attended law school and opened a legal office in 1823. As his practice flourished, however, he never forgot his struggle to go to school, and the memories influenced his activities for the rest of his life. Over the 1830s, Mann served in both houses of the Massachusetts legislature, and while in the Senate he was able to give concrete form to his concerns. He worked on behalf of a bill creating a State Board of Education, and served as secretary of the new agency for over a decade (1837–48). It was during his tenure in the post that Mann instituted the educational reforms that changed the nature of American schooling. Among these reforms were a minimum school year of six months, the establishment of fifty new schools, a significant increase in schoolteachers' salaries, reformed curriculum and teaching methods, a doubling of appropriations for public education, and improved professional training for teachers. In 1839, he established the first normal school in the United States. During the course of this revolution in education, Mann wrote extensive and numerous reports, along with creating and editing the *Common School Journal*, which spread his educational theories and practices around the country and indeed the world. In 1848, Mann left the Board of Education to take the vacant House of Representatives seat of John Quincy Adams. He held it until 1853 (like Adams, he was a committed abolitionist), when he lost an election for governor of Massachusetts. After his defeat, he left politics, and from 1853 until his death in 1859 he served as president of Antioch College in Yellow Springs, Ohio.

While Mann's chief claim to fame was his work in education, he was in fact a dedicated champion of other reform causes as well. He was a pioneer advocate of more enlightened treatment for the mentally ill, a firm and unswerving enemy of slavery, and an opponent of the public lottery system. He was also an enthusiastic temperance worker. Drink, he believed, was a major source of personal dissolution and social disruption—all contrary to the better society he hoped his educational reforms would help create. Thousands of drunkards would never have become so, he wrote, if liquor was simply not available to them. In his first years in the state legislature, he favored laws restricting the availability of liquor through sales limitations; and as an initial step, he proposed a ban on all Sunday liquor sales. He fought for the Sunday closing law for seven years, virtually alone at the start of his career, and finally had the satisfaction of seeing it passed. The great reformer was also a proponent of legally enforced prohibition, believing that the elimination of the liquor traffic was the only real way to eliminate the evils of drink. It was his ultimate goal, although he knew that prohibitionist sentiment in Massachusetts was not strong enough to carry the measure in the 1830s and 1840s. Yet he watched the progress of the battle for the Maine Law and realized correctly that it was a sign of things to come for the rest of the country. "The faith is now in a forward state of realization," he confided to his diary as the struggle in Maine reached its critical pass, "and what a triumph it will be." When the Maine Law actually went on the statute books in 1851, Mann joined other temperance men in celebration. Had he not left for his duties at Antioch College, in Ohio, shortly thereafter, one wonders what role he would have played in the movement that subsequently brought prohibition to Massachusetts.

### Bibliography:

A. *Slavery: Letters and Speeches* (1851; New York, 1969); *The Institution of Slavery: A Speech . . .* (Boston, 1852); *Lectures on Education* (1855; New York,

1965); *The Republic and the School: The Education of Free Men*, ed. Lawrence A. Cremin (New York, 1960); *Horace Mann on the Crisis in Education*, ed. Louis Filler (Yellow Springs, OH, 1965).

B. SEAP 4, 1685–86; WW H, 401; Mary Mann, *Life of Horace Mann* (Boston, 1865); Jonathan Messerli, *Horace Mann: A Biography* (New York, 1972); Louise Hall Thorp, *Until Victory: Horace Mann and Mary Peabody* (Boston, 1953); Edward Irwin Franklin Williams, *Horace Mann: Educational Statesman* (New York, 1937).

**MANN, Marty**    (15 October 1904, Chicago—22 July 1980, Bridgeport, CT). *Education*: studied at Santa Barbara Girls Sch., CA, 1921–22; studied at Montemare Sch., NY and FL, 1922–24; studied at Miss Nixon's Sch., Florence, Italy, 1924–25; studied at Yale Summer Sch. of Alcohol Studies, 1944. *Career*: assistant editor, *International Studio*, 1928–30; writer, *Town and Country Magazine*, 1929–34; partner in photography business, London, 1930–36; fashion publicity, R.H. Macy, Inc., NY, 1940–42; research director and radio script author, American Society of Composers, Authors, and Publishers, 1942–44; founder and executive director, National Committee for Education on Alcoholism (later National Council on Alcoholism), 1944–68; founder-consultant, National Council on Alcoholism, 1968–80.

In the aftermath of National Prohibition, it took considerable time and effort to rebuild public support for dealing with alcohol problems. Among those who labored to create an "alcoholism movement" (the modern attempt to treat alcoholics and to research the nature of alcoholism), few names stood higher than Marty Mann's. Once she had become interested in the problems of the alcoholic, Mann devoted her career to the popularization of the disease conception of alcoholism, to efforts to lessen the stigma surrounding the condition, and to marshalling support for alcoholism treatment. Her commitment to these activities was intensely personal: After working successfully in editing and writing for some years, Mann became an alcoholic herself, thus she knew the tribulations of alcoholism firsthand. She recovered with the aid of Bill "W" (Wilson),* one of the founders of Alcoholics Anonymous, and was credited with being one of the first women to stay sober in AA. From AA, Mann went on to study at the Summer School of Alcohol Studies, then at Yale University, where she began thinking about a means to stimulate public discussion on the alcoholism problem without reigniting the old and emotionally-charged wet–dry controversy. With the assistance of some of the summer school faculty, including E. M. Jellinek* and Selden Bacon,* Mann founded (1944) the National Committee for Education on Alcoholism, a voluntary organization dedicated to the propositions that alcoholics were sick, that they could be helped, and that alcoholism was a public health problem deserving public attention. At the same time, she began organizing the first of a network of community-based local chapters whose job it was to spread this gospel in the press, the schools, the churches, anywhere they might influence popular sentiments. The group later changed its name to the

National Council on Alcoholism, and by the mid-1950s its local chapters had spread across the nation. Marty Mann, as executive director, could justly take credit for much of the growth and for a great deal of the consequent American willingness to start facing up to alcohol-related issues once more.

The administration of the National Council of Alcoholism, however, was only one facet (albeit an important one) of Mann's work. As NCA spread, so did popular recognition of its founder, and she became one of the most sought after speakers in the country. For some thirty-five years, she travelled the nation and a good deal of the world lecturing and teaching. She averaged some two hundred lectures per year, appearing in front of forums ranging from professional organizations and college auditoriums to official government bodies. In addition, she wrote extensively. Her publications were among the best known in the field and were extremely popular with the public (some of them were translated into several languages). In 1948, the State Department asked Mann to represent the United States at the Twenty-third International Congress on Alcoholism at Lucerne, Switzerland. Her tireless advocacy of aid for the alcoholic, a labor brought into bold relief by the example of her own struggle with the bottle, won her widespread admiration. In the 1950s, for instance, news correspondent Edward R. Murrow listed her among his choices for the ten greatest living Americans. Over the years, Mann was also the recipient of numerous awards and honorary fellowships and degrees. Mann gave up the directorship of NCA in 1968, but she remained active with the organization on a consulting basis and maintained her activities as a proponent for the field generally. She served in various capacities with a number of important national groups dealing with alcohol problems, including the National Institute on Alcohol Abuse and Alcoholism (where she was special consultant to the director) and the National Commission on Alcoholism and Other Alcohol-Related Problems. At all times, Mann was especially sensitive to the special difficulties facing women alcoholics, and she urged particular attention to efforts to bring them into treatment. When she died, still actively campaigning, the alcoholism field mourned the passing of one of its most influential pioneers.

**Bibliography:**

A. *Alcoholism: America's Public Health Problem No. 4...* (Columbia, SC, 1946); *Primer on Alcoholism* (New York, 1952); *Alcoholism and You* (New York, 1956); *New Primer on Alcoholism: How People Drink, How to Recognize Alcoholics, and What to Do* (New York, 1968); *Marty Mann Answers Your Questions About Drinking and Alcoholism* (New York, 1970).

B. NYT, July 24, 1980; *Who's Who of American Women* 8th ed. (Chicago, 1973); "A Tribute to Marty Mann: She Opened America's Eyes," *Alcoholism: The National Magazine* 1, No. 2 (1980):11–19.

**MARSH, John**    (12 April 1788, Wethersfield, CT—5 August 1868, Brooklyn, NY). *Education*: graduated from Yale Coll., 1804; private study of theology,

1804–9; D.D. (honorary), Jefferson Coll., 1852. *Career*: licensed to preach as Congregationalist minister, 1809; preaching in various churches, CT, 1809–18; ordained, 1818; minister, Haddam (CT) Congregational Church, 1818–33; secretary and general agent, Connecticut Temperance Society, 1829; agent, Baltimore Temperance Society, 1831; agent, American Temperance Union, 1833–36; editor, *Journal of the American Temperance Union*, 1837–65.

The son of a pious and devout Connecticut family, John Marsh studied theology at home before embarking on his career in the service of the Congregational Church and the Temperance Movement. He was a hard-working minister who recalled a life of almost daily preaching in his various pulpits as well as unceasing pastoral calls on the families of his congregations. Indeed, he had a fine and deserved reputation as a clergyman. Yet he was seldom at ease: We gather from his autobiography and accounts of his life that the Reverend Marsh was a man who brooded on the sins and shortcomings of the world. Most particularly, he brooded on the evils of drink, which he saw at the root of so many of society's other ills. The liquor problem, in fact, had been much on his mind since his school days at Yale, when in a moment of weakness he admitted having raised a glass of wine with horrific results: "As I went out of the Hall," he related, "I saw the buildings moving round and discharged the contents of my rebellious stomach." It left an indelible impression on the young man, and he never touched another drop. Nor did he want others to, and he made temperance the crux of his preaching and pastoral messages. In this stance, Marsh was fighting the prevailing mores of the day, and he recognized that most of his parishioners were "hard drinkers" (many of whom, he claimed, "filled drunkards' graves"). Even religious ordinations, to his infinite disgust, sometimes ended up with clergymen deep in their cups. Reverend Marsh, however, resolved to fight back and in 1828 joined a local temperance society; from that point on, he was drawn steadily into the thick of the organized war on the liquor traffic, and he emerged as one of its most effective and dedicated warriors.

The activities that eventually took Marsh out of the ministry and into full-time temperance work began the following year (1829), when the Connecticut Temperance Society chose him as its secretary and general agent. Given the fact that he was still pastor at the Haddam Congregational Church, the new post was an enormous burden. But the ardent reformer loved the work. He lectured all over the state and authored numerous tracts (one of which, *Putnam and the Wolf*, became a Temperance Movement classic, with a total printing of some 150,000 copies). In 1831, he agreed to conduct a three-month temperance campaign for the Baltimore Temperance Society, and while speaking in the nation's capital on its behalf, he was instrumental in persuading a number of legislators to found the Congressional Temperance Society. At this point, Marsh's antiliquor campaigning made it impossible for him to continue as a pastor, and he resigned his pulpit in 1833. His career became that of a professional reformer, and he did his work well. In the early 1830s, he helped to organize the first National Temperance Convention, out of which came the American Temperance Union

(1833). Serving as its agent and editor of its *Journal*, he took charge of the union's affairs, maintained its reports and correspondence, and published them under the title of *Permanent Temperance Documents* (1836). (The volume remains a standard source on the history of the antebellum Temperance Movement.) Marsh also received credit for directing the union onto a firmly total abstinence path and away from the moderationist outlook that many temperance workers preferred. Over his many years with the organization, the former minister became one of the most visible antiliquor proponents in the nation, so much so that another prominent reformer, looking back in 1865, proclaimed that Marsh "for the past twenty-five years has *been* the American Union—its body, its soul, its spirit, its president, its executive committee, its energy and its everything." He was also its driving force during the Civil War, when he struggled to keep the temperance flame alight as public attention shifted to the armed struggle and later to Reconstruction. In ill health as the war was fought, Marsh managed his last major effort as a dry crusader when he arranged a temperance propaganda effort for the Union armies. When he died at age seventy-eight, the Temperance Movement lost one of its most dedicated and accomplished crusaders.

## Bibliography:

A. *Hannah Hawkins: The Reformed Drunkard's Daughter* (New York, 1843); *Temperance Hymn Book and Minstrel . . .* (New York, 1844); *The Boy's Temperance Book* (New York, 1848); *Temperance Recollections, Labors, Defeats, Triumphs: An Autobiography* (New York, 1867); *The Temperance Speaker . . .* (New York, 1868); *Putnam and Wolf, The Fool's Pence, The Poor Man's House Repaired, and Jamie* (New York, 187-?).

B. SEAP 4, 1694–95; WW H, 404; Daniel Dorchester, *The Liquor Problem in All Ages* (Cincinnati, OH, 1884).

**MARSHALL, Thomas Francis**    (7 June 1801, Frankfort, KY—22 September 1864, near Versailles, KY). *Education*: studied law with John J. Crittenden, 1820s. *Career*: admitted to the bar, KY, 1828; legal practice, KY, beginning 1828; member, Kentucky House of Representatives, 1832–36, 1838–39, 1854; member, U.S. House of Representatives, 1841–43; captain, U.S. Army in Mexican War, 1846–48; legal practice, Chicago, 1856; legal practice, KY, 1860s.

A nephew of John Marshall, chief justice of the Supreme Court from the Federalist to the Jacksonian eras, Thomas Francis Marshall began his own legal career in the office of John J. Crittenden, the Kentucky senator who authored the last-minute compromise efforts to avert the Civil War. Thomas, while a successful practitioner at the bar in his own right, never achieved the status of his uncle or teacher; yet he was noted for his forensic skills and he was at least an earnest legislator. Indeed, he emerged as a reformer and a popular lecturer on the issues of the day. Marshall's reform views began almost as a "conversion" experience: A strong drinker while serving in the national legislature, he felt himself slipping into alcohol addiction. Panic-stricken, he asked another member of the Congress to swear him to a pledge of total abstinence. Thus converted to the temperance cause, he supposedly never touched another drop. In fact, he sought to bring other legislators into the fold. Marshall took the lead in reorganizing the Congressional Temperance Society along total abstinence lines. The old society, he claimed, which had been moderationist in tone, had "died of intemperance, holding the pledge in one hand and the champagne bottle in the other."

After leaving the House of Representatives his career as a public speaker gathered momentum. He toured the Eastern section of the nation, speaking on temperance and other current subjects (at least reportedly) to enthusiastic audiences. During the Mexican War he served as a captain of volunteers, stories of which later enriched his lecture schedule. Marshall was never in the first rank of the dry reform, nor did he affiliate with any mass temperance group; yet his example of an evidently sincere conversion in the face of alcoholism, and his efforts to advance the total abstinence cause in the halls of the nation's capital, won him the admiration of later generations of antiliquor reformers.

### Bibliography:

A. *Speech...on Fashionable Wine Drinking* (n.p., 1842?); *The Speeches of Hon. Thomas E. Marshall on Alcohol and Intemperance...* (New York, 1842); *Substance of an Address on Temperance...* (New York, 1842); *Temperance Address...* (New York? 1842); *Speech of Hon. Thos. F. Marshall, in Opposition to the Principles of the Know-Nothing Organization* (Versailles, KY, 1855); *Speeches and Writings*, ed., W. L. Basse (Cincinnati, OH, 1858).

B. SEAP 4, 1696–97; WW H, 405.

**MARTIN, John Alexander**    (10 March 1839, Brownsville, PA—2 October 1889, Atchison, KS). *Career*: printer's apprentice, PA, 1850s; publisher, *Squatter Sovereign* (under several names, finally *Atchison Champion*), Atchison, KS, 1858–89; chairman, Central Republican Committee, KS, 1859–61, 1864–84; member, Kansas Senate, 1858; officer, Union army, 1861–64; mayor, Atchison, KS, 1865; member, Republican National Committee, 1868–84; governor of Kansas, 1884–88.

Journalist and politician, John Alexander Martin got his start in life as an apprentice to a printer, where he developed an interest in the publishing business. He was nothing if not talented and ambitious, and when only eighteen he moved to Kansas Territory and bought a weekly newspaper, the Atchison *Squatter Sovereign* (1858). Shortly thereafter, he changed the name to *Freedom's Champion*, then the *Champion*, and finally the *Atchison Champion*. But whatever its name, Martin's journal was a leading voice for the antislavery cause in the territory and proclaimed loyalty to the Union during the troubled years before the Civil War when the area was known as Bleeding Kansas. Using the paper as a power base, Martin rose quickly to political prominence in Kansas Territory, playing a crucial role in Republican Party affairs and working as secretary to the antislavery Wyandotte state constitutional convention and as a senator in the first legislature. After serving with distinction as an officer in the Union army during the War Between the States, Martin resumed his political activities and made little secret of his desire for the governorship. As chairman of the Republican state organization, he was able to secure the GOP nomination in 1884 and 1886 and to win both elections. His campaigns served to demonstrate how important the prohibition issue had become to the electorate. In 1880, Martin had openly and staunchly opposed prohibitory legislation; but upon running for governor he came out in support of a dry amendment to the Kansas constitution. Somewhere between 1880 and 1884, Martin had seen the antiliquor light, and in planning his victorious campaign, he ran hard for the temperance vote. Indeed, the man who raised one of the strongest regional cries against slavery was now to do the same against the liquor traffic.

Martin's reasons for his rather sudden zeal for the temperance crusade were rooted in several quarters. No doubt he was aware of the growing popularity of the dry position; in fact, Kansas was a leader in post–Civil War prohibitionism, and to oppose the drys had become politically risky by the 1880s. Part of Martin's conversion, however, seems to have been sincere. The experience of his own town of Atchison with prohibition, as well as other parts of the state, had proven beneficial in his view and had made a believer of him. Having found the faith, Martin pursued it with a vigor, berating saloon keepers, whom he characterized as "a lot of shameless ingrates, who were not only opposed to prohibition, but to any and all restraint on their dirty business." So enthusiastic was he in persecuting purveyors of alcoholic beverages that he was later to claim that the "most wonderful era of prosperity, of material, moral and intellectual development, of growth in country, cities and towns ever witnessed on the American Continent" had come about because of his endeavors. Martin, however, was not a one-issue politician. He supported reforms in legal procedures and in the judicial system of Kansas, along with improvements in correctional institutions, railroad regulations, and labor arbitration. In short, he anticipated many of the Progressive reforms, and he considered prohibition as of a piece with these other changes. Together, they would make post–Civil War industrial America work for everyone's benefit, freeing it from poverty and corruption. After his second term as governor (in which some of his reform program proved out of step with the more conservative elements of his party), Martin retired from politics and returned to journalism.

**Bibliography:**

A. *Annual Address Before the Editors' and Publishers Association of the State of Kansas* (Atchison, KS, 1869); *Military History of the Eighth Kansas Veteran Volunteer Infantry* (Leavenworth, KS, 1869); *The Wyandotte Convention: An Address...* (Atchison, KS, 1882); *Address...at the Quarter-Centennial Cele-*

*bration of the Admission of Kansas as a State* (Topeka, KS, 1886); *Addresses* (Topeka, KS, 1888).

B. DAB 12, 341–42; SEAP 4, 1697–98; WW H, 405–6.

**MASON, Lewis Duncan**    (20 June 1843, Brooklyn, NY—12 June 1927, Brooklyn, NY). *Education*: special diploma, New York Univ., 1863; M.D., Long Island Hosp. Coll., NY, 1866. *Career*: clinic surgeon, Long Island Hosp., Brooklyn, NY, 1866–75; surgeon and instructor in surgery, Long Island Coll. Hosp., 1875–82; visiting and consulting physician, Fort Hamilton Inebriates Home, 1866–94.

Lewis Duncan Mason seems to have had little doubt that alcoholism was a disease. Indeed, from the beginning of his long and distinguished medical career, he devoted much of his time to the treatment and research of alcohol addiction, or "inebriety," as Mason and his colleagues generally called it. The medical community was never (and has never been) in full agreement on the nature of alcoholism, but Mason's longstanding identification with the disease conception lent considerable weight to that view. For the Brooklyn doctor's reputation was first-rate. Educated in Brooklyn, New York, where he made his home all of his life, Mason began practicing surgery in 1866 and a decade later was teaching the subject at his alma mater. Over the years, he was one of the most sought-after surgeons in the New York City area and a respected member of the American Medical Association and the New York Academy of Medicine. Yet as soon as he finished medical school, the young surgeon also became affiliated with the Fort Hamilton Inebriates Home (in Brooklyn), where in over thirty years of work he treated thousands of alcoholics, compiled masses of case study data on alcoholism, and emerged as a pioneer advocate of special institutions—"inebriate asylums"—for drug and alcohol addicts. (In this, he may have been influenced by his father, T. D. Mason, also a proponent of the disease conception.) The asylum idea had been popularized in great measure through the work of Dr. Joseph E. Turner* and in the early 1860s had resulted in the opening of the New York State Inebriate Asylum in Binghamton. That first venture was plagued with difficulties, but Mason and others kept the idea alive in similar institutions (such as the Fort Hamilton Home), and through the formation of the Association for the Study and Cure of Inebriety. Mason was a charter member of the association and its president for a number of years. With his colleagues he led the fight for the scientific investigation and treatment of addictions, as well as public support for the construction of asylums. He was also a member of the British Society for the Study of Inebriety, reflecting the international interest the disease conception of alcoholism had aroused by the late nineteenth century.

While Mason gave his time generously in the service of these organizations, his personal interests lay in the study of the effects of alcohol on the human system. Over the years, he wrote numerous articles on alcohol-related conditions, the different types of addicted states, and how physicians could deal with them. He spoke widely on these topics as well, becoming a familiar figure at medical conferences and at meetings dealing specifically with alcohol problems in both the United States and Europe. Significantly, Mason grasped some of the essentials of alcoholism treatment that remain standard in the late twentieth century: Treatment outcome, he believed, had to be total abstinence, as any return to social or moderate drinking on the part of an alcoholic would eventually lead to a relapse into addiction and injury. In short, he was convinced, as many modern alcoholism treatment specialists are also convinced, that even nondrinking alcoholics retained their potential for addiction, that "they are fighting a diathesis, a tendency" toward inebriety that was always with them, and that their only escape was to make "their principal ambition" an effort "to live sober lives and sober deaths." In all of this, Mason kept a humane outlook on his work, viewing the victims of alcoholism with compassion and loathing the liquor traffic as an enemy of mankind. Nor did he confine his reform sentiments to alcohol problems. A deeply religious man, he also was active in the Brooklyn City Bible Society (of which he was president for some years), a director of the American Bible Society, and an honored member of the local Mission Society. As a doctor, Mason was as much concerned for the spiritual health of his fellow man as he was for his physical welfare.

### Bibliography:

A. *Alcoholic Anaesthesia* (Hartford, CT, 1882); "A Study of the Social Statistics of 4,663 Cases of Alcoholic Inebriety," *Journal of the American Medical Association* 14(1890):822–24; *The Pauper Inebriate: His Legal Status, Care and Control* (Hartford, CT, 1899); *Inebriety a Disease* (Hartford, CT, 1903); *The Psychic Treatment of Inebriety and Its Relation to So-called Cures* (Chicago, 1907); *The Present Status of the Results of the Study of Alcohol in America* (Brooklyn, NY, 1925).

B. NYT, June 13, 1927; SEAP 4, 1705–6; WW 1, 786; Leonard U. Blumberg, "The American Association for the Study and Cure of Inebriety," *Alcoholism: Clinical and Experimental Research* 2(1978):234–40; T. D. Crothers, ed., *The Disease of Inebriety* (New York, 1893); Arnold Jaffe, *Addiction Reform in the Progressive Age: Scientific and Social Responses to Drug Dependence in the United States, 1870–1930.* Addiction in America Series, Gerald Grob, series ed. (New York, 1981).

**MATHER, Increase**    (21 June 1639, Dorchester, MA—23 August 1723, Boston, MA). *Education*: B.A., Harvard Coll., 1656; M.A., Trinity Coll., Dublin, 1658. *Career*: chaplain to British garrison, Guernsey, 1659–61; preacher in MA (sometimes with his father, Richard Mather), 1661–64; ordained, 1664; minister, Second Congregational Church, Boston, 1664–1723; president, Harvard Coll., 1685–1701; Massachusetts agent in negotiations for colonial charter, London, 1688–91.

Drinking and alcohol were integral parts of society in colonial America. Liquor was a dietary staple at most tables, and it generally appeared at social affairs from militia musters to church gatherings. Alcohol, in short, was not recognized as a major problem of the era; although that is not to say that intemperance, when it did occur, was condoned or went without criticism. Drunkenness did draw fire and none stronger than that leveled in the strictures of the Reverend Increase Mather. Mather was the epitome of a Puritan minister: The son of Richard Mather and father of Cotton Mather, he was thus part of the greatest clerical family in colonial Massachusetts. Strong in his personal faith, he devoted his career to sustaining the influence of the church and traditional moral norms in Puritan society. To that end, he was active not only in the pulpit but also in the highest circles of government and as a commentator on most aspects of Massachusetts life. As a theologian, Mather was a bulwark of Puritan orthodoxy, although over the years he was able to accommodate demands for more liberal standards of church membership (if only to maintain the social and political importance of the church). Politically, he acted whenever possible to preserve the independence of the colony, in which cause he skillfully negotiated with two British kings (1688–91) for a new Massachusetts charter; and he was a confidant of Governor Phips, which enabled him to render good service in ending the witchcraft trials at Salem. Mather also spoke out forcefully on behalf of established morality, launching powerful jeremiads against sins ranging from declining religious observance to "vain and promiscuous dancing" to drunkenness. Indeed, his *Wo to Drunkards* (1673) was one of the first great denunciations of intemperance in American history. At all points, then, and in all spheres, he sought to resist the decline of what he saw as a divinely-appointed social and religious order.

Mather's attacks on drinking excesses, which he considered especially insulting to both God and God-fearing Puritans, won the applause of later generations of temperance workers, who saw the great divine as an intellectual ancestor. Like them, Mather saw alcohol problems as morally degrading and socially disruptive, as well as productive of other mischief. Too much time spent in taverns, for example, led to neglect of more important duties. Too much alcohol, he charged in addition, could enflame the passions and provoke deadly violence. King Philip's War, Mather was sure, started as a result of liquor sales to the Indians. Thus drink and misanthropy seemed to go hand in hand for both Mather and nineteenth- and twentieth-century drys. But beyond these obvious concerns over drinking excesses the comparison breaks down, for Mather's views had nothing to do with prohibition. While he abhorred intemperance, he had nothing against alcohol itself, a position clearly expressed in *Wo to Drunkards*: "Drink is in itself a good creature of God, and to be received with thankfulness, but the abuse of drink is from Satan, the wine is from God, but the Drunkard is from the Devil." At no time did Mather suggest getting rid of the "good creature"; nor, moreover, was he interested in consigning problem drinkers to hell. On the contrary, the community standards he sought to uphold were ready to welcome a penitent sinner back into the fold. Puritan society required public recognition of its values, not necessarily punishment. Colonials were generally successful in obtaining that during Mather's lifetime, and as long as these prevailing norms remained intact, they never considered it necessary to attack alcohol generally or to class drinking as a major social problem. And although these values felt the stress of new political and social forces by the early eighteenth century, Mather defended them with vigor until the end of his days.

## Bibliography:

A. *The Life and Death of. . .Richard Mather* (Cambridge, 1670); *Wo to Drunkards. . .* (Cambridge, 1673); *A Brief History of the War with the Indians* (Boston, 1676); *The Call from Heaven* (Boston, 1679); *New England Vindicated* (London, 1688); *Cases of Conscience Concerning Evil Spirits* (Boston, 1693).

B. DAB 12, 390–94; DARB, 296–97; NCAB 6, 412–13; SEAP 4, 1726–27; Mark Edward Lender, "Drunkenness as an Offense in Early New England: A Study of 'Puritan' Attitudes," *Quarterly Journal of Studies on Alcohol* 34(1973):353–66; Mason I. Lowance, Jr., *Increase Mather* (New York, 1974); Cotton Mather, *Parentator: Memoirs of. . .Increase Mather* (Boston, 1724); Robert Middlekauf, *The Mathers: Three Generations of Puritan Intellectuals, 1596–1728* (New York, 1971).

**MATHEW, Theobald**   (10 October 1790, Thomastown House, Ireland—8 December 1856, Queenstown, Ireland). *Education*: studied at St. Canice's Acad., Kilkenny, Ireland; studied at the Royal Coll. of St. Patrick, Maynooth, 1807; studied for priesthood in Capuchin Order, Dublin, 1808–14. *Career*: mission work in Kilkenny and Cork, 1814–38; temperance campaigns, 1838 to 1850s.

From beginning to end, a deep sense of Christian humility, gentleness, and compassion marked the labors of Father Mathew. Distressed by the poverty of many of his countrymen, he worked selflessly to mitigate the lot of the poor during his mission work in Cork. He played an active role in the city's religious life and successfully sponsored a number of educational projects for the poor. His efforts endeared him to the populace, although his personal generosity to those in need soon had him deep in debt, a situation which plagued him throughout his career. His allegiance to temperance grew out of his work with the poor: While tending the sick during Cork's severe cholera epidemic in 1832, a Quaker, William Martin, convinced Mathew of the deleterious effects of intemperance on Ireland. And after repeated exhortations from Martin and others, the priest founded the Cork Total Abstinence Society in 1838. Thereafter, he campaigned extensively throughout Ireland and Britain and by the mid-1840s had induced close to five million people to sign a pledge of total abstinence, including many non-Catholics. His efforts earned him social and church plaudits, although some churchmen remained skeptical of his techniques. Occasionally assailed by Protestant extremists as threat to their creed or as anti-British, Mathew kept his movement largely removed from politics and even put it aside for a time to assist in relief efforts during the Great Famine in the late 1840s.

Mathew had long wanted to carry his crusade to the United States, although the 1844 anti-Catholic riots in Philadelphia discouraged him. But after an invitation from American bishops and Protestant-dominated temperance societies (his trip was financed in part by the staunchly Protestant American Temperance Union), he arrived in New York in 1849 to a tumultuous welcome. His tour carried him next to Boston, Philadelphia, and Washington, D.C., where he was honored by the president and the Congress. The rest of his trip was spent almost exclusively in the South; and before returning to Ireland in 1851, he visited over three hundred cities and towns in twenty-five states and pledged over 600,000 Americans to total abstinence. As in Ireland, Mathew relied on the pledge as the means of advancing temperance, and he did not directly endorse the prohibitionist goals of many Americans (although late in life he eventually conceded that the prohibitory ''Maine Law'' was probably a necessary adjunct to his type of temperance activity). While successful, though, Mathew's tour did generate some antagonism, notably from anti-Catholic American nativists and from those involved in the debate over slavery. He courageously defended his faith against the few anti-Catholic barbs openly directed at him; although he had expressed some antislavery views in Ireland, he tried to avoid the American sectional controversy, but extreme proslavery Southerners denounced him nevertheless and extreme abolitionists (many of whom were also temperance workers) railed at him for not endorsing their position. The work of Father Mathew, however, clearly established the groundwork needed for others to advance the temperance cause among Catholics both in the United States and Ireland, and his American visit gave impetus to the growth of the Catholic Total Abstinence Union.

**Bibliography:**

B. DBTB, 87; SEAP, 4, 1727–30; Joan Bland, *Hibernian Crusade: The Story of the Catholic Total Abstinence Union of America* (Washington, DC, 1951); *Congressional Globe*, 31st Cong., 1st sess., (Washington, DC, 1849), 51–59; Cuthbert A. Goeb, ''The Journey of Father Theobald Mathew to America, 1849–1851'' (MA Thesis, Catholic University of America, 1922); Rev. Father Augustine J. Osgniach, *Footprints of Father Theobald Mathew* (Dublin, 1947); Rev. P. Rogers, *Father Theobald Mathew* (Dublin, 1944).

**MATHEWS, George Martin**   (22 August 1848, Hamilton Co., OH—3 April 1921, Dayton, OH). *Education*: B.S., Otterbein Univ., 1870; studied at Lane Theological Sem., 1879–80; studied at Union Biblical Sem., 1881–82; D.D. (honorary), Lane Univ., 1896; LLD. (honorary), Otterbein Univ., 1912. *Career*: ordained, United Brethren ministry, 1882; minister, Cleves, OH, 1880–81; minister, Dayton, OH, 1881–89, 1894–98; presiding elder, Miami Conference, OH, 1889–94; editor, *United Brethren Quarterly Review*, 1893–99; associate editor, *Religious Telescope*, 1899–1902; bishop, United Brethren Church, beginning 1902.

Bishop George Mathews was one of the numerous Protestant clergymen of high standing in their denominations who made the work of the Temperance

Movement the work of their church. We know little of his early interest in the dry crusade, but he was of a pious frame of mind and likely approached the liquor problem with the same view to Christian morality and values that prompted so many other Americans to war on the "demon rum." As a churchman, he devoted much of his preaching to the temperance issue, and his views carried increasing weight in the denomination as he rose progressively in its ranks. Indeed, a good deal of Mathews' career was spent out of the pulpit in positions where he could act as a spokesman for the United Brethren as a whole: For years, he was both an editor of the church's publications and an administrator, culminating in his election as bishop in 1902. In addition to exhorting his listeners and readers away from the bottle, however, the reforming bishop took a direct hand in organized antiliquor activities. As a young minister in Ohio, he had been an enthusiastic member of a number of local temperance societies, and he devoted many hours to campaigns against the traffic in his home areas of Cleves and Dayton. Later, Mathews expanded his antiliquor role, sitting for a number of years as chairman of the United Brethren Temperance Committee and representing the denomination on the larger Temperance Committee of the Federal Council of Churches of Christ in America. As bishop, he willingly used his influence in political efforts against drink. He served as a chairman of the Illinois Anti-Saloon League and then as a vice president of the Anti-Saloon League of America, where he earned a reputation as a judicious and effective planner. That description seemed to match the bishop's character generally, for although a committed temperance leader and a deadly foe of the liquor traffic, there was nothing of the fanatic in Mathews. In his eyes, temperance was a boon to humanity, a cause worthy of Christian endeavor, not a means of forcing the benighted or the evil to heal. His work, both as a church leader and as a reformer (he was also active in United Brethren missionary and charitable enterprises), made him beloved of his denomination, and he was honored with two honorary degrees. Remembered by other drys for his effective work on the temperance campaign circuit and for "his wisdom in council," he died in 1921, when it at last appeared that the battle for a sober America had been won.

### Bibliography:

A. *A Century... of the Church of the United Brethren in Christ* (Dayton, OH, 1901); *Justification* (Dayton, OH, 1902); *The Church in Earnest...* (Dayton, OH, 1908); with others, *The Call of China and the Islands...* (Dayton, OH, 1913?); *Christ in the Life of Today* (Dayton, OH, 1916).

B. SEAP 4, 1730; WW 1, 788.

**MAUS, Mervin Louis**    (8 May 1851, Burnt Mills, MD—3 August 1939?). *Education*: studied at St. John's Coll., MD, 1870s; M.D., Univ. of Maryland, 1874; postdoctoral studies, Pasteur Inst., Paris, and European clinics, 1890–91. *Career*: army officer, Medical Corps, 1874–1907 (ultimately colonel, assistant surgeon general); commissioner of public health, Philippine Islands, 1900s; chief surgeon, Central Division, 1911; department surgeon, Department of the East, 1912–15; secretary, Kentucky Tuberculosis Commission, 1915–17; department surgeon, Western Department, and Council of National Defense, 1917–19.

The high esteem in which the American public held Dr. Mervin Maus for his outstanding service as a military surgeon lent extra weight to his addresses and writings on temperance issues. Maus was among an extraordinary generation of army doctors, which included other such notables as Walter Reed and Leonard Wood, that brought acclaim to the service while vastly improving its professional capabilities. A well-trained physician, Maus compiled an admirable service record. His long tenure in uniform included duty in the Reconstruction South, on the Great Plains (where in 1877, in the war against the Sioux of Sitting Bull and Crazy Horse, he was recommended for the Congressional Medal of Honor for exceptional gallantry), in the Spanish-American War and the Philippine Insurrection, and in a variety of important staff positions. He won major acclaim serving as public health commissioner in the Philippines under Governor William Howard Taft. In a monumental effort, which easily rivaled the work of the doctors battling the problems of yellow fever and malaria in the Panama Canal Zone, Maus made vast improvements in the health of the islands. Instituting changes in public sanitation, his efforts reduced mortality, virtually eliminated bubonic plague in the Manila area, reduced cholera, and nearly eradicated small-pox. Throughout these activities, and during his other assignments, he also devoted considerable attention to the reform of army medical services, urging measures to promote better hygiene among the troops, to improve the delivery of health care, and to institute higher standards of efficiency generally in the military. Indeed, Maus's ideas on army reform closely reflected the efforts of the Progressive reformers then active in civilian America; and like so many of his civilian counterparts, Maus saw temperance as a central concern, necessary if other reforms were to be effective.

Long a total abstainer himself, Maus was convinced that drinking had no place in a modern, complex industrial society. He wrote frequently on the liquor question in the United States, arguing that the issue went far beyond the personal health problems inherent in alcoholism. Multiply the personal problems by thousands of drinkers, and intemperance also became a major public health matter. Indeed, it was a doubly grave affair in that the functioning of modern industry demanded that everyone concerned—workers and managers—be at their best. Impaired by alcohol, no work force could produce efficiently or avoid waste. Maus made this case repeatedly and insisted that it was especially important in the military context. Soldiers and sailors could not perform their tasks, nor could officers properly exercise the responsibilities of command, with their minds clouded by drink. In a very real way, the implication of this position was that booze was a threat to national security; and if Maus only hinted at this conclusion himself, the Temperance Movement later used his writings on the subject to make the point expressly. Maus, however, did urge specific steps the military could take to protect itself: Officers, he wrote, should abstain, as even moderate drinking was a danger to health and efficiency, and he campaigned heatedly against the sale of alcohol beverages in army canteens. The celebrated army doctor belonged to no temperance organization, but the antiliquor reform nevertheless enjoyed his support and derived the benefit of his many speeches and writings on alcohol problems.

**Bibliography:**

A. *An Army Officer on Leave in Japan...* (Chicago, 1911); *Alcohol and Officials: Does the Moderate Use of Alcohol Lower Health and Efficiency...?* (Washington, DC, 1912); *Sanitary and Economical Improvement in the Philippines Since American Intervention...* (New York, 1912); *The Sanitary Conquest of the Philippine Islands* (New York, 1912); *Prophylaxis of Venereal Diseases in the Army and Navy* (Washington, DC, 1913); *Injurious Effects Resulting from the Moderate Use of Alcohol* (n.p., 1941).

B. SEAP 4, 1733; WW 1, 791.

**MERRICK, Caroline Elizabeth Thomas**    (24 November 1825, East Feliciana Parish, LA—19 March 1908, New Orleans, LA). *Education*: privately educated by family governesses. *Career*: occasional charitable and philanthropic work, 1855–79; reform organizing on behalf of woman's suffrage and temperance, 1879 to 1900s.

In a brief account of Caroline Merrick's long life, one biographer put the following construction on Merrick's career: ''She demonstrated that a woman could be 'actively interested in public and benevolent activities' without abandoning 'her position as leader of the domestic circle.' She forms a significant link between the Old South and the New.'' The ''position'' referred to here was that of wife of a Louisiana Supreme Court justice, Edwin Thomas Merrick, whom Caroline Thomas had married in 1840 at age fifteen. In the earlier years of her marriage she adhered closely to the routines of antebellum domesticity in a wealthy, plantation-owning family—gardening, household management, a bit of the charities and culture. The only major disruption in Merrick's life was the Civil War, from which the family emerged with its properties and position intact. But in 1878, when she was fifty-two, tragedy brought a deep change to her tranquil existence. Her oldest daughter died of yellow fever, and Merrick was beside herself with grief. Searching for a way to console her and take her mind off of her loss, Judge Merrick recommended that she work out her sadness by attacking the problem of women's legal rights in Louisiana. Mrs. Merrick had recently complained to him about the issue, which had angered her when the St. Ann's Asylum for Women and Children (of which she was secretary) lost a considerable inheritance because the will of the donor had been witnessed only by women. Somewhat reluctantly at first, then, Caroline Merrick became enmeshed in the movement for women's suffrage. The following year, she and two other suffragettes addressed the Louisiana Constitutional Convention; and although that body did little to remove restrictions on women's rights, the fact that the women spoke at all generated considerable public comment. They were the first to do so on the subject in the history of the state.

Merrick's suffrage work drew her steadily into other reform efforts as well. Seeking to take advantage of Merrick's regional influence on behalf of the Woman's Christian Temperance Union, the organization's first president, Annie Wittenmyer,* invited her to enlist in the war against drink. Merrick politely refused, but several years later (in 1882) she did agree to make speaking arrangements in New Orleans for Frances E. Willard,* Wittenmyer's successor at the helm of the WCTU. When in the city, Willard was also a house guest of the Merricks. At this point, the Temperance Movement seemed to reach out to Mrs. Merrick despite her hesitations about becoming involved. While Willard was still in New Orleans, the city's WCTU chapter elected the suffrage leader as its president—even though she was not a union member. Not surprisingly, she quickly declined the office, but Willard and Judge Merrick soon convinced her to serve. Even so, she later recalled that she had no "deep conviction of duty on the temperance question." Yet tragedy again pushed her toward vigorous participation in reform work: In August of 1882 her youngest daughter died of Bright's disease, which caused Merrick to devote long hours to WCTU affairs. Once more, intense activity was a way to forget: "This temperance work has come to me like a beam of heavenly sunshine in the great darkness of my grief." Merrick proved an effective and energetic dry leader. She founded a state chapter of the union and sat as its president for a decade (1883–84), and she became a familiar figure in the state capital where she emerged as a persistent lobbyist for temperance legislation. Her particular interest in this regard was "scientific temperance instruction," and along with Mary Hunt* (who campaigned for the issue nationally), she succeeded in having such teaching required in the public schools. Her initial reluctance aside, then, Merrick was one of the most highly regarded temperance leaders in the South.

Throughout her temperance efforts, however, Merrick reserved most of her time for the fight for women's rights. She continued to organize on behalf of her sex and in the 1890s was elected president of the first Louisiana woman's suffrage association. In this capacity she also sought political change in the state, and although progress was never dramatic, her efforts kept the issue in front of the public. In 1898, although still refusing to grant full suffrage, the state did agree to allow women taxpayers to vote on tax measures. Merrick also lobbied on a national basis, speaking before a number of reform conventions and the Senate in the nation's capital. While committed to reform, however, she was never a zealot. Indeed, one of her chief contributions to the suffrage and temperance struggle was the social prestige she brought to them. Beyond that, she clearly demonstrated that women could play an important leadership role in the New South.

**Bibliography:**

A. *Old Times in Dixie Land: A Southern Matron's Memories* (New York, 1901).

B. NAW 2, 530–31; NCAB 10, 147–48; Frances E. Willard, *Woman and Temperance* (Hartford, CT, 1883); Frances E. Willard and Mary A. Livermore, eds., *A Woman of the Century* (New York, 1893).

**MERRICK, Frederick**     (29 January 1810, Wilbraham, MA—5 March 1894, Delaware, OH). *Education*: studied at Wesleyan Univ., 1833–34. *Career*: partner in retail business, Springfield, MA, 1825–33; principal, Amenia Sem., NY, 1834–38; professor of natural science, Ohio Univ., 1838–41; minister, Methodist Church, Marietta, OH, 1842–43; ordained in Methodist Church, 1843; professor of natural science, Ohio Wesleyan Univ., 1845–51; professor of moral philosophy, Ohio Wesleyan Univ., beginning 1851; president, Ohio Wesleyan Univ., 1860–73.

Frederick Merrick is one of the great names in the history of the spread of Methodism into the American West. At the same time, he pioneered the rise of organized temperance sentiments in the Ohio region. His early career plans included neither religion nor reform; rather, he had a partnership in a store and seemingly had a secure future as a retailer. In 1829, however, he experienced a religious conversion and sought a life in the pulpit. While pursuing his religious education, Merrick was licensed as a local Methodist preacher and then left his studies to teach in a Methodist school, Amenia Seminary. His reputation for probity and dedication next brought a call from Ohio University, where his teaching and preaching made him a well-known and respected figure in regional church and educational circles. Taking time off from his teaching just before being formally ordained in 1843, he served a pastorate for two years in Marietta, during which time he became a central figure in the effort to found a Methodist university in the region. The new college, Ohio Wesleyan University, opened in 1844, and Merrick once more went back into the classroom as a professor and administrator. For the rest of his life, the minister-teacher was associated with Wesleyan, instructing students, raising funds, establishing new departments and facilities, and building further denominational and public support for the school. Between 1860 and 1873 he was president of the institution, and after failing health compelled him to give up the burdens of leadership, he remained on the faculty until his death. Merrick's commitment to the university was total. He turned down other opportunities that would have taken him away, including a missionary venture in China that he found tempting, always placing the needs of Wesleyan first. Few individuals, then, did more than Merrick to establish Methodism as a cultural force in the area.

During most of the nineteenth century, many Americans considered work on behalf of religious denominations and education to be fully in step with the reforming spirit of the era. Certainly Merrick did, and his dedication to the affairs of the college mirrored his regard for social reform generally. Service to God required service to man, and the Methodist educator did not shrink from what he saw as his duty. As the Civil War approached, he was militantly antislavery, and he ran a station on the Underground Railroad. Similarly, he was a staunch friend of the Temperance Movement. The liquor traffic, Merrick insisted, was an implacable foe of mankind, and he warned his students, his fellow Methodists, and people in general away from beverage alcohol. Methodists had been among the earliest to avoid distilled liquor as a matter of faith—a legacy of John Wesley—and the Ohio college president inveighed strongly for total abstinence. His personal example in this regard, and his effective and consistent preaching on the subject, did much to stimulate popular sentiments against alcohol and to establish the Midwest (and especially Ohio) as one of the most fertile grounds for temperance work in the nation. It was no coincidence that the Woman's Crusade, the Woman's Christian Temperance Union, and the Anti-Saloon League all had their beginnings in the state. Merrick, and others of his mind, had done their work well. But his was no shrill voice. Indeed, he was better noted for his reasonableness and his steady faith that the Lord would act through men for the betterment of all. An elder statesman of Methodism in his later years, Merrick remained active in the affairs of the church, and he acquired an unmatched reputation for piety and gentleness.

### Bibliography:

A. *Formalism in Religion* (n.p., 1865); *Religion and the State: A Centennial Sermon* (Cincinnati, OH, 1875).

B. DAB 49, 555–56; WW H, 425; J. W. Bashford, "Frederick Merrick," *Annual Report of the President to the Trustees of Ohio Wesleyan University* (Delaware, OH, 1894); Isaac Crook, *The Great Five: The First Faculty of the Ohio Wesleyan University* (Delaware, OH, 1908); E. T. Nelson, ed., *Fifty Years of History of the Ohio Wesleyan University* (Delaware, OH, 1895); W. G. Williams, "Frederick Merrick," *Methodist Review* (May–June, 1895).

**MERWIN, James Burtis**    (22 May 1822, Cairo, NY—3 April 1917, Brooklyn, NY). *Career*: journalist and educator, beginning 1840s; founder and editor, *American Journal of Education*, beginning 1879; public lecturer on Shakespeare, education, and reform subjects.

Few temperance advocates could claim the active support of an American president, though many had at least tacit approval. But such was the claim of James B. Merwin, sometime educator and journalist. While addressing audiences on literary matters, including Shakespeare, he had developed an effective speaking style. Furthermore, his work as publicist and educator (he had founded the *American Journal of Education* in 1879) had prepared him for the effort that was soon to become the major preoccupation of his life. Merwin had met Abraham Lincoln during the campaigns for state prohibition in Illinois in the 1850s. And while Lincoln was never a prohibitionist, he did have a friendly relationship with the dry reformer. Upon Lincoln's election as president, Merwin visited him a number of times in Washington, D.C., and when the Civil War broke out, he approached him again with a proposal he considered crucial for improving the morale and efficiency of the Northern troops: What this lifetime teetotaler and prohibition campaigner suggested was that he be permitted to travel among the troops and spread the gospel of temperance. In July 1861, by Merwin's account, Lincoln gave him carte blanche to deliver temperance lectures to the soldiers, an activity which seems to have had the support of Generals Winfield Scott and Benjamin F. Butler.* Actually, Merwin seems to have been relatively effective. We know little of what the troops thought of him, but he lectured to thousands of men, won the applause of many officers and civilian leaders, and had the satisfaction of seeing a number of active temperance societies formed in some regiments. Soldiers have seldom enjoyed being lectured on morality, but the Illinois reformer seems to have evoked little overt hostility, which is more than could be said for some speakers (including some generals) who addressed the Union rank and file. At any rate, Merwin did nothing to antagonize the president, with whom he remained friendly. His last meeting with Lincoln was for dinner in the White House—after which the leader of the Union left for Ford's Theater. Despite later Temperance Movement claims, Merwin's association with the martyred president did not signify Lincoln's approval of prohibitionist policies. More likely it was simply Lincoln's way of staying in touch with an old and apparently fairly pleasant acquaintance, while keeping his finger on the pulse of temperance sentiments and strength.

**Bibliography:**

B. SEAP 4, 1745; *Who's Who in America*, 1916–17; Ervin Chapman, *Latest Light on Abraham Lincoln* (New York, 1917); William E. Johnson, *The Federal Government and the Liquor Traffic* (Westerville, OH, 1911).

**MILLER, Emily Clark Huntington** (22 October 1833, Brooklyn, CT—2 November 1913, Northfield, MN). *Education*: A.B., Oberlin Coll., 1857; A.M. (honorary), Oberlin Coll., 1893; LHD. (honorary), Northwestern Univ., 1909. *Career*: teacher, OH, 1857–60; editor, *Little Corporal*, 1865–71; trustee, Northwestern Univ., 1873–85; dean of women, Northwestern Univ., 1891–98; assistant professor of English, Northwestern Univ., 1891–1900; active writing on various subjects, 1870s–1900s.

Emily Huntington was the daughter of a venerable Connecticut family. Her father was a prosperous doctor and Baptist minister, while her grandfather was Revolutionary War general Jedediah Huntington. Raised in relative affluence, then, she had fine educational opportunities and was encouraged to pursue a career. After graduation from Oberlin College in Ohio (1857) and several years of teaching at her alma mater, she married John Edwin Miller, another educator. Until 1870, the Millers moved frequently as John took a succession of teaching and administrative jobs in Illinois and Ohio. They finally settled in Evanston, Illinois, when he became co-owner of the *Little Corporal,* a juvenile magazine. As John travelled throughout the Midwest to promote the publication, Emily became actively involved in the editorial side of the business (which she handled by herself after 1871); at the same time she began writing short, generally moralizing pieces for young readers. It was the start of a writing career that later brought her considerable public recognition and wealth. Eventually, she turned out over a dozen books (mostly on moral and social themes and poetry), and many articles for such magazines as *Cosmopolitan*, *Atlantic Monthly*, *Scribner's*, and *Ladies' Home Journal* (where she spent some years as an associate editor). In the 1870s, however, when she was not working on the *Little Corporal*, she lent much of her time to editing for the Temperance Movement. An earnest reformer, Miller had been active in Methodist educational and mission affairs, and she extended her interests to the dry reform when the Woman's Crusade spread through the region in 1873 and 1874. Beginning in 1874, she put out the *Call*, a dry newsletter that soon evolved into *Our Union* (and then the *Union Signal*), the official organ of the new Woman's Christian Temperance Union. While never a major leader in the WCTU, Miller did good service in helping to start its publication efforts. For a time, she also penned a short column, "Home Talks," for the paper, which brought her to the attention of a national temperance audience.

That Miller did not become more deeply involved with the WCTU is perhaps worth further mention. Certainly she had skills the union needed (indeed, her fame as an author was growing all the time), and her dedication to reform was never in doubt. Her low profile in the organization may have stemmed, however, from her relationship to Frances E. Willard,* corresponding secretary of the National WCTU in 1875 and president beginning in 1879. Prior to either woman's involvement in the temperance movement their paths had crossed at Northwestern University. Between the 1870s and 1890s, Miller was associated with the school as a trustee, dean, or professor; even earlier, she had been a founder of the Evanston College for Ladies, of which Willard was president. In 1873, the college merged with Northwestern, with Willard becoming dean of women. Following a controversy over separate rules of conduct for women, however, with Willard insisting on a separate social life for women, Willard resigned. Miller, as a trustee, was on a select committee having to decide whether to accept the resignation. Miller, and most of the rest of the other trustees, believed that women should be integrated into the student body without special rules and voted to let Willard go. While Willard later had kind words for Miller in a number of publications, the two were never close, and other WCTU members, probably out of loyalty to their beloved president, evidently remained aloof as well. Later, when Miller became dean of women at Northwestern, the position had few duties and she spent more time in teaching and writing. She left the university in 1900, and until she died in 1913 at age eighty, she remained active on the lecture circuit and a firm partisan of the causes she had espoused during her long and productive career.

### Bibliography:

A. *The Royal Road to Fortune* (New York, circa 1869); *The Parish of Fair Haven* (St. Paul, MN, 1886); *Captain Fritz: His Friends and Adventures* (New

York, 1887); *Little Neighbors* (New York, 1887); *What Tommy Did* (New York, 1893); *From Avalon, and Other Poems* (Chicago, 1896).

B. DAB 12, 613–24; NAW 2, 541–42; NCAB 10, 305–6; NYT, Nov. 5, 1913; WW 1, 840; Frances E. Willard, *Woman and Temperance* (Hartford, CT, 1883).

**MILNER, Duncan Chambers**    (10 March 1841, Mt. Pleasant, OH—18 March 1928, Mount Dora, FL). *Education*: A.B., Washington and Jefferson Coll., 1866; studied at Union Theological Sem., 1866–68; D.D. (honorary), Coll. of Emporia, KS, 1883. *Career*: officer, Union army, 1861–65; ordained in Presbyterian Church, 1868; minister, various pastorates in MO, KS, IL, 1868–1915; president, Ottawas (KS) Chautauqua Assembly, 1882–99; moderator, Synod of Kansas, 1883–84; editor, *Kansas Presbyter*, 1883–84; president, Kansas State Temperance Union, 1893–94; associate minister, Ravenswood Presbyterian Church, Chicago, beginning 1915.

Raised in rural Ohio, Duncan Milner set his course on a career in the pulpit, only to have his ambitions obstructed by the outbreak of the Civil War in 1861. He promptly rushed to the colors and was mustered into service as a sergeant major of the Ninety-eighth Ohio Infantry, ultimately being promoted to first lieutenant and regimental adjutant. The young volunteer did not see easy duty. His unit was involved in some tough actions, not the least of which was the murderous Battle of Chickamauga in northwest Georgia in 1863. Milner was wounded in the arm in the Union debacle and was crippled the rest of his life. Soon after the conflict, the still young veteran resumed his pursuit of the ministry and upon completing his undergraduate and theological studies was ordained in the Presbyterian Church in 1868. There followed a succession of pastorates in the Midwest, most of them in Kansas, but ultimately the associate minister's post with the large Ravenswood Presbyterian Church in Chicago. During his many years in the pulpit, Milner emerged as a steadfast enemy of the liquor traffic. Long a total abstainer, he urged others to the same course on a personal basis as well as organizing local prohibitionist activities. So vehement were his strictures on drinking that he aroused the special hatred of many wets, and on one occasion in Atchinson, Kansas, a drunkard attacked him on the street. Not to be bested, the old combat veteran fended off his assailant with his one good arm—a staunch campaigner indeed.

Combat, however, was not a usual part of Milner's temperance work. But he did emerge as an effective organizer. He was a member of the Kansas Temperance Union and its president from 1893 to 1894, as well as an officer of the state Chautauqua association, which sponsored temperance speakers on a regular basis. Once settled in Chicago, Milner continued his reform activities without interruption, maintaining his fire on the "demon rum" and denouncing the doings of the Ku Klux Klan as well. During National Prohibition, he served as director of the Chicago Law and Order League, a group dedicated to the enforcement of antiliquor laws; and in Chicago, that was no mean task. In addition, he authored a number of titles on temperance and other reform problems. He was probably best known for his *Lincoln and Temperance* (1926), yet another dry attempt to place the martyred president in the prohibitionist camp. To the end of his eighty-seven years, Milner was proud of his life of service: He had fought hard and well for the Union (indeed, he was active for years in veterans groups), worked until late in life for his church, and just as importantly in his eyes, labored tirelessly for the cause he thought would rid his country of a host of social and moral ills. Few citizens could boast of more.

**Bibliography:**

A. *The Original Ku Klux Klan and Its Successor. . .* (Chicago, 1921); *Lincoln and Temperance* (Chicago, 1926).

B. SEAP 4, 1775; WW 1, 347.

**MINER, Alonzo Ames**    (17 August 1814, Lempster, NH—14 June 1895, Boston, MA). *Education*: A.M. (honorary), Tufts Coll., 1861; STD. (honorary), Harvard Univ., 1863; LLD. (honorary), Tufts Coll., 1865. *Career*: school-teacher, 1830–34; managed Cavendish (VT) Acad., 1834–35; principal, Unity (NH) Scientific and Military Acad., 1835–39; ordained in Unitarian Church, 1839; minister, Methuen and Lowell, MA, 1839–48; minister, School Street Church, Second Universalist Society of Boston, 1848–91; president, Tufts Coll., 1862–74.

A Universalist minister of great renown and a dedicated advocate of the struggle against drink, Alonzo Ames Miner grew up in a family estranged from the religion of their New England neighbors. His parents rejected strict Calvinism, preferring a more liberal view of man's relationship to the Almighty, and young Miner inherited the family penchant for questioning prevailing community norms, religious or otherwise. He had no higher education, but intelligent and well-read, he began teaching at sixteen years old and then took positions managing private New England academies. Miner moved away from education for a time after his ordination in 1839; but he always retained a strong interest in the subject, and during his academy years he had learned much that he was to put to good use later when he served (without salary) as president of financially troubled Tufts College and became a leading promoter of the establishment of other schools. Yet Miner's goal was the pulpit, not the classroom. He was preaching in local Universalist congregations even before ordination, and afterward he steadily climbed to prominence in his denomination. He was an effective speaker, and he excelled in public debate with more orthodox clergy. Once drawn into the public arena he became actively involved in the reform battles that marked the antebellum social and political scene. He emerged as a passionate champion of the Temperance Movement, urging his parishioners and society in general to total abstinence (indeed, he was a pioneer of this extreme position), and he was a firm antislavery man. As one of his biographers has noted, however, he was not willing to sacrifice his church on the altar of reform, and he passionately opposed the attempts of some reformers (including William Lloyd Garrison*) to lead sympathetic members out of established churches when entire congregations refused to adopt a reform posture. To do so, in Miner's view, was simply to invite the social disorder that would make effective reform even more difficult.

The battle to defend established congregations from extremist advocates of reform, however, never stopped Miner from pursuing his vision of the good society. In this effort, he always placed great emphasis on temperance work. Both in Lowell and in Boston, the reform-minded minister waged a relentless war on the liquor traffic, castigating taverns and saloons as sink-holes of corruption, sources of monumental waste, and productive only of misery. Government, he insisted, had not only the right but the responsibility to attack the evil for the good of society. In the antebellum years, he was active in attempts to deny the issuance of local liquor licenses as a means of drying out municipalities, and he favored state-wide prohibition efforts when the Maine Law controversy erupted in the 1850s. Nor did he confine his efforts to his home region: For more than fifty years, Miner carried the prohibitionist gospel throughout the rest of the New England states, to a good deal of the rest of the nation, and to several Canadian provinces. After the Civil War, Miner joined the Prohibition Party at its inception, and he campaigned under its banner repeatedly, twice as a candidate. In 1878, he ran for governor of Massachusetts, and in 1893, still ardent in the cause only two years before his death, he made a run for the Boston mayoralty. He stood little chance, he knew, in either contest; but he was determined to give the Prohibitionist platform a public hearing, and he did accomplish that. In addition to his work for the party, Miner was also the president of the Massachusetts Temperance Alliance, a post he held for some twenty years. Yet this dedication to a cause in which he believed was typical of his character; he served in other fields to equal effect. Indeed, upon his death at eighty-one, his church and state lost one of their most distinguished servants.

**Bibliography:**

A. *Bible Exercises*... (Boston, 1865); *Shall Criminals Sit on a Jury?* (Boston, 1865); *The Right and Duty of Prohibition*... (Manchester, England, 1867); *The Old Forts Taken: Five Lectures on Endless Punishment and Future Life* (Boston, 1878); *Is Prohibition the True Legislative Policy?* (n.p., 187–?).

B. DAB 13, 21–22; SEAP 4, 1776; WW H, 429; G. H. Emerson, *Life of Alonzo Ames Miner* (Boston, 1896); A. B. Start, *History of Tufts College* (Boston, 1896).

**MOODY, Dwight Lyman**    (5 February 1837, Northfield, MA—22 December 1899, Northfield, MA). *Career*: shoe clerk, Boston, 1854–56; shoe salesman, Chicago, 1856–61; agent, Christian Commission, 1861–65; officer, Chicago Sunday School Union, Young Men's Christian Association, 1865–71; revivalist preacher and organizer, 1871–99.

"The prominent revival men in the Old World and the New," proclaimed one address at the Centennial Temperance Convention in Philadelphia in 1876, "are temperance men." He continued that "our great modern evangelist, D. L. Moody, in whom the revival spirit is incarnated, who has stirred two continents and been a wonder unto many, is known to be a sworn foe of the drinking usages." The speaker did not exaggerate: Moody was one of the most powerful evangelicals of his generation, and his revivalism lent undeniable power to the temperance cause. The great itinerant preacher had no formal theological training. Indeed, his initial background was that of a shoe clerk and salesman. But he had a deeply spiritual side and became active in lay church activities, emerging as a tireless proponent of the Sunday school movement in the Chicago area. For years, he also worked for the Young Men's Christian Association, proving himself in all of these capacities an effective organizer and executive. He was in addition, a fine speaker, a talent he developed during his efforts on behalf of the YMCA. By the 1870s, his impact on listeners was electric. Moody's first great successes came in Great Britain, where his simple message eschewed all denominational orthodoxy and stressed adherence to Christian virtues (in which he included temperance) and personal salvation. He drew enthusiastic audiences, and upon his return to the United States his fame spread in similar fashion among his countrymen. Over his more than two decades of revivalist preaching, he toured most of the important urban centers of the North and Midwest; millions heard his preaching and legions professed conversion to Christ as a result. At the same time, he gave renewed stature to evangelical religion in America, and his spiritual influence on many social and reform leaders of the era was profound. Frances E. Willard,* for example, president of the Woman's Christian Temperance Union, as well as many other dry crusaders, found his messages deeply moving. In order to further his work and to provide guidance for the converted, Moody also established a number of successful schools and a Bible institute. His institutional efforts, however, never diverted him from his original mission of revivalism and conversion.

If Moody never tied his gospel to any denomination, neither did he link it to any political or social cause. Yet his preaching reflected his personal views on many of the issues of the day, especially when they touched on what the evangelist believed to be central Christian values. Such was the case with the temperance question. Moody belonged to no specific antiliquor organization, and he considered intemperance only one of many affronts to virtue, but he recognized its prominence in public concern and its complicating role in other problems. Accordingly, there were times when he gave the issue particular attention. At one point, he set aside one day of preaching per week to deal with temperance problems. In response, the rank and file of the Temperance Movement counted him among their members, and there is no doubt that he was an important inspiration to some of the most effective work in rehabilitating alcoholics. These efforts came under the heading of "gospel temperance." Taking their cues from Moody's appeals to receive Christ, a fair number of antiliquor ministers held forth gospel temperance as the best means of reclaiming the drunkard, although members of the WCTU probably did the most in this regard. The appeal was simple: In addition to making the standard revivalist pleas to repent of evil ways and be saved, gospel temperance used the same opportunity to induce the convert to sign a total abstinence pledge. The technique could boast some success. Thousands took the pledge, professing that their religious experience had enabled them to lay down the bottle where all other means to that end had failed. In fact, such spiritual appeals to the alcoholic were probably as effective an approach as any (and arguably still are); certainly temperance leaders thought so. Moody himself always took a dim view of pledge-signing, trusting only to "the sovereign Grace of God" to break the chains of alcohol addiction. As for preventive measures, the evangelist hoped to see the day when American churches would cleanse themselves of any compromise on the liquor question—when they would not accept members who worked in the beverage traffic or condone moderate drinking. And if they did not fight the evil, Moody firmly believed that good Christian "men and women will get out of the Church as Lot did out of Sodom."

**Bibliography:**

A. *How to Study the Bible* (New York, 1875); *Selected Sermons* (Chicago, 1881); *The Way to God* (Chicago, 1884); *Prevailing Prayer* (New York, 1885); *Bible Characters* (Chicago, 1888); *The Great Redemption* (Chicago, 1889).

B. DAB 13, 103–6; NYT, Dec. 23, 1899; R. F. Burns, "Temperance as Related to Revivals," 151–63, in *Centennial Temperance Volume...* (New York, 1877); Richard K. Curtis, *They Called Him Mr. Moody* (Garden City, NY, 1962); W. H. Daniels, *The Temperance Reform and Its Great Reformers* (Cincinnati, OH, 1878); James F. Findlay, *Dwight L. Moody: American Evangelist, 1837–1899* (Chicago, 1969); William R. Moody, *The Life of Dwight L. Moody* (New York, 1900); Emma M. Powell, *Heavenly Destiny* (Chicago, 1943).

**MOORE, Edward Jay**    (6 September 1861, near Norwich, NY—19 December 1935, Columbus, OH). *Education*: graduated from Bloomsburg (PA) State Normal Sch., 1882; A.B., Univ. of Puget Sound, 1891; A.M., Allegheny Coll., 1892; Ph.D., Allegheny Coll., 1893; D.D., Univ. of Puget Sound, 1913. *Career*: Methodist minister, LaConner, WA, 1886–90; minister, Tacoma, WA, 1890–94; minister, Cleveland, OH, 1894–99; minister, Ravenna, OH, 1899–1901; district superintendent of Cincinnati, Anti-Saloon League of Ohio, 1901–6; assistant state superintendent, Anti-Saloon League of Ohio, 1906–8; state superintendent, Missouri Anti-Saloon League, 1908–12; state superintendent, Pennsylvania Anti-Saloon League, 1913–16; assistant general superintendent, Anti-Saloon League of America, 1916–25; state superintendent, Anti-Saloon League of Ohio, 1925–31; secretary, Ohio Dry Federation, 1931–32.

A clergyman and a lifetime temperance worker, Edward Jay Moore was another example of the connections between the Methodist Church and the dry crusade. He seems to have grown up a solid temperance enthusiast and to have set his sights early on a career in the ministry, although at one point he apparently considered teaching. Ordained in 1888, he spent the next thirteen years in pulpits in Washington State and Ohio, where his congregations heard him expound on the merits of prohibition. Indeed, as the years went by, Moore spent an increasing amount of his time on temperance work, and in 1901 he left the ministry in order to pursue the reform crusade full time. He took a position with the Anti-Saloon League of Ohio as superintendent of the Cincinnati District, and until he retired in 1932 he was one of the organization's most effective and energetic stalwarts. After Cincinnati, he took on assignments of steadily greater responsibility, and he served in league superintendent's jobs at the state level in Ohio (assistant superintendent, 1906–8, and state superintendent, 1925–31), Missouri (state superintendent, 1908–12), and Pennsylvania (also state superintendent, 1913–16) and on the national level in the league bureaucracy from 1916 to 1925. Sharpening his skills in the legislative and political battles inherent in the anti-liquor controversy, the former minister studied law as well during these years and was admitted to the bar in Ohio and Missouri. His record as an activist paralleled that of the dry movement itself. He did well in Ohio, for example, appreciably building the strength of the league there. In Missouri, however, heavy wet opposition checked him in a premature attempt to orchestrate a winning drive for state prohibition in 1910, although three years later he produced a dramatic victory for a local-option bill in the state. During World War I, Moore also went to England and France to study the morale of the American Expeditionary Force. On balance, then, all of his assignments helped the league in its organizing efforts, and Moore entered the years just prior to National Prohibition as a highly regarded dry champion.

His career after the coming of the Eighteenth Amendment, however, also reflected the course of general movement fortunes. At first he stayed active enough, attending two major conclaves on alcohol problems: the Fifteenth International Congress Against Alcoholism in Washington, D.C., in 1920; and the 1922 International Convention of the World League Against Alcoholism in Toronto, Canada, where he was a featured speaker. But as public enthusiasm for the "noble experiment" began to wane in the middle and late 1920s, neither Moore nor anyone else was able to stem the adverse tide. In 1925, he left his position as assistant general superintendent of the National Anti-Saloon League and returned to head the state organization in Ohio. There he resumed the methods that had brought dry victories to the league in the past: direct political lobbying, urging ministers to exhort their congregations in the antiliquor gospel, and bringing out the vote for pro-dry candidates. But the old magic was gone. From his headquarters in Columbus, Moore watched dismayed as prohibitionist support eroded throughout the state; and although the league remained a political force to be reckoned with, by the end of the decade it lacked its former influence. Moore himself was aging by this time and simply did not have the personal reserves of energy that had carried him through the battles of the previous years. Finally, in 1932, he gave up his personal crusade and retired—the victory of

Franklin D. Roosevelt in the presidential election, and thus the sure repeal of National Prohibition, perhaps being the last straw for the old campaigner. Nor did he long outlive the Eighteenth Amendment, as he died in 1935 at age seventy-four.

**Bibliography:**

A. With James Cannon, Jr., *Official Report of Special Commissioners (of the Anti-Saloon League of America) to Great Britain and France...Vital Facts About Vice and Drinking Amongst U.S. Soldiers Abroad, with Special Recommendations* (Westerville, OH, 1918).

B. SEAP 4, 1817–18; WW 1, 859.

**MOORE, Henrietta Greer**    (2 September 1844, Newark, OH—28 January 1940, Pasadena, CA). *Education*: private tutoring, 1850s. *Career*: teacher and school principal, OH, beginning 1859; ordained, Universalist Church, 1891; minister, Church of the Good Shepherd, Springfield, OH, and Church of Divine Love, Dayton, OH, 1891–1904; lecturer, National WCTU, 1885–95; trustee, American Temperance Univ., Harriman, TN, 1893.

Active in the Temperance Movement for almost seven decades, Henrietta Greer Moore was as dedicated a prohibitionist as ever took up the cause. A gifted young woman, she had some education in Ohio public schools and with private tutors but lacked the means to pursue formal secondary studies. Nevertheless, she began teaching at age fifteen and several years later worked as a school principal. She was also active in religious affairs. Moore, who never married, became a mainstay of the regional Universalist Church, for years serving with the Women's Universalist Missionary Association and as a trustee of the denomination's Buchtel College in Akron, Ohio. Her interest in work with the young (demonstrated through her teaching) and her deep spirituality found Moore receptive to the message of the post–Civil War antiliquor reform. The liquor traffic, or so went the arguments of the 1870s, posed a direct threat to the American home, the nation's families and children, and consequently the very moral fiber of the republic. Thus when the Woman's Crusade exploded across Ohio—and then much of the rest of the country—with its appeals to Christian concern for the sanctity of the family and the preservation of the public welfare, Moore was quick to enlist. Throughout 1873 and 1874 she marched with the bands of women praying in front of saloons and putting the alleged evils of drink under the spotlight of national publicity. When the crusade coalesced into the more formally organized Woman's Christian Temperance Union in late 1874, Moore stayed with the movement as secretary of the Ohio chapter of the new group. She was soon to emerge as one of the most energetic reformers ever to serve under the WCTU banner.

Moore balanced her temperance work with a continuing commitment to the Universalist Church. Indeed, in 1891 she was ordained and for the next thirteen years had the simultaneous charge of pulpits in two Ohio towns. Making her home in one of them, Springfield, Reverend Moore carried her zeal for the battle against alcohol into local politics. In a staunchly Republican area, she ran for a seat on the school board in 1895 as a member of the Prohibition Party, winning the endorsement of the Populists as well. To the joy of her party, which seldom fielded winning candidates, she carried the vote over two male opponents, becoming the first woman elected to such a post in the town's history. She remained active in the party for years thereafter and was acknowledged as one of its most effective champions. During these years Moore also proved an indefatigable lecturer for the National WCTU. In fact, between 1885 and 1895 her itinerary was extraordinary. She traveled some 150,000 miles, with speaking engagements in every state and territory in the continental United States and in most of the Canadian provinces. In all, she gave around 3,200 speeches, damning the "demon rum" and praising the merits of prohibition and woman's suffrage. It was a public speaking record that few other temperance workers ever matched. For a year (1893) she added to her busy schedule duties as a trustee of the short-lived American Temperance University in Harriman, Tennessee; and throughout the 1890s and 1900s she was president of the largest suffrage organization in Ohio. By the 1920s, however, with the victories of her chosen reform—temperance and suffrage—Moore ended her days as an active crusader. She had fought the good fight well into her seventies, and she retired to the warmer climate of California to spend the later part of her ninety-six years.

**Bibliography:**

B. SEAP 4, 1818; WW 1, 860.

**MORROW, George Washington** (27 May 1863, Champaign Co., IL—24 June 1934, Detroit, MI). *Education*: graduated from Christian Biblical Inst., NY, 1889; D.D. (honorary), Defiance Coll., OH, 1915. *Career*: ordained in "Christian" ministry, 1889; minister, St. Johnsville, NY, 1889–90; minister, Randolph, VT, 1891–99; superintendent, Vermont Anti-Saloon League, 1899–1905; superintendent, Michigan Anti-Saloon League, 1905–13; secretary, Anti-Saloon League of America, 1913–21; national lecturer, Anti-Saloon League of America, 1922–25; lecturer, World's League Against Alcoholism, beginning 1915.

Active over a period of more than a quarter century in temperance work, George W. Morrow brought the evangelical zeal of his religion to the aid of the antiliquor crusade. Ordained a "Christian" minister in 1889, he held three pastorates in New York State and Vermont, where he was active in interdenominational affairs. His primary interest, however, seems to have been the liquor question, as he left the pulpit for full time service in the Temperance Movement when the opportunity presented itself in 1899. That year, he joined the Vermont branch of the Anti-Saloon League, newly organized in the state, as superintendent. Using the contacts he had established as a minister, he was able to link many congregations around the Granite State into an effective voting bloc against the liquor traffic. Indeed, Morrow did so well that National League authorities chose him for the tougher job of leading the prohibitionist fight in Michigan, where wet strength was considerable. At the head of the Michigan League he began a step-by-step assault on the traffic and orchestrated one of the movement's classic local-option campaigns. From 1905 to 1913, the former pastor supervised the growth of dry counties from one to thirty-four, a process which included the closing of almost two thousand saloons. This performance secured his reputation with the National League, which called him to work as league secretary and as a lecturer. He toured the country several times, berating the liquor traffic (which was supposedly dying when Morrow was lecturing in the 1920s) and exhorting the populace on the benefits of the Eighteenth Amendment. On his travels, he spoke with some of the giants of the dry reform, including John G. Woolley,* William ("Pussyfoot") Johnson,* William Jennings Bryan,* and Richmond P. Hobson.* Morrow also won an appointment from the governor of Michigan to represent the state at the International Convention of the World's League Against Alcoholism in Toronto, Canada, in 1922. Later, he lectured on behalf of the World's League. In retrospect, Morrow was never a temperance leader of originality or statesmanlike reputation. But he was active and diligent, and his career exemplified the importance of good field leaders in the battle against the traffic. Morrow was a fine local organizer who brought results; and repeated across the nation in other regional campaigns, his story told a good deal of how, at least for a time, the Anti-Saloon League swept its opposition before it.

**Bibliography:**

B. SEAP 4, 1826; WW 1, 869.

**MOTT, Lucretia Coffin**   (3 January 1793, Nantucket, MA—11 November 1880, Roadside, PA). *Career*: minister, Society of Friends, PA, 1818–20; Hicksite group, Society of Friends, 1821–80; president, Philadelphia Female Anti-Slavery Society, beginning 1833; president, American Equal Rights Association, 1866–69.

One of the pioneer women reformers in American history, Lucretia Mott (born Coffin) was born on Nantucket Island, Massachusetts, a descendant of one of the original purchasers of the island. Her life combined deep piety with a zealous determination to serve others and to right society's wrongs. It was an activism born of her Quaker faith. Mott had begun preaching in meeting, becoming an "acknowledged minister" in 1818. In 1821, however, she and her husband broke with their orthodox society to join the more liberal meeting of Elias Hicks, who emphasized good works and the daily application of Christian teachings rather than theology. In keeping with this view, Mott became directly involved in reform causes ranging from antislavery and temperance to women's rights and world peace. She played an especially distinguished role in the fight against slavery, a subject on which she preached widely throughout the antebellum period. A friend of William Lloyd Garrison,* Mott also stood for immediate emancipation, opposition to the fugitive slave acts, and, after the Civil War, a continuing commitment to the civil rights of the blacks. The Quaker minister fought just as hard for the rights of women. She had been personally affronted when a London antislavery convention in 1840 refused to seat her and other women delegates from the United States; she had also seen women teachers paid half the salary of men simply because they were women. Allowed equality in the Quaker meeting, she refused to accept less than the same status in society. She spoke eloquently and at length against discrimination against her sex, organized (along with Elizabeth Cady Stanton) the women's rights convention at Seneca Falls, New York, in 1840, and did her best to ease factionalism within the ranks of the reform effort itself. Few worked harder or achieved more in her day, and she managed all of it while maintaining a home and raising five children.

While devoting most of her considerable energy to the problems faced by women and blacks, Mott nevertheless paid important attention to the temperance question. As a Quaker, she had grown up an abstainer and a foe of the liquor traffic. Yet her aversion to drink went deeper than the observance of denominational practice. The same faith that drove her to action on behalf of her other causes also compelled her to act against "the demon." She believed in the innate goodness of man, that humanity could be purged of its evils—indeed, that people should strive toward perfection. And if any obstacle stood in the way of human perfection, it was drunkenness as much as the enslavement of blacks or the oppression of women. Temperance, then, was a vital contribution to the betterment of mankind, and she spoke from the heart when she urged her listeners to give up the bottle and to persuade others to do likewise. Mott, however, did not cast herself in the role of temperance leader. Her services to the cause were substantial and her sympathies for it deep, but she never assumed the organizational responsibilities in the battle against drink that she took on in the abolitionist and feminist reforms. The dry rank and file, though, always considered Mott one of their own, and justifiably so. For she characterized much of the perfectionist strain in the early Temperance Movement, and her reputation as a faithful champion of virtue always reflected credit on any cause she espoused.

### Bibliography:

A. *The Liberty Bell* (Barton, PA, 1846); *Discourse on Woman...* (Philadelphia, 1849); *A Sermon to the Medical Students...* (Philadelphia, 1849); *Letter to William Lloyd Garrison* (Roadside, PA, 1876?); *Slavery and the "Woman Question": Lucretia Mott's Diary of Her Visit to Great Britain to Attend the World's Anti-Slavery Convention of 1840*, ed. Frederick B. Tolles (Haverford, PA, 1952).

B. DAB 13, 288–90; DARB, 319–20; NAW 2, 592–95; SEAP 4, 1828–29; WW H, 441; Otelia Cromwell, *Lucretia Mott* (Cambridge, 1958); Anna D. Hallowell, ed., *James and Lucretia Mott: Life and Letters* (Boston, 1884); Lloyd C. M. Hare, *The Greatest American Woman: Lucretia Mott* (New York, 1937).

**MOTT, Valentine** (20 August 1785, Glen Cove, NY—26 April 1865, New York, NY). *Education*: studied medicine in office of Dr. Valentine Seaman, NY, 1804–7; M.D., Medical Dept. of Columbia Coll., 1806; studied medicine with Dr. Astley Cooper, London, and in Edinburgh, Scotland, 1807–9. *Career*: medical practice, New York City, beginning 1809; professor of surgery, Columbia Coll. (merged with Coll. of Physicians and Surgeons after 1813), 1811–26, 1830–35; co-editor, *Medical Magazine*, 1814–15; co-editor, *Medical and Surgical Reporter*, 1818–20; founder and faculty member, Rutgers Medical Coll., 1826–30; travel in Europe, Africa, and Asia, 1835–41; professor of surgery and surgical anatomy, Univ. of City of New York, 1841–50; European travel, 1850–52; professor emeritus (although with teaching assignments), Coll. of Physicians and Surgeons, 1852–65; president, New York State Inebriate Asylum, 1861–65.

Well educated, humane, widely-traveled, and a dedicated teacher, by all accounts Valentine Mott was one of the most brilliant surgeons of his time. Over his long and distinguished career, Mott was credited with introducing numerous innovative surgical techniques, including pioneering approaches to combatting aneurism and dealing with vein surgery and amputation problems. He operated nearly a thousand times—more operations, by one contemporary estimate, than any surgeon in local memory. His reputation was such that the famous sought his services with some frequency: At one point, while on vacation in Europe, he was asked to operate on the Sultan of Turkey. Mott began his practice before the introduction of anesthesia into surgery in the 1840s. He was quick, however, to recognize its value, and he rapidly became a leading authority on its use. During the Civil War, he employed his expertise on behalf of the national Sanitary Commission, writing a report on *Pain and Anaesthetics* (1862) in order to bring Union army doctors up to date on the subject. Throughout his years as a surgeon, he was also a leader in medical education, helping to found two medical schools, including that of the University of the City of New York. And in his long association with the College of Physicians and Surgeons of Columbia University, he taught hundreds of medical students. Vigorous and innovative into his old age, he taught until the end of his life and was still operating only days before his death. Ever anxious to serve his colleagues, he left his personal medical library, one of the finest in the East, to the profession.

Reflective of Mott's surgical innovations was his receptiveness to new medical ideas. His views on the problems posed by intemperance were a prime example in this regard. The great physician was an early advocate of the disease conception of alcoholism, and he found the time to explore actively treatment ideas. As early as 1845, he endorsed the plans of Dr. Joseph E. Turner* to hospitalize alcoholics in special asylums. He also spoke in favor of Turner's theories on the physical effects of alcohol. When Turner began his campaign for state support for a New York Inebriate Asylum, Mott publicly lobbied for the plan, and his influence was telling. The legislature issued a charter, and Mott assisted in the organization of the new institution at Binghamton, sitting as president from 1861 to 1865. No medical facility, he proclaimed at the opening ceremonies in 1861, including the schools he had founded, were "ever founded upon a greater necessity." With the asylum functioning, Mott continued to consult with the state legislature on temperance matters. Temperance workers and other reformers sought his endorsement in pressing their measures on the lawmakers, and he was generally obliging. His primary concern, however, was the New York Asylum. It faced operating difficulties in its early years, and Mott was able to secure help from the state to rescue the venture more than once. His death robbed the institution of a needed patron, and in later years it ultimately failed as an alcohol treatment center. Yet the effort—thanks in large measure to Mott's help—had set a valuable precedent, and similar facilities succeeded based on what was learned at Binghamton.

### Bibliography:

A. *Travels in Europe and the East*. . . (New York, 1842); *Inaugural Discourse Before the Trustees of the New York Inebriate Asylum*. . . (Binghamton, NY, 1862); *Pain and Anaesthetics* (Washington, DC, 1862); *On Hemorrhage from Wounds, and the Best Means of Arresting It* (New York, 1863).

B. DAB 13, 290–91; SEAP 4, 1829–30; S. W. Francis, *Memoir of Valentine Mott* (New York, 1865); S. D. Gross, *Memoir of Valentine Mott* (New York, 1868); *Lancet* (London), May 20, 1865; Alexander B. Mott, *Catalogue of the Surgical and Pathological Museum of Valentine Mott*. . . (New York, 1858); J. E. Turner, *History of the First Inebriate Asylum in the World*. . .(New York, 1888).

**MUIR, Robert Valentine ("Father Muir")**    (23 October 1826, Scotland—4 February 1917, Brownsville, NB). *Career*: farmer and real estate interests, 1852–1917.

A Scotch immigrant of headstrong determination, Muir helped settle the Nebraska frontier in the early 1850s. Joining with a small group of other Scots, he founded the town of Table Rock, where he initiated his life-long campaign against intemperance. The town fathers, holding title to all tracts in the municipality, forbade the sale of liquor on any parcel sold by the original owners. Should a buyer enter the beverage trade the sale was void and the tract forfeited to the town. Muir was the driving force behind this policy, which made Table Rock the first dry locality in Nebraska. After selling his holdings in the town, Muir moved on to help establish the municipality of Brownsville, where he lived for the rest of his days. In his new home, the ardent Scotsman proved as bitter a foe of drink as ever. He fought not only to keep Brownsville dry but also to carry the antiliquor banner to other parts of the territory. He became a noted speaker on temperance questions, and eastern Nebraska newspapers frequently carried his literary assaults on the "demon rum." Zealous and tireless, the crusader sustained his attacks for well over fifty years, earning the sobriquet "Father Muir" from two generations of prohibitionists. He was anything but fatherly toward the traffic, however, as his attacks on the saloon and wets dripped with venom. Some of his diatribes even rage of a crude nativism (a real irony from the pen of an immigrant) as he lashed out at the signers of a wet petition: Among them, Muir noted, were "foreigners who" brought "their debauched ideas from Europe." He helped lead the fight for prohibition in Nebraska, which became part of the state constitution shortly before his death in 1917 (although the measure did not become effective until three months later). A dedicated if caustic reformer, Muir's career demonstrated the continuing presence of the antiliquor crusade in the settling of the American frontier and its enduring influence as stability and development came to the Great Plains.

**Bibliography:**

B. SEAP 4, 1833–34.

**MUNNS, Margaret Cairns**   (10 August 1870, Fairbury, IL—3 September 1957, Burlingame, CA?). *Education*: studied at Colfax Coll., WA, 1887–90; A.B., California Coll., 1891; M.A., California Coll., 1894. *Career*: schoolteacher, Vancouver and Snohomish, WA, 1891–95; various local WCTU offices, WA, 1891–95, 1899–1915; part-time teaching, Seattle, WA, 1899–1915; treasurer, National WCTU, 1915–46; treasurer, World's WCTU, 1925–53.

The career of Margaret Munns demonstrates something of how the Woman's Christian Temperance Union was able to manage its internal affairs and to project its influence so effectively in the years leading to National Prohibition. It may also hint, however, at one of the reasons why the WCTU was unable to maintain its membership and power in the years following the end of the "noble experiment." Like a number of other WCTU leaders, Munns (born Cairns) had considerable experience as an educator, which evidently served to heighten her interest in social problems and reform. She was also a confirmed total abstainer, and after completing her college studies (1891) she joined the West Washington chapter of the WCTU. Within the organization she discovered talents of working effectively with others and local leadership, and Cairns (she was not yet married) shortly rose to the presidency of the local union and to the office of treasurer in the county unit. In 1895, her marriage to Horace Munns interrupted her growing antiliquor involvement. The new couple moved to California, but Mrs. Munns returned to Washington after the death of her husband in 1899, settling in Seattle. She returned to the WCTU as well, once more becoming an officer in both the local and county organizations. She worked continuously with these groups, helping to plan their activities, editing their publication (*White Ribbon Bulletin*), and providing continuity of leadership until 1915, when she left to become treasurer of the National WCTU. While Munns was also active in the affairs of the state and city Federation of Women's Clubs (1911–15) and taught classes in parliamentary law, the WCTU had otherwise become a full-time career, and she had advanced steadily up the ladder of responsibility.

At the national level, Munns proved fully up to her job and gradually assumed other duties as well. For several years, she held the superintendency of the WCTU's Department of Institutes, in which she arranged special lectures and training for the organization's personnel. Still later (1925), she was elected treasurer of the World's WCTU, an office she held until 1953. In many ways, Munns was a fairly typical WCTU national leader: She had a proven local and state record before holding a post with national headquarters, and she brought a long-term commitment to the group. Women like Margaret Munns, in other words, knew their jobs—they were in fact skilled reform administrators—and they provided a stable core of leadership. Turnover in key offices was not especially rapid: Munns, for example, was national treasurer until 1946, and world treasurer for well over twenty-five years. In the struggle for National Prohibition, this experienced and tried leadership was a reform advantage that wets could not immediately match. After the Eighteenth Amendment became law, however, and the battle to enforce it grew in intensity over the later 1920s, the continuity in leadership may have proved a two-edged sword. By then, the opposition had put able spokesmen in the field as well, individuals who exploited every weakness they could find in the "noble experiment." On the other hand, temperance workers, who had long held the initiative in the debate over the liquor, seemed unable to adjust to the counterattack or to changing public perceptions of Prohibition. Too many reformers relied on old ideas, insisted on rigid adherence to dry statutes in spite of some glaring weaknesses and inequities in the enforcement effort, or failed to convince the public that the cause deserved undiminished support. Whether new blood in temperance leadership could have stemmed the wet tide, or at least have compromised with it, is open to serious question; but the fact remains that most important temperance leaders, like Munns, did not make way for new ideas or personnel and remained in office as the nation grew increasingly frustrated with the Volstead Act. Even after Repeal, WCTU leadership gave little sign that it was aware of how far from public favor it had fallen. Perhaps, after having given so much to the organization and to the cause, Munns and others like her felt they had nowhere else to go, so they hung on long after they were capable of keeping vitality in the movement.

**Bibliography:**

B. SEAP 4, 1835–36; WW 3, 625.

**MURPHY, Francis**   (24 April 1836, Wexford, Ireland—30 June 1907, Los Angeles, CA). *Career*: itinerant laborer, 1852–56; farm hand, NY, 1856–61; enlisted man, Union army, 1861–64; proprietor, Bradley Hotel, Portland, ME, 1865–70; prison, 1870; temperance evangelist, beginning 1871; chaplain, Fifth Pennsylvania Volunteers (Spanish-American War duty), 1898.

One of the most celebrated evangelists of his day, and certainly one of the best-known temperance spokesmen, Francis Murphy was born, raised, and educated in Ireland. Although he was widely acclaimed in his later years, his road to prominence was long and hard. His formal schooling was limited to the parish schoolhouse, an experience which he was later to claim was "far from happy." While still a youngster he left school to work for his family's landlord, which he found more to his liking. His chief ambition, however, was to leave Ireland and make his fortune in the United States. This he did when he was sixteen years old, by which time, he later recalled, he already had acquired the "cursed habit of drink." In the United States, the young immigrant found, as most did, that the streets were not paved with gold. He made no fortune to send home to his mother (his announced intention); instead, he eked out a meager existence as a transient laborer in New York State. And a good deal of the little he earned went toward drink as he and fellow Irish frequently continued some of the heavy drinking they had known in the old country. At eighteen, he married a New York farmer's daughter, although the couple were separated when Murphy enlisted in the Union army during the Civil War. After his discharge, with the financial backing of his older brother, he became proprietor of a Portland, Maine, hotel. The venture proved tragic. He not only fell to heavy drinking again but afoul of the law as well. Arrested for illegal liquor sales at his establishment, Murphy went to jail in 1870, and the event was to change his life. In prison, he received a visit from a religious sea captain, one Cyrus Sturdevant, who prevailed upon him in a prayer meeting to give his "heart to Christ" and to sign a pledge of total abstinence. Sturdevant, who apparently was a volunteer evangelist, also helped Murphy back on his feet financially upon his release. The family needed the assistance: The Murphys were destitute, and Mrs. Murphy, her health broken, died within months. But once out of jail, Francis Murphy was a new man. He not only kept his own pledge of abstinence but resolved to help others do the same.

It was the start of an extraordinary career. The reformed alcoholic and prisoner gave his first temperance lecture (April 3, 1871) at the request of a group of Portland citizens who hoped his message of conversion and recovery would prove instructive to others. It was a great success, and Murphy repeated the performance all over New England. To his gratification, he found that people— especially drinkers—would listen to him, based on his having experienced alcoholism, whereas the pleas of other temperance lecturers often fell on deaf ears. The situation was analogous to the modern use of recovered alcoholics serving as alcoholism counselors; having "been there," they are arguably better able to deal with those still drinking than are other treatment personnel. At any rate, as Murphy's reputation spread, Frances Willard,* the later president of the Woman's Christian Temperance Union, invited him to give a series of thirty-two lectures in Chicago in late 1874. His reception there was phenomenal, and from that point on the "Murphy Movement" spread nationally. Uncounted thousands signed the "Murphy Pledge" (one estimate put the figure as high as twelve million worldwide), and he was greeted by the great and near great. At the Centennial Exhibition in Philadelphia in 1876, for example, he met with John Wanamaker; while in Britain he was received by Queen Victoria. Yet Murphy took his success in stride. He remained earnest and sincere in his work and was justly noted for his tolerance and personal warmth. While he was a firm Protestant, he never sought ordination (although the Methodists offered it), and he enjoyed working with clergy of all denominations. Murphy was also lukewarm about prohibition, and he never joined in the activities of the Prohibition Party or the Anti-Saloon League. Legislation, he was sure, would not cure alcoholism. Only conversion could, as well as subsequent participation in a Reformed Men's Club, akin to modern Alcoholics Anonymous. Over the years, the evangelist had the devoted help of two of his sons and of his second wife, the former Rebecca Johnstone Fisher, a WCTU leader. His final triumph also involved his family: It came, he related, when his "sweet-faced little mother" journeyed from Ireland to witness the public acclaim of the son she had not seen in years.

**Bibliography:**

A. [Address on Gospel Temperance], 232–36, *Centennial Temperance Volume*... (New York, 1877); *Talks by Francis Murphy*, ed. Lenore H. King (Los Angeles, 1907).

B. DAB 13, 349–50; SEAP 4, 1838–40; WW 1, 882; W. H. Daniels, *The Temperance Reform and Its Great Reformers* (Cincinnati, OH, 1878); Daniel Dorchester, *The Liquor Problem in All Ages* (Cincinnati, OH, 1888); Charles P. Hower and J. L. Linton, comp., *Francis Murphy Gospel Hymns, with a Sketch of the Great Reformer's Life* (Philadelphia, 1877); Rebecca Fisher Murphy, *Memoirs of Francis Murphy, the Great Temperance Apostle, by His Wife* (Long Beach, CA, 1907?); "The Reform Club Movement," 758–69, *Centennial Temperance Volume*...(New York, 1877).

**MURRAY, William Henry**   ("Alfalfa Bill") (21 November 1869, Collinsville, TX—15 October 1956, Tishomingo, OK). *Education*: B.S., College Hill Inst., TX, 1889. *Career*: laborer and farm worker, early 1880s; schoolteacher, circa 1886–91; reporter, *Fort Worth Gazette*, 1891?; editor, *Farmer's World*, Dallas, TX, 1891; editor, *Daily News*, Corsicana, TX, 1894–95; admitted to bar, TX, 1895; legal practice, Fort Worth, TX, 1896–98; legal advisor, Chickasaw Nation, Indian Territory, 1898–1901; ranching business, beginning 1903; speaker, Oklahoma House of Representatives, 1907–9; member, U.S. House of Representatives, 1913–17; governor of Oklahoma, 1931–35; chairman, Oklahoma Code Commission, 1931–35; retired 1935.

The "Sage of Tishomingo," William Murray grew up the hard way in the Texas of the late nineteenth century, and little in his background pointed toward a future role as a temperance champion. When he was twelve, his mother died and young Murray ran away from home. The boy was apparently nothing if not capable and ambitious: During several years as a transient laborer and farm hand, when he worked picking cotton, chopping cordwood, and making bricks, he managed to educate himself and go on to work five years as a schoolteacher while earning a college degree. Years afterward, when he had achieved wealth and public recognition, Murray looked back with considerable pride at his early struggle to make something of himself. (Later, much to the delight of the Temperance Movement, he attributed his success in great measure to his aversion to "saloon beverages or saloon support" for anything he did.) With college behind him, Murray tried his hand at journalism, working with a number of Texas newspapers while studying for the bar. After briefly practicing law he left his native state in 1898, settling in Tishomingo, Indian Territory (later the state of Oklahoma), where he lived for the rest of his life. There he became heavily involved with the affairs of the Indians resident in the territory, and consequently with the economic interests and politics of the region as a whole. He was legal advisor to the Chickasaw Nation and chairman of the Choctaw-Chickasaw Coal Commission. Murray also had his own ranch, on which he specialized in raising alfalfa: thus the nickname by which he was best known, "Alfalfa Bill." His various activities and personal associations gradually made the rancher and lawyer one of the most politically popular men in the territory. In 1906, he was elected president of the Oklahoma Constitutional Convention, and after statehood he rose steadily through the state legislature, the national Congress, and finally the governorship.

Having avoided the evils of liquor as a youth (or so the story went), the mature "Alfalfa Bill" was a consistent temperance man. Over the years, he made his sympathies known in a number of ways and with undeniable political impact. At the Oklahoma Constitutional Convention, for example, he took a strong stand in support of a popular referendum on a dry amendment to the state charter and heavily influenced the committee that actually drew the amendment. When Oklahoma was in fact, as one historian put it, "born sober," Murray deserved a good deal of credit. In Congress, the Sooner State dry continued a firm enemy of the liquor traffic. He worked for the passage of the Webb-Kenyon Act, which sharply limited the interstate liquor business, and four years later cast his vote for the Eighteenth Amendment. Still later, while back home as governor, Murray pledged himself to the active and efficient enforcement of the state liquor statutes and to the ratification of National Prohibition. He saw all of this effort as a chance to foster the industry and thrift—on a national basis—that he insisted lay at the root of his own rise in life. The saloon, he argued, was productive of only waste and corruption. During his years in public office, we should also note, Murray's interests ranged well beyond the temperance issue: He was also a dependable advocate of farmer and Western concerns, as well as something of a continuing student of political theory and religious affairs. He authored many books and papers on these and other topics; thus, in addition to "Alfalfa Bill," he was also remembered as the "Sage of Tishomingo."

**Bibliography:**

A. *The Speeches of William Henry Murray*, comp. A. L. Beckett, intro. Victor E. Harlow (Oklahoma City, OK, 1931); with Anson B. Campbell, *The Presidency of the Supreme Court and Seven Senators* (Boston, 1939); *Rights of Americans Under Constitution of the Federal Republic . . .*, 3rd ed., rev. (Boston,

1940); with Anson B. Campbell, *Uncle Sam Needs a Doctor* (Boston, 1940); *The Negro's Place in the Call of Race* . . . (Tishomingo, OK, 1948); *Adam and Cain* . . . (Tishomingo, OK, 1952).

B. SEAP 4, 1840; WW 3, 628; Keith L. Bryant, *Alfalfa Bill Murray* (Norman, OK, 1968); Jimmie Lewis Franklin, *Born Sober: Prohibition in Oklahoma, 1907–1959* (Norman, OK, 1971).

**MUSSEY, Reuben Dimond**    (23 June 1780, Pelham, NH—21 June 1866, Boston, MA.), *Education*: A.B., Dartmouth Coll., 1803; M.B., Medical Dept. Dartmouth Coll., 1805; M.D., Univ. of Pennsylvania, 1809; LLD. (honorary), Dartmouth Coll., 1854. *Career*: medical practice, Salem, MA, 1809–14; professor of materia medica, therapeutics, obstetrics, anatomy, and surgery, Dartmouth Coll., 1814–38; lecturer in anatomy and surgery, Bowdoin Coll., 1831–35; professor of surgery, Ohio Medical Coll., 1838–52; president, American Medical Association, 1850; founder and professor, Miami Medical Coll., Miami, OH, 1852–58; retired 1858.

Born the son of a country doctor, Reuben Mussey rose to become one of the most distinguished physicians and medical educators of his generation. In addition to his private practice—and his skills as a surgeon were always in demand—Mussey devoted much of his time to medical research and inquiry. He made early investigations of the value of sanitation, the absorptive nature of human skin, and intracapsular fracture. Mussey was also one of the first American doctors to use ether and chloroform as anesthetics, and was actually the first to tie the carotid arteries successfully. His was a brilliant mind, and his accomplishments earned him one of the finest medical reputations in the country while he was still a relatively young man. As a result, Mussey was in great demand as a teacher, and except for the first five years of his career, he was constantly working on the faculty of some medical school, where he imparted his skills to hundreds of medical students over the years. He was honored as few other men of his field were, and his colleagues frequently turned to him for professional leadership. For several years he served as president of the New Hampshire Medical Society, and in 1850 he was elected president of the American Medical Association. Until he retired in 1858, moving to Boston to live with his daughter, probably only a handful of other American doctors could command such respect: When Reuben Mussey spoke, the medical community listened.

To the delight of the Temperance Movement, one of the topics Mussey spoke on most frequently was the liquor question. Indeed, aside from his advocacy of medical research and education, the hard-working surgeon devoted most of his time to expounding on the evils of drink. He was a total abstainer who touched neither alcohol nor tobacco (nor, for that matter, meat), and he urged others to the same course at every opportunity. Moderate drinking attracted his special scorn. It was only the first step, he warned, on the road to destruction. He adamantly opposed the use of alcohol as a medicine, and he persuaded a number of medical societies to pass resolutions against the practice. He lectured on temperance problems for some thirty years, starting long before there was an organized antiliquor crusade in the country, and he wrote voluminously on the subject. His 1835 tract, an *Essay on Ardent Spirits and Its Substitutes as a Means of Invigorating Health*, was for years considered a temperance classic on the medical aspects of alcohol abuse. Nor would the famed surgeon shy away from a professional fight. When the surgeon general of the United States issued an opinion holding that beverage alcohol was a food that could be safely consumed, Mussey replied with a stinging counterattack, *What Shall We Drink?* (1862). He regularly attended temperance meetings and once spoke in London at the World's Temperance Convention in 1846. To the end of his days, Mussey was staunch in the cause, his reputation lending prestige and credence to the antiliquor movement.

### Bibliography:

A. *An Address on Ardent Spirit* (Boston, 1829); with Harvey Lindsly, *Temperance Prize Essays* (Washington, DC, 1835); *An Essay on the Influence of Tobacco Upon Life and Health* (New York, 1854); *Alcohol in Health and Disease* (Cincinnati, OH, 1856); *Health: Its Friends and Its Foes* (Boston, 1862); *What Shall We Drink?* (Boston, 1862).

B. *Boston Transcript*, June 25, 1866; DAB 13, 372–73; SEAP 4, 1841–42; A. B. Crosby, *An Address Commemorative of Reuben Dimond Mussey* (Boston, 1869); J. B. Hamilton, "Life and Times of Dr. Reuben D. Mussey," *Journal of the American Medical Association*, April 4, 1896.

# N

---

**NATION, Carry Amelia Moore** (25 November 1846, Garrard Co., KY—9 June 1911, Leavenworth, KS). *Education*: teaching certificate, State Normal Sch., Warrensburg, MO, circa 1869. *Career*: schoolteacher, circa 1869–75; temperance agitator and lecturer, 1888–1911.

Throughout her crusade for temperance, Carry Nation stood out as a dry spearhead and a highly controversial figure. Her aggressive and unorthodox methods of closing "joints" always gained widespread notoriety and aroused public opinion against saloons; but her violent approach to the liquor question (and particularly her hatchet-swinging image) and the legal complications that often followed hindered her from ever receiving the public support of any national temperance body—including her beloved WCTU. She had a tumultuous childhood. The daughter of a slaveowning family whose fortunes declined steadily during the Civil War, Carry lived variously in Kentucky, Missouri, and Texas until she was sixteen. Her mother was insane, and Carry herself was a semi-invalid, plagued by digestive trouble and prone to religious excitement and visions. When her family returned to Missouri in 1865, she met and married Dr. Charles Gloyd two years later. Gloyd was an alcoholic, and he quickly drank himself to death despite his wife's efforts to reform him. Shattered by the experience (her parents finally persuaded her to leave Gloyd shortly before he died) and deeply embittered against the liquor traffic, Carry was forced to support her physically and emotionally impaired daughter alone. In 1877 she married David Nation, an ineffectual lawyer, minister, and sometime newspaper editor. For ten years they tried vainly to establish themselves in various Texas towns, with Mrs. Nation—now frequently claiming religious visions—often carrying the burdens of family support. They finally settled in Medicine Lodge, Kansas, when Nation became pastor of a local church (a position he soon resigned to practice law). It was here that she emerged as a temperance crusader.

Although Kansas had adopted a state prohibition amendment in 1880, which apparently did dry up many localities, some towns enforced the law only laxly. Illegal "joints" did a thriving business in these areas—and Medicine Lodge was one of them. Vehemently opposed to the drink trade and convinced the Lord was with her, Mrs. Nation helped organize a local WCTU chapter and declared war on the local joints. Along with a companion, she made her first attack in

1899, smashing up a drug store that did a sideline business in illegal whiskey. The results encouraged her to mount additional assaults—a course she believed had both legal and moral sanction. The saloons were in operation contrary to law, she noted in justification of her course, and thus their owners had "no rights that anyone is bound to respect." Besides, she claimed that another vision from heaven directed her to expand her crusade. In her first solo foray, she bombarded a number of Kiowa saloons with a basketful of rocks in June 1900, after which she moved into high gear. She now had national recognition and had aroused the antipathy of Kansans against the saloons; and when she demolished several Wichita bars (including that of the opulent Hotel Carey) later in the year, causing thousands of dollars in damage, her fame became international. Despite jailings after most of her raids, not to mention physical assaults against her, she then carried her program of "hatchetation" (her term, derived from her favorite tool of mayhem) to major cities from Washington, D.C., to San Francisco. Arrested over thirty times, she paid her numerous fines through donations from sympathizers, lecture fees, and the sale of souvenir hatchets. Convinced that she was about the Lord's work, she described herself as "a bulldog running along at the feet of Jesus, barking at what He doesn't like."

Although the fees from her lecture appearances were substantial—she usually attracted large audiences—Carry never sought personal wealth from her crusade. She supported a number of charities, including a home she established in Kansas City for the families of drunkards; at other times she simply gave money outright to those who claimed a need. Additional funds went into the publication of her short-lived tracts, such as *The Smasher's Mail*, *The Hatchet*, and *The Home Defender*. Zealous to the end, she spent her later years lecturing at several American universities and in Britain. More often than not, her student listeners—whom she felt she had a special mission to "save"—greeted her with sarcasm and hostility. She finally retired to a farm in Arkansas, and after her mental powers began to fade, Mrs. Nation spent her last five months in a Leavenworth, Kansas, hospital. While she was alive, her violent methods—though they sometimes inspired others to similar escapades—were matters of dispute; but after her death, few could argue with the inscription on her Belton, Missouri, grave: "Faithful to the cause of Prohibition, 'She hath done what she could.'"

**Bibliography:**

A. *The Use and Need of the Life of Carry A. Nation* (Topeka, KS, 1905, and many later editions).

B. DAB 13, 394–95; NYT, June 10, 1911; SEAP 4, 1851–52; Herbert Asbury, *Carry Nation* (New York, 1929); J. L. Dwyer, "The Lady with the Hatchet," *American Mercury* (March 1926); Robert Lewis Taylor, *Vessel of Wrath: The Life and Times of Carry Nation* (New York, 1966).

**NEWKIRK, Matthew**    (31 May 1794, Pittsgrove, NJ—31 May 1868, Philadelphia, PA). *Career*: dry goods business, Philadelphia, 1816–39; assistant to

Nicholas Biddle, Bank of the United States, 1828–29; president, Wilmington and Baltimore Railroad, with interest in Cambria Iron Works, PA, beginning 1854; president, Female Medical Coll., PA, 1850s?; trustee, Coll. of New Jersey (now Princeton Univ.), 1830s–1860s.

Around 1838 (the date is not certain) the Philadelphia press reported considerable astonishment and public comment upon the occasion of a banquet in honor of Senator Henry Clay. The issue was not Henry Clay; rather, the excitement stemmed from the menu, for there was no alcohol. For prominent businessmen, clergy, and politicians to sit down at a formal dinner without the almost obligatory drinks of the era was something of an event. The host at this affair (which the Temperance Movement chose to look back on as a milestone in changing American attitudes away from social drinking) was Philadelphia businessman Matthew Newkirk, who had neglected the booze in order to demonstrate his antiliquor sympathies. There is no question that the banquet for Clay reflected a growing uneasiness in the public over temperance questions, and by the late 1830s the nation's liquor consumption was indeed levelling off, if not starting to fall. The fact that some members of the country's business elite, such as Newkirk, had been abstainers themselves and were willing to press the temperance cause on public opinion was a sign of the times. Newkirk in particular knew how to make the point. Beyond his dry banquet, he also ended the practice of "treating" (with alcohol) his customers in his dry goods business, going so far as to publicly destroy his stocks of liquor. He spoke out forcefully on the temperance question for over forty years, beginning as a pioneer of the movement in the late 1820s, and for a considerable period served as president of the Pennsylvania Temperance Society. When he decided that coffee, tea, and lemonade were better drinks than liquor for banquet guests, then, he was acting fully in character.

Yet Newkirk's reform sympathies reflected more than a personal preference for abstinence. As the nineteenth century advanced, more than views on drinking in social life was in flux. The problems of intemperance in an industrializing workplace were also becoming evident for the first time. The everyday workings of business and industry, many Americans became convinced, were more vulnerable to the effects of drinking problems than was the agricultural economy. Certainly Newkirk thought so. When he poured out his liquor and stopped treating, he was making an economic as well as a personal statement—he was protecting the efficiency and productivity of his business. Later, when he became head of the Wilmington and Baltimore Railroad, he saw the dangers of alcohol problems in even bolder relief: The consequences of having a brakeman or an engineer intoxicated on the job were too appalling to ignore, and Newkirk supported vigorous regulations against employees drinking while on duty. In this respect, he was fully in accord with a great many other railroad executives of the era. (We should note that, as well as pioneering safety regulations, Newkirk was the man who instituted the modern system of railroad baggage checking.) Indeed, the economic and safety arguments, which became standard Temperance Movement messages over the 1840s and 1850s, made believers of many of

America's rising industrial leaders. Newkirk never expressed any doubts on the subject, and he used whatever forum he could to express his opinion (thus the Henry Clay banquet). As a longtime presiding elder in the Presbyterian Church, he also worked to keep his denomination in the vanguard of temperance activity. In Matthew Newkirk, then, we see the rise of the view that temperance was not only necessary to public and personal health and morality but also an economic imperative if the new industrial society was ever going to be a fit place to live.

**Bibliography:**

B. SEAP 4, 1914; WW 1, 1347; *A Memorial of Matthew Newkirk* (Philadelphia, 1869).

**NEWMAN, Angelina French Thurston Kilgore**    (4 December 1837, Montpelier, VT—15 April 1910, Lincoln, NB). *Education*: studied at Lawrence Univ., WI, 1857–58. *Career*: schoolteacher, VT, circa 1850–51; Western secretary, Women's Foreign Missionary Society, Methodist Episcopal Church, 1871–79; superintendent of prison and jail work, National WCTU, 1870s–1900s; secretary, Mormon Bureau, Woman's Home Missionary Society, 1880s–1890s; lobbyist for interests concerning Utah women, Washington, DC, 1885–91; military hospital inspector, Hawaii, circa 1899.

Having moved with her family from Vermont to Wisconsin when she was fifteen years old, young Angelina ("Angie") Thurston married Frank Kilgore in 1856, only to see him die several months later. Marrying David Newman in 1859, she eventually set up home with him in Lincoln, Nebraska, where the couple moved in 1871. These had not been easy years for Mrs. Newman. In addition to the moves and the death of her first husband, she had also suffered from a debilitating disease since 1862, which medical attention had proved unable to help. Yet, as the story was recounted later, after long years of prayer she recovered through what she firmly believed was divine intervention. Thereafter, it was not surprising to find Newman devoting much of her time to church affairs, and she was an enthusiastic member of the Methodist Women's Foreign Missionary Society. As she helped direct the operations of this group, however, she quickly discovered that some of the best opportunities for mission work existed not overseas but much closer to home, in Utah Territory. Newman professed horror at the polygamous marriages condoned by the Mormons and expressed a special concern for the rights and condition of Mormon women. The Mormon Church, the charged, had degraded them by the "substitution of the *Harem* for the *Home*." Utah, she insisted, was as fertile a field for conversion as the Orient. (Newman habitually referred to the inhabitants of Salt Lake City as "foreign.") As an officer in the Woman's Home Missionary Society and as superintendent of the Mormon Department of the Woman's Christian Temperance Union, she conducted a highly visible campaign against polygamy throughout the 1880s (the practice was illegal under federal law as of 1882, but the Mormon Church renounced it only in 1890). As part of this effort, she was a prominent contributor to the Home Missionary Society's official publication, the *Heathen Woman's Friend*, and a central figure in a successful lobbying effort to obtain federal funding for a home to support "refugee" Mormon wives and their children.

Throughout her years of activity on behalf (as she saw things) of Mormon women, Newman had the support of the WCTU. Not only did the union create a special department for work among the Mormons (who, somewhat ironically, were dry as a part of their faith), but it widely publicized Newman's labors in Utah. Newman also headed another WCTU department concerned with carrying the temperance gospel into prisons, serving as superintendent for over a quarter of a century. Her diverse reform activities were reflective of the "Do Everything" policy stressed by the union's president, Frances E. Willard.* Indeed, Willard and Newman were fairly close friends. At one point, the two crusaders led a test of male dominance of the Methodist Church. Both were extremely devout, and in 1887 they were among the first five women ever elected as representatives to the Methodist General Conference, the governing body of the church. When the General Conference actually convened in 1888, however, the ministers and lay delegates refused to seat the women. Yet Willard, Newman, and the others had made their point, and the issue would not die. The Methodists finally allowed women representatives in 1904. Newman continued to speak and write on reform and political subjects (she was an ardent Republican) well into advanced age. She even served briefly as a hospital inspector in Hawaii just after the Spanish-American War. Contemporaries remembered her as tireless, eloquent, and devoted to her work, which she was convinced fully was the work of the Almighty.

**Bibliography:**

A. *A Scene in Salt Lake City* (Salt Lake City, UT, 1884?); *Memorial of Mrs. Angie F. Newman, Demonstrating Against the Admission of Utah Territory Into the Union...* (Washington, DC, 188–?); *McKinley Carnations of Memory...* (New York, 1904).

B. NAW 2, 620–22; *Nebraska State Journal*, April 16, 1910; SEAP 4, 1914–15; WW 1, 894; Laura Tomkinson, *Twenty Years' History of the Woman's Home Missionary Society of the Methodist Episcopal Church, 1880–1900* (Cincinnati, OH, 1903); Frances E. Willard and Mary A. Livermore, eds., *A Woman of the Century* (New York, 1893).

**NICHOLSON, Samuel Edgar**     (29 June 1862, Azalia, IN—17 April 1934, Media, PA). *Education*: studied at Friends' Sem., IN, 1880s; A.B., Earlham Coll., 1885; LLD. (honorary), Friends' Univ., KS, 1916. *Career*: recording clerk, Friends Western Yearly Meeting, 1890–99; Quaker minister, beginning 1891; publisher, *Russianville* (IN) *Observer*, 1891–93; publisher, *Kokomo* (IN) *Times*, 1893–94; member, Indiana House of Representatives, 1895–99; president, Indiana Good Citizens' League, 1895–98; field secretary, Indiana Anti-Saloon League, 1898–99; superintendent, Maryland Anti-Saloon League, 1900–1903; superintendent, Pennsylvania Anti-Saloon League, 1904–10; secretary,

Anti-Saloon League of America, 1898–1931; legislative superintendent, Anti-Saloon of America, 1910–12; manager and editor, *The American Friend*, 1913–17; head of Quaker relief mission to the Soviet Union, 1923–24; associate superintendent, New York Anti-Saloon League, 1926–31.

A pious Quaker minister who devoted long years to the service of his denomination, Samuel Edgar Nicholson was also one of the Temperance Movement's consummate organizers in the late nineteenth and early twentieth centuries. His faith included a strong commitment to the social gospel of the era, and he campaigned tirelessly not only for temperance but also for international peace and hunger relief efforts. Nicholson first became interested in temperance in the early 1870s as a result of the Woman's Crusade, although at the time he was too young to become involved. Later, however, as editor and publisher of the *Kokomo* (Indiana) *Morning Times* in the mid-1890s, he came out zealously for the antiliquor cause. The reform-minded editor took the liquor traffic to task as the major root of corruption and misery in the state. Partly as a result of Nicholson's efforts, Kokomo elected a temperance mayor, who promptly found he could do little against "the demon" because of state laws protecting the beverage trade. Outraged, Nicholson ran for the legislature himself in 1894, won, and upon taking his seat in 1895 quickly became active in mounting legal challenges against drink. Lacking the votes for outright state prohibition, he did successfully sponsor a bill for the strict control of alcohol distribution and consumption. When passed, it was known as the Nicholson Law after its author, who followed it with another even tighter limit on consumption in 1897. While still sitting in the legislature, he organized and led the Indiana Good Citizens' League in an effort to enforce the new laws. Concentrating his activities at the local level (a technique anticipating the methods of the Anti-Saloon League), he was generally successful and emerged with a reputation as one of the most effective dry crusaders in the Midwest.

Thereafter, Nicholson began a steady climb to national temperance leadership. The vehicle for his rise was the Anti-Saloon League, which established a chapter in Indiana in 1898. Nicholson merged the Good Citizens' League with it and went full time into reform work as the Indiana League's first field secretary. Later the same year, the Quaker minister (who throughout these years remained active in a variety of Friends activities) won election as secretary of the national Anti-Saloon League, a post he held for more than thirty years. His talents as a field organizer, however, kept him involved at the state level, as national headquarters sent him on administrative missions to key regions. He did good work as superintendent of the Maryland and Pennsylvania leagues between 1900 and 1910, and as associate superintendent of the New York League in the late 1920s and early 1930s. After World War I, the tireless campaigner worked with the legislative department of National League headquarters in Washington, D.C., lobbying for the ratification of the Eighteenth Amendment, and toured New England in the same cause. His only major time away from the temperance struggle came in the early and mid-1920s. Appalled by the carnage of the World

War, and a pacifist as part of his Quaker faith, Nicholson agreed to serve as secretary of the National Council for the Prevention of War in 1922 and 1923, when he also led a Quaker mission to Russia to combat the starvation then prevalent in that war-torn nation. Upon his return, though, he was as effective as ever. His success in bringing out the vote against wet candidates in New York State won him a rare special commendation from the league in 1926. He supported National Prohibition to the bitter end, remaining one of the Anti-Saloon League's most faithful leaders until his retirement from active service in the 1930s. After Repeal, however, living in Media, Pennsylvania, he largely dropped out of the public eye.

**Bibliography:**

A. *The Liquor Program: The Friends of Prohibition Must Rally to Enforce the Burial of Rum*, Pamphlets on Prohibition in the United States, No. 73 (Westerville, OH, n.d.).

B. NYT, April 18, 1934; SEAP 4, 1982–83; WW 1, 898.

**NICHOLSON, Thomas**    (27 January 1862, Woodburn, Ontario, Canada—20 December 1947, Indianapolis, IN). *Education*: graduated from Toronto Normal Sch., 1883; A.B., Northwestern Univ., 1892; STB., Garrett Biblical Inst., 1892; A.M., Northwestern Univ., 1895; postgraduate study at Univ. of Chicago, 1890s; D.D. (honorary), Iowa Wesleyan Univ., 1898, and Garrett Biblical Inst., 1906; LLD. (honorary), Cornell Coll., IA, 1907, Northwestern Univ., 1912, and Allegheny Coll., 1915. *Career*: schoolteacher, MI, 1878–83; minister, various Methodist churches, MI, 1884–89, 1893–94; professor and principal, Acad. at Cornell Coll., IA, 1894–1903; president and professor of philosophy, Dakota Wesleyan Univ., 1903–8; general corresponding secretary, Board of Education, Methodist Episcopal Church, 1908–16; bishop, Methodist Episcopal Church, beginning 1916; resident bishop, Chicago, 1916–24; resident bishop, Detroit, 1924–32; president, Anti-Saloon League of America, 1921–32; retirement, 1932.

Thomas Nicholson was yet another Methodist clergyman to rise to distinction in the ranks of the Temperance Movement. His years in the pulpit were relatively few, but thereafter he compiled an impressive record as an educator. Nicholson, throughout his career, placed great emphasis on the value of Christian education for the future of the country, and he spoke and wrote frequently on the subject. Indeed, his most important experience as an administrator before his election as a bishop (1916) came in denominational schools and on the Methodists' Board of Education. (He was also instrumental in the establishment of the Association of American Colleges.) The Methodist minister was also a dedicated reformer beyond his work in education. He was always active in the affairs of his church, holding many clerical offices, and a firm supporter of the growth of Sunday schools, foreign missions (he helped to organize the Korean Methodist Church in 1930), and the deep Methodist commitment to the struggle against the liquor traffic. Over the years, beginning with his initial pulpits in Michigan in the

1880s, Nicholson urged all who would listen to the path of total abstinence and prohibition. He strongly endorsed the call for National Prohibition when the Anti-Saloon League began its drive for the measure in the 1890s, and his position as bishop lent added credence to his message. In fact, the league considered Nicholson to be one of its most valuable allies.

Temperance work ultimately allowed the bishop to combine his talent for administration with his devotion to reform in a major position. In 1921, Nicholson was chosen president of the Anti-Saloon League of America, a position in which he served until 1932. For the league, this was something of a coup: The new president was not only a bishop, and thus highly regarded by much of the public (especially Protestants), but he was also an urban bishop. Nicholson's residence was in Chicago, and he later worked in Detroit, all of which enabled the league to increase its base of support in America's populous urban centers. On his part, Nicholson was proud to serve. The office of league president was not especially demanding, as most of the organization's day-to-day efforts were directed by its various departmental superintendents and its permanent staff. The president generally restricted his activities to presiding over national league meetings, representing the group in public, helping to formulate league policies and programs, and overseeing administrative arrangements in support of the superintendents' labors. Nicholson was good at all of this, and his duties with the league did not impinge on his responsibilities as bishop. As a dry spokesman, he displayed a fairly astute grasp of national affairs, especially as they related to National Prohibition. The battle against drink had not been won, he warned, with the ratification of the Eighteenth Amendment. The final victory, which he regarded as the most significant in the affairs of mankind since the crucifixion of Christ, would not come until dry values slowly took hold "down to the last man." It would be no "easy task," and he predicted "greater fighting, I think, than any we have yet gone through." He was right, at least, in the latter observation, although when he made it (1922), he was unaware of the coming debacle for the antiliquor cause. He retired in 1932, the same year that Franklin Roosevelt's election as president sealed the doom of the dry experiment for which the bishop had worked so long.

**Bibliography:**

A. *The Necessity for the Christian College* (n.p., 1904); *Studies in Christian Experience* (n.p., 1907).
B. SEAP 4, 1983–84; WW 2, 397.

**NICHOLSON, Timothy**   (9 November 1828, Belvidere, NC—15 September 1924, Richmond, IN). *Education*: studied at Belvidere Acad., NC, 1840–47; studied at Friends Sch. (now Moses Brown Sch.), RI, 1847–48. *Career*: principal, Belvidere Acad., 1848–55; instructor, preparatory department, Haverford Coll., PA, 1855–61; principal, bookselling and stationery business, Nicholson & Brother, 1861–1924; president, Nicholson Printing and Manufacturing Company, 1860s to 1924; trustee, Earlham Coll., 1862–77; trustee, Indiana State Normal Sch., 1880–1924; member, Indiana State Board of Charities, 1879–1924; active in affairs of Quakers and reform organizations, 1840s–1920s.

Timothy Nicholson may well have held the record for longevity in the service of the Temperance Movement. He signed a pledge of total abstinence at the age of eight and remained true to it for eighty-eight years before he died at ninety-six in 1924. Moreover, they were an eventful eighty-eight years. After finishing his education in 1848, he taught or administered programs at Belvidere Academy in North Carolina and at Haverford College in Pennsylvania before setting up in the bookselling, stationery, and printing businesses with his brother in Richmond, Indiana (1861). He remained in those lines, and in Richmond, for the rest of his life, acquiring a national reputation in the trade. A devout and active member of the Society of Friends (Quakers), Nicholson held a sincere passion for reform and human betterment, which found expression in any number of charitable and philanthropic activities, not the least of which was temperance. Always interested in the liquor question, the reform-minded Quaker was moved to action when the Woman's Crusade spread out of Ohio to the Richmond area in the early 1870s. He took part in crusade meetings and provided the women with material support, as well as heading local committees which circulated prohibition petitions and brought pressure to bear on Richmond's illegal saloons. Nicholson's reform vision found other outlets as well. He had gone South after the Civil War to provide aid for the newly-freed former slaves; and for much of the late nineteenth century he took a prominent part in the work of the Friends' Indiana Yearly Meeting committee. The committee's efforts bore fruit in the establishment of state schools for delinquent boys and girls, a woman's prison, and a State Board of Charities (on which he did good service for many years). Nicholson also donated his time to campaigns for world peace, to reforms in education, and to the governance of Earlham College in Richmond, of which he was long a dedicated trustee. As his biographer put it aptly, Nicholson was a "master Quaker," as service to God and to others was at the heart of his character.

The reform movements of the late nineteenth and early twentieth centuries often sparked considerable bitterness between their advocates and opponents, especially when the antiliquor crusade was involved. Yet throughout, Nicholson was a gentleman, ever courteous, never mean. This was true even as he led the Indiana Anti-Saloon League, of which he was president from its inception in 1898 until his death. In keeping with his Quaker persuasion, Nicholson eschewed the tough talk of many other league officials; whenever criticizing anyone, he preferred, as he put it, "to dip my sword in oil in order that it may heal as well as cut." This trait was not lost on the public, including the wets. When Indiana instituted state-wide prohibition, a cause for which Nicholson had worked hard, he experienced perhaps the ultimate compliment: The following day, a Richmond brewery manager stopped in at his bookstore to congratulate him. While the reformer had put him out of business, the brewer felt compelled to say that "all these years your consistent course has been such as to command the profound respect of the community.'' Thus with his gentle approach and genuine concern for the feelings of even his opponents, Timothy Nicholson was probably one of the few advocates of National Prohibition to avoid the deep-seated enmity of wets that dogged the careers of other temperance leaders. It was in keeping with the pious Quaker's view of reform: He intended it not to smite his enemies but to ameliorate the condition of humanity.

**Bibliography:**

A. *Administration of State Institutions: The Indiana System. . .* (Richmond, IN, 1917).

B. *American Friend*, Sept. 25, 1924; DAB 13, 507–8; SEAP 4, 1984; WW 4, 703; W. C. Woodward, *Timothy Nicholson: Master Quaker* (Richmond, IN?1923).

**NOON, Alfred**   (8 December 1845, Elstead, Surrey, England—28 February 1926, Boston, MA). *Education*: A.B., Wesleyan Univ., 1872; Ph.D., Mc-Kendree Coll., IL, 1890. *Career*: ordained in Methodist Episcopal Church, 1871; minister, various pastorates in MA, IA, 1871–86, 1888–93; president, Little Rock Univ., AR, 1886–88; secretary, Massachusetts Total Abstinence Society, 1891–1913; secretary, National Board of Directors, Anti-Saloon League of America, 1895–1926.

Alfred Noon's career was the familiar one of a dedicated, tireless, and largely unsung activist—the type of worker without whom the Temperance Movement could have done little either locally or nationally. A devout Methodist minister who served pastorates for many years in Massachusetts and Iowa, Noon fully reflected the antiliquor sentiments of his denomination. Little is known of his pastoral career, although his pulpits were most likely forums for admonitions against "the demon," and we do know that he joined the fraternal Independent Order of Good Templars as early as 1866. Active with the Templars for years, he also affiliated with the Sons of Temperance in 1879. With his zeal against drink, Noon rose steadily in the hierarchy of the organization, winning election as grand worthy patriarch of Massachusetts and becoming a familiar figure in the national affairs of the order. In 1912, the Sons chose him as most worthy patriarch, the highest post in the country. In that capacity, he toured the nation (and also made a visit to Glasgow, Scotland, on Templar business), speaking repeatedly on the evils of drink and the benefits of abstinence. In addition, the ardent pastor served for more than two decades as president of the Massachusetts Total Abstinence Society, in which role he emphasized spreading the dry gospel to Bay State youth. Noon enjoyed addressing audiences in the public schools, and he induced upwards of 200,000 pupils to sign a dry pledge. His efforts over the years did not go without notice. Recognized nationally (although never accorded the attention of many other dry leaders), Reverend Noon was welcomed as a delegate to the 1895 organizing convention in the nation's capital that established the Anti-Saloon League of America. The gathering elected the Massachusetts reformer secretary of the new league's National Board of Directors, a post he held proudly through the battles leading finally to the advent of National Prohibition. At his death in 1926, the league, and the Temperance Movement generally, noted the loss of a crusader who exemplified the stalwart service that, however briefly, had made the "noble experiment" a reality.

**Bibliography:**

A. *The History of Ludlow, Massachusetts...*, 2nd ed., rev. (Springfield, MA, 1912); ed., *The School Guard* (Boston, n.d.).

B. SEAP 5, 1994–1995.

**NORTHEN, William Jonathan** (9 July 1835, Jones Co., GA—25 March 1913, Atlanta, GA). *Education*: A.B., Mercer Univ., 1853; LLD. (honorary), Mercer Univ., 1892, Richmond (VA) Coll., 1894, Baylor Univ., 1900. *Career*: public school education in Hancock Co., GA, 1854–74; farmer, 1874–90; member, Georgia House of Representatives, 1877–78, 1880–81; member, Georgia Senate, 1884–85; governor of Georgia, 1890–94; manager, Georgia Immigration and Investment Bureau, from 1895.

Raised in a strict Southern Baptist family, Northen's personal religious and ethical values were strongly reflected throughout his varied career. Upon graduation from Mercer University in 1853, he turned first to education; and both prior to and after the Civil War—during which he bore arms for the Confederacy—he either taught or served as principal in a local high school. He began a rise to public prominence, however, when he took up farming in the 1870s. He became a leader in Georgia cattle breeding and an outspoken advocate for state agricultural interests. These concerns ultimately led Northen to the presidency of both his county and state agricultural societies and, at various periods in the 1870s and 1880s, to run successfully for terms in the Georgia House of Representatives and Senate. His campaigns for governor in 1890 and 1892, as a Democrat, were also marked by strong farm support. None of these activities, however, diverted his attention from church duties, and he took a prominent role in Baptist affairs—at one point serving as president of the National Baptist Congress. He had long supported the dry sympathies of his denomination, and it was no surprise that he sought to give them concrete form during his political career.

A highly respected member of the legislature, and a forceful governor, Northen openly proclaimed the dry cause while in office. His first major contribution to the Temperance Movement was his sponsorship in the House of an Atlanta WCTU petition for a state local option law in 1881. The Atlanta women had labored for months in compiling their document, which contained almost sixty thousand signatures and unrolled to a length of six hundred feet. In a strident address, Northen urged the House to receive the petition—which was then unrolled in the aisles to thunderous applause. For Northen, it was a personal triumph; and when the local option bill subsequently failed, he forcefully argued for it in following legislative sessions until 1885. Then, as a state senator, he saw the measure become law. His support for the measure never wavered in succeeding years, and state temperance workers considered it a milestone. Northen's many interests, however, led him away from active antiliquor work after the close of his electoral career, and he instead pursued projects in Georgia history and agricultural, educational, and religious affairs. But he was a strong proponent of prohibition, and until his death he lent whatever moral support he could to those who championed the dry cause.

**Bibliography:**

A. ed., *Men of Mark in Georgia*, 6 vols. (Atlanta, GA, 1907–12).

B. DAB 13, 564; SEAP 5, 2016–17; WW 1, 904; H. A. Scomp, *King Alcohol in the Realm of King Cotton* (Chicago, 1888).

**NOTT, Eliphalet**    (25 June 1773, Ashford, CT—29 January 1866, Schenectady, NY). *Education*: M.A., Rhode Island Coll. (now Brown Univ.), 1795; LLD. (honorary), 1828; D.S. (honorary), Coll. of New Jersey (now Princeton Univ.), 1805. *Career*: teacher and principal, local schools, CT, circa 1790–94; minister, Presbyterian Church, Cherry Valley, NY, 1796–98; minister, First Presbyterian Church, Albany, NY, 1798–1804; president, Union Coll., Schenectady, NY, 1804–66.

A man of varied talents and towering intellect, Eliphalet Nott left his mark prominently in a number of fields. His diverse interests, coupled with his strong religious faith, were typical of much of the pre–Civil War temperance leadership. He left an early career as a teacher in order to study theology, and in 1796 he received a license to preach from the New London Congregational Association. Serving as a pastor in upper New York State, where he simultaneously founded and operated another school, Nott's clerical reputation grew quickly; within two years he became minister of the First Presbyterian Church in Albany, won acclaim for his manner in the pulpit, and was honored with preaching a sermon upon the death of Alexander Hamilton. In 1804, however, he gave up the Albany pulpit for the presidency of Union College, which he held until his death in 1866. Through extraordinary labors, Nott built the financially-ailing school into a sound institution noted for its academic excellence. An educational innovator, under his guidance Union became one of the first American schools to complement the normal classical curriculum with scientific courses; he also freed Union's students from many of the administrative regulations on their conduct found in most other schools of the period. Nott himself reflected the interests he hoped to build in his students: He became an inventor of note, with over thirty patents to his credit (primarily in aspects of steam heat and power); he remained active in church affairs and remained an admired preacher; and he was a leading national voice in educational reform. As a reformer, he put Union on record against slavery, and he strenuously inveighed against liquor. In fact, he emerged as one of the most influential temperance advocates of his day, and his addresses and writings on the subject commanded national attention.

Nott's arguments against intemperance derived from a number of quarters. As a teacher and college president he was particularly concerned with the impact of alcohol on the young. He also drew on his own scientific background in insisting that teetotalism was a key factor in human health and longevity; and he was among the most articulate in describing the social and familial disruption drunkenness could wreak on a community. This aspect of the problem he found so upsetting that he once appealed directly to taverners to examine the consequences of their business (a tactic which fast became part of other dry orators' stock and trade). Nott became best known, however, for his initiating role in the "Bible Wine" controversy. He became convinced through Scriptural study that the Bible permitted the use of only "unfermented" wine, and that the "wines" mentioned in Scripture thus were nonalcoholic. As other temperance advocates adopted this opinion it sparked one of the most intense controversies the movement had ever induced. Dry sympathizers argued the point among themselves, while wets used the situation to attack the temperance cause generally; and some clergymen, otherwise inclined toward dry positions, found the "unfermented wine" argument theologically offensive (particularly as it related to communion wine). The issue far outlived Nott himself and over succeeding generations continued to produce considerable heat well into the twentieth century. Ultimately, the argument drew in some of the best theological and scientific minds concerned with the temperance question in the United States and Western Europe.

### Bibliography:

A. *A Discourse...Occasioned by the Ever to Be Lamented Death of General Alexander Hamilton* (Albany, NY, 1804); *Miscellaneous Works* (Schenectady, NY, 1810); *Ten Lectures on the Use of Intoxicating Liquors* (Albany, NY, 1846); *Lectures on Temperance* (Albany, NY, 1847); *Lectures on Biblical Temperance* (Albany, NY, 1863).

B. DAB 13, 580–81; WW H, 453; Codman Hislop, *Eliphalet Nott* (Middletown, CT, 1971); Norman Kerr, *Wines: Scriptural and Ecclesiastical* (London, 1881); G. W. Samson, *The Divine Law as to Wines* (New York, 1880); Cornelius Van Stanvoord and Taylor Lewis, *Memoirs of Eliphalet Nott* (New York, 1876); E. A. Wasson, *Religion and Drink* (New York, 1914).

# O

**O'CALLAGHAN, Peter Joseph** (6 August 1866, Mulford, MA—11 August 1931, Temperance, MI?). *Education*: A.B., Harvard Univ., 1888; studied at St. Thomas Coll., Catholic Univ. of America; D.D., St. Mary's Sem., 1919. *Career*: ordained in Paulist Order, 1893; assistant, Church of St. Paul the Apostle, NY, 1893–95; missions preacher, 1895–1903; novice master of Paulists, St. Thomas Coll., 1898–99; treasurer, then pastor and superior of Paulist Fathers, St. Mary's Church, Chicago, 1904–15; rector, Apostolic Mission House, Catholic Univ. of America, 1915–18; rector, Church of Our Lady of Angels, San Diego, CA, 1918; editor, *Missionary Magazine* (Washington, DC), 1915–21.

The biographical legacy of Father O'Callaghan is a most impressive list of offices held and religious societies founded. Deeply concerned since the beginning of his pastoral career with mission and charitable work among the poor and imbued with the "social gospel" of the era, he was a leader in organizing and administering Catholic relief agencies in urban areas. Throughout the late nineteenth and early twentieth centuries, New York, Chicago—both with large Roman Catholic populations—and Washington, D.C., proved fertile ground for his efforts, and contemporary sources lauded him as doing "much to improve the condition of the working classes." An able manager, he supervised the affairs of a number of churches and religious orders during his stays in various cities; and between 1915 and 1921 he also found time to edit *Missionary Magazine*, a Washington, D.C., Catholic monthly. Not noted for theological innovation, his considerable attainments were the results of his leadership abilities and personal commitments to reform within the religious, political, and social structures of the day.

O'Callaghan's involvement with temperance organizations stemmed from his work in other areas of reform. Convinced that urban poverty was in great measure attributable to the liquor traffic, temperance seemed a necessary corollary to his other work. He turned his attention to the Catholic Total Abstinence Union of America and served various terms as its president between 1909 and 1926. He had an uphill fight among his fellow Catholics, most of whom did not share his dry sympathies. While he candidly admitted the difficulties of his task, his spirit seldom flagged, and he was a central figure in building the union to respectable numbers. At the same time, his efforts also helped identify his order, the Paulists, with the temperance (although not necessarily prohibitionist) cause. O'Callaghan earned prominent recognition in non-Catholic dry circles as well. He was an American delegate to the International Congress Against Alcoholism at its meetings at The Hague (1911), Milan (1913), Washington, D.C. (1920), and Copenhagen (1923), and then served as a permanent member of the congress. He was also vice president of the National Temperance Council, and during World War I directed temperance activities in the military. He played leading roles in other temperance groups as well, and the Paulist priest deserves ranking among the most active temperance men of the period. Although the Temperance Movement was often characterized as Protestant-dominated and even anti-Catholic, Father O'Callaghan's role in it demonstrated something of its appeal to many non-Protestant Americans as well.

**Bibliography:**

B. SEAP 5, 2040; WW 1, 910; Joan Bland, *Hibernian Crusade: The Story of the Catholic Total Abstinence Union of America* (Washington, DC, 1951).

**O'NEALL, John Belton**   (10 April 1793, Bush River, SC—27 September 1863, near Newberry, SC). *Education*: graduated from South Carolina Coll., 1812. *Career*: legal practice, from 1814; member, South Carolina House of Representatives, 1816, 1822–28 (as speaker of the House); judge, State Circuit Court, 1828–30; judge, State Court of Appeals, 1830–35; judge, State Court of Law Appeals, 1835–63; president, Court of Law Appeals and Court of Errors, 1850; chief justice of South Carolina, 1859–63.

In what may be construed as an ironic twist of fate, John Belton O'Neall—who ultimately became one of the foremost figures in the annals of South Carolina jurisprudence—was the child of a man who deserted a British ship and probably assumed the O'Neall name to avoid capture. But the deserter's son proved a quick study and after obtaining a college education began a notable rise in society. Admitted to the bar in 1814, and active in politics—he was elected to the legislature when only twenty-three—he received his first judicial assignment on the circuit court in 1828. While on the bench, he took to denouncing both drinking and the liquor traffic, often pointing out to juries the relationships of alcohol to crime and other social maladies. O'Neall's repugnance was apparently first evoked by the steady stream of rum customers he encountered while working in his father's grocery store as a boy. When drunkenness finally brought the father himself to ruin, O'Neall was moved to a permanent commitment. In 1832, at the age of thirty-nine, he signed a pledge against liquor and another one against smoking the next year. He also joined a local temperance society, which became involved with the outpouring of antiliquor enthusiasm generated by the Washingtonian temperance revival of the early 1840s. O'Neall himself earned a considerable reputation as a dry speaker.

By this time his judicial career was well under way. Despite some political setbacks, his thirty-year climb to the position of South Carolina's chief justice was generally steady. Almost simultaneously with his official career he rose to the presidencies of the South Carolina Temperance Society (1841), the state Sons of Temperance organization (1850), and the Sons of Temperance of North America (1852); and for a time he also wrote a weekly column, "The Drunkard's Looking-Glass," in the *South Carolina Temperance Advocate*. Other channels extended his leadership even further: He was active in Baptist denominational work (though his parents were Quakers), served as a trustee of South Carolina College, and took a prominent and forceful role in opposing nullification in the 1830s. In addition to having a natural facility for writing—and he was indeed prolific in essays, letters, and longer works—O'Neall is said to have been blessed with the other personal graces of good looks and a clear voice and eloquent speaking style in which to express his numerous opinions on the law, drink, and other matters wide and various. Moreover, posterity's judgement upon his deeper qualities, his essential motivations, seems emphatically in his favor; he has been described as "a true philanthropist" and a man who "strove to leave the world better than he found it." Finally, it may not be irrelevant to our sense of him that by the age of thirty-two he had attained the rank of major general in South Carolina's militia: Like his efforts in jurisprudence, temperance, and Baptist religion, this suggests in yet another way his powerful impulse to leadership, discipline, and order.

**Bibliography:**

A. *The Negro Law of South Carolina* (Columbia, SC, 1848); *The Annals of Newberry, Historical, Biographical and Anecdotal* (Newberry, SC, 1859); *The Biographical Sketches of the Bench and Bar of South Carolina*, 2 vols. (Charleston, SC, 1859).

B. DAB 4, 42–43; SEAP 5, 2065; WW H, 457–58; *Cyclopedia of Eminent and Representative Men of the Carolinas in the Nineteenth Century...*, vol. 1 (Madison, WI, 1892).

**OSGOOD, Joshua Knox**    (11 November 1816, Gardiner, ME—28 January 1885, Gardiner, ME). *Career*: merchant and auctioneer, Gardiner, ME, 1840 to 1870s; Reformed Men's Club organizer, 1872–85.

Not much is known of Osgood's early years, only that he apparently became a moderately successful merchant and auctioneer in his home town of Gardiner, Maine. He also drank a lot—that much is certain. In fact, it was his drinking that ultimately led to his reputation as a temperance leader. By 1872, his alcoholism had reduced Osgood and his family to poverty; it was a familiar story, with the formerly successful businessman falling from social respectability to "the lowest grade of drunkenness." In desperation, he reportedly experienced a religious conversion and was able to keep a resolve to stop drinking. To save himself, however, was not enough, and Osgood pushed on to help other problem drinkers as well. Working with three friends, at least one of whom was also a former alcoholic, he issued a call for all "occasional drinkers, constant drinkers, hard drinkers, and young men who are tempted to drink'' to attend a meeting in the Gardiner City Hall on January 19, 1872. At the gathering, which was well attended, Osgood issued a general call for individual reform and was chosen president of the Gardiner Temperance Reform Club. The new group soon had more than a hundred members, all of whom related some past difficulty with the bottle. The club was intended to give drinkers a source of mutual support in their efforts to stay dry and in some respects functioned in a manner similar to the modern Alcoholics Anonymous. Soon after the founding of the Gardiner club, Osgood spread the idea across the state of Maine, and his mission was a major success. Within months, dozens of "Reformed Men's Clubs" had enrolled thousands of members, and Osgood, the former sot, was a Temperance Movement celebrity.

With Maine singing his praises, Osgood set his sights higher. Moving his base of operations to Massachusetts, the enthusiastic reformer began to proselytize under the aegis of the Massachusetts Temperance Alliance. He was a powerful and eloquent speaker and over several months was able to found some forty clubs in the Bay State. These new clubs were similar to those in Maine, although there were differences between individual groups. Some admitted women, for example, while others restricted membership to men. A few memberships used their clubs to further temperance politics, while others eschewed politics in favor of drinking issues. As a whole, however, the Reformed Club phenomenon generated important publicity for the dry cause and led to further club activity on the part of still other recovered alcoholics. For instance, Osgood's example paved the way for the work of Henry A. Reynolds,* another Maine reformer who managed to quit drinking and to launch a Reformed Club movement of his own. By the late 1880s, the combined efforts of Reynolds, Osgood, and Francis Murphy* (another Reformed Club champion) had drawn tens of thousands of American men and women into a nationwide network of clubs. Osgood, though, never lived to see the clubs reach their peak of effectiveness: He died in 1885, leaving the growth of the movement to Reynolds and Murphy.

### Bibliography:

B. SEAP 6, 2086; W. H. Daniels, *The Temperance Reform and Its Great Reformers* (New York, 1878).

**OSTLUND, David** (19 May 1870, Orebro, Sweden—?). *Career*: ordained by Seventh Day Adventists, 1897; minister, Iceland, 1897–1915; converted to Baptist Church, 1909; immigrated to United States, 1915; minister to Scandinavian population, MI, 1915–16; superintendent, Scandinavian Department, Anti-Saloon Leagues of Michigan and Minnesota, 1915–19; superintendent, Anti-Saloon League of Norway, 1925–27.

Throughout the many years of the temperance reform, there were ministers who made antiliquor work their special province, often devoting virtually full-time careers to the issue. The dry movement derived enormous benefits from this kind of activity, and also from the fact that some of these ministers selected specific target populations for their proselytizing. Among these was the Reverend David Ostlund, an ordained Seventh Day Adventist minister who early in his career donned a Baptist collar. Born in Sweden, he took his theological training in Denmark and Norway and upon his ordination in 1897 took up ministerial duties in Iceland. It was there that he emerged a zealous antiliquor reformer. He had been a member of the Independent Order of Good Templars as a student, and in 1901 he was elected grand chaplain of the Iceland Grand Lodge. He led the fight against drink in his small adopted land in the pulpit and in front of civic audiences, and he represented Icelandic Templars at a number of the lodge's international gatherings. During his years in Iceland, he also edited and published *Frackorn* (Seed Corn), a family-oriented paper stressing the moral verities in which he further pursued his temperance arguments. Thus when he left the North Atlantic island for the United States in 1915, Scandinavia, at least for a time, lost one of its most enterprising antiliquor crusaders.

If he had left Scandinavia, however, Ostlund did not leave Scandinavians. He settled first in Michigan, which, like neighboring Minnesota, had a large Scandinavian immigrant population. Ostlund's fluency in English and the various Scandinavian tongues made him a welcome member of this ethnic community, which became his special concern when he revived his struggle against drink. Indeed, he wasted no time in that regard. Working with the Michigan Anti-Saloon League, and heading its Scandinavian Department, he labored diligently to win his ethnic countrymen to the side of temperance. While not heavy drinkers, the Scandinavians of the region were not dry either; their European heritage, while disapproving drunkenness, was wet. Yet the Icelandic minister made converts, and when the Michigan electorate voted the state dry after a heated campaign in 1916, the league publicly credited Ostlund with helping to bring about the victory. Shortly thereafter he moved to Minnesota, where he worked in a similar capacity until 1919. That year took him back to Scandinavia as a representative of the World League Against Alcoholism. From that time until 1927, our latest point of knowledge about the man, he held a series of important posts in the Scandinavian Temperance Movement. Beginning in 1920, he was superintendent of the Anti-Saloon League of Sweden, which he had helped to found, and he simultaneously occupied the same office in Norway from 1925 to 1927. He proselytized all over Northern Europe and frequently attended international temperance conferences. One of these, in 1917, brought him briefly back to the United States. During his many years as a temperance leader, he also wrote widely on reform matters, and his two histories of the antiliquor crusade in America were extremely popular among European drys.

### Bibliography:

A. *Amerikas Helige Krig* (America's Holy War) (Stockholm, 1919); *48 Forbudsstaler* (48 Prohibition States) (Stockholm, 1921).

B. SEAP 5, 2026–87.

**OWEN, Robert Latham**    (2 February 1856, Lynchburg, VA—19 July 1947, Washington, DC). *Education*: A.M., Washington and Lee Univ., Lexington, VA, 1877; LLD., Washington and Lee Univ., 1908. *Career*: began legal practice in OK, 1880; federal Indian agent, 1885–89; president, First National Bank of Muskogee, 1890–1900; business interests in OK, early 1900s; member, U.S. Senate, 1907–25; law practice and active retirement, 1925–47.

Raised and educated in Maryland and Virginia, where he grew up in the shadow of Reconstruction and memories of the "lost cause," Owen moved West to make his mark in life in 1879. Settling in Salina, Indian Territory, with his mother—who was part Cherokee—he took an early interest in Indian affairs, which became a life-long concern. He began teaching at an Indian school soon after his arrival, but his capacities as an organizer and administrator soon led him to the front of a variety of political and reform movements—which included advocacy of territorial prohibition and organizing the local Democratic Party in 1892. Upon passing the bar, he served as Indian agent or as legal counsel for the Five Civilized Tribes from the late 1880s to the turn of the century, when he effectively represented their interests in Washington, D.C. In this regard, he was instrumental in securing national citizenship for the Territory's Indians and in bringing the area under the jurisdiction of the National Banking Act, a move many considered essential to the Indian Territory's economic growth. At the same time, Owen also became one of the region's leading businessmen, with interests in farming, cattle, and banking. His prominence was such that when the Territory entered the Union as Oklahoma in 1907 (an event he had worked hard to bring about), the new state sent him back to Washington as one of its first senators.

Owen's senatorial career demonstrated how temperance and other reform legislation often intertwined. Identified with the progressive wing of the Democrats, he strongly supported the program of Woodrow Wilson's "New Freedom." He was, however, considerably more enthusiastic about National Prohibition than his party's leader. He had fought to keep the old Indian Territory dry and applauded Oklahoma's constitutional prohibition when it attained statehood. Indeed, on the eve of statehood Owen had served as an advisor to the local Anti-Saloon League and thus had a direct role in giving Oklahoma its antiliquor status. In the Senate, he supported the Webb-Kenyon Act of 1913, which banned the transport of alcoholic beverages from wet to dry states; and in 1917 he voted in favor of the resolution calling for a prohibition amendment to the federal Constitution. His popularity with temperance forces and other reform groups, however, was not enough to assure Owen's continued political success. In the 1920s the Ku Klux Klan entered Oklahoma politics, and Owen, who opposed the Klan, was not sure he could win reelection in 1924. Under the circumstances he declined to run, although he remained in Washington to pursue a legal career and, thereafter, an active retirement.

**Bibliography:**

A. "The True Meaning of Insurgency," *Independent*, June 30, 1910; "Progressive Democracy," *Independent*, April 18, 1912; "Cloture in the Senate,"

*Harper's Weekly*, Nov., 27, 1915; "The Restoration of Popular Rule," *Arena* (June 1918).

B. DAB Supp. 4, 640–42; SEAP 5, 2089; WW 2, 408; Wyatt W. Belcher, "The Political Theory of Robert L. Owen" (M.A. thesis, University of Oklahoma, 1932); Jimmie Lewis Franklin, *Born Sober: Prohibition in Oklahoma, 1907–1959* (Norman, OK, 1971); Edward E. Keso, *The Senatorial Career of Robert Latham Owen* (Nashville, TN, 1937).

# P

---

**PALMER, Bertha Rachel** (31 August 1880, Graham Lakes, MN—15 December 1959, Evanston, IL). *Education*: graduated from State Teachers Coll., ND, 1903; graduate study, Univ. of Minnesota, 1900s; graduate study, International Training Sch. for Sunday Sch. Leadership, WI, 1922. *Career*: schoolteacher, ND, 1898–1915; assistant to superintendent of schools, ND, 1915–18; superintendent of field workers, State Sunday School Association, ND, 1918; assistant superintendent of public instruction, ND, 1919–24; field agent, Council of Religious Education, ND, 1924–26; superintendent of public instruction, ND, 1927–32; research activities, Research Library of Scientific Temperance Federation, 1933; director, Department of Scientific Temperance Instruction, National WCTU, beginning 1933; head, Bureau of Scientific Research, National WCTU, beginning 1944.

A devout Presbyterian and an accomplished educator, Bertha Palmer combined her love for her church and for teaching in a single career. She began teaching at Devil's Lake, North Dakota, in 1898, before finishing her education. But she completed her undergraduate work in 1903, and enrolled for further study at the University of Minnesota shortly thereafter. In the meantime, she steadily compiled an impressive record of service in the North Dakota public school system. Between 1898 and 1933 she worked not only in the classroom but as an administrator as well, ultimately becoming state superintendent of public instruction. As such, Palmer was one of the most important figures in public education in the West. When not involved with North Dakota schools, she labored on behalf of religious education. Palmer was a central force in the regional Sunday school movement (she even took a training course on the subject in 1922) and for a time worked for the North Dakota Council of Religious Education. For a number of years Palmer was also director of education at her church. At the same time, she was a firm temperance enthusiast as well, convinced of the antiliquor movement's duty to rally Christian virtue in defense of home and community. Given the nature of her religious and professional inclinations, the appeal of temperance, particularly as embodied in the Woman's Christian Temperance Union, was perhaps not surprising in Palmer's case. Indeed, when the WCTU offered her a post in which she could use her talents as an educator on behalf of the cause, she took the opportunity to embark on a full-time reform career.

Palmer's new field was "scientific temperance instruction." The WCTU had stressed it for years and under the able direction of Mary Hunt* had supported a national campaign to have such alcohol education introduced into the public schools. The effort met great success in many areas, although with the coming of National Prohibition—which was supposed to make alcohol abuse a thing of the past—the union put less emphasis on such work. Repeal, however, changed that view, once more raising concerns over what the nation's youth were taught about "the demon." Temperance forces hoped not only to turn back the wet tide by shaping the attitudes of school children (who would, if the temperance forces had any luck, grow up sober and later reinstitute Prohibition), but also fight off a challenge from nontemperance alcohol educators. Supported initially by the Yale Center of Alcohol Studies and later by other groups, new ideas on alcohol instruction began to penetrate the curriculum—ideas which avoided the scare tactics and emphasis on the evils of drink that permeated much of the dry teaching effort. Palmer took over the WCTU Department of Scientific Temperance Instruction in 1933 (the same year as Repeal) and later the union's alcohol research program. She worked hard at devising curriculum materials, lecturing, and trying to interest school officials in the services of the WCTU, which was willing to send members into the schools to teach. For the most part, it was a frustrating battle. Temperance-oriented instruction remained in some areas, but its value-laden content gradually lost favor over the 1940s and 1950s. Certainly it never provided the spark for a rejuvenated Temperance Movement. Palmer, though, remained committed to the end. She never went back to North Dakota and instead took up residence in Evanston, Illinois, home of the National WCTU, where she spent her final years crusading in a lost cause.

## Bibliography:

A. *Alcohol* (Evanston, IL, 1934); *What Is Alcohol and What It Does: An Elective Course* (Evanston, IL?, 1934); *How I Taught Alcohol Education...* (Evanston, IL, 1935); *The Bible and the Use of the Word "Wine"* (Evanston, IL, 1937?); *A Syllabus in Alcohol Education*, 7th ed., rev. (Evanston, IL, 1943); *Teaching Plan for Alcohol Education...* (Evanston, IL?, n.d.).

B. WW 3, 661; Mark Edward Lender and James Kirby Martin, *Drinking in America: A History* (New York, 1982); Gail Gleason Milgram, "A Historical Review of Alcohol Education: Research and Comments," *Journal of Alcohol and Drug Education* 21(1976): 1–16.

**PALMER, Norman Austin**    (3 February 1853, Pataskala, OH—11 November 1926, Allentown, PA). *Education*: studied at DePauw Univ., IN, circa 1884. *Career*: owned farm implements (corn planters) business, beginning 1870s; manufactured telephones of private patent, beginning 1870s; licensed to preach, Methodist Episcopal Church, circa 1885; minister, various pastorates, OH, 1880s to 1905; superintendent, Anti-Saloon League of Minnesota, 1905–9; superintendent, Anti-Saloon League of Kentucky, 1909–23; retirement, 1923.

Born in Ohio, Norman Palmer did his most effective temperance work in his native Midwest and in Kentucky. We know little of his youth or of what prompted him to enlist in the dry crusade; we can surmise, however, that his Methodist faith and the rise in antiliquor sentiments in the region as he entered his young manhood probably helped to shape his views on the subject. At any rate, Palmer apparently was a total abstainer, and he clearly was a devout Methodist. In fact, after some five years of operating his own small manufacturing businesses, he pulled up stakes in Ohio and entered DePauw University in Indiana to study religion. He began preaching about a year later (probably late 1885) and over the next twenty years ministered to a number of Ohio Methodist congregations. Palmer was evidently not an especially distinguished pastor (he was licensed to preach but not, so far as is known, formally ordained), although he emerged as a consistent and dedicated temperance advocate. Indeed, he was regarded better as a reformer than as a preacher, and he readily left the pulpit in 1905 when offered the state superintendency of the Minnesota Anti-Saloon League. There, he proved effective in rallying local churches behind the antiliquor cause, and he was so successful in turning out the local vote for prohibition that the league selected him for a tougher assignment. In 1909, Palmer took the league superintendency in Kentucky, considered a staunchly wet state whose dry forces needed a skilled and firm leader. It was a challenge, and Palmer rose to the occasion. Using the Anti-Saloon League's proven technique of local organizing (starting with church congregations), he gradually marshalled public support for dry laws and then translated these popular sentiments into legislative action. Thanks in good measure to Palmer's tireless and patient work, the Blue Grass State was the first wet state (one that previously had not enacted state-wide prohibition) to ratify the Eighteenth Amendment, and it did so by a sizable margin. The former preacher also led a fight to secure a prohibitory amendment to the Kentucky Constitution and then laws to crack down on moonshining operations. His effectiveness brought Palmer a national reputation in temperance circles, and for some years he represented Kentucky on the Anti-Saloon League's National Board of Directors. With major victories behind him, but with the fight to make the Volstead Act and the Kentucky dry laws fully effective still ahead, Palmer's health gave out in the early 1920s. He retired from the league in 1923, and in 1924 moved to Allentown, Pennsylvania, where he spent his final two years.

**Bibliography:**

B. SEAP 5, 2095–96.

**PARKER, Willard**    (2 September 1800, Lyndeborough, NH—25 April 1884, New York, NY). *Education*: A.B., Harvard Univ., 1826; M.D., 1830; M.D., Berkshire Medical Inst., circa 1836; LLD. (honorary), Princeton Univ., 1870.

*Career*: professorships in surgery and anatomy, institutions in VT, NY, OH, 1830–37; professor of principles and practice of surgery, Coll. of Physicians and Surgeons in New York City in 1839, he had already compiled an impressive and Surgeons, 1870–84.

Parker was one of the most eminent American physicians of the nineteenth century. When he became a professor of surgery at the College of Physicians and Surgeons in New York City in 1839, he had already compiled an impressive record as a teacher and practitioner; and his subsequent career fulfilled its early promise. His practice grew steadily, as did his professional renown as he dealt successfully with some of the most difficult surgical problems of his era. He operated five times for aneurism in 1864, and in 1867 he was the first American doctor to successfully remove an abscessed appendix. Parker was also an able spokesman for his profession: He served a term as president of the New York Academy of Medicine and became a prominent advocate of public health measures. His concern for public health led him as well into an active temperance role. A moderate drinker himself, he believed that alcohol was an addicting poison and that alcoholism was a distinct (and treatable) disease. He lent his support to the growing post–Civil War dry movement and, with the assistance of Dr. Joseph Parrish* and others, helped found the American Association for the Study and Cure of Inebriety in 1870. He served as the president of the new organization, which advocated the medical treatment of alcoholics and drug addicts and the construction of special inebriate asylums for that purpose. Parker's prestige as a surgeon and medical teacher added credence to the association and did much in the late nineteenth century to popularize the disease concept of alcoholism.

Parker's interest in alcoholism treatment led him to endorse the plans of Dr. J. E. Turner* for the construction of the first inebriate asylum. When Turner's dream became a reality in the 1860s with the opening of the New York State Inebriate Asylum in Binghamton, Dr. Parker agreed to sit as one of the new institution's trustees. In 1865 he became president of the facility, which turned out to be anything but a tranquil position. Parker and Turner, who as superintendent was in charge of asylum operations, differed over management practices and over treatment methods. Parker was critical of Turner's financial appropriations and held that patients should receive considerable freedom to come and go while in treatment. Turner, on the contrary, claimed that successful alcoholism treatment demanded strict patient discipline, lest they slip off and resume drinking; he also charged that Parker was simply using his financial criticisms as a cover for a conspiracy to seize full control of asylum operation for himself. Their feud became bitterly personal, and members of the staff and board of trustees were eventually drawn in. In a showdown vote, the board voted to remove Turner in 1867 and finally conveyed ownership of the facility (which was not showing a profit) to the state. Turner and Parker were never reconciled, and acrimony and litigation (Turner sued to overturn the actions of the trustees) dragged on for years. The affair was a serious setback for those trying to establish medical institutions for alcoholics, although it appears that Parker's difficulties with Turner—however unfortunate their results—stemmed initially from sincere differences over how best to cure the drunkard.

**Bibliography:**

A. "A Thesis on Nervous Respiration" (M.D. thesis, Harvard Univ., 1830); "Practical Remarks on Concussion of the Nerves," *New York Medical Journal* l(1856):189; "Ligature of Subclavian Artery for Axillary and Subclavian Aneurysm," *Medical Record* 2(1867):97; "Operation for Abscess of the Appendix Vermiformis Caeci," *Medical Record* 2(1867):169; *Cancer: A Study of 397 Cases of Cancer of the Female Breast, with Clinical Observation*, comp. Willard Parker (New York, 1885).

B. DAB 14, 242–43; SEAP 5, 2104–5; J. Parton, "Inebriate Asylums, and a Visit to One," *Atlantic Monthly* 22(1868):385–404; John Ruhrah, "Willard Parker," *Annals of Medical History* 5(1933):205–14, 376–89, 458–83; Senta Rypins, "Joseph Turner and the First Inebriate Asylum," *Quarterly Journal of Studies on Alcohol* 10(1949):127–34; J. E. Turner, *A History of the First Inebriate Asylum in the World* (New York, 1888).

**PARRISH, Joseph**    (11 November 1818, Philadelphia, PA—15 January 1891, Burlington, NJ). *Education*: M.D., Univ. of Pennsylvania, 1844. *Career*: medical practice, Burlington, NJ, 1844–55; founder and editor, *New Jersey Medical and Surgical Reporter*, beginning 1848; professor of obstetrics, Philadelphia Medical Coll., 1855–56; travel in Europe, 1856–57; superintendent, Pennsylvania Training Sch. for Feeble-Minded Children, 1857–61; service in U.S. Sanitary Commission, 1861–65; proprietor, alcoholism and addiction asylum, Media, PA, 1867–73; superintendent, Maryland Inebriate Inst., 1873–75; proprietor, inebriate asylum, Burlington, NJ, 1875–91.

Temperance advocate and physician, Joseph Parrish helped pioneer the medical treatment of addiction in the United States. After a decade of general medical practice in New Jersey and a brief period as a medical school professor, he travelled to Europe to observe medical conditions and practices there. While in Rome, he was appalled at the treatment accorded the mentally ill, and by dint of his personal intervention with Pope Pius IX the American physician was able to secure some improvements in the situation. At the same time, he formed a life-long interest in psychological matters and for the rest of his career was recognized as an alienist. Following this new direction upon his return home in 1857, he secured appointment as head of a Pennsylvania school for "feeble-minded children," a post he held until the Civil War, when he left for service in the U.S. Sanitary Commission. After the conflict, Parrish's interest in mental problems led him to inquiries on the nature of addiction, especially alcoholism (*inebriety* was the general term of the era). He was aware of the efforts of Dr. Joseph E. Turner* and others to interest the public and the medical community in the treatment of addiction problems, and in the construction of "inebriate asylums'' for that purpose. Indeed, Parrish had done some work himself at the Jeffersonian Home in Philadelphia, which had been founded in the aftermath of the Washingtonian temperance revival of the 1840s. The home, however, was more a center for rest and recuperation and had emphasized spiritual renewal rather than the disease conception of alcoholism that Turner advocated. Yet Parrish became an enthusiastic proponent of alcoholism treatment and was affiliated with treatment facilities for the rest of his life. In 1867, he established and directed an asylum for opium and alcohol addicts in Media, Pennsylvania, where he remained until 1873, when he left to run a similar institution in Maryland. Finally, in 1875 he returned to Burlington, where he opened yet another asylum, and where he lived until his death in 1891.

Parrish's efforts in the treatment of inebriety were extensive and went well beyond asylum administration. He was one of the original members of the American Association for the Study and Cure of Inebriety, and he played an active role in its affairs. The association sought public support for asylum construction and the disease conception of addictions, for which Parrish became an articulate proponent. He wrote widely on the subject and showed a continuing interest in the psychological aspects of the issue. In 1876, he chaired an association committee that launched the *Quarterly Journal of Inebriety*, the nation's first journal devoted to the study and treatment of alcoholism and addictions. Parrish's reputation as an authority in the field grew considerably over the years. By the early 1870s, he was being called regularly to testify before governmental bodies on matters concerning alcohol problems (including, in 1872, the British House of Commons). He was also a firm proponent of temperance. Parrish saw little sense in working solely to treat alcoholism; rather, he advocated the antiliquor cause as a means of preventing drinking-related problems in the first place. The dry movement, in turn, considered that Parrish's help lent it credence in its battle against alcohol, as indeed, it probably did. Despite his concentration on inebriety, however, Parrish never became divorced from the rest of the medical profession. To the end, he was active in any number of other professional groups and maintained a lively interest in the progress of medicine as a whole.

## Bibliography:

A. *Intemperance and Disease* (Harrisburg, PA? 1868); *The Probe: An Inquiry Into the Use of Stimulants and Narcotics, the Social Evils Resulting Therefrom and Methods of Reform and Cure* (Philadelphia, 1869); *The Classification and Treatment of Inebriety* (New York, 1871); *The Philosophy of Intemperance* (Philadelphia, 1871); *Alcoholic Inebriety from a Medical Standpoint* (Philadelphia, 1884); *Inebriety and Homes for Inebriates in England. . .* (Hartford, CT, 1886).

B. SEAP 5, 2107–8, Arnold Jaffe, *Addiction Reform in the Progressive Age: Scientific and Social Responses to Drug Dependence in the United States, 1870–1930.* Addiction in America Series, Gerald Grob, series ed. (New York, 1891).

**PATTON, Robert Howard**   (18 January 1860, Auburn, IL—12 March 1939, Springfield, IL). *Education*: B.S., Illinois Wesleyan Univ., 1883; M.S., Illinois Wesleyan Univ., 1885. *Career*: legal practice, Springfield, IL, beginning 1885.

After being admitted to the Illinois bar at the age of twenty-five, Patton embarked on a career combining the life-long practice of law in the state capital with a diligent dedication to the advocacy of temperance and National Prohibition. He was a staunch member of the Prohibition Party, and over the years he was a six-time delegate to its national convention. But his commitment to the Prohibitionist cause was characterized by a certain failure of nerve, or at least an aversion to involvements beyond Illinois. He possessed a strong local orientation, and he achieved a certain prominence at the state level. He drafted its local-option law in the early 1900s, for example, and he ran for governor on the Prohibition ticket in 1904. Patton also chaired the party's state committee between 1912 and 1918, but he shrank back from seeking national office. It was not that he lacked the support and confidence of others. He was nominated three times for top positions in the national party, yet three times he indicated his reluctance to embark on a national campaign. At the 1896 Pittsburgh convention, for which he had drafted and moved the "single-issue" platform, he declined to stand for vice president. In 1904, after having been elected national chairman of the party, he refused to accept the position. And at the 1908 Columbus, Ohio, convention, at which he acted as temporary chairman (eight years later he served as permanent chairman), he again declined a nomination, this time for the presidency. Whatever the reasons behind his reticence, however, there was no questioning Patton's dry idealism, and he certainly sought no personal advancement through his reform activities.

Patton's career with the party, though, local as it generally was, did reflect a significant aspect of temperance history. In particular, his role in the 1896 party convention brought him a moment of considerable national attention. That year, Prohibitionists fought a bitter internal struggle over the party platform. One faction sought a "broad-gauge" plank: a stance favoring a gamut of reforms including free silver, labor legislation, temperance, women's suffrage, and others. On the other hand, "narrow-gauge" party members resisted the effort to broaden the party's base through addressing other issues: The party would rise or fall, they insisted, on the prohibition question alone. Patton, who had favored the broad-gauge position at first, feared that the acrimony of the debate would destroy the party. Consequently, he advanced the "single-issue" platform, which threw the convention into turmoil. Finally, adopted, it confined the Prohibitionist campaign, with Joshua Levering* of Maryland as its presidential candidate, to the drink question alone. While the measure carried the majority of delegates, however, it failed to heal the wounds engendered by the controversy. Several hundred broad-gauge delegates walked out of the convention, founded yet another dry political group, the National Party, and put forward their own platform and candidates. As a result, the Prohibitionists, never a powerful political force, went down to one of their worst defeats. Later, Patton returned to his broad reform outlook, which he maintained in his race for the Illinois governorship in 1904. But he always hesitated to stray too far from thecentral dry question, fearing even that working with the Anti-Saloon League—which made an art of political compromise—would lead to a weakening of principles. It was an outlook which may have preserved conscience but which at the same time did much to consign the Prohibition Party to the political wilderness.

**Bibliography:**

B. SEAP 5, 2114; WW 1, 944; Jack S. Blocker, Jr., *Retreat from Reform: The Prohibition Movement in the United States, 1890–1913* (Westport, CT, 1976).

**PAYNE, Charles Henry** (24 October 1830, Taunton, MA—5 May 1899, Clifton Springs, NY). *Education*: A.B., Wesleyan Univ., CT, 1856; preparation for ministry, Biblical Inst., NH, 1856–57; D.D. (honorary), Dickinson Coll., 1871; LLD. (honorary), Ohio State Univ., 1875. *Career*: minister, various Methodist pastorates, MA, NY, PA, OH, 1857–76; president, Ohio Wesleyan Univ., 1876–88; corresponding secretary, Board of Education, Methodist Episcopal Church, beginning 1888.

Ordained at the age of twenty-seven into the Methodist Episcopal Church, the Reverend Charles Payne spent two decades ministering to congregations in New England, New York City, Philadelphia, and Cincinnati. An effective speaker and a dutiful pastor, toward the end of this period his good works received due recognition when he was awarded two honorary doctorates and soon after chosen as president of Ohio Wesleyan University, a denominational school. He held the post with distinction for the next twelve years, while also playing an active role in the national and international conferences of Methodism over the 1880s. Payne then returned to the East in 1888, maintaining his interest in Methodist education by taking a post as corresponding secretary of the church's Board of Education, with headquarters in New York City. A deeply pious man with a profound concern for ameliorating the social problems of his day, Payne travelled extensively in Northern Europe, the Mediterranean countries, and the Middle East to observe religious conditions and evaluate other nations' attempts to improve social welfare. Back home, he was drawn to a number of reform causes; but like so many other Methodists, he had a special affinity for the Temperance Movement. He lectured and wrote widely on the liquor question, which he saw at the base of a gamut of other social disorders. At all times, he insisted that the pulpit take the van against the evil and argued forcefully that addressing the alcohol problem should constitute a central part of the Christian ministry. In politics, Payne generally supported the Republican Party, although he grew disenchanted with it over the years as it refused to take a consistently prohibitionist direction. Eventually, the reform-minded minister left the GOP for the Prohibition Party, which, while never a major threat to the two largest parties, at least hewed to a solidly dry course. Once in Prohibitionist ranks, Payne's level of political activity grew apace. He participated vigorously in a number of electoral campaigns during the 1880s and early 1890s. Never one of the chief leaders of the antiliquor movement, Payne nevertheless made effective contributions and clearly demonstrated the dedication of the Methodist clergy to the battle against the "demon rum."

## Bibliography:

A. *The Social Glass and Christian Obligation* (New York, 1868); *Daniel, the Uncompromising Young Man* (New York, 1883); *Guides and Guards in Character-Building* (New York, 1883); *Sermon on the Universal Triumph of Christianity . . .* (Chicago, 1895); *The American Sabbath: Shall It Be a Holyday or a Holiday?* (New York, 189-?); *Duty of the Pulpit Against the Liquor Traffic* (New York?, 189-?).

B. SEAP 5, 2115–16; WW 1, 946.

**PEARSON, Samuel Freeman**    (16 July 1841, Roxbury, MA—6 August 1902, Portland, ME). *Education*: studied at business coll., Boston, 1860s? *Career*: enlisted man, Union army, 1862–65; merchant and real estate broker, 1865 to 1870s; missionary work with alcoholics, beginning circa 1874; proprietor, Gospel Temperance Mission, Portland, ME, beginning 1878; ordained, interdenominational "Gospel" ministry, 1879; travel in Great Britain, 1886–87; sheriff, Cumberland Co., ME, 1900–1902.

Samuel Pearson knew well the evils of the "demon rum." A self-confessed drunkard, he had endured watching his profitable business and real estate interests go to ruin on the shoals of alcoholism. Pearson grew up in eastern Massachusetts, getting a public school education and some business training before enlisting in the Union army during the Civil War. After the Confederate surrender, his business ventures in Boston prospered, and the successful veteran and his bride (he married Elvira Merrill in 1865) seemed economically secure. By his telling, however, a woman friend convinced an otherwise abstinent Pearson to take a drink at a party—an event which sent him on the road to intemperance and degradation. Although his wife stood by him, he subsequently lost everything because of his drinking, which apparently went out of control in 1865. It was the start, as he described it later in a popular pamphlet, of "seven years in hell." His recovery began in 1874 in Portland, Maine, where an acquaintance persuaded him to attend a religious service; it led to his signing the pledge, a spiritual conversion, and a new life as a missionary to the alcoholic. He worked closely for a time with Reformed Men's Club organizer J. K. Osgood,* also a recovered alcoholic, helping to establish a number of such groups in various sections of New England. After parting with Osgood, Pearson and his wife began their own program of "gospel temperance," preaching salvation to the intemperate if they would take the pledge and accept the Lord. The Pearsons were effective proselytizers and in 1878 opened their own modest Gospel Temperance Mission in Portland. It soon became a haven not only to the intemperate but to the poor and sick of the city as well. The fame of the mission spread throughout the region, and in recognition of his labors Pearson received an interdenominational ordination in 1879.

After having run the Gospel Mission for eight years, Pearson's career took a new and, eventually, more militant turn. In 1886, he travelled to Great Britain, where he conducted a well-received dry revival. He lectured to the English, the Scots, and the Welsh and reportedly succeeded in gathering over 100,000 pledges. Returning home, evidently in a fighting mood after his blows against "the demon" in Britain, he accepted the nomination of the Prohibition Party for the office of county sheriff. He campaigned on a promise of strict enforcement of Maine's prohibitory law and won a narrow victory by less than five hundred votes. He then proceeded to do battle with the liquor traffic. Organizing a posse of deputies, the crusading sheriff engaged in a series of nocturnal raids on illegal stills, wine cellars, and caches of hidden booze. The liquor men took none of this lying down. They did their best to smuggle new supplies into the county, bribed Pearson's deputies, and planted informers in the locale to report on his movements. But in his two years in office Pearson was relentless, serving no less than 4,816 search warrants and seizing 6,566 gallons of beer and ale and another 2,987 gallons of whiskey. By the time he was through, drinks were hard to come by in Cumberland County, and fines assessed against the guilty had enriched the county by over $25,000. Pearson's health, however, gave out under the strain of his activities, and he died in 1902.

**Bibliography:**

A. *Seven Years in Hell* (Portland, ME, 1874?).
B. SEAP 5, 2116–17.

**PERHAM, Sidney**    (27 March 1819, Woodstock, ME—1907, Portland, ME?). *Career*: schoolteacher and farmer, ME, 1830s–1850s; member, Maine State Board of Agriculture, 1852–53; member, Maine legislature, 1855; clerk, Supreme Judicial Court, Oxford Co., ME, 1858–62; member, U.S. House of Representatives, 1863–69; governor of Maine, 1871–74; appraiser, port of Portland, ME, beginning 1877.

From his humble origins in rural Maine, Perham advanced through a political career that culminated with his election to the governorship of the state. He showed enough promise during the course of his brief immersion in the elementary education provided by his local public school to be retained as a teacher, an activity he found sufficient energy to combine with his duties on the farm. In his early adulthood, he acquired an active interest in Democratic politics but broke with the party as the agitation over the Temperance Movement spread throughout Maine. Perham's motives for enlisting under the dry banner are unknown, but once committed, he was a firm advocate of the reform. He left the Democrats when they refused to support Neal Dow's* prohibitory measures. On the other hand, Perham considered Dow a genuine statesman and vigorously championed the Maine Law. In order to rally support for the legislation, he not only spoke widely on the issue but founded a temperance society in his home town. His first official duties in public life came with his election to the State Board of Agriculture in 1852. Increasingly, however, he became identified with the Temperance Movement rather than with farming interests. He campaigned vigorously, for example, on behalf of the temperance-minded gubernatorial candidate in 1853, A. P. Morrill; and after the repeal of the Maine Law in 1855, he visited and spoke at some two hundred local community gatherings in a campaign on behalf of the State Temperance Union to spur support for its reenactment. In fact, his role as temperance activist was largely responsible for the further distinction thrust upon him two years later. Not only did he win election to the state legislature, but, largely because of the respect he had earned for his labors on behalf of prohibition, he gained the unprecedented honor of being selected, on the first day of the session, to the speakership of the lower house. Later he served as a judicial official in Oxford County before being elected to Congress in 1862, where he sat until 1869. (He was a Republican, having joined the party at its inception.) Thereafter he was nominated for the governorship of Maine and was elected in 1870. In both his congressional and gubernatorial campaigns he continued to place the issue of prohibition, on which his early reputation was founded, at the forefront of his platform. Following his retirement from the governorship he was appointed appraiser of the port of Portland, Maine. His energies during his later years were given over to a lively interest in charitable organizations and the field of education.

**Bibliography:**

B. SEAP 5, 2135–36; WW 1, 959.

**PHILLIPS, Wendell**    (29 November 1811, Boston, MA—2 February 1884, Boston, MA). *Education*: graduated from Harvard Univ., 1831; graduated from Cambridge (now Harvard) Law Sch., 1834. *Career*: legal practice, Boston, 1834–39; lecturer and pamphleteer on abolition, 1837–65; lecturer and writer on various reform subjects, 1830s–1880s; president, American Anti-Slavery Society, 1865–70.

Born into a patrician old-stock Boston family, whose wealth matched its elevated social standing, Wendell Phillips emerged as one of the most prominent American reformers of the nineteenth century. Called ''the foremost orator of the anti-slavery movement'' by one biographer, Phillips demonstrated his rhetorical skills early, winning acclaim for oratory and public debating while still at the Boston Latin School and at Harvard. After three years at what is now Harvard Law School, he was admitted to the bar and embarked on a legal career whose challenges were no match for Phillips' considerable talents and sense of public duty and whose material rewards paled into insignificance alongside his generous personal fortune. Hence it required no great renunciation of either prestige or wealth for him to terminate his duties of professional advocacy in

1839 by refusing to swear the oath of loyalty to the federal Constitution that was a prerequisite for continued legal practice. This gesture was symbolic, a repudiation of the Supreme Court's constitutional interpretations in support of slavery. Indeed, Phillips was one of the bitterest foes of the South's "peculiar institution." He was an early member of the American Anti-Slavery Society and a zealous ally of William Lloyd Garrison.* Speaking and writing widely (often contributing pieces to Garrison's *Liberator*), the Massachusetts radical not only damned the Constitution but urged a division of the Union, if necessary, to divest the United States of slave territory. During the Civil War, he frequently criticized Abraham Lincoln's moderate policies, and he even argued with Garrison after the conflict over the continuing necessity of abolitionist activities. Phillips insisted that they were still needed and replaced Garrison at the head of the Anti-Slavery Society in 1865. All the while, he had been building a second fortune in lecture fees, to which he added substantially by diversifying his lecture topics in the postbellum period. While speaking on women's rights, prison reform, labor legislation, the plight of the Indians, and other subjects, Phillips also held forth as a powerful champion of temperance.

Phillips was no stranger to the Temperance Movement. He had long favored many of its goals, although he had focused his energies on antislavery in the first half of his career. Even so, as he told the first national convention of the Prohibition Party in 1872, he had been "a temperance man of nearly forty years' standing." Earlier, however, he had not necessarily been a prohibitionist. He was a teetotaler himself but questioned the effectiveness of a legal assault on alcohol. His antislavery experiences, though, had made him more appreciative of the powers of governmental coercion, and by the early 1870s he was fully converted. Indeed, as early as 1870 he ran for governor of Massachusetts at the head of the Labor and Prohibition parties, urging the abolition of the drink trade in a campaign that tallied some twenty thousand votes. Yet he always maintained a distinction (not always firm) between the public and private aspects of drinking. The latter, the reformer argued, was under the realm of individual conscience, while the former fell under the governance of the legal system. "The use of intoxicating liquor rests with each man's discretion," he told Boston journalists in 1870. "But the trade in them comes clearly within the control of the law." A decade later, his views had not altered. "We don't care what a man does in his own parlor. He may drink his champagne or whiskey, and we don't care. But the moment a man opens his shop, and sells, we will interfere." There had to be a complete prohibition of alcohol sales, however, for any regulation was pointless in his view. "License has been tried in every shape," he noted. "You can't execute a license law." He took a similarly hard line on the pledge of abstinence, opposing, in what was later regarded as a classic statement on the position, the views of those less strident reformers who favored moderate alcohol use in socially sanctioned settings. Thus Phillips' views on the "temperate" and "intemperate" paralleled one that saw the "saved" and the "damned." They were hard and fast categories. The latter could enjoy the privilege of resisting salvation if their lack of moral fiber so dictated. The former, however, could entertain no truck with the "devil" alcohol. External constraints, therefore, in the form of institutional safeguards, combined with an internal commitment in the form of the pledge ("a solemn assertion") were absolute requirements. Thus if Phillips was a moral crusader on behalf of Prohibition, it was as much a reflection of a concern for the continuation in a state of grace of the elect as it was for a proselytizing mission among the infidels.

**Bibliography:**

A. ed., *The Constitution: A Pro-slavery Compact...* (1844; New Haven, 1969); *Review of Lysander Spooner's Essay on the Unconstitutionality of Slavery* (1847; New York, 1969); *The Maine Liquor Law in Massachusetts...* (Manchester, England, 1865); *Speeches, Lectures and Letters* (1891; New York, 1969); *Two Sides of One Canvas: The Right of Prohibition* (New York, 18—?); *Wendell Phillips on Civil Rights and Freedom*, ed. Louis Filler (New York, 1965).

B. DAB 14, 546–47; SEAP 5, 2157–58; WW H, 480; George Lowell Austin, *The Life and Times of Wendell Phillips* (1884; Chicago, 1969); McAlister Coleman, *Pioneers of Freedom...*(New York, 1929); Ralph Korngold, *Two Friends of the Man: The Story of William Lloyd Garrison and Wendell Phillips, and Their Relationship with Abraham Lincoln* (Boston, 1950); Lorenzo Sears, *Wendell Phillips: Orator and Agitator* (1909; New York, 1967); Oscar Sherwin, *Prophet of Liberty: The Life and Times of Wendell Phillips* (New York, 1958).

**PIERPONT, John**    (6 April 1785, Litchfield, CT—27 August 1866, Medford, MA). *Education*: graduated from Yale Coll., 1804; graduated from Litchfield (CT) Law Sch., 1812; graduated from Harvard Divinity Sch., 1818. *Career*: private tutor, SC, 1805–9; legal practice, Newburyport, MA, 1812; merchant (dry goods), Boston and Baltimore, MD, 1814–16; minister, Hollis Street Church (Unitarian), Boston, 1819–45; travel in Europe and Palestine, 1835–36; minister, Unitarian Church, Troy, NY, 1845–49; minister, First Congregational Church (Unitarian), West Medford, MA, 1849–58; clerk, U.S. Treasury Department, 1861–66.

If the character of financial mogul J. P. Morgan's grandfather had to be summarized in one sentence, it would be that it was composed of a firm conscience embedded in a highly diffused personal identity. A man of assuredly brilliant but somewhat eccentric intellect, Pierpont successively turned his hand to education, to the law, to business, to religion, and, at the age of seventy-six, to the federal civil service bureaucracy. But far more than any of these, it was from his avocation of poetry and of zeal for reform that he gained his reputation. After completing his education and passing four years as tutor to a South Carolina family, Pierpont opened a law office in Newburyport, Massachusetts. He was less than successful: In fact, he had so few clients that he was able to begin the writing career that continued throughout his years as a minister and reformer.

The unhappy lawyer next tried his hand as a dry goods merchant, and, testimony to his lack of business acumen, found that he still had plenty of time to write. Pierpont finally found his professional niche in the ministry (he was ordained at age thirty-five) and took up the pulpit of the Hollis Street Church (Unitarian) in Boston in 1819. It was during this Hollis Street period that he emerged as a proponent of a gamut of contemporary reforms. He became an ardent spiritualist and believer in phrenology; he advocated the abolition of the state militia, of imprisonment for debt and of slavery; and he labored as a zealous propagandist for pacifism and temperance. As an antiliquor man, Pierpont gained a certain fame as a radical. He insisted early that the Temperance Movement openly declare itself a political effort and that it make every attempt to vote the alcohol traffic out of existence. A powerful speaker at temperance conventions and before popular audiences, the crusading reverend had little patience with timidity in fellow campaigners, and he constantly urged more concerted attacks on "the demon" rather than gradualist reform methods.

Pierpont's reform ideals, however, were not uniformly popular with his congregants. His antiliquor zeal in particular met determined resistence in some quarters. The church members included several liquor dealers, and the congregation also rented out part of the church basement to a rum merchant for storage. In 1838, the minister's enemies launched what became known as the "Seven Years' War" to oust him. But Pierpont fought back gamely, refusing to be shouldered aside and adamantly clinging to his temperance beliefs. Finally, after vindication in an ecclesiastical hearing and earning the respect of many for his pluck, he resigned honorably in 1845. He moved to Troy, New York, where he ministered to another Unitarian church for four years before returning to a Boston-area congregation (West Milford) in 1849. Still maintaining his reforming enthusiasm, he ran for governor and for Congress during these years at the head of antislavery tickets, and his poetry continued its abolitionist and antiliquor themes. Pierpont finally left the pulpit in 1858 at age seventy-three; but retirement, he found, had little appeal. He remarried and in 1861, with the outbreak of the Civil War, volunteered as chaplain of a Massachusetts infantry regiment. He found his strength not up to the rigors of the field, but he stayed active nevertheless. The old reformer finally moved to the nation's capital and took up duties for the last five years of his life as a Treasury Department functionary. It was in the Boston suburb where he held his last pastorate, however, that he died in the late summer of 1866.

## Bibliography:

A. *The Portrait* (Newburyport, MA, 1812); *Airs of Palestine* (Baltimore, MD, 1816); *The Anti-Slavery Poems of John Pierpont* (Boston, 1843); *The National Reader: A Selection* (Philadelphia, 1854); *The Young Reader...* (Philadelphia, 1859?); *The American First-Class Book...* (Philadelphia, 1860).

B. *Boston Transcript*, Aug. 27, 1866; DAB 14, 586–87; SEAP 5, 2161–62; A. A. Ford, *John Pierpont: A Biographical Sketch* (n.p., 1909); O. B. Frothingham, *Boston Unitarianism, 1820–1850* (Boston, 1890); S. K. Lothrop, *Proceedings of an Ecclesiastical Council in the Case of the Proprietors of Hollis-Street Meeting-House and the Rev. John Pierpont* (Boston, 1841).

**PINCHOT, Gifford**    (11 August 1865, Simsbury, CT—4 October 1946, New York, NY). *Education*: attended private schools in New York and Paris; A.B., Yale Univ., 1889; postgraduate study of forestry, French National Forestry Sch., Nancy, and elsewhere in Western Europe, 1889–90; A.M. (honorary), Yale Univ., 1901, and Princeton Univ., 1904; ScD. (honorary), Michigan Agricultural Coll., 1907; LLD. (honorary), McGill Univ., 1909, Pennsylvania Military Coll., 1923, Yale Univ., 1925, and Temple Univ., 1931. *Career*: forester, Phelps, Dodge & Co., 1890–91; forester, Biltmore, NC, 1892; private forestry consulting, 1890s; member, National Forest Commission, National Academy of Sciences, 1896–98; chief, Division of Forestry, U.S. Department of Agriculture, 1898–1910; president, National Conservation Association, 1910–23; nonresident professor of forestry, Yale Univ., 1903–36; Pennsylvania commissioner of forestry, 1920–22; governor of Pennsylvania, 1923–27, 1931–35.

From his genteel patrician origins, Pinchot (named by his father after Sanford Gifford, the landscape artist) acquired not only a commitment to high culture in general (and Francophile tastes in particular) but also a keen sense of the duties that he saw as corollary to the privileges of his inherited position. The best known of these was his life-long dedication to the conservation of America's forests. Before entering government service, he was arguably the nation's first professional and systematic forester; afterward, with the strong backing of President Theodore Roosevelt, he almost singlehandedly created the U.S. Forestry Service and played a major role in shaping policies for the federal regulation of natural resources. In addition to his forestry service, however, Pinchot was also a dedicated Progressive reformer, fully in favor (like Roosevelt) of using the power of government to solve a variety of social problems. Over the years, he espoused government regulation (and sometimes ownership) of railroads, public utilities, mines, and forests; he also advocated the reorganization of government to increase its efficiency and public spending to improve rural life. He was, as well, a firm and committed prohibitionist. In 1912, he joined the Progressive Party in order to back Roosevelt's presidential bid (indeed, it may have been Pinchot who first suggested the Roosevelt campaign credo of the "New Nationalism"); but thereafter he devoted most of his attention to political affairs in Pennsylvania, where he had made his home. Viewed as a maverick by the Republican Party, he established a solid reputation as state forestry commissioner; and when the factionalized GOP could not agree on a gubernatorial candidate in 1922, Pinchot won the nomination by a thin plurality. He went on to victory in the general election, and while unsuccessful in later contests for the national Senate, he won a second term in the statehouse in 1930. To no one's surprise, he was an avid reformer in office, a stance consistent with his previous conduct and his long-held views on the obligations of public service.

Of all of the issues pursued by Governor Pinchot, perhaps none better demonstrated his reform zeal, or stirred more controversy, than his devotion to
National Prohibition. A personal abstainer, the great forester had seen the bottle
as a prime source of all manner of social ills. His marriage to Cornelia Elizabeth
Bryce (1914) confirmed his views on the matter: A firm dry herself (she was a
member of the Woman's Christian Temperance Union), as well as an astute
reformer generally, she became one of the governor's closest political advisors.
The Pinchots publicly announced that their family would keep the governor's
mansion dry and that the enforcement of the Volstead Act in Pennsylvania would
top the new administration's priorities list. It was no idle talk. Pinchot appointed
no one to a judgeship without being satisfied of the nominee's position on
National Prohibition. In his efforts to banish the saloon (one of his campaign
pledges), he also posed a tough state law to combat violations of the federal
Volstead statutes. The State Senate passed it easily, but the Assembly produced
a majority of only two votes. Then the legislature balked, withholding funds
from an enforcement effort for the new law. Undaunted, the governor put the
administrative machinery in motion anyway using monies raised and donated by
the Pennsylvania WCTU. Pinchot was, in fact, one of the firmest political friends
of the Temperance Movement, and even as popular sentiments began to shift
away from the "noble experiment," he never lost the faith. As late as 1928, he
told a dry audience that "notwithstanding all the handicaps, all the treachery,
all the lawbreaking, Prohibition is a blessing to the people of the United States."
While there was no denying his sincerity on the matter, when he had to, Pinchot
made his peace with the man whose election meant the death of the Eighteenth
Amendment—Franklin D. Roosevelt. The Pennsylvania governor recognized the
dangers of the Great Depression and did his best to make the most of New Deal
funds in the state. Still later (1940), he openly declared for Roosevelt as the
man best able to lead the nation in the face of the gathering threat of foreign
war. He never turned his back on Prohibition, but he considered the calamities
of the economy and fascism to have a greater call on public attention.

## Bibliography:

A. *A Primer of Forestry* (Washington, DC, 1903); *The Conservation of Natural
Resources* (Washington, DC, 1908); *The Fight for Conservation*, intro. Gerald
D. Nash (1910; Seattle, WA, 1967); *The Power Monopoly: Its Make-up and Its
Menace* (Milford, PA, 1928); *The Training of a Forester*, rev. ed. (Philadelphia,
1937); *Breaking New Ground*, intro. James Penick, Jr., (1947; Seattle, WA,
1972).

B. DAB Supp. 4, 663–66; SEAP 5, 2162–63; WW 2, 425; Martin L. Fausold,
*Gifford Pinchot: Bull Moose Progressive* (Syracuse, NY, 1961); Martin Nelson
McGeary, *Gifford Pinchot, Forester-Politician* (Princeton, NJ, 1960); James
Pernick, Jr., *Progressive Politics and Conservation: The Ballinger-Pinchot Affair*
(Chicago, 1968); Harold T. Pinkett, *Gifford Pinchot: Private and Public Forester*
(Urbana, IL, 1970).

**PLUMB, Preston Bierce**    (12 October 1837, Delaware Co., OH—20 December 1891, Washington, DC). *Education*: studied law, Cleveland, OH, 1860. *Career*: editor, *Xenia* (OH) *News*, 1854–56; ran arms to antislavery forces, KS, 1856; founder and editor, *Kansas News*, 1857; antislavery political activity, KS, 1857–60; admitted to bar, OH, 1861; reporter, Kansas Supreme Court, 1861; member, Kansas House of Representatives, 1862, 1867–68; officer, Union army, 1862–65; resumed legal practice, 1865; founder and officer, Emporia National Bank, beginning 1865; member, U.S. Senate, 1877–91.

Senator Preston B. Plumb of Kansas epitomized the self-made Western man. He rose to public attention soon after moving to Kansas Territory from Ohio, becoming embroiled in the struggle against slavery. He became a leading member of the Free Soil faction, smuggling weapons into the region, editing an antislavery journal, serving in various political posts, and, finally, fighting against Southern guerillas. During the Civil War (for which "Bleeding Kansas" had been something of a grim rehearsal) he entered Union ranks as a major in the Eleventh Kansas Cavalry. The young officer spent most of the conflict in northwestern Arkansas chasing Confederate irregulars, including the notorious William Quantrill, and did good service in helping to clear most of them out of the area. With the return of peace, Plumb quickly established himself as one of the leading citizens of the state. He made a fortune in banking and in cattle and mining investments and served briefly but with distinction in the Kansas legislature. A reformer, he supported the rise of political prohibition, although, unlike some especially zealous drys who bolted to the Prohibition Party when it became active, he always remained an orthodox Republican. Still, with the advent of state-wide prohibition in Kansas, he praised it as beneficial and castigated those (including some in the GOP) who would have allowed the return of the traffic. Elected to the national Senate in 1876 (and remaining in office for the rest of his life), he continued as a reformer and a spokesman for Western interests. He sponsored land law reform, tariff revisions favorable to the West, the free coinage of silver, and conservation projects. In his time, Plumb was counted an intelligent and useful legislator, one who was responsive to his constituents and who thoroughly enjoyed his role as senator.

Plumb's services to the Temperance Movement, while ignored by some of his biographers, were nevertheless important. While Kansas fought its internal temperance question, dry sentiments were also growing nationally. By the 1880s, many states were witness to bitter struggles between antiliquor and wet partisans. These battles, however, were at the state level; the federal government had not yet played a major role in the fray. Senator Plumb was one of the first dry legislators to try to change that. In early 1881, he introduced a resolution into the Senate formally proposing a prohibitory amendment to the Constitution. The Kansan's measure called for the abolition of the manufacture and sale of intoxicating beverages, and it went to the Senate Judiciary Committee on the same day that Senator Henry Blair* of New Hampshire submitted a bill to amend the Constitution along similar lines. Neither senator's proposal made any headway, although their constituents (and, of course, most temperance workers) seemed pleased enough. Plumb was evidently so happy with the reception of his resolution back home that between 1882 and 1885 he submitted the proposal three times more—with an equally cold reception in the nation's capital. Nevertheless, the consideration of prohibitory amendments was a sign of things to come, and they did serve to further public discussion of the liquor question. By 1885, Plumb was responding to a constituency beyond Kansas: His last resolution went to the Senate at the request of the National Temperance Union, and he was happy to oblige. Temperance laws, though, were never among the many successful pieces of national legislation the Kansas senator initiated. Yet the antiliquor crusade honored him for his attempts, and Plumb was listed as a pioneer of the prohibitory amendment that became part of the Constitution a generation after his death.

### Bibliography:

A. *A New Treatise on the Law Relating to the Powers and Duties of Justice of the Peace...in...Kansas...* (Cincinnati, OH, 1872); *The Blair Education Bill, Speech...* (Washington, DC, 1890); *Coin and Currency, Speech...* (Washington, DC, 1891).

B. DAB 15, 10–11; SEAP 5, 2170; WW H, 486; William Elsey Connelley, *The Life of Preston B. Plumb, 1837–1901, United States Senator from Kansas...* (Chicago, 1913); W. H. Michael, *Memorial Address on the Life and Character of Preston B. Plumb...* (Washington, DC, 1892).

**POLING, Daniel Alfred**   (30 November 1884, Portland, OR—7 February 1968, Philadelphia, PA). *Education*: A.B., Dallas Coll., OR, 1904; A.M., Dallas Coll., 1906; graduate study, LaFayette Sem., OR, and Ohio State Univ., 1907–8; LLD (honorary), Albright Coll., 1916, Temple Univ., 1937; Litt.D. (honorary), Defiance Coll., 1921, Norwich Univ., 1952; D.D. (honorary), Hope Coll., 1925, Univ. of Vermont, 1934, Phillips Univ., 1939, William Jewell Coll., 1960; STD. (honorary), Syracuse Univ., 1927; LHD. (honorary), Bucknell Univ., 1946, Bates Coll., 1951; HHD. (honorary), Huntington Coll., 1952? *Career*: ordained, Reformed Church in America, 1908; secretary, Flying Squadron of America, 1914–15; vice president, Anti-Saloon League of America, 1914–18; member, Headquarters Committee, Anti-Saloon League of Massachusetts, 1915–20; vice president, Intercollegiate Prohibition Association, 1920–21; minister, Marble Collegiate Church, New York City, 1922–30; editor, *Christian Herald*, beginning 1927; minister, Baptist Temple, Philadelphia, 1936–48; active writing on reform and religious subjects, 1900s–1960s.

In the mind of the Reverend Daniel Poling, prohibition was the reform that was going to save the moral fiber and social structure of America. As long as the liquor traffic existed, he believed, social ills would persist and the people of the United States could never realize their full potential. This was not an especially novel line of thought, but Poling espoused it with a passion and effectiveness that few others could rival over his many years as a dry crusader. Poling grew up dry and entered antiliquor politics even before he was old enough to vote. In 1904, at twenty years old, he was a delegate to the national convention of the Prohibition Party, a position he filled every four years until 1916. Indeed, he devoted a major share of his time to party affairs as a young man, serving as a member of its National Executive Committee and, in 1912, running as its candidate for governor of Ohio. Ordained in 1908 in the Reformed Church, he had no time for pastorates as his work with the Temperance Movement was in fact a full-time career. When not tending to Prohibitionist activities, he was involved with other dry organizations, sometimes working in more than one capacity simultaneously. At various times, he was secretary of the Flying Squadron, which sent a battery of speakers across the nation on behalf of the temperance gospel, vice president of the Intercollegiate Prohibition Association, which tried to rally dry enthusiasm on campus, and the Anti-Saloon League. In all of his posts, he had a reputation for dedication and effectiveness. He was also practical: While always loyal to the Prohibition Party, his work with the Anti-Saloon League demonstrated that, unlike some other Prohibitionists, Poling could co-operate with the major political parties in the interest of furthering dry legislation. His name was familiar in print as well, for in addition to his other pursuits he was a prolific writer on religious and reform topics. Thus by the time National Prohibition became the law of the land, Poling had a reform reputation of considerable stature.

With the achievement of the Eighteenth Amendment, however, Poling devoted less time directly to organized antiliquor work. For the first time, he assumed prestigious pulpits, serving as pastor of Marble Collegiate Church in New York City (1922–30) and of the Baptist Temple in Philadelphia (1936–48). He also edited the *Christian Herald* during these years. He never lost faith in Prohibition, and he continued to speak and write actively on its behalf. Yet during the later 1920s there was a sense of change in Poling's career. He would still belabor the drink trade for its sins, but he knew that all was not right with the Volstead Act. As public disenchantment with the ''noble experiment'' grew, so did his dismay with the social turmoil engendered by the dry enforcement effort. Poling had been a firm temperance man, but in the end he evidently knew when to let go of the measure. He did not defend Prohibition to the last, and he chose not to be embittered at the final dry defeat. Rather, the end of the dry era signaled a new and creative time for the hard-working minister. Poling was deeply involved with church and civic affairs, plus his almost constant writing, and the dry debacle seems not to have affected his activities greatly. Over the three decades after Repeal, he served not only in the pulpit but as a military chaplain and a central figure in efforts on behalf of the Boy Scouts, the state of Israel, Bucknell University, and other groups and causes. His talents proved extremely diverse, and his services as a citizen were repeatedly honored by academic institutions, professional organizations, civic associations, and government. In reviewing his varied accomplishments, one is tempted to observe that Poling did not really tap his full range of interests until he had put his involvement with the liquor question behind him. Sincere as he was in his dry conviction, however, we can also doubt that he would have seen things that way.

**Bibliography:**

A. *Hats in Hell* (Boston, 1918); *The Furnace* (New York, 1925); *John of Oregon* (New York, 1928); *The Romance of Jesus* (1931, as *Between Two Worlds*; New York, 1953); *A Preacher Looks at War* (New York, 1943); comp., *A Treasury of Great Sermons* (New York, 1945).

B. SEAP 5, 2175–76; WW 5, 575.

**POLLACK, Charles Andrew**    (21 September 1853, Elizabethtown, NY—11 July 1928, Fargo, ND). *Education*: A.B., Cornell Coll., IA, 1878; A.M., Cornell Coll., 1881; LLB., Iowa State Univ., 1881; LLD. (honorary), Cornell Coll., 1908. *Career*: legal practice, Fargo, Dakota Territory, beginning 1881; district attorney, Cass Co., Dakota Territory, 1885–89; district court judge, ND, 1897–1917.

Charles Pollack began his legal career while the Dakotas were still a territory, and his actions there testified to the ability of the Temperance Movement to shape the moral and political course of frontier society. If there was indeed a period when the West was "wild," there were generally always forces present striving to establish stable institutions and cultural norms, and men like Pollack supported them. As an agent of the law, whether acting as a lawyer, prosecutor, or judge, he sought to restrain the excesses of frontier life and to create a Dakota Territory (and later a state of North Dakota) of orderly and secure farms and communities. Like many others of his generation, he located the source of a great deal of societal disorder in drink, and he turned to the antiliquor crusade as a means of bringing civilization to the West. As a citizen, he called regularly for the legal restraint of the liquor traffic, and on the bench he was noted for his strict enforcement of the local and state liquor laws. Indeed, while he served as a district attorney in the late 1880s, a state temperance convention elected him chairman of a committee to draft what became North Dakota's state prohibition law. He joined the Anti-Saloon League of America at its inception shortly thereafter and for years served as one of its vice presidents. In that capacity he made a number of speaking tours on behalf of prohibition in the United States, Canada, and Europe. Pollack aroused considerable support in his home state and throughout the rest of the West, clearly demonstrating that the reform crusade was as much a part of the region's formative years as were the more picturesque cattle drives and cavalry charges.

Pollack's attachments to the antiliquor cause, however, had deeper roots than the desire to bring order to the Dakotas. He was also a highly religious man and prominent in the lay affairs of the Methodist Church. Thus his belief in total abstinence and prohibition also mirrored his denominational creed. In fact, he worked hard to increase the effectiveness of Methodism in the war against drink.

A frequent lay delegate to the General Conferences of the church, in 1916 a gathering of his churchmen elected him chairman of the Methodist Committee on Temperance, Prohibition, and Public Morals. At the time, this was one of the more active and important units of the denomination's bureaucracy, and Pollack quickly moved to increase its political stature nationally. Under his lead, the committee shifted its headquarters from Kansas to Washington, D.C. "Most of the West has already gone dry," was the explanation; "and Kansas needed" the dry Methodist group "the least of any state in the Union." The final battle would come in the East "and center in Washington." It was an astute tactical assessment, and the committee eventually became one of the most influential lobbying groups in the nation's capital. While fighting to reform his country, we should note in closing, Judge Pollack also made significant contributions to the reform of his church. Over the years, he served diligently on committees trying to reunite the Civil War–inspired split between the Northern and Southern factions of Methodism.

## Bibliography:

A. *Prohibition Law of North Dakota* (Fargo, ND? 1889); *Manual of Prohibition Law of North Dakota* (n.p., 1910).
B. SEAP 5, 2179; WW 1, 980.

**POLLARD, William Jefferson**    (1 May 1860, Kingston, MO—12 December 1913, St. Louis, MO). *Education*: private study of law, 1890s. *Career*: messenger, Western Union Telegraph Co., 1880s; grocery business, circa 1889–97; admitted to bar, MO, 1897; justice of the peace, St. Louis, MO, 1900s; judge, public court, St. Louis, MO, 1903–13.

Local jurist and minor politician in Missouri, William Jefferson Pollard pioneered American efforts to remove the public inebriate from the prison system. Indeed, what began as an attempt to deal with repeat drunkenness offenders in the St. Louis municipal police courts won international recognition for the Missouri judge. Pollard grew up in the state, with any early interest in the Temperance Movement he may have had escaping biographical accounts. No reformer, he worked as a grocer before reading law and passing the bar. Meanwhile, he had also become something of a local Democratic Party activist, and he played helpful roles in state campaigns over the 1880s and 1890s (he was also a delegate to the 1896 Democratic National Convention). His appointment as a St. Louis justice of the peace and, beginning in 1903, public court judge, was probably a reward for his work on behalf of the party. Certainly there was nothing in Pollard's background to suggest that he would quickly emerge as a judicial reformer. Yet service on the bench made an impression on the man. The police court traditionally dealt with such street crime as public disorder, assault, and intoxication. And just as often, especially with drunkenness, many of those arrested were repeat offenders; the legal system had little permanent impact on their drinking. Pollard saw the futility of arresting the same individuals over and over again, and about 1905 he devised an alternative approach to the problem which soon became known as the Pollard Plan. Under its provisions, instead of arrest, drunkards brought into court would be offered a chance to sign a pledge of total abstinence for a year. If they broke the pledge within the year, offenders would then be committed to a public workhouse for the crime that had originally brought them into the hands of the law. The idea was to assist alcoholics to reform as well as to remove some of the burden on the court and prison system. In its essentials, then, the Pollard Plan was not unlike a number of modern efforts to get the alcoholic out of the legal system.

At the time, however, Judge Pollard's approach was novel enough to create a stir in reform circles. In practice, it never worked perfectly, and Pollard never claimed that it could. But it apparently did have some positive effects on the court system (although exact statistics are lacking on the subject), and other states and even countries expressed an interest in the idea. In 1906, Pollard travelled to Great Britain, where he explained the plan to a number of temperance gatherings; he also attended the Twelfth and Thirteenth International Congresses on Alcoholism (London, 1909, and The Hague, 1911) for the same purpose. In 1910, the St. Louis judge also spoke before the National German Abstinence Convention in Augsburg. In each case, his audiences accorded him an enthusiastic hearing. His message was always the same: "A judge of a court should exhaust every means to reform a victim of drink before he sends him to jail." Following the St. Louis example, the state of Vermont, Great Britain, and Victoria, Australia, enacted similar plans, and initial reports on their effect seemingly confirmed Pollard's observations. Indeed, the delegates at both the 1909 and 1911 International Congresses expressed overwhelming approval of the Pollard Plan based on evidence gathered from areas where it operated. "The possibilities of this wise and beneficent policy are so great," proclaimed the 1911 delegates, "that we desire to commend its adoption throughout the world." Most of the world, however, was not ready for anything of the sort, and with Pollard's death in 1913 the idea lost its most visible advocate. Still, the Pollard Plan had made its mark, and interest in it never completely died; it was an initial step in society's dealing with alcoholism in other than punitive ways.

**Bibliography:**

B. SEAP 5, 2177–78; WW 1, 979.

**POTTER, Alonzo**   (6 July 1800, Beekman, NY—4 July 1865, San Francisco, CA). *Education*: graduated from Union Coll., NY, 1818; D.D. (honorary), Kenyon Coll., 1834, Gambier Coll., 1834, and Harvard Univ., 1846; LLD. (honorary), Union Coll., 1846. *Career*: bookseller, Philadelphia, 1818; tutor, Union Coll., 1819–22; professor of mathematics and natural philosophy, 1822–26; ordained a priest in Protestant Episcopal Church, 1824; rector, Saint Paul's Church, Boston, 1826–31; professor of philosophy and political economy, Union

Coll., 1831–38; vice president, Union Coll., 1838–45; bishop of Pennsylvania, 1845–65.

As a bishop of the Protestant Episcopal Church, Alonzo Potter's temperance and antislavery enthusiasms demonstrated something of the contributions of even the moderate religious denominations to the reform movements of the nineteenth century. Indeed, the Potter family itself generated enough activity to qualify as a small crusade: In addition to Alonzo's work, Horatio Potter, his brother, was an ardent reformer as bishop of New York, while still later, Henry Codman Potter, Alonzo's son and a committed temperance man, succeeded to his father's bishopric in Pennsylvania. Thus the family played visible roles through the reform upheavals which gripped the nation well past the turn of the century. Alonzo Potter, rising to bishop after a distinguished career in education and in the pulpit, formed his judgments on intemperance and slavery in reference to standards natural for a man of his calling: Both were evils which degraded humanity and were thus affronts to the Lord. With regard to slavery, he participated in the debate over whether the Bible supported human bondage. He argued vigorously that it did not, even to the point of a public exchange with another bishop. Considering drink, Potter's language frequently avoided direct appeal to religion and cited instead the sanctions of "self-evident" reasoning. Nonetheless his argument for total abstinence depended upon a Biblical purism: If alcohol offended the social body—and for that matter if it posed even the slightest threat to personal well-being—then it ought to be eliminated altogether. "If there were no temperate drinking," he insisted, "there would be none that is intemperate." The consequences of drink—the "debauch," "error," or "crime" which would follow one "with shame and sorrow all his days"—were sufficient to negate whatever good might seem to come from even the most innocent-seeming use. And as long as he lived, he saw no reason to change his mind on the subject.

Potter's stance on the reform questions of his day was indicative of his many interests in life as well as his belief that the church had to assert itself in the affairs of contemporary society. As an individual, he would most likely have come out for abolitionism and temperance even without a clerical collar. His many and perceptive writings on philosophy, politics, and education revealed a mind eager to improve the state of mankind and hopeful of a society in which drunkenness and chattel slavery would have no place. As a churchman, and especially as a bishop, Potter felt an added responsibility to the cause of reform. He saw the church as a bulwark of social decency, a trait which compelled it to become involved in secular affairs and to take positions on particular issues. Thus while Potter devoted years to the strengthening of ecclesiastical bodies and to founding new churches, so far as it was in his power he also had the church sponsor hospitals, higher education, and social reform. Throughout his tenure as bishop, he lectured and wrote on behalf of these causes and had the satisfaction of receiving the plaudits of many reform groups in return. While he was forceful and persistent in his views, however, Potter was not a zealot. Tolerant of other views whenever possible, and preferring logic and reason to strident emotionalism, he demonstrated the importance and appeal of temperance in the thinking of many nonevangelical Americans. His son, Bishop Henry Codman Potter, while also an implacable foe of the liquor traffic, reflected this same inclination to nonradical reform approaches.

**Bibliography:**

A. *The Christian Bishop...* (New York, 1851); *The Drinking Usages of Society* (Boston, 1854, and subsequent editions); *The Principles of Science Applied to the Domestic and Mechanic Arts...*, rev. ed. (New York, 1860); *Handbook for Readers and Students...* (New York, 1870); *The School and the Schoolmaster...* (New York, 1873); *Political Economy: Its Objects, Uses, and Principles...* (New York, 1892).

B. DAB 15, 124–25, 127–28; SEAP 5, 2189–90, 2190–91; WW H, 491; George Hodges, *Henry Codman Potter, Seventh Bishop of New York* (New York, 1915); Mark Antony DeWolfe Howe, *Memoirs of the Life and Services of the Rt. Rev. Alonzo Potter, D.D., LL.D., Bishop of the Protestant Episcopal Church...* (Philadelphia, 1871); Henry Codman Potter, *The Drink Problem in Modern Life* (New York, 1905); William Bacon Stevens, *A Discourse Commemorative of the Rt. Rev. Alonzo Potter...* (Philadelphia, 1866).

**POWER, Frederick Dunglison**    (23 January 1851, Yorktown, VA—14 June 1911, Washington, DC). *Education*: A.B., Bethany Coll., WV, 1871; A.M., Bethany Coll., 1874; LLD. (honorary), Bethany Coll., 1890. *Career*: ordained in Disciples of Christ, 1871; minister, Vermont Avenue Christian Church, Washington, DC, 1875–1911; chaplain, Forty-seventh Congress, 1881–83.

The Disciples of Christ, while not as large a denomination as the ubiquitous Methodists, constituted one of the most important Protestant churches in the nineteenth century. Emphasizing the common aspects of Christian faith and consciously trying to avoid the doctrinal disputes that separated the various churches, the Disciples grew quickly in the first half of the century under the guidance of Thomas Campbell (1763–1854) and his son Alexander (1788–1866). While never as united on the issue of prohibition as the Methodists, the Disciples had many dry members and produced some reform leaders of considerable note. One of the most prominent of these was the Reverend Frederick Power, who took an influential part in the affairs of his denomination and in the Temperance Movement. Preaching initially in rural Virginia pulpits, he emerged as a speaker of genuine power and displayed a talent for writing and scholarship (for a time, he taught ancient languages on an adjunct basis at his alma mater, Bethany College in West Virginia). In 1875, he became pastor of the Vermont Avenue Church in Washington, D.C., where he remained for the next thirty-five years (until his death). There, Power's abilities came to full flower as he steadily increased his congregation, took a hand in establishing eight more Disciples' churches, sat as a Bethany College trustee, and became a key figure in quickening the pace of Disciples' missionary activities. In addition, he was an intimate friend of James A. Garfield, who attended the Vermont Avenue Church, and Power preached at the assassinated president's funeral; he also served as chaplain of the Congress from 1881 to 1883. Hard-working and highly visible as he was, his denomination could hardly have asked for a better representative in the nation's capital.

Nor could the Temperance Movement. Power being a prominent minister in a large denomination, an intimate of a president and other national figures, and an acknowledged spiritual leader in Washington, the dry crusade was more than happy to list him as one of its own. As he maintained the rest of his busy schedule, Power devoted considerable attention to the struggle against drink. He inveighed against booze from the pulpit, served as the last president of the Congressional Temperance Society, and lent his voice to the call that led to the organizing convention of the Anti-Saloon League of America. Out of regard for his dedication and the example he set for the rest of the nation's clergy, the league repeatedly elected him one of its vice presidents. At the same time, Power worked actively with the league's District of Columbia branch, in which he was a member of the executive committee. In that role, he became a prime mover in attempts to dry out the capital city. Reverend Power died some nine years before National Prohibition became the law of the land, but while he lived, he did yeoman service in bringing the Disciples into the temperance fold and in carrying the dry gospel to the national legislature.

**Bibliography:**

A. *Bible Doctrine for Young Disciples* (St. Louis, MO, 1889); *Sketches of Our Pioneers* (Cleveland, OH, 1898); *Life of William Kimbrough Pendleton, LL.D., President of Bethany College* (St. Louis, MO, 1902); *Thoughts of Thirty Years...of Frederick D. Power...*, intro. Frances E. Clark (Boston, 1905).

B. *American Issue* (Maryland ed.), July 8, 1911; DAB 15, 155–56; SEAP 5, 2192–93; WW 1, 989.

**PRICE, Hiram** (10 January 1814, Washington Co., PA—30 May 1901, Washington, DC). *Career*: storekeeper, Davenport, IA, 1844 to 1850s; local offices (school fund commissioner, recorder, treasurer, tax collector), Davenport, IA, 1847–50s; railroad executive, 1850s; branch manager, State Bank of Iowa, 1858–60; president, State Bank of Iowa, 1860–65; paymaster general, Iowa troops, 1861–63; member, U.S. House of Representatives, 1863–69, 1877–81; commissioner of Indian affairs, 1881–85; president, Anti-Saloon League of America, 1895–1901.

Starting life with a minimal formal education from local country schools in Pennsylvania, Hiram Price steadily climbed the ladder of economic success. After working as a store clerk and farmer, he married in 1834 and a decade later moved to Davenport, Iowa, where he went into business for himself. He was soon involved in local civic affairs, first as school fund commissioner and then as recorder and treasurer of Scott County. From these foundations Price rose in prominence and emerged in the 1850s as a financier of some importance. Indeed, he made a fortune in banking and railroading, having played a key role in the construction of the first rail line in the state. Throughout his rise, Price was a firm temperance man, to which fact he attributed much of his success. His views on the liquor question were fully representative of the sentiments of many early business leaders who saw drink as productive of waste and detrimental to progress. This was especially true among railroad executives, who feared the potential disruption and mayhem that could come from besotted train crews. Even before moving to Iowa, Price had been an active member of the fraternal Sons of Temperance and, so far as is known, was a teetotaler all of his adult life. In Iowa, he eventually was elected head of the state branch of the order, a position he held for many years. During the prohibition controversy of the 1850s, when agitation for ''Maine Laws'' was embroiling state legislatures throughout the nation, Price carried his reform views into politics. He played a central role in drafting Iowa's prohibitory statute, and when it became law in 1855 he was among the most ardent proponents of a strict enforcement effort. His work in this regard won him a reputation as one of the most zealous reform advocates in the region.

Price had equally pronounced views on other issues of the day, not the least of which was the preservation of the Union. Originally a Democrat, he broke with the party in 1856 as the sectional crisis loomed and joined the new Republican organization. Outraged at Southern secession, he personally raised and equipped some five thousand Iowa volunteers and maintained them at his own expense until they mustered into the Union army. Later, he was elected to several terms in Congress (1863–69, 1877–81), where, putting his financial acumen to good use, he actively pursued monetary reform measures. Yet he never let go of the temperance issue. In Congress, Price was a dedicated member of the Congressional Temperance Society, and friends of the dry movement found him ever willing to speak on the matter. As the Temperance Movement regained momentum after the Civil War, Price gave it whatever support he could, either in politics or through his participation in the affairs of the Methodist Church, of which he was a generous and devout member. Even out of elective office, however, Price still battled ''the demon'' whenever he could. He was eighty-one years old when the Anti-Saloon League of America was organized in 1895, and such was dry regard for the old reformer that the league named him its first president. When he died in 1901, he was still in office.

## Bibliography:

A. *Constitution of the Freedman! Speech. . . (Washington, DC, 1864?); A Printed Letter to Some of My Friends in Book Form* (Washington, DC, 1889); ''Government and the Indians,'' *Forum* 10 (1890):708; *A Scrap Book. . .* (Washington, DC, 1895).

B. DAB 15, 212–13; SEAP 5, 2198–99; WW 1, 994; B. F. Gere, ''The Public

Services of Hiram Price," *Annals of Iowa* (Jan. 1895); S. S. Howe, "Biograph-ical Sketch of Hiram Price," *Annals of Iowa* (Jan. 1864).

**PRIME, Nathaniel Scudder**    (21 April 1785, Huntington, NY—27 March 1856, Mamaroneck, NY). *Education*: graduated from Princeton Univ., 1804; D.D. (honorary), Princeton Univ., 1848. *Career*: licensed to preach, Presbyterian Church, 1805; minister, Cutchogue, NY, 1805–6; minister, Sag Harbor, NY, 1806–8; ordained in Presbyterian Church, 1809; minister, Smithtown, NY, 1809–11; minister, Cambridge, NY, 1813–30; principal, Washington Acad., NY, 1821–30; minister, Sing Sing, NY, 1830–35; headmaster, Mt. Pleasant Acad., NY, 1830–43.

The American Temperance Movement always put particular pride in its his-tory. It had a keen sense of mission, and many of its rank and file saw their reform as advancing inexorable historical forces that would carry the republic to a destiny (which some saw as divinely predestined) of greatness and perfection. Thus temperance workers made special efforts to record the contributions of the movement's pioneers—a category in which they included many men and women who, by the more exacting standards of the later nineteenth and early twentieth centuries, contributed relatively little to the cause. In large measure, such was the case with the Reverend Nathaniel Scudder Prime. Prime was a well-travelled Presbyterian minister in the eastern New York area: Between 1805, when he received his license to preach, and 1835, when he finally left the pulpit, he had charge of five congregations. In addition, he ran two private schools over the years and sat as a trustee at Williams College in Massachusetts (1826–31) and Middlebury College in Vermont (1822–26). He had a reputation as a forceful speaker and a man who never hesitated to denounce evil as he saw it. In the eyes of the Reverend Prime, intemperance was evil in one of its most monstrous forms. A firm total abstinence man himself, he urged others to the same course on any number of occasions.

All of this marked the reform-minded minister as a man ahead of his time. In 1805, when he took his first pulpit in Cutchogue, New York, there was no Temperance Movement. Indeed, the social norms of the day permitted consid-erable drinking, even among the clergy. It was in this atmosphere that Prime raised his objections. His most memorable contribution came in 1811, when, probably influenced by the temperance preaching of like-minded churchmen, he delivered a sermon on the Biblical passage, "Who hath woe?. . . They that tarry long at the wine" (later reprinted as *The Pernicious Effects of Intemperance* in 1812). It was one of the first major calls for concerted action against intemper-ance, and the regional presbytery called for its publication and distribution. The group also asked all Presbyterians to leave off supplying their guests with liquor as a part of hospitality. Prime's own congregation passed similar resolutions, and, if dry accounts are accurate, the neighborhood's drinking habits became noticeably more temperate. Two years later, having moved to Cambridge, New York, the reforming reverend added organization to exhortation. He organized his new congregation, mostly local farmers, into a temperance society. Thus if there was no formal Temperance Movement before Prime began his work, he clearly helped to point public sentiments in that direction. Indeed, by the time he died, the seeds he had planted had taken firm root, and prohibition had become one of the chief issues of the day in New York State.

**Bibliography:**

A. *A Collection of Hymns...* (Sag Harbor, NY, 1809); *The Pernicious Effects of Intemperance in the Use of Ardent Spirits and the Remedy for the Evil...* (Brooklyn, NY, 1812); *The Year of Jubilee: But not to Africans!* (Salem, NY, 1825); *A History of Long Island...* (New York, 1845).

B. SEAP 5, 2199–200; Daniel Dorchester, *The Liquor Problem in All Ages* (New York, 1888).

**PRINGLE, Coleman Roberson**    (1830s, Monroe Co., GA—1905, Sandersville, GA). *Career*: farmer, GA, 1850s to 1861; mayor, Sandersville, GA, 1871; member, Georgia House of Representatives, 1882–85; member, Georgia Senate, 1886–87; president, Sandersville Railroad, 1880s–1900s.

Born sometime during the 1830s in Monroe County, Georgia, Coleman Pringle spent the first eighteen years of his life working the family farm. Other than these sketchy facts, we know little of his background. After his marriage in 1861, he moved to Sandersville, Georgia, and went into business. He prospered in his new home, and the son of a poor farmer began a rise to economic and political success. For somewhere along the way, success in business led to an interest in local government, and in 1871 Pringle won election as the first mayor of Sandersville. Soon after, he also served as president of the county commissioners and then as president of the Sandersville Railroad for some eighteen years. Over these years, he developed a deep interest in forestry as well. He became an authority on the subject, and in fact won recognition as one of the South's most accomplished foresters. In sum, Pringle emerged as a pillar of his community and state, with an established reputation as a local and regional leader. Thus, when he sought a place in the state legislature, his victory was not surprising. Pringle served for five years, three in the House of Representatives and two in the Senate. Although he addressed other matters, his interests as a lawmaker focused mainly on the liquor question, and he emerged as one of the state's most vocal champions of legal prohibition. His constituents probably expected it, for Pringle's dry sentiments were no secret. In 1883, in fact, he became president of the Georgia Prohibition Association, a post he held until his death in 1905. In this capacity, he proved an enthusiastic scourge of the drink trade, and he spoke widely around the state on behalf of the antiliquor reform. During his remaining years in the legislature, the zealous crusader devoted himself almost exclusively to temperance matters. He served as a chairman of temperance committees in both houses, where his record of productivity verged on the extraordinary. In his relatively short legislative career, Pringle saw some three hundred antiliquor bills voted out of his committees, the majority of which he drafted himself. His signal triumph came in 1885, when he was successful in guiding a local-option bill through the Georgia House; the measure failed later in the Senate, however. Yet Pringle was not overly disappointed. Prohibitionist sentiment was slow in forming in Georgia, where the movement had not been especially strong earlier in the century. His work did much to popularize the issue, and there is little question that he helped lay much of the foundation for later efforts that finally brought Georgia into the dry camp. His career illustrated the indefatigable activities that not only kept temperance issues almost constantly before the public in the later nineteenth and early twentieth centuries but also kept the liquor interests on the defensive. Writ large, the Coleman Pringles of the nation, working at the state and local level, gave the Temperance Movement most of its considerable influence in the highest councils of the land.

**Bibliography:**

B. SEAP 5, 2201; WW 1, 997.

**PUGH, Esther**    (31 August 1834, Cincinnati, OH—28 March 1908, Phila-delphia, PA). *Career*: schoolteacher, OH, 1850s?; editor, *Our Union* (later the *Union Signal*), 1870s to 1890s; treasurer, National Woman's Christian Tem-perance Union, 1878–93.

So far as can be determined, Esther Pugh had but one interest in life, the Temperance Movement. She never married and evidently chose to pour all of her energy into a career in reform. After teaching in Ohio public schools for several years, she settled in Waynesville, Ohio, where she spent most of her life. In her new home, Pugh became involved with the Woman's Crusade when it spread over the state in 1873 and 1874. Indeed, the women of Waynesville elected her their leader as they organized to pray in front of the saloons and conduct other demonstrations against the liquor traffic. The nature of Pugh's activities in the mid-1870s are unclear, although she apparently remained active in the movement after the spontaneous crusade had coalesced into the formally organized Woman's Christian Temperance Union. In 1878, Pugh emerged as treasurer of the National WCTU, an office that would have gone to a woman only with a distinguished local record. As a national officer, the Ohio crusader proved industrious and capable and was, so far as is known, content in her efficient and necessary, although largely unsung, role. Pugh worked directly with WCTU president Frances E. Willard* and did a creditable job in managing the group's finances in its crucial early years. It was not spectacular work, but it was essential to the union's success as it built itself to a position of national influence. Perhaps more important, Pugh was a central figure in the union's effort to establish a national publication. She was editor and publisher of *Our Union*, which served to carry the WCTU message to the public and to keep local chapters and individual members abreast of temperance affairs across the nation. In 1883, *Our Union* merged with another dry journal to become the *Union*

*Signal*, which ever since has been the official organ of the WCTU. Pugh resigned from her position with the organization in 1893 when she was fifty-nine and eventually moved to Philadelphia to live her final years with her sister. Never a temperance leader of the first rank, or often in the public eye, she nevertheless did faithful and important service when the WCTU had good need of it.

**Bibliography:**

B. SEAP 4, 2225–26.

# R

**RANDALL, Charles Hiram** (23 July 1865, Auburn, NB—1951, Los Angeles, CA). *Career*: editor, *Observer*, NB, 1885; editor, various weekly newspapers, 1880s to 1906; editor, *Highland Park* (CA) *Herald*, 1906–15; member, California House of Representatives, 1911–12; member, U.S. House of Representatives, 1915–21; member, Los Angeles City Council, 1925–28.

A career in journalism ultimately led Charles Randall to politics. He had watched reform affairs as editor of the *Highland Park Herald*, a Los Angeles, California, newspaper; and imbued with the Progressive spirit of the day, he plunged into the political arena himself. After service on a city commission (for parks, 1909–10), Randall won a seat in the state legislature, where he emerged as an articulate proponent of reform generally and of the Temperance Movement in particular. He played a key role in framing local-option legislation which dried out hundreds of towns. His advocacy of the dry cause broadened his political base: He was a Democrat, but the small—although active—Prohibition Party also found the crusading editor an attractive candidate. With temperance support, then, Randall was able to score his most notable political successes on the national level. Running on the combined Democratic and Prohibition ticket in 1914, he was elected to Congress from the Sixty-fourth Congressional District (Los Angeles). He was thus the first person to be elected to Congress by the Prohibition Party, albeit on a hybrid ticket. His performance in the House was such that two years later he secured the nomination for a second term from the Republican, Democratic, Progressive, and Prohibition parties. He won easily. Randall continued to serve in the House until 1921 (he was, afterward, a member of the Los Angeles City Council from 1925 to 1928).

Randall's multipartisan support says much of the popularity the antiliquor cause enjoyed as the country moved toward National Prohibition. Elected as a temperance champion, the California congressman fully reflected this dry surge as he went about his duties in the nation's capital. Indeed, he won high praise from reformers as he established himself as a major thorn in the side of the liquor traffic. He was the moving force behind the Jones-Randall Law, which made it illegal to send liquor advertisements through the mails (it won approval as a rider on a post office appropriation measure). In addition, Randall sponsored the War Prohibition Amendment to the Food Production Bill during World War

I. War Prohibition was a body blow to the liquor industry, which found it impossible to fight a temperance measure wrapped, in effect, in the flag. To have resisted the law would have seemed an unpatriotic act in time of war. Randall also vigorously supported the eighteenth Amendment, which he saw as the first step in the elimination of a host of social and political evils. In addition to his political activities, he also served as vice president of the National Board of Temperance, Prohibition, and Public Morals of the Methodist Episcopal Church.

**Bibliography:**

B. *Biographical Directory of the American Congress, 1774–1971* (Washington, DC, 1971); SEAP 5, 2251; WW 4, 775.

**REED, Seth**    (2 June 1823, Hartwick, NY—24 March 1924, MI). *Education*: legal study in private law firm, MI, 1843; private study for ministry, 1840–44; D.D. (honorary), Albion Coll., 1907. *Career*: schoolteacher, NY, MI, 1840–44; licensed to preach as Methodist, 1844; served various Methodist pastorates, MI, 1844–62; ordained, 1848; duty with U.S. Sanitary Commission, 1862; minister, Edgarton and Providence, RI, 1863–67; fiscal agent, Albion Coll., MI, 1868; minister, various pastorates, MI, 1869–93 (part-time service after 1893); directed Methodist retirement home, 1906–7.

Surely one of the longest-lived of temperance advocates, New York-born Seth Reed gave the greatest part of his one hundred-plus years to the service of his church and to the abolition of the liquor traffic. Largely self-educated, he taught school periodically in both New York and Michigan before studying for the bar at age seventeen. It was not the law, however, but the pulpit that really attracted him. Raised a Universalist, Reed had converted to Methodism in 1840 and soon developed a serious interest in the ministry. Shortly thereafter, he witnessed the spread of the Washington temperance revival and became a fast adherent of the dry reform. This antiliquor sentiment was amplified by his devout Methodist faith, and he reportedly began giving temperance lectures at age eighteen. By 1844, having been licensed to preach (although he was not formally ordained until 1848), he took charge of a number of small congregations in the Flat River circuit of Michigan. Full of zeal as he was, the busy preacher did not seem to mind the salary he later described as "hay, oats, socks, mittens, and cash," all worth less than sixty dollars a year. With the coming of the Civil War, Reed ministered to the spiritual needs of wounded Union soldiers, chiefly in Tennessee. After the Civil War, for reasons unknown, he went East and served four years as a pastor in New England before returning to Michigan, where he spent the rest of his long life. His many years in the service of his beloved church earned him the well-merited accolade of the "Grand Old Man of Michigan Methodism."

Reed had much the same status with the Temperance Movement. Once he had set foot on the antiliquor path, he never questioned his course. Throughout his career in the ministry, his pulpits rang with denunciations of drink, and his fame as a scourge of the traffic spread well beyond Michigan. Reed, however, did more than preach his hatred of drink. During his sojourn in New England, he worked in league with the Temperance Committee of Rhode Island. Canvassing the state in a lengthy speaking tour, he induced some seven thousand citizens to take the pledge. Reed's accomplishment won high temperance honors, as Rhode Island was not a dry stronghold over the years. Back in Michigan, the tireless clergyman continued to support the cause, even into old age. At the age of seventy, Reed capped his long service in the reform crusade by sitting among those in the nation's capital in 1895 who founded the Anti-Saloon League of America. In his autobiography, he noted the event with particular pride. Still vigorous in his hundred and first year, Reed died in 1914 as the result of a fall. In retrospect, we can note that other dry reformers made contributions of greater importance to the movement; few, however, could boast of having labored for so long.

**Bibliography:**

A. *A Discourse Delivered on the Occasion of the Funeral Obsequies of President Lincoln...* (Boston, 1865); *The Gains and Losses of Fifty Years: A Sermon...* (Huron, MI, 1910?); *The Story of My Life* (Cincinnati, OH, 1914).
B. SEAP 5, 2255–56.

**REEVE, Tapping**   (October 1744, Brookhaven, NY—13 December 1823, Litchfield, CT). *Education*: graduated from the Coll. of New Jersey (now Princeton Univ.), 1763; study of law under Judge Root, Hartford, CT, 1771–72; LLD. (honorary), Middlebury Coll., 1808, Princeton Univ., 1813. *Career*: schoolteacher, 1763–69; tutor, Coll. of New Jersey, 1769–70; admitted to bar, CT, 1772; legal practice, Litchfield, CT, beginning 1772; service in Continental army and on state committee to rally support for the Revolution, CT, 1776–77; founder and instructor, Litchfield Law Sch., 1784–98; state's attorney, CT, 1788; member, Connecticut Legislature and Council, 1790s; judge, Superior Court, 1798–1814; chief justice, Supreme Court of Errors, 1814–16.

Born the son of a Presbyterian minister, Tapping Reeve graduated from the College of New Jersey (now Princeton) in 1763 and went on to teach for seven years, two of them at his alma mater. In 1771, however, he left New Jersey for Connecticut, where he stayed for the remainder of his life. He studied law in the office of a Judge Root in Hartford before passing the bar and setting up his own legal practice in Litchfield in 1772. The new lawyer rose quickly in his profession, and his social stature was such that with the outbreak of the American Revolution the Connecticut government offered him a Continental army commission (although he never saw active duty) and asked him to serve on a special committee to rally his fellow citizens to the colors. After the war, Reeve was politically active as a member of the Federalist Party, and while he won election to a number of state offices, he could display a rather prickly disposition in dealing with his opponents. He wrote avidly for local journals on political subjects, often flaying his political enemies, and he wrote numerous scurrilous pamphlets in the style of the time, using classical pseudonyms. On one occasion he went too far, and a federal grand jury indicted him for libeling President Thomas Jefferson. But Reeve escaped prosecution, owing probably to Jefferson's wishes. In his less combative periods, though, Reeve made significant contributions to the growth of legal education, most notably the founding of the Litchfield Law School, the first independent institution of its kind in the United States (1784). For the first fourteen years, Reeve was its only faculty member, teaching some two hundred students in all. When he was appointed to the Connecticut bench he put James Gould in charge of the school, and under Gould's hand it became the premier law school in the country.

While pursuing his other activities, Reeve also emerged as a leading social and moral advocate. Arguably, Reeve's views on reform were indistinguishable from his politics: He believed in the dominance of the nation's (and especially New England's) established cultural and social elite. From this perspective, reform was a means of bringing others into line with cultural orthodoxy and checking ideas and tendencies (including, in Reeve's mind, excessive democracy) threatening social disruption. In this cause, he helped found the Society for the Suppression of Vice and Promotion of Good Morals and took part in the establishment of a number of temperance groups. In 1789 he was one of the signers of the Litchfield Agreement, in which local farmers agreed to end the practice of supplying liquor rations to their hired hands. (Reeve was no farmer and evidently signed as an expression of sentiment.) He also was a central figure in the rise of the Connecticut Temperance Society and for years served as president of the local Litchfield Temperance Society. The reformer-lawyer spoke widely on the drink question as well and while on the bench often agreed to hear dry challenges to various aspects of the liquor business. His actions won the praise of other reformers, who appreciated not only his zeal but the prestige his efforts lent to their moral and social causes. Reeve, in conjunction with his reform work, was also a pillar of his church. He fostered the career of Lyman Beecher* and for a time served as a local agent for the state Bible society.

## Bibliography:

A. *The Law of Baron and Femme...* (1816; New York, 1979); *A Treatise on the Law of Descants in the Several United States of America* (New York, 1825); *Domestic Relations*, ed. James W. Eaton, Jr., 4th ed. (Burlington, NJ, 1846); *Reeve's and Gould's Lectures in the Litchfield Law School* (n.p., 18—?).

B. DAB 15, 468–70; SEAP 5, 2258; WW H, 507; Charles Beecher, ed., *Autobiography, Correspondence, Etc., of Lyman Beecher, D.D.*, 2 vols. (New York, 1864–65); D. S. Broadman, *Sketches of the Early Lights of the Litchfield Bar* (1860); Samuel H. Fisher, *The Litchfield Law School, 1775–1833* (New Haven, CT, 1933).

**REGAN, Frank Stewart**   (3 October 1862, Rockford, IL—24 July 1944, Rockford, IL). *Education*: private study of law, 1890s. *Career*: admitted to bar, 1895; legal practice, Rockford, IL, beginning 1895; member, Illinois legislature, 1898–1900?; active Chautauqua and lyceum speaker, 1890s–1930s.

Little is known of Frank Regan's youth, except that he grew up in an apparently staunchly prohibitionist family. We do know that his dry upbringing influenced his adult views on the liquor question and brought him a certain distinction among temperance workers: In 1898, Regan was probably the first American to be elected to a state legislature (in this case, Illinois) by virtue of being the nominee of the Prohibition Party. If the party never had any real political muscle on the national level, Regan's career demonstrated that at times, in local contests, the Prohibitionists could make an impact. The Rockville lawyer began his anti-liquor work early. Before completing his legal studies he won election as a local alderman, making temperance his campaign issue. He served for two years in this capacity, while at the same time heading the Young People's No License League, an organization fighting the town's policy of issuing liquor licenses. With the league and other drys behind him, Regan successfully orchestrated an effort to elect a prohibitionist mayor and six more antiliquor aldermen in 1893. Rockville had been noted as a wet stronghold, willing to make liquor dealers buy licenses, but not to challenge the existence of the drink trade. Thus Regan's activities brought him celebrity stature among Illinois drys and a reputation as a dedicated and capable reformer with much of the citizenry generally. When he joined the small Prohibition Party in 1896, the group's members saw him as a natural candidate, and he did not disappoint them. He won his seat in the legislature handily and demonstrated that the Prohibitionists were not necessarily interested in just the fight against drink. Regan also supported efforts to reform the state property tax laws, transit fares, court procedures, and certain advertising practices.

Throughout his years in politics, Regan was also active on the public lecture platform. Indeed, if his political efforts brought him a regional visibility, his speaking tours brought him national recognition. Regan traveled the Chautauqua and lyceum circuit for more than forty years. He was, by all accounts, an enthralling speaker, and his denunciations of booze and other social ills drew large and enthusiastic audiences. Having a facility for rapid sketching, he was best known for his "chalk talks," something of a novelty on the podium of the era. His standard subjects, besides prohibition, included tax reform ("The Fool Taxpayer" was one of his favorite speeches) and exposés of corruption. On the latter, he was able to establish that some German-owned breweries had evaded American taxes, and his presentation, which he repeated again and again, allowed him to combine the rhetoric of tax reform, temperance, and even patriotism during World War I. The dry orator's most popular talk, however, was "What Is Wrong with Prohibition?" It was a rhetorical question, for Regan's answer was a loud "nothing!" He used the speech often in defense of National Prohibition during the 1920s, and he believed his own arguments until the end of the "noble experiment." As a Prohibitionist, though, Regan went down fighting: His last political effort was a run for the vice presidency on the party ticket, after which he largely dropped out of public view.

**Bibliography:**

A. *Can Chicago Live Without Saloon Revenue?* (Chicago, 1910).
B. SEAP 5, 2260–61; WW 2, 442.

**REYNOLDS, Henry Augustus**   (9 November 1839, Bangor, ME—13 February 1922, Worcester, MA). *Education*: graduated from Medical Dept. of Harvard Univ., 1864. *Career*: assistant surgeon, First Maine Regiment of Heavy Artillery, 1864–65; medical practice, Bangor, ME, 1865 to 1870s; founder and organizer of Red Ribbon Movement (Reform Clubs), beginning 1875; editor, *Living Issues*, 1892–97.

The son of a middle-class family with sufficient resources to send him to Harvard, Reynolds seemed destined for a promising medical career. After service with Maine troops during the Civil War, he set up practice in his home town of Bangor and quickly established a solid professional reputation. He also traveled in social circles, as one biographical account noted, that included fine wine and champagne as normal aspects of dining and entertaining. And it was only after making such friends that the successful young doctor found that he was, in his words, "one of the unfortunate men who inherited an appetite for strong drink." Within short years his drinking was out of control, and alcoholism soon cost him his practice. At times he was barely able to function: "A periodical drunk with me," he later recalled, "usually lasted six weeks." Yet Reynolds still had friends who urged the physician to lay aside the bottle, and in 1875 he was able to do so. He did not take the step alone, however. He took the pledge at a temperance meeting sponsored by women "crusaders"—those who banded together against alcohol as a result of the original "Woman's Crusade" launched in Ohio in 1873. Grateful for his reformation, Reynolds not only dedicated the rest of his life to the salvation of the drunkard but, learning from the women who had helped him, proposed to expand upon their "gospel temperance" techniques. He was also convinced that, as a former alcoholic himself, he could persuade those still suffering to organize on their own behalf (much as the Washingtonians had done in the 1840s or Alcoholics Anonymous in the twentieth century).

The result of Reynolds' planning was the Red Ribbon Movement, or alternatively, the Red Ribbon Reform Clubs. The idea was fairly simple: Reynolds wanted to organize clubs (known generally as Reformed Men's Clubs) of alcoholics who would support one another in efforts to stop drinking. Hearing the antiliquor message from themselves, the doctor believed, would do more good than lectures or strictures from temperance workers. At the same time, club members would strive for Christian renewal, which would sustain them in their fight against alcohol. As a mark of identity club members wore a piece of red ribbon—thus the name of the movement. The approach was not especially novel, as Dr. J. K. Osgood* and Francis Murphy,* both recovered alcoholics as well, were also organizing reform clubs along similar lines, as was the Woman's Christian Temperance Union. Nevertheless, Reynolds' effort flourished. In Maine alone he attracted some 46,000 members, and he proselytized successfully in Massachusetts, Michigan (where he eventually settled), Mississippi, and several other states besides. Tens of thousands took the pledge at his urging, and his fame spread across the land as one of the premier temperance reformers of his day. In Maine, the former alcoholic was honored by the state legislature, which asked him to hold a club meeting on the floor of the House of Representatives; other states passed special resolutions endorsing his campaign. Reynolds frequently worked with the WCTU over the years, often cooperating in the founding of Reformed Men's Clubs. Indeed, it was the Red Ribbon leader who, in 1876, suggested that the union adopt the white ribbon as its official badge. Later, he edited the official publication of the Prohibition Party in Michigan (*Living Issues*). While he worked hard on behalf of prohibition, however, and lived to see it adopted, Reynolds was always best remembered as a man who reached out to help the alcoholic—whose plight had done so much to spark the temperance reform in the first place.

**Bibliography:**

A. [Address Before the National Temperance Convention, 1876], 237–43, in *Centennial Temperance Volume . . .* (New York, 1877).

B. SEAP 5, 2268–69; W. H. Daniels, *The Temperance Reform and Its Great Reformers* (Cincinnati, OH, 1878); Daniel Dorchester, *The Liquor Problem in All Ages* (New York, 1888); "The Reform Club Movement," 758–69, in *Centennial Temperance Volume . . .* (New York, 1877).

**ROSS, William**    (25 December 1812, London—18 December 1875, Dover, IL). *Education*: private study of medicine, 1840s? *Career*: temperance and reform lecturer, 1840s to 1870s.

Born in England in 1812 and raised the son of a British soldier in Canada, Ross grew up in a family that drank heavily. His early years were marked by wild drinking sprees and probably by alcoholism. So dissolute did he become that by the time he was twenty years old Ross literally had to be rescued from the gutter into which an irate saloonkeeper had thrown him. He seemed headed for a drunkard's grave, but a drinking-related injury that almost cost him a hand and a family incident in which his twin sister was killed during a drunken brawl by her own husband shocked Ross back into sobriety. Indeed, he became sober with a vengeance, pledging himself to a life of total abstinence and opposition to the liquor traffic. With his still unhealed arm in a sling, he gave his first temperance lecture in Rochester, New York, probably in the early 1840s, when the Washingtonian temperance revival had created a hospitable climate for itinerant dry speakers in the United States. He was a major success, as audiences at lecture after lecture flocked to hear his firsthand stories of the horrors of drink. Taking time off to study medicine, he then expanded his talks to include material on the pathology of alcoholism; he also took to carrying a small still with him in order to demonstrate how the beverage industry might "adulterate" liquor. Thus armed with a ready store of lectures, he ranged up and down the public platforms of the Atlantic coast and by the 1860s had pushed as far west as Missouri with his speeches. Known now as "Doctor" Ross, he was clearly one of the most popular temperance lecturers of his day.

Although he made handsome profits from his appearances, there is little question that Ross's devotion to the reform cause was sincere. When he might otherwise have spent his time on the fee-paying podium, he gave a great deal of attention to prohibitionist political work, which was often a frustrating business. A Republican during the Civil War, he found that the party would not take a firm stand on the liquor question, which convinced the zealous lecturer of the need for an independent reform party. While Ross believed in reforming individual drunkards, he also held that the traffic had to be legislated out of existence if the nation was ever going to decisively defeat "King Alcohol." Thus in 1868 he urged the Illinois State Temperance Convention to pass a resolution in favor of a separate Prohibition Party as a means of challenging the liquor interests at the polls. The measure carried, and with the aid of other temperance workers the national Prohibition Party was established in Illinois the following year. While Ross took no direct hand in the party's leadership, the Temperance Movement looked back on his work in 1868 as one of the key steps in its birth.

**Bibliography:**

B. SEAP 5, 2308; David Leigh Colvin, *Prohibition in the United States: A History of the Prohibition Party and of the Prohibition Movement* (New York, 1926).

**ROUNDS, Louise S. Jones**  (6 July 1839, Heuvelton, NY—27 September 1918, Clifton Springs, NY). *Career*: schoolteacher, NY, circa 1850s to 1864; various offices, National and Illinois WCTU, 1877 to 1900s.

Little is known either of the youth of Louise S. Jones or of her reasons for allying herself with the Temperance Movement. We may suppose that she shared the same fears of the liquor traffic that drew millions of other Americans into the ranks of the antiliquor reform. At any rate, after teaching in the New York State public schools for several years, she married one Freeman Rounds in 1864 and moved with him to Chicago, where she made her home for the next thirty-five years. She apparently became involved with the Woman's Crusade, which erupted in the Midwest in 1873. Her exact role is obscure, but she evidently won a modest reputation as an effective public speaker and for "thoroughly uncompromising hostility to the liquor traffic." She must have developed some leadership qualities as well, for when the Woman's Christian Temperance Union emerged from the crusade in 1874, Rounds was elected secretary of the local

Chicago branch. In that capacity, she organized daily "gospel temperance" meetings, in which WCTU members tried to lead drunkards to abstinence and spiritual rebirth. By 1877 Rounds, by this time an experienced veteran, won election as secretary of the National WCTU. Her duties in the office were routine, but she played a key role in one decision that dramatically affected the course of the union and consequently the movement generally. As secretary, she had worked closely with Frances E. Willard,* then the organization's corresponding secretary. Many in the WCTU considered Willard, former dean of women at Northwestern University and a woman of broad reform interests, to be the best choice as the next president of the group. But sentiment for Willard was not unanimous, as some union members preferred a narrow concentration on temperance issues and prohibition rather than involvement with additional causes. Willard was not sure about fighting for the job and was in fact considering a return to education. It was Rounds who was the central figure in persuading her to stand for election, and Willard began her long tenure as WCTU president in 1879. The union itself evolved into one of the most effective broad-based reform organizations in the country.

After performing this service, the rest of Rounds' career in the Temperance Movement was largely anticlimactic. She continued, however, to do good if unspectacular service. Rounds maintained her office as national secretary until the death of her husband in 1883, when she was overwhelmed with grief. In 1884, reportedly to help escape her sorrow, she took post as an itinerant evangelist for the Illinois WCTU, the duties of which put her on a busy lecture schedule throughout the state. The change apparently helped, for she recovered her stride and even took on more responsibility two years later, when she was chosen president of the state union. For the next fifteen years, the Illinois WCTU was her life. She served it well, guiding it through political campaigns and directing its affairs across the state. Throughout, she also continued her evangelical touring. Finally, too tired to continue in all of her duties, she declined to stand again for the state presidency in 1901, although she retained her position as evangelist until old age and health problems took her off the circuit. She was a woman of solid achievements: At the state level, she provided stalwart, if generally unsung leadership, the kind necessary to the success of any cause at the grassroots; and, at a critical time, her friendship and counsel to Frances Willard had resulted in a service of the first magnitude to the dry crusade as a whole.

**Bibliography:**

B. SEAP 5, 2314–15.

**RUSH, Benjamin**    (24 December 1746, Philadelphia, PA—19 April 1813, Philadelphia, PA). *Education*: graduated from Coll. of New Jersey (now Princeton Univ.), 1760; studied medicine with Dr. John Redman, Philadelphia, 1761–66; attended medical lectures, Philadelphia Medical Coll., 1760s; studied at Univ. of Edinburgh, Scotland, 1768; hospital experience, London and Paris,

1760s. *Career*: medical practice, Philadelphia, beginning 1769; professor of chemistry, Philadelphia Medical Coll. (later merged with Univ. of Pennsylvania), 1769–91; member, Continental Congress, 1776–77; signer of Declaration of Independence, 1776; surgeon general, Middle Department, Continental army, 1777; lecturer, Univ. of Pennsylvania, 1780; physician, Pennsylvania Hosp., 1783–1813; founder, Philadelphia Dispensary, 1786; active in Pennsylvania constitutional politics, 1787, 1789; co-founder, Philadelphia Coll. of Physicians, 1787; port physician, Philadelphia, 1790–93; professor, Univ. of Pennsylvania, beginning 1792; treasurer, U.S. Mint, 1797–1813.

Ardent Revolutionary politician, signer of the Declaration of Independence, one of the premier medical men of his era, and briefly a surgeon general of the Continental army, Benjamin Rush was a man of broad learning and interests and possessed of a zealous concern for political and personal "virtue." The fate of the young republic, he believed, hinged on purging evil from society and government; and with this end in view he advocated a range of reforms, including medical education, constitutional revisions, treatment of the mentally ill, antislavery, and other causes with the same vigor he had devoted to the struggle for American independence. Over time, however, Americans came to know him best for his efforts on behalf of temperance. Rush had spoken out against the use of distilled liquors since at least 1772, but his masterpiece on the subject was *An Inquiry Into the Effects of Ardent Spirits on the Human Mind and Body* (1785). The tract was a radical challenge to the traditional dictum that drinking was a positive good. Rush had no quarrel with wine and beer, but he pointed out that most Americans were drinking distilled beverages and that consumed over time these drinks were lethal. Indeed, in this connection the Philadelphia doctor was the first American to call chronic drunkenness a distinct disease. He described it as an addiction process and specifically identified alcohol as the addictive agent. Once an "appetite" or "craving" for spirits had become fixed, he claimed, a drinker was helpless. In these cases, drunkenness was no longer a vice, for the imbiber no longer had any control over his drinking. In Rush's view, the old colonial idea that drunkenness was a personal failing was valid only in the early stages of the disease, when a tippler might still pull back. Once addicted, even a saint was in trouble.

The *Inquiry* was a powerful indictment, and it conveyed a sense of urgency. The threat of hard liquor, Rush believed, called for immediate action. As a doctor, he was genuinely concerned about personal health. Drinking habits as they were, many people did risk addiction and a host of related medical complications. Longstanding friendships with Anthony Benezet* and early Methodist leaders had also convinced Rush of the moral and social threats posed by hard liquor. His political ideology, moreover, had so affected his reactions to public behavior that he saw clearly in American drinking patterns what others had only hinted at: As American preferences had shifted away from traditional beers, cider, and other lighter alcoholic drinks (and the social norms that controlled their use) to distilled spirits, no new social standards had arisen to limit drinking excesses associated with the new beverages. Not only was there more drunkenness in the postrevolutionary era, but with the loosening of old behavioral norms as the populace moved to the frontiers and adjusted to independence from Britain, more people seemed to care less about such formerly unacceptable behavior. The traditional consensus on how to handle drinking, or so it appeared to Rush, had broken down and nothing had taken its place. The prospect was societal anarchy, civil discord, and political corruption and chaos. Allow drunkenness, with its attendant social and economic problems, to flourish, he cautioned, and the Revolution would have been fought in vain. "Our country would soon be governed by men chosen by intemperate and corrupted voters," rather than by citizens of virtue. "From such legislators the republic would soon be in danger." To avert such a calamity, Rush urged personal abstinence from distilled liquor (but not from wines and beers) and strong social action against drunkenness.

But the Philadelphia doctor harbored few illusions. Americans loved their whiskey, and anyone telling them to forgo it would be waging an uphill battle. Still, stubborn and zealous as he was, Rush was willing to try: The very fate of the new republican nation—the great legacy of the Revolution—depended upon it. Before his death in 1813, Rush thus labored mightily to spread his gospel. He had thousands of reprints of the *Inquiry* distributed nationally, and in a later edition he attached a "Moral and Physical Thermometer" to illustrate the progressive nature of alcohol addiction, outlining the disease's social, medical, and moral complications. Rush wrote other tracts on temperance, and he made some headway in pressing his views on the Protestant churches. Some of the early temperance efforts of such crusaders as Lyman Beecher,* for example, came as a direct result of Rush's pleas. But the real impact of Rush's work lay years in the future, although he did more than anyone of his generation to point out the dire implications inherent in the way Americans drank. Later generations of temperance workers, however, honored his memory, according him the status of "father" of the movement.

## Bibliography:

A. *A Syllabus of a Course of Lectures on Chemistry* (Philadelphia, 1770); *An Address to the Inhabitants of the British Settlements, on the Slavery of the Negroes in America, etc.* (Philadelphia, 1773); *An Inquiry Into the Effects of Ardent Spirits Upon the Human Mind and Body* (Philadelphia, 1785, and many later editions); *Medical Inquiries and Observations Upon the Diseases of the Mind* (Philadelphia, 1812); *The Autobiography of Benjamin Rush: His Travels Through Life Together with His Commonplace Book for 1789–1813*, ed. George W. Corner (Westport, CT, 1970).

B. SEAP 5, 2323–24; Winthrop Neilson and Frances Neilson, *Verdict for the Doctor: The Case of Benjamin Rush* (New York, 1958); Carl Alfred Lenning Binger, *Revolutionary Doctor: Benjamin Rush, 1746–1813* (New York, 1966); Donald J. D'Elia, *Benjamin Rush: Philosopher of the American Revolution* (Philadelphia, 1974); David Freeman Hawke, *Benjamin Rush: Revolutionary*

*Gadfly* (Indianapolis, IN, 1971); Mark Edward Lender and James Kirby Martin, *Drinking in America: A History* (New York, 1982); Sarah Regal Riedman, *Benjamin Rush: Physician, Patriot, Founding Father* (London, 1964).

**RUSSELL, Howard Hyde**    (21 October 1855, Stillwater, MN—30 June 1946, Westerville, OH). *Education*: studied at Griswold Coll., IA, 1870–72; LLB., Indianola Coll., 1877; B.D., Oberlin Theological Sem., 1888; A.M. (honorary), Oberlin Theological Sem., 1895; D.D. (honorary), Ohio Wesleyan Univ., 1896, Oberlin Theological Sem., 1921; LLD. (honorary), Otterbein Coll., 1922; LHD. (honorary), Otterbein Coll., 1935. *Career*: clerk, Rock Island Arsenal,1872–73; cowboy, 1874; schoolteacher, IA, 1874, 1875–77; editor, *Adams County* (IA) *Gazette*, 1875; admitted to bar, IA, 1878; legal practice, 1878–83; school superintendent, Adams Co., IA, 1881–82; minister, North Amherst and Berea, OH, 1883–88; ordained, Congregational Church, 1885; minister, Tabernacle Congregational Church, Kansas City, MO, 1888–91; minister, Armour Mission, Chicago, 1891–93; superintendent, Anti-Saloon League, OH, 1893–97; general superintendent, Anti-Saloon League of America, 1895–1903; superintendent, Anti-Saloon League of New York, 1901–9; associate general superintendent and other offices, Anti-Saloon League of America, beginning 1909.

The man who founded the Anti-Saloon League, Howard Hyde Russell, was born the son of an Episcopal minister. He went to school in three different states, showing no particular direction in life, and then drifted from job to job working as a clerk, cowboy, schoolteacher, and editor of a small-town Iowa newspaper. At age twenty, however, he began studying law, was admitted to the bar in 1878, and quickly built a successful legal practice in Corning, Iowa. The prosperous lawyer, though, gave up his business after a religious conversion experience in 1883. Entering Oberlin Theological Seminary, Russell served two Ohio pulpits while a student and received a Congregational ordination in 1885. At Oberlin, he also earned a considerable reputation as a temperance reformer. Working with local dry groups in 1888, he organized a successful local-option campaign, driving booze out of Beatty Township and testing the local organizing techniques that the Anti-Saloon League would later use to such effect. He took his reform ideas with him to Kansas City, Missouri, where he went the same year to found what became a thriving congregation at the Tabernacle Church. In 1890, the antiliquor reverend called a state-wide convention of church delegates, seeking to form a movement that would sweep the saloon out of Missouri by main force. The result was the Anti-Liquor League of Missouri, with Russell as president. When he moved to Chicago the following year, the organization declined, but its founder was satisfied that, with proper leadership, it was possible to establish a league of churches. That lesson, coupled with his knowledge of local-option work, gave Russell the experience he needed to launch the most influential antiliquor group in American history.

In 1891, Russell moved on to the Armour Mission in Chicago, where he brought vitality and organizing genius to his pastoral responsibilities. It was in this post that he, with his wife, believed he "received a divine call" to wage war on the saloon as a life's work. He discussed his ideas with friends back at Oberlin in 1893, and with their encouragement and further consultation with the divinity he officially established the Anti-Saloon League on May 21 of that year. Russell's strategy had two components: He intended to organize churches as the league's basic units; he then wanted to use the congregations to build local-option campaigns to dry out Ohio town by town. He also intended to generate as much political leverage as possible, and toward that end the league adopted a nonpartisan stance. It would support candidates of either party provided they voted dry, and as time went on Russell and his colleagues proved repeatedly that they could effectively marshall voters for or against candidates. Over the 1890s, league tactics began to tell. Ohio, little by little, went dry, and Russell's organization captured national attention. It also attracted talented and devoted reform workers: During these early years, Russell was able to recruit the likes of Edwin Dinwiddie* and Wayne B. Wheeler,* who would soon take the league to the heights of political influence in the struggle for National Prohibition.

In 1895, the league was reorganized on a national basis as the Anti-Saloon League of America. Russell was general superintendent from 1895 to 1903, during which time he travelled some fifty thousand miles in helping to found chapters in thirty-six states. Considering New York a critical state, he personally headed the New York League from 1901 to 1909, after which he returned to national headquarters in Washington, D.C., taking on a succession of leadership assignments. He toured the country extensively on behalf of prohibition and represented the United States several times at international temperance gatherings. With the advent of the Eighteenth Amendment, the daily affairs of the league, including its massive lobbying efforts, fell largely to the management of younger men. Many of these, like Wheeler, owed their posts to Russell, whom they honored at a special ceremony in 1925 as the official founder of the organization. To further recognize his contributions, in 1927 the league placed a granite marker on the site of his birthplace in Stillwater, Minnesota. Even after Repeal, the old reformer never lost the faith; to the end, he believed that the war against drink was a struggle on behalf of the Lord.

## Bibliography:

A. *The Conversion of Children*... (Oberlin, OH, 1887); *The Lincoln-Lee Legion: The Story of Its Beginning* (New York, 1903); *The New Trilly-Wainwright...Local Option Bill: The Full Text, a Brief on Its Fairness and Fitness*... (New York, 1906); *A Lawyer's Examination of the Bible*... (Westerville, OH, 1935); *The White Thread Box: A Christmas Narrative*... (Westerville, OH, n.d.).

B. SEAP 5, 2324–27; WW 2, 463; Ernest H. Cherrington, *History of the Anti-Saloon League* (Westerville, OH, 1913); Norman H. Dohn, "The History of the Anti-Saloon League" (Ph.D. diss., Ohio State Univ., 1959); Peter H.

Odegard, *Pressure Politics: The Story of the Anti-Saloon League* (New York, 1928).

**RUSSELL, John**   (20 September 1882, Livingston Co., NY—3 November 1912, Detroit, MI). *Career*: ordained, Methodist Episcopal Church, 1845; minister, pastorates in Port Huron, Romeo, Ypsilanti, Flint, Pontiac, Marguette, Detroit, MI, 1845 to 1900s; editor, *Penninsular Herald*, 1867.

Born in New York State, Russell was educated in local schools until moving to Michigan with his family at age sixteen. The Russells were evidently strict Methodists and drys, and while little else is known about John's youth, it seems that he decided early on a career in the ministry and a life dedicated to the antiliquor reform. He started to preach in 1843, and after ordination in 1845 he took pulpits in a number of Michigan towns over the years. Something of a church activist, he ultimately held important posts in the regional Methodist hierarchy as well. He was district superintendent in the Detroit Conference for eight years, a delegate to the church's General Conference on two occasions, and in 1891 a representative to the Methodist Second Ecumenical Conference. In all of these positions, and especially in his preaching, Russell sought to advance the fortunes of the Temperance Movement. The battle against drink, in his mind, was an integral part of the Christian life. For many years he served as a temperance agent in the Detroit Conference, lecturing on the liquor question and organizing dry partisans for the struggle in the cause of reform. Russell was also a leader of the region's fraternal temperance effort. For twelve years he was head of the Michigan lodge of the Independent Order of Good Templars, a lodge lecturer (with the grandiloquent title "right worthy grand lodge lecturer") for two years more, and head of the order's world organization for two years beyond that. In this latter capacity, the reforming reverend travelled extensively on behalf of the order, appearing before Templars and popular audiences across the United States and abroad in Great Britain, Canada, and France. By the late nineteenth century he was unquestionably one of America's best-known temperance speakers.

Russell's chief claim to fame as a reform leader, however, came well before he rose to the highest ranks as a Templar or clergyman. Rather, as early as 1867, as editor of a prohibitionist journal, the *Penninsular Herald*, he issued the first call for the formation of a separate prohibition political party. The Republicans and Democrats, he argued, had too many ties to the liquor in history to allow them to face the drink question squarely. Reformers, Russell insisted, therefore had to go their own way. In the *Herald*, generally considered the leading antiliquor journal of its day, he repeatedly challenged drys to organize the new party; and he took the lead himself in founding the Prohibition Party of Michigan in 1867. Two years later, he served as temporary chair of the convention which established the national Prohibition Party. Russell was jubilant at the event, and the new party honored him by naming him chairman of its National Committee. All of this won the Michigan preacher the sobriquet "Father of the Prohibition

Party.'' In the Prohibitionists' first presidential election, Russell joined the ticket as the dry candidate for vice president, running with James Black.* They were smothered in the election by Republican Ulysses S. Grant, but they had successfully launched the antiliquor crusade into the contest for the highest elective office in the land.

**Bibliography:**

A. *The Funeral Discourse and Obituary of the Late Rev. Abel Warren* (Romeo, MI, 1863); *An Appeal to Christian Men in Behalf of the Temperance Cause* (Detroit, MI, 1867?); *Plea for a National Temperance Party!* (Detroit, MI, 1868?); *Is a Prohibition Party a Feasible and Reliable Agency for Securing the Enactment and Execution of Prohibitory Laws?* (n.p., 187-?); *The Liquor Traffic Versus Political Economy* (n.p., 187-?).

B. SEAP 5, 2327–28; David Leigh Colvin, *Prohibition in the United States: A History of the Prohibition Party and of the Prohibition Movement* (New York, 1926).

# S

---

**ST. JOHN, Charles Henry**   (18 September 1843, near Auburn, NY—10 February 1904, Salina, KS). *Education*: Ph.B., Illinois Wesleyan Univ.; M.D., Kansas City Univ. (KS), 1896; D.D. (honorary), Kansas Wesleyan Univ., 1900. *Career*: Methodist minister, IL, until 1881; lawyer, CO, KS, CA, 1881–1904; active reform lecturer, 1882–1904.

St. John's career was fairly typical of those who organized and led the zealous but largely ineffectual Prohibition Party in the late nineteenth and early twentieth centuries. His first calling was that of a Methodist minister in Illinois, where he made no particular mark. In 1881 he moved to Colorado for reasons of health, and there he gave up the ministry to study law. He quickly gained admission to the Colorado bar, and over the 1880s he established a successful law practice in several Western states. At the same time, St. John assumed an active role in Colorado civic affairs and, reflecting his Methodist background and his family's dry sentiments, became involved in reform causes as well. Living in Denver in 1882, he was a founder of the State Temperance Union of Colorado, of which he then served two terms as president. Unable to convince either of the major political parties to adopt strong prohibitionist stances, St. John, like others of similar feelings throughout the nation, then became involved in a third-party movement. Relying on his influence in regional temperance circles, he took the lead in organizing a Colorado branch of the Prohibition Party; and in 1884 he led his state's delegation to the national party convention in Pittsburgh, Pennsylvania. He supported the presidential nomination of his cousin, former Kansas Governor John P. St. John,* and then campaigned actively on behalf of his more famous relative. After the campaign, he returned to reform work, maintaining an active lecture schedule in the United States, Canada, and Europe. While he devoted most of his energy to the prohibitionist cause, he also remained interested in church affairs, serving in 1889, along with his wife, as a delegate to the World's Sunday-School Convention in London. In 1896 he received a medical degree from Kansas City University, after which he added lectures on narcotics, physiology, and other health-related topics to his repertoire. Never in the first rank of temperance leaders, his reform labors did earn him considerable recognition, especially in the West, and in 1900 Kansas Wesleyan University presented him with an honorary D.D. degree.

**Bibliography:**

B. SEAP 6, 2341.

**ST. JOHN, John Pierce**    (25 February 1833, Brookville, IN—31 August 1916, Olathe, KS). *Education*: private study of law, 1850s; study of law, offices of Starkweather and McLain, Charleston, IL, 1860. *Career*: store clerk, 1840s; joined Gold Rush to California, circa 1851; fought Indians, CA, OR, 1852–53; seaman, shipped to Latin America, South Pacific, 1856–60; law partner, Starkweather and McLain, 1860–61; officer, Union army, 1861–65; legal practice, Independence, MO, 1865–69; legal practice, Olathe, KS, beginning 1869; member, Kansas Senate, 1873–74; governor of Kansas, 1879–83; lecturer, National Prohibition Lecture Bureau, 1884–97; mining and real estate ventures, Olathe, KS, 1897–1916.

John P. St. John, one of the most colorful advocates of political prohibition of the post–Civil War period, started life with a meager education of only a few years in a one-room schoolhouse. He also grew up with a loathing of drink: When he was only a boy, he watched as his father drank himself to a drunkard's grave. As a youth, St. John led a peripatetic existence including immigration to California in the famous Gold Rush, a spell as an Indian fighter, and a lengthy voyage on a merchant ship. He returned to Illinois in 1860 to pursue a legal career, but service during the Civil War intervened and it was not until 1869 that he finally settled permanently in Olathe, Kansas, where he established a successful law office. Entering the State Senate as a staunch Republican in 1873, he stood firmly for temperance, and, buoyed by the rise of the Woman's Christian Temperance Union and other antiliquor groups, he campaigned successfully on the prohibition issue for governor in 1878. True to his word, after a bitter struggle he was able to submit a prohibitory amendment to the Kansas Constitution to the electorate, which approved it in 1880. His was the first such amendment in any of the states (the antebellum Maine Laws had been only statutory legislation), and its passage made St. John a national figure and a Temperance Movement hero. It also enraged the wets, as well as Republican officials concerned that the liquor question would create party discord; an alliance of these figures frustrated the governor's hopes for a third term in 1882, but the dry amendment (which was reasonably well enforced) remained in effect.

St. John had hoped that the Republican Party would ultimately endorse prohibition. In this he was disappointed and even somewhat embittered when his inflexible support of temperance laws and his contest for a third term resulted in his virtual exile from the Kansas GOP. Thus, after some initial hesitation the former governor accepted the nomination of the Prohibition Party for the presidency at its 1884 convention in Pittsburgh. St. John, an excellent speaker and dynamic campaigner, fought hard to carry the dry message to the people. He also bore up well under an absolutely vile smear effort directed at him by the Republicans. The GOP was right to fear the man: Although St. John had no chance to win, he did drain off enough votes from Republican James G. Blaine to tip the election to Democrat Grover Cleveland. Even in defeat, however, St. John flourished. He had done better than any previous Prohibition Party candidate, and over the next decade he was one of the most sought after lecturers in the country. He emerged as more than a single-issue reformer. His speeches endorsed women's rights, tariff reform, "free silver," and a host of other causes— all of which eventually got him into trouble with the Prohibition Party as well. At its 1896 convention he was among a large group of party members to protest the official platform, which confined itself solely to the prohibition issue. Like other "broad-gaugers," St. John wanted the party to address other reforms, and he walked out with the dissenters to form a short-lived rival National Party. Retiring from the lecture circuit in 1897, St. John pursued mining and real estate investments in Kansas and enjoyed celebrity stature until the end among opponents of the "demon rum."

### Bibliography:

A. *Prohibition in Kansas* (New York, 1882); *Prohibition: A Constitutional Law . . .* (Philadelphia, 1883); *Why St. John Will not Withdraw* (n.p., 1884); with others, *The White Angel of the World, that Foretells the Freedom of the Nations from the Evils of Strong Drink* (Lynn, MA, 1893).

B. DAB 16, 303–4; SEAP 5, 2341–42; WW 1, 1168; Jack S. Blocker, Jr., *Retreat from Reform: The Prohibition Movement in the United States, 1890– 1913* (Westport, CT, 1976); Edna Tutt Frederikson, "John P. St. John: The Father of Constitutional Prohibition" (Ph.D. diss., Univ. of Kansas, 1931).

**SANDERS, Newell**  (12 July 1850, Owen Co., IN—26 January 1939, Chattanooga, TN). *Education*: B.S., Indiana State Univ., 1873; LLD. (honorary), Indiana State Univ., 1931. *Career*: merchant, Bloomington, IN, 1873–77; plow manufacturer, Chattanooga, TN, 1878–82; president, Chattanooga Plow Company, 1882–1901, 1915–19; president, Newell Sanders Plow Company, beginning 1901; interests in banking and railroads, 1900s; member, U.S. Senate, 1912–13.

A successful manufacturer and businessman for over sixty years, Newell Sanders led the battle for state-wide prohibition in Tennessee. As the first Republican senator from the state in sixty years, he also carried the antiliquor crusade onto the floor of the national legislature. We know little of the origins of Sanders' prohibitionist sympathies, as he apparently devoted his earlier years to establishing his various business enterprises rather than to reform activities. But with his rise in the state Republican Party, he also emerged as an antiliquor champion of unquestioned sincerity. Republicans were a minority in formerly Confederate Tennessee, but Sanders worked hard to build the party's strength, and he frequently held important posts within the GOP. For years he served as chair of the state party's executive committee (1894–98, 1906–12), was a national convention delegate six times, and between 1912 and 1916 sat on the Republican National Committee. Even if Republicans were not often elected in the state, then, Sanders was still politically well placed to take advantage of any opportunities that chance brought his way. It came in 1912, largely through a chain of events that Sanders' temperance efforts had set in motion. He pushed a dry Republican platform through the state committee, which precipitated a bitter split between GOP wets and drys. However, the Republican nominee for governor, a firm dry, captured enough antiliquor Democratic votes to beat his wet opponent in the general election. It was a hard-fought campaign, and the victorious governor was largely beholden to Sanders not only for his nomination but also for the businessman's effective campaign work. (Sanders had gone so far as to buy one of the principal Democratic newspapers and merge it with a prohibitionist journal.) Thus when it came time in 1912 to fill an unexpired vacancy in the Senate, Sanders took the seat on April 8.

The Tennessee Republican would be "Senator Sanders" for less than a year, as his term ended on February 2, 1913. But he made the most of his months in the nation's capital. He was in great measure responsible for the success of the first federal attempt to limit the interstate traffic in alcoholic beverages, a legislative initiative that wets had been able to bottle up in House and Senate committees since 1911. After some tricky parliamentary maneuvering, however, Sanders was able to get a compromise bill, which forbade the shipment of liquor across state lines for illegal purposes, voted on favorably. This was the Webb-Kenyon Act. President William Howard Taft, who made no secret of his distaste for legal prohibitionism, then promptly vetoed the bill. Not to be discouraged, Sanders quickly rounded up enough dry members of both houses of Congress to override the veto. (Sanders later claimed that Taft told him in private that he had come to consider the veto an error.) It was a significant dry victory, and it pointed the way toward more effective laws against the drink trade. In retrospect, many dry leaders considered the Webb-Kenyon law a giant step in the direction of National Prohibition, with reformers thus in the debt of the short-term senator from Tennessee for his labors in bringing it into existence. Upon his return home in 1913 he resumed the active management of his business interests.

**Bibliography:**

B. SEAP 5, 2358; WW 1, 1076.

**SARGENT, Lucius Manlius**    (25 June 1786, Boston, MA—2 June 1867, West Roxbury, MA). *Education*: studied at Harvard Coll., circa 1804–7; A.M. (honorary), Harvard Coll., 1842. *Career*: admitted to bar, 1811; active writing on reform subjects, fiction, nonfiction, poetry, and translation, circa 1807 to 1860s.

Born to a Boston family of considerable means, Sargent received one of the finest educations available to a young man of his region: secondary schooling at prestigious Phillips Exeter Academy and study at Harvard College. He did not graduate from Harvard, however, as he left precipitously in 1804 after an angry dispute over the quality of food the school served to its undergraduates. It was a telling incident: Sargent liked nothing better over the years than a good argument. Failure to get a Harvard degree did not prevent him from studying the law, though, and he was admitted to the Massachusetts bar in 1811. Yet the economic status of his family did not require Sargent to practice his profession for a living, and he turned to the more leisurely pursuit of a literary career. Sargent was both prolific and bright, and he wrote occasional poetry and translated Virgil with genuine accomplishment. But chiefly he was a journalist and popular writer. He used the pseudonym "Sigma" for his pieces in the *Boston Transcript*, which were generally on the subject of temperance reform. Just how Sargent came upon the issue is not known, but there is little doubt that he was vehement and uncompromising in his opposition to liquor. Indeed, "harsh prejudices" is how one obituary later described his views on matters generally. The observation was very much on the mark, for he was a considerable polemicist. In all of his writings, whether he was flaying the liquor traffic, attacking the British coolie trade in India, castigating Thomas Babington Macauley for allegedly defaming William Penn, or denouncing Ralph Waldo Emerson and other abolitionists for their views, he lashed out with abandon and vim. Above all else, noted one biographical sketch, Sargent "was preeminently a good hater."

Polemicist and hater or not, however, Sargent made substantial contributions as a reformer. While he wrote widely on temperance issues, his most popular titles were his series of Temperance Tales, which he penned in the 1830s and 1840s. Twenty-one stories with titles like, "My Mother's Gold Ring," "Groggy Harbor," and "I Am Afraid There Is a God," portrayed the inevitable downfall into besottedness, impecuniousness, degeneracy, and oblivion that was the lot of those who came under the malevolent spell of "demon rum," wine, and beer. These tales were highly popular with the public and sold enormously. They were one of the chief means in the early days of the Temperance Movement of dramatizing the antiliquor message and of explaining to the general public the movement's conception of the addictive and disease nature of alcohol and alcoholism. After Sargent (and a few others, notably Timothy Shay Arthur*) led the way, a legion of dry authors exploited the Temperance Tales genre over the mid- and late nineteenth century. Few of these imitators, however, did as well as Sargent with his original Tales, one collection of which went through 130 editions and was translated into a number of foreign languages. He was also a dynamic speaker and enjoyed haranguing audiences on the evils of booze and the merits of prohibition. For all of his prickly nature, though, he did have his less strident side. If he delighted in berating his antagonists, he was also gracious to his friends and close to his family. He even admitted at least one mistake: He had probably gone too far in his undergraduate protest at Harvard, he conceded, and in 1842 the school awarded him an honorary A.M., signifying the end of the quarrel.

### Bibliography:

A. *Translations from the Minor Latin Poets* (Boston, 1807); *Address Before the Massachusetts Society for the Suppression of Intemperance* . . . (Boston,

1833); *The Temperance Tales*, 2 vols. (Boston, 1848, and many following editions); *Dealings with the Dead* (Boston, 1856); *Reminiscences of Samuel Dexter* (Boston, 1858); *The Ballad of the Abolition Blunder-buss* (Boston, 1861).

B. *Boston Daily Advertiser*, June 4, 1867; DAB 16, 367–68; SEAP 5, 2362; WW H, 78; Mark Edward Lender and Karen R. Karnchanapee, "'Temperance Tales': Antiliquor Fiction and American Attitudes Toward Alcoholics in the Late 19th and Early 20th Centuries," *Journal of Studies on Alcohol* 38(1977):1347–70; E. Pearson, *Queer Books* (Garden City, NY, 1928); J. H. Sheppard, *Reminiscences of Lucius Manlius Sargent* (Boston, 1871).

**SAVAGE, John**    (22 February 1779, New York, NY—19 October 1863, Utica, NY). *Education*: graduated from Union Coll., NY, 1799; private study of law, 1800; LLD. (honorary), Union Coll., 1829. *Career*: admitted to bar, 1800; legal practice, Salem, NY, beginning 1800; district attorney, 1806–11, 1812–13; member, New York Assembly, 1814; member, U.S. House of Representatives, 1815–19; district attorney, Washington Co., NY, 1819–20; New York state comptroller, 1821–23; chief justice, New York Supreme Court, 1823–26.

John Savage was among the first American proponents of total abstinence. Over the years he was adamant on the subject, refusing to tolerate the liquor traffic and belaboring those who sought the compromise position of "moderate" drinking. When Savage went on record with his views in the early 1800s there was no Temperance Movement, and the fact that organized antiliquor groups were firmly established in New York State (and neighboring regions) by the 1820s owed quite a bit to the early spadework of the zealous reformer and his colleagues. Savage was not only pronounced in his views, he was also a man whose ideas commanded respect—or at least a thorough hearing. A successful lawyer and district attorney, he won election as a Democrat to the New York Assembly in 1814, where he stayed only briefly before moving on to the national Congress the following year. He served until 1819, when he returned to New York again for another tour as a district attorney and state comptroller. From 1823 on, however, Savage was chief justice of the State Supreme Court. Throughout his service in these posts he remained an active figure in Democratic Party affairs. He was an elector in the presidential victory of James K. Polk and was highly enough regarded by the administration to be offered the position of assistant U.S. treasurer for New York (he turned down the job). Thus in New York, when John Savage spoke, people generally paid attention. And he spoke forcefully and at length on the liquor question.

As a firm abstainer himself, Savage helped in the dry effort to define the word *temperance* as excluding moderation. The roots of the reforming justice's total abstinence beliefs are not clearly evident. Religion played no certain role, and the fact that Savage was a Democrat of the Jacksonian persuasion suggests that the moral stewardship of some reform advocates also had little bearing on the issue. Rather, there was something of an egalitarian ethos in his sentiments: Moderation, he claimed, was really an elitist perspective on the drink question.

"You condemn the poor man's alcohol," he once charged, "and say nothing against the rich man's wine." If the motive of temperance were genuinely a social reformation, this view held, *everyone* had to leave off drinking. In a democratic society, drinking could not be permitted to one class while placed off limits to another. If reformers would adopt that position, Savage noted, "then I am with you, and not till then." He was as good as his word, refusing to join the New York Temperance Society while it endorsed moderation. In this stand he was closely allied with other dry luminaries such as Edward C. Delavan,* with whom he worked closely. When total abstinence became the prevailing policy, however, Savage readily joined dry organizations. He was president of the state bar's temperance society, sat for many years as president of the New York Temperance Society (then cleansed of its moderationists), and for a year (1855) headed the American Temperance Union. No doubt he would have appreciated Delavan's comments upon his death in 1863: "He would not tolerate half-way measures; he was always ready to strike the blow best fitted to destroy the evil, and at once."

**Bibliography:**

B. SEAP 5, 2370; WW H, 536.

**SCANLON, Charles**    (5 October 1869, Three Churches, WV—21 March 1927, Pittsburgh, PA). *Education*: B.S., Valparaiso Univ., 1895; A.M., Valparaiso Univ., 1899; studied at Univ. of Minnesota, 1901; LLD. (honorary), Coll. of Wooster, OH, 1916. *Career*: teacher and principal, WV, VA, 1890–94; ordained, Presbyterian Church, 1895; minister, Wheaton, MN, 1895–99; minister, Minneapolis, MN, 1899–1903; full-time temperance work with various groups, beginning 1903.

Scanlon went into full-time temperance campaigning after a relatively brief career in the pulpit as a Presbyterian minister and following several years as a professor at Manchester College in St. Paul, Minnesota. He had long been interested in the antiliquor crusade and had made opposition to drink an important part of his preaching. Indeed, he was an ardent member of the Prohibition Party, and he took an active part in its affairs. In 1900, Scanlon ran as the party's candidate for Congress (representing the St. Paul area), and as its standardbearer for governor in 1902. In both cases he campaigned vigorously but to little avail. In 1903, the former minister went to work for the Prohibition Party as a national lecturer. He held the position for some twenty-five years, touring the country and denouncing "the demon" at every opportunity. And while he was able to do little to further the popularity of the Prohibition Party itself, his efforts gained him considerable personal recognition in reform circles. Scanlon was viewed, as one dry source put it, "as one of the most prominent men in the American temperance movement." He earned the honor mostly through persistence and dedication: His ideas were not novel, but he never tired of conveying the orthodox messages of the crusade and serving generally as a movement workhorse.

Active as he was in these areas, however, Scanlon's forte was perhaps his executive ability. He helped to organize or to administer any number of temperance groups. In 1908, he was elected permanent chair of the Prohibition Party National Convention, while even earlier (1904) he accepted appointment as general secretary of the Board of Temperance of the Presbyterian Church, a post he filled until his death. He was one of the founders of the National Dry Federation and its secretary. In addition, he was the official U.S. delegate to the International Congresses Against Alcoholism, held variously in London, 1909, The Hague, 1911, Milan, 1913, and Lausanne, 1921. He represented the American section at the Fifteenth Congress (Washington D.C., 1920) of the World Prohibition Federation. Scanlon also held office in the National Temperance Society, National Interchurch Temperance Federation, National Prohibition Association, Intercollegiate Prohibition Association, National Temperance Council, Scientific Temperance Federation, Committee of Sixty on National Prohibition, and National Legislative Council. In effect, Scanlon was a career reform bureaucrat— a man who kept the organizational machinery of the dry movement running and maintained. He also edited two religious publications, *Moral Welfare* (Pittsburgh) and the *National Advocate* (New York).

**Bibliography:**

A. ed., *Social Facts: A Handbook of Information . . .* (Pittsburgh, PA, 1925).
B. SEAP 5, 2371–72; WW 1, 1084.

**SCOTT, Richard Hugh**   (23 July 1869, Renfrew Co., Ontario, Canada—11 March 1944, Lansing, MI). *Career*: apprentice and machinist, Paige Tube Co., OH, 1886–98; superintendent, Olds Gas Engine Works, Lansing, MI, 1899– 1904; officer, Reo Motor Car Co., 1904 to 1930s (president and general manager after 1917).

A successful career in the automobile industry gave Richard Scott an appreciation of the value of safety and efficiency in the workplace and in business generally. His perspectives as an executive, however, were not new; even as a young apprentice Scott had noted the special demands and risks inherent in working in a highly sophisticated industrial environment. Carelessness resulted not only in waste and financial loss but also in injury. Early in his career, Scott located a chief source of such disruption in the saloon. Catering to the industrial workforce, as Scott saw it, the saloons cared little if men reported to work under the influence of alcohol, to the detriment of both worker and employer. His reaction was not only personal abstinence but a resolve to fight the saloon on an organized basis as well. After his marriage in 1898 and his move to a new job with the Olds Gas Engine Company in Lansing, Michigan, he began a long formal affiliation with the Temperance Movement. He worked on a local campaign to dry out his home township in 1910 and made a rather detailed (for its day) study of the effects of drinking problems in the automobile industry. Writing in the *Scientific Temperance Journal* in 1912, he noted that after payday, work absences and declines in on-the-job performance reached alarming levels due to drinking problems. His conclusion was pronounced: The saloon not only induced men to squander their wages, but due to its relation to work performance it was also a threat to American industry. It was the kind of thinking that made many of the nation's business leaders into firm prohibitionists, and Scott was a typical case.

Scott's concern over the saloon was expressed in political action. Along with other automobile executives, including Henry Ford, he encouraged the growth of temperance organizations and lent his personal prestige to the drive for both state and national prohibition. Scott, however, also became personally involved in national prohibition. Scott, however, also became personally involved in temperance organizing. In 1912 he won election as president of the Michigan Anti-Saloon League and served for some thirteen years (until 1925). During most of this time he was also a member of the National Board of Trustees of the Anti-Saloon League of America. And Scott was an activist. He worked with genuine zeal during the campaign for state-wide prohibition in Michigan in 1916, and when the populace voted approval of the measure in the November election, the reformer-executive received a great deal of the credit. Scott also believed in educating the public. He was among the first to introduce alcohol education into the workplace, using corporate funds and allowing time off for workers to attend lectures on the personal and social impact of intemperance. During National Prohibition, Scott continued with the Michigan League as a member of its headquarters committee, although his active participation was minimal during the 1930s, when the Great Depression drove his Reo Motor Car Company to its demise.

**Bibliography:**

B. SEAP 5, 2400; WW 2, 476.

**SHAW, Anna Howard**    (14 February 1847, Newcastle-upon-Tyne, England— 2 July 1919, Moylan, PA). *Education*: studied at Albion Coll., MI, 1873–75; graduated from Boston Univ., 1878; M.D., Boston Univ., 1886; D.D. (honorary), Kansas City Union, 1902; LLD. (honorary), 1917. *Career*: schoolteacher, MI, 1860s; licensed to preach, Methodist Church, 1871; pastor, Hingham, MA, 1878; pastor, East Dennis, MA, 1878–85; ordained, Methodist Protestant Church, 1880; lecturer, Massachusetts Woman's Suffrage Association, 1885; national superintendent, Franchise Dept., WCTU, 1888–92; vice president at large, National American Woman Suffrage Association, 1892–1904; president, NAWSA, 1904–15; chair, Woman's Committee, U.S. National Defense Council, 1917–19.

Primarily a suffragist with a peripheral interest in temperance, Anna Shaw's work nevertheless demonstrated the frequently close relationship between the fight for women's rights and the struggle against alcohol. The daughter of British immigrants, Shaw learned many of her reform sentiments at home. During the

1850s, her father used their house in Lawrence, Massachusetts, as a station on the so-called Underground Railroad to assist the flight of escaped Southern slaves. In 1859, the elder Shaw moved his family to Michigan as part of an effort to found a frontier colony; but he soon returned to Lawrence, leaving his family in the care of his wife, who had a breakdown in the face of the rigors of frontier life. Anna took charge of the family. She later wrote of her unhappiness during her years on the frontier and noted that the experience left her with an unflattering view of men. She became a voracious reader and out of her loneliness developed a "desire to talk to people, to tell them things." In fact, it was a desire to preach. And to the dismay of her Unitarian family, Shaw decided to pursue a pastoral calling as a Methodist minister. After doing some local speaking, she was licensed to preach in 1871; she then used her fees to study for formal ordination. The Methodist hierarchy, however, with some exceptions, did not favor the ordination of women. Nevertheless, with the encouragement of a number of Methodist women and of Mary Livermore,* a noted temperance speaker and organizer, Shaw first entered Albion College in 1873 and then completed her religious studies at Boston University in 1878 (having been the only woman in her class). She began her ministerial career the same year in the pulpit of the Methodist Church of Hingham, Massachusetts, but the New England Methodist Conference still refused to ordain her. To add insult to injury, they soon after also revoked her license to preach. In 1880, however, the Methodist Protestant Church agreed to ordination, and for the next seven years she led the congregation of the East Dennis, Massachusetts, Methodist Church as well as the pulpit of a nearby Congregational church. She was finally a minister, but it had been a grueling fight.

While in the pulpit, however, she found that she was not satisfied with her role in society. Her reform instincts, latent while she fought her personal battle for ordination, now flourished, and she began to speak out on the liquor question and on women's suffrage. She also decided that she could be of more service to women as a physician than as a minister, and in 1883 she enrolled in the medical school of Boston University; after part-time study she graduated in 1886. But it was still not enough. By now she had become convinced that there was "but one solution for women"—the vote. Giving up her religious and medical work, Shaw now gave her life to women's issues. She became a lecturer for the Massachusetts Woman Suffrage Association in 1885, and, with Frances Willard's* blessing, she served as superintendent of the Franchise Department of the Woman's Christian Temperance Union, a position she held from 1888 to 1892. In the course of her lecturing for the WCTU, however, Shaw met Susan B. Anthony* (a former temperance worker as well), who had little difficulty in persuading her to work exclusively for the suffrage movement. By 1892, Shaw had left the WCTU and become an officer in the National American Woman Suffrage Association, an event which started a new phase in her career. She worked tirelessly for the organization, becoming one of Anthony's closest aides. Shaw ascended to the association presidency in 1904; but over the years her shortcomings as an administrator led to considerable disaffection within the group, and in 1915 she chose not to stand for reelection. Yet she remained active in women's issues. With America's entrance into World War I, she did a commendable job as chair of the Woman's Committee of the U.S. Council of National Defense, for which she won the Distinguished Service Medal. In July of 1919 she contracted pneumonia and died at age seventy-two.

**Bibliography:**

A. "Rest" (M.D. thesis, Boston Univ., 1878); with Alice Stone Blackwell, *The Yellow Ribbon Speaker...*, comp. Lucy Elmira Anthony (Boston, 1901); *Passages from Speeches of Dr. Anna Howard Shaw* (New York, 1915); *What the War Meant to Women* (New York, 1919); with Elizabeth Jordan, *The Story of a Pioneer...* (New York, 1929).

B. DAB 17, 35–37; NAW 3, 274–77; NYT, July 3, 1919; SEAP 5, 2427; WW 1, 1110.

**SHELDON, Charles Moore**    (26 February 1857, Wellsville, NY—24 February 1946, Topeka, KS). *Education*: B.A., Brown Univ., 1883; B.D., Andover Sem., 1886; D.D. (honorary), Temple Univ., 1898, Washburn Coll., 1900, Brown Univ., 1923. *Career*: ordained, Congregational Church, 1886; minister, Waterbury, VT, 1886–88; minister, Central Congregational Church, Topeka, KS, 1889–1919 (at-large status, 1912–15); editor, *Christian Herald*, 1920–25 (contributing editor after 1925); active writing on religious and reform subjects, 1890s–1940s.

Born the son of a Congregational minister who served in parishes across the country, Charles Sheldon spent much of his boyhood in South Dakota. His education, however, came at some of the best schools in the East: Phillips Academy, Brown University, and Andover Theological Seminary. Ordained in 1886, his years in the pulpit revealed him as a sincere believer in uncomplicated Christian verities. He applied them without hesitation to the major reform issues of his era, asking his listeners to react as Christ might to such matters as urban poverty, ethnic intolerance, political corruption, intemperance, and other social ills. It was hardly original theology, but it made Sheldon one of the nation's best-known voices of the "social gospel." He wrote widely on religious and social affairs, but one volume in particular struck the popular imagination. In 1897 he published *In His Steps*, based on a series of earlier articles, in which a minister and several of his congregation agreed to live a year strictly according to the example of Christ. It sold millions of copies, establishing Sheldon as one of American Protestantism's premier voices of reform. None of his thirty-odd other books were received nearly as well, but he was in great demand as a lecturer and spokesman for various reform causes.

Sheldon devoted particular attention to the Temperance Movement over the course of his career. Like many other reformers of the Progressive period, he saw the antiliquor crusade as an integral part of the wider effort to right social wrongs. He campaigned actively against the liquor traffic for some twenty-five years, both in the United States and abroad. In 1900, at the invitation of British temperance leaders, he made a lecturing tour of the United Kingdom; and in 1915 he made a similar visit to New Zealand. Sheldon's reputation as a dry campaigner was such that between 1912 and 1915 his church (the Central Congregational Church, in Topeka, Kansas) gave him special leave to work against the liquor traffic. He spent the final year of this period as a member of the Flying Squadron of America, a group of temperance advocates who criss-crossed the nation speaking on the evils of drink and the promise of prohibition. He was one of the central figures in the Kansas State Temperance Union and during World War I worked with government authorities to "protect" the morality of American troops. With the ratification of the Eighteenth Amendment, Sheldon welcomed the coming of what he and his fellow reformers hoped would be a new age of social justice. As such, he defended the measure against wet assaults, remaining a vigorous proponent of the dry laws to the end.

### Bibliography:

A. *The Crucifixion of Philip Strong* (Chicago, 1894); *In His Steps* (Chicago, 1897, and many following editions); *The Redemption of Freedom* (London, 1899); *The Twentieth Door* (New York, 1899); *Born to Serve* (Chicago, 1900); *Charles M. Sheldon: His Life Story* (New York, 1925).

B. DAB 24, 740–42; DARB, 408; NYT, Feb. 25, 1946; SEAP 5, 2429–30; WW 2, 483.

**SHELTON, Emma Frances Sanford**    (?, Montrose, VA—14 July 1926, Chevy Chase, MD). *Career*: recording secretary, Washington, DC, WCTU, 1874–94; financial secretary, building fund, Washington, DC, WCTU, 1901; president, Washington, DC, WCTU, 1912–26.

Putting all one's eggs in one basket was not a policy that Emma Shelton favored or followed. Living practically all her life in Washington, D.C., Shelton had a hand in numerous campaigns for reform and was instrumental in the fight against what she saw as evils ranging from liquor to narcotics to cigarettes. She was a charter member of the Woman's Christian Temperance Union in the nation's capital, joining in 1874. Over the years, she proved one of the organization's most active and dedicated adherents, serving as recording secretary for more than two decades and briefly as legislative superintendent of the National WCTU. Her most significant contribution, however, came as the head of the National Union's effort against narcotics. In this role she reflected Frances Willard's* characterization of the WCTU's crusade as constituting a "fight for the clear mind," not just a war on alcohol. Shelton's interest in addictive substances of all types led her to champion anticigarette legislation, prohibiting the sale of cigarettes to anyone under the age of sixteen in the District of Columbia. In this endeavor, she managed to secure the assistance of the Washington medical community, who were more concerned with the health aspect of the issue than the moral problem. Petitions from medical men, school superintendents, ministers of the gospel, and other community leaders made a profound effect upon the U.S. Senate, where the Committee on Washington soon enacted the desired legislation. It was a modest law, but it did serve to demonstrate the growing political acumen of the WCTU and to enhance the group's visibility in the capital. Such was the WCTU's regard for her abilities, that when the organization decided to construct a building in Washington, it gave Sheldon a central role in the building effort, which she carried out successfully. She became president of the Washington, D.C., WCTU in 1912, and in that capacity was an active participant in the lobbying effort for National Prohibition, a cause she also served as a member of the local chapter of the Anti-Saloon League. Sheldon's reform interests, however, reached beyond the Temperance Movement. During World War I she was president of the Board of Management of the Soldiers and Sailors Recreation Rooms in Washington, D.C., as well as a member of the International Council of Women for Christian and Patriotic Service. Yet she was always best known as one of the most tireless dry workers active on the capital scene, and she continued her temperance work up to the year of her death in 1926.

**Bibliography:**

B. SEAP 5, 2430–31.

**SHEPPARD, Morris**    (28 May 1875, Wheatville, TX—9 April 1941, Washington, DC). *Education*: A.B., Univ. of Texas, 1895; LLB., Univ. of Texas, 1897; LLM., Yale Univ., 1898; LLD. (honorary), Southern Methodist Univ. *Career*: legal practice, Pittsburg, TX, 1898–99, legal practice, Texarkana, beginning 1899; member, U.S. House of Representatives, 1902–13; member, U.S. Senate, 1913–41.

Morris Sheppard, Yale Law School graduate, millionaire developer of Texas real estate, and Democratic senator for virtually three decades, is remembered primarily as the man who introduced the Eighteenth Amendment to the Constitution of the United States. After practicing law for several years, he entered politics at the age of twenty-seven in 1902, elected to fill the unexpired House term of his father, Congressman Levi Sheppard, who had died in office. Subsequently reelected in his own right, he served until 1913, when he resigned to take another unexpired seat, this time in the Senate. He remained there, winning reelection with the regularity of the seasons until his death in 1941. Throughout his long years in the national legislature the Texas lawmaker had a generally progressive reputation and was an especially active enemy of the liquor traffic. He sponsored some of the earliest measures to curtail the interstate commerce in alcoholic beverages and was instrumental in framing local-option laws for the District of Columbia and the territory of Hawaii. Sheppard's efforts won high praise from the Temperance Movement, which looked to him as one of "the most aggressive men" in the ranks against drink. And while he was indeed staunchly against the liquor traffic (especially the saloon), Sheppard held no

particular brief against individual drinking. His hesitations on that score, however, generally went overlooked as the Texan led the vanguard in the advance
toward a National Prohibition amendment.

Sheppard's role in framing the Eighteenth Amendment began as early as 1913.
In league with Alabama Congressman Richmond Hobson,* he introduced the
Hobson-Sheppard Resolution, which called for a prohibitory addition to the
Constitution. The original measure, however, was not strictly dry: It aimed at
eliminating sales, not actual drinking. The resolution demanded the abolition of
"the sale, manufacture for sale, transportation for sale, importation for sale, and
exportation for sale of intoxicating liquors" anywhere in the United States. In
1914, the measure won a majority in the House, but not the two-thirds vote
necessary for passage. On the Senate floor, the resolution was stymied until
Sheppard took a legislative gamble. He accepted a proposal by wet Congressman
Boies Penrose of Pennsylvania, who proposed that the amendment die unless
ratified by the requisite number of states (thirty-six) within six years. Wets
thought the time limit posed an impossible barrier; Sheppard and other drys were
willing to risk it, and the revised measure cleared Congress and went to the
states. However, there had also been another change. Wayne Wheeler,* of the
Anti-Saloon League, had convinced Congress to remove the term "for sale"
from Sheppard's original resolution. Thus the amendment, as approved, was a
truly dry statute. And to the dismay of wets, the states took scarcely a year to
ratify the measure, which mandated the start of National Prohibition in January
of 1920.

Sheppard, like other drys, took heart at the demise of the traffic, but he still
had some reservations about the "noble experiment" as a whole. In particular,
he wondered about the wisdom of the National Prohibition Act—the Volstead
Act—with its narrow definition of an intoxicating beverage. It seemingly attacked
any and all drinking, and Sheppard was uneasy. As late as May 1919, he stated,
"I am not a prohibitionist in the strict sense of the word. I am fighting the liquor
traffic. I am against the saloon." But he was not, he added, "in any sense
aiming to prevent the personal use of alcoholic beverages." (It was just as well,
because only a few months later it was disclosed that a 130-gallon-per-day-
capacity still had been found on one of his Texas properties.) Three years after
the passage of the Volstead Act, Sheppard furnished the Anti-Saloon League
with a glowing assessment of the impact of Prohibition: "Long live Prohibition!"
he wrote. It had led to better health, greater savings, and an improved way of
life "for the mothers and children of America"; all of this would become even
more apparent, he concluded, as the years gave citizens a chance to reflect on
"the nation's shame and misery" when the drink trade was legal. Nevertheless,
Sheppard soon after told a reporter that he never intended "to stop the making
of liquor in homes" or the private use of alcohol "unless these things were done
for commercial purposes." The social revolution his legislative actions had
fostered, though, had run beyond his control. Yet as popular sentiments shifted
against Prohibition, the Texas senator defended it, and after Repeal he continued

to speak out for federal controls on the beverage trade. He never relented in his belief that Americans would be better off without the liquor industry, and until his death the ebbing Temperance Movement considered him one of its greatest public advocates.

**Bibliography:**

A. *The Work of the League of Nations: Speech*... (Washington, DC, 1912); *Fraternal and Other Addresses*, 2nd ed. (Omaha, NB, 1914); *Speeches of Morris Sheppard*, 2 vols. (Washington, DC, 1907–41 [reprints of the *Congressional Record*]).

B. SEAP 5, 2431–32; WW 2, 484; Norman Clark, *Deliver Us from Evil: An Interpretation of American Prohibition* (New York, 1976); *Memorial Services Held in the House of Representatives and Senate... in Eulogy of Morris Sheppard...* (Washington, DC, 1943).

**SHUMAKER, Edward Seitz**    (30 July 1867, Greenville, OH—25 October 1929, Indianapolis, IN). *Education*: A.B., DePauw Univ., 1918. *Career*: ordained, Methodist Episcopal Church,1890; minister, various pastorates, IN, 1890–1903; field agent, Indiana Anti-Saloon League, 1903–7; state superintendent, Indiana Anti-Saloon League, 1907–29; editor, *American Issue* (Indiana edition), 1907–16, 1919–29; member, Executive Committee, National Anti-Saloon League, 1925–27.

Born in Ohio just after the Civil War and growing up in Illinois, the Reverend Edward Seitz Shumaker decided early on a ministerial career. He began to preach as a Methodist while still in college and between 1890 and 1903 held five pastorates in the Hoosier State. As part of his attachment to Methodism, Shumaker was also a confirmed temperance man even before the start of his days in the pulpit. He had belonged to a number of juvenile dry groups while still a boy, and while a teenager he had served as president of the Young Men's Temperance League of Effingham County (Illinois). But he came into his own as a reformer only upon entering the ministry. Indeed, he used each of his pastorates as a forum to blast the "demon rum" in a style that made him a local dry hero. He was a tireless and implacable foe of drink, and he became embroiled in temperance fights in every town he served. Shumaker led aroused drys in campaigns that closed illegal saloons, passed Sunday closing laws, and, in his Maple Avenue Church in Terre Haute, Indiana, solicited funds in 1902 to install a memorial stained-glass window in honor of Woman's Christian Temperance Union president Frances Willard.* Throughout, he was anything but gentle in his assaults on wets: For Shumaker, liquor and liquor men were evils, to be fought without remorse or compromise. It surprised no one, then, when he left the ministry in 1903 to work full time as a field agent and, after 1904, as a local officer in the Indiana chapter of the Anti-Saloon League. Nor did it surprise anyone when he proved good at his job and in 1907 secured the superintendency of the state organization.

As an officer of the Indiana League, Shumaker demonstrated just how effective a well-led reform organization could be. When he became state superintendent, Indiana had only two dry counties, and most of its larger cities were notoriously wet. The former minister played a critical role in marshalling a remarkable popular effort to reverse the situation. Beginning in 1905 (when he was still field agent), the league successfully lobbied for legislation that closed almost two thousand saloons (1905), established local option (1917), strengthened dry enforcement statutes over the 1920s, mandated serious penalties against drunken driving, and dried out seventy counties well before the ratification of National Prohibition. In the course of his war on alcohol, however, Shumaker's abrasive public statements made him few friends outside of the dry camp. In fact, they made him quite a number of powerful enemies. In 1926, in a series of remarks about members of the State Supreme Court, whom the Anti-Saloon League leader considered soft on the liquor traffic, he finally went too far. Cited for contempt of court, he faced either a sixty-day jail sentence or a $250 fine; and in order to avoid the expenses of an appeal (and, one suspects, to garner sympathy as a reformer) he chose to serve his sentence. Upon arrival at the state penal farm in 1928, he found that the Indiana governor had pardoned him—although when the attorney general ruled the pardon invalid, Shumaker served his sixty days in 1929. A crowd of sympathizers greeted him on his release, and upon his death later in the year, still in office, he was the longest serving state superintendent in the ranks of the league.

### Bibliography:

A. with Amos Keller, eds., *Descendants of Henry Keller of York County, Pennsylvania and Fairfield County, Ohio* (Indianapolis, IN, 1924); *What Medicinal Value Has Wiskey? An Array of Facts by Competent and Expert Witnesses*, 3rd ed. (Westerville, OH, 192-?).

B. SEAP 5, 2436; WW 1, 1123.

**SIBLEY, Frank J.**    (11 August 1847, Royalton, NY—?). *Career*: general manager and president, Copper Creek Mining Company, AZ, beginning 1880s; general manager, Minnesota-Arizona Copper Company, AZ, 1880s; secretary and founder, Demorest Land Company, beginning 1888; publisher, *New Republic*, 1880s; publisher, *Northeast Georgian*, 1890s.

A mining engineer whose career led him to take up residence in seven states during the course of his life, Sibley spent his youth in upper New York State. Largely self-taught (he complemented his meager public school instruction with correspondence courses in science and engineering), he rose to prominence in his field. He managed mining concerns successfully in Arizona, serving for years as president of the Copper Creek Mining Company in that state (then still a territory). In the late 1880s, the prosperous mining executive diversified his holdings, becoming a founder and principal of a real estate company and establishing several newspapers, including the *New Republic* in Nebraska and the

*Northeast Georgian*. Throughout his years in business, Sibley was also deeply involved in temperance activities. His initial interest in the liquor question evidently stemmed from his distaste for the waste and inefficiency associated with intemperance, but later he denounced drink as the root of an entire gamut of social evils. He was a familiar speaker in temperance circles for over thirty years, and he wrote a number of books on the subject as well. His dedication to the dry crusade amply demonstrated the strong alliance between the Temperance Movement and important sectors of the business community.

Originally a Republican, Sibley became impatient when the GOP refused to come out unequivocally for prohibition. He quickly found a new political home in the fledgling Prohibition Party in 1874, two years after its first national convention in Chicago, and a year after the "Woman's War" had burst upon the nation. Amid the growing public interest in temperance, Sibley devoted considerable time to party affairs in the states to which his business responsibilities carried him. He was secretary to the party's Central Committee in New York from 1877 to 1879, and in Kansas in 1880. From there he moved to Nebraska, where, from 1881 to 1886, he held the leading position in that state's Grand Lodge of the International Order of Good Templars. That organization, more than any other, had been responsible for the founding of the Prohibition Party, and over the years Sibley was a loyal member of the order. While he was in Nebraska, the dry business leader also took a leading role in establishing a state branch of the party (1884), and he later served on the party's National Committee. As secretary and general manager of the Nebraska Prohibitory Amendment Association, he continued, with some success, a line of action he had initiated in Kansas in 1879 and 1880. In that earlier campaign, he had spoken in forty counties, urging support for state-wide prohibition; after the measure became law, Sibley launched some of the first prosecutions of violators. Later in the 1880s, he managed a string of prohibition lecturers who carried the dry gospel to five states, as well as continuing his political work. In the 1890s and early 1900s, he served with the Prohibition Parties of Georgia and California; and while his party won no victories, the indefatigable (and well-travelled) temperance worker had the satisfaction of seeing the dry cause as a whole make great strides. After the loss of his first wife, at age fifty-five he married Mary Charlton Edholm, herself an active antiliquor crusader.

**Bibliography:**

A. *What Prohibition Did for Kansas* (n.p., 1886); *John B. Finch: His Life and Work* (New York, 1888); *The Templar at Work...* (Madison, WI, 1888).
B. SEAP 5, 2437–38; WW 3, 785.

**SIDES, Johnson**   We know virtually nothing of most of the life of Johnson Sides, a dearth which includes even the dates of his birth and death. An American Indian raised in the Nevada area, Sides was probably born before the mid-nineteenth century and died near its end. In between, he was noted as a friend of white immigrants, acting as a guide for parties making their ways to California and as a peacemaker with the local tribes. As the Nevada area saw permanent white settlement itself, Sides evidently became one of the most active Indian negotiators with the newly-arriving Americans and won the friendship of many of them. The whites apparently appreciated his willingness to treat with them, although there is no evidence of what other Indians thought of his actions—or even if he was actually in a leadership position. At any rate, Sides did react against some of the detrimental effects of white civilization, especially the impact of drinking on Indian society. He became an ardent temperance advocate, even though he had occasional trouble with the bottle himself. Sides ranged across Nevada in the last quarter of the century, speaking repeatedly against alcohol and warning of the violence and disruption that too frequently accompanied drunkenness. At one point, he was arrested himself for public intoxication; but due to his standing in the white community he received a fine of only a dollar. Still, his stock as a temperance lecturer fell considerably, as did his pride. He appealed to a friend in the Nevada legislature for redress (a Senator Doolin), who arranged for the passage of a resolution in the State Senate: "*Resolved*, By the Senate, the people of the State of Nevada, concurring, that the drink of whisky taken by John Sides on the 17th day of September, in the city of Virginia, county of Story, be and is hereby declared null and void." As the story went, Sides was satisfied and returned to his crusade against drink, while whites had a laugh at his expense. Indeed, it appears that Sides, while no doubt sincere in his efforts to combat the ravages of alcoholism among the Indians, found little real white support for his mission. Local annals recorded his activities more out of regard for his drinking having been "declared null and void"—a distinction perhaps unique in history—than because of any concern for the tribes. In fact, the accounts of Johnson Sides appeared fully within the context of the stereotype of the "drunken Indian," which characterized the tribes as hopelessly unable to tolerate the white man's "firewater" and dangerous under its influence. Nevertheless, despite white views, Sides was a reformer whose efforts, even if of doubtful success, raised serious questions on the nature of alcohol in Indian societies in America.

**Bibliography:**

B. Norman B. Wood, *Lives of Famous Indian Chiefs* (Aurora, IL, 1906).

**SILKWORTH, William Duncan**    (22 July 1877, Brooklyn, NY—22 March 1951, New York, NY). *Education*: A.B., Princeton Univ., 1896; M.D., New York Univ., Bellevue Medical Sch., 1899. *Career*: psychiatric staff, U.S. Army Hosp., Plattsburgh, NY, 1917–19; associate physician, Neurological Inst., Presbyterian Hosp., New York City, 1919–29; physician-in-charge (later medical superintendent), Charles B. Towns Hosp., New York City, 1932–51; director of alcoholism treatment, Knickerbocker Hosp., New York City, 1945–51.

Bill W., the co-founder of Alcoholics Anonymous, once described William

Silkworth as "the benign little doctor who loved drunks." Silkworth had little evident interest in alcoholism early in his career, which had a psychiatric emphasis. Indeed, he was fully fifty-nine years old by the time he became physician-in-chief at the Charles B. Towns Hospital in New York, where he became deeply involved with addictions and alcohol-related problems. The Towns Hospital was largely a detoxication institution for the well-to-do. It had been founded in 1901 by Charles Towns, who at one point had garnered national attention through his claims to have found a cure for addiction, the so-called Towns Cure. By the 1930s he was out of the public eye; but he was still a firm believer in a physiological, medical model of addiction, although he denied that alcoholism per se was a disease. Silkworth ultimately disagreed with his employer, arguing that certain individuals were "constitutionally susceptible to sensitization by alcohol" and that drinking sparked an allergic reaction. This made it physically impossible for the alcoholic to tolerate alcohol, the doctor argued, a fact that problem drinkers had to learn and accept as part of their treatment. It was this point that Silkworth drove home to William Wilson*—"Bill W."—when he was in treatment at the Towns Hospital, and which later became a cornerstone in the founding and growth of Alcoholics Anonymous.

Silkworth's relationship with Alcoholics Anonymous was both deep and emotional. Bill W. was forever grateful for the treatment he received at the doctor's hands when he sought help for his drinking problems. But his contributions went beyond helping Wilson in his hour of need. During the early years of AA, Silkworth was one of the first medical voices to publicly attest to its effectiveness. Still later, when Wilson and others founded the Alcoholic Foundation to raise funds for AA activities, the New York physician agreed to serve as one of the foundation trustees. He remained with the group until his death in 1951. In addition, Silkworth also continued the active treatment of alcoholics. After 1945, while remaining the chief medical officer at the Towns Hospital, he took charge of alcoholism treatment at the Knickerbocker Hospital (also in New York City). Over the years, he received credit for aiding some seven thousand alcoholics, many of whom went on to participation in AA. Not a prolific author, Silkworth nevertheless devoted five of his eight articles to AA, including the introduction he contributed to Bill W.'s book, *Alcoholics Anonymous*. Near the end of his days, Wilson, who later on called Silkworth "the first friend and perhaps the greatest friend" of AA, sponsored a fund-raising drive to provide for the doctor's retirement. Silkworth, however, died before retiring, still holding his posts at the Towns and Knickerbocker hospitals.

**Bibliography:**

A. "Alcoholism a Manifestation of Allergy," *Medical Record* (NY) 145 (1937):249–51; "Reclamation of the Alcoholic," *Medical Record* (NY) 145 (1937):321–24; "New Approach to Psychotherapy in Chronic Alcoholism," *Journal-Lancet* 59 (1939):312–15; "Psychological Rehabilitation of Alcoholics," *Medical Record* (NY) 150 (1939):65–66; "Highly Successful Approach to Alcoholic Problems Confirmed by Medical and Sociological Results,'' *Medical Record* (NY) 154 (1941):105–7; "The Doctor's Opinion," 1–9, in, Bill W., *Alcoholics Anonymous* (New York, 1946); with M. Texon, "Chloride Levels in the Blood of Alcoholic Patients in Relation to the Phenomenon of Craving," *Quarterly Journal of Studies on Alcohol* 11 (1950):381–84.

B. NYT, March 23, 1951; Leonard Blumberg, "The Ideology of a Therapeutic Social Movement: Alcoholics Anonymous," *Journal of Studies on Alcohol* 38 (1977):2122–43; *Journal of the American Medical Association* 146 (1951):489; Robert Thompson, *Bill W.* (New York, 1975).

**SKELTON, Henrietta**   (5 November 1842, Giessen, Germany—22 August 1900, San Francisco, CA). *Education*: studied at Collegiate Inst., Heidelberg, 1850s. *Career*: German teacher, Bishop Strasy's Young Ladies Coll., 1858–59; lecturer and organizer, National WCTU, 1880s to 1900.

Henrietta Skelton was the daughter of a prominent German academic family. Her father was president of Heidelberg University, and she was educated at the Collegiate Institute in that city. When she was fifteen years old her father died, and she emigrated to Toronto, Canada, to live with an uncle. For two years the young immigrant taught German at a private religious school for women and in 1859 married Samuel Murray Skelton, traffic superintendent of the Northern Railroad of Canada. For the next fourteen years, she led an apparently secure existence as the wife of the well-to-do rail executive's wife. Skelton's life, however, was not uneventful. She had to manage an invalid child (a son) while she also became active in the Canadian branch of the Woman's Christian Temperance Union. The roots of her interest in the Temperance Movement (which had considerable strength in Canada) are obscure, but it may have reflected her desire for social participation outside of the home, or something of her husband's views. As a railroad executive, Samuel Skelton could hardly have been unaffected by his industry's concerns over drinking by railroad workers. Her temperance role, however, was not particularly prominent, and despite her genuine interest in the reform she did not have credentials as an important dry leader. But personal tragedy was to change all of that. Samuel Skelton died in 1873, and his saddened widow moved to California, where her son died the following year. Distraught, Mrs. Skelton turned to reform work as a means of diverting herself from her troubles.

She joined the local WCTU and soon found employment with the National Union as a full-time lecturer. Skelton specialized in carrying the dry gospel to German-Americans. The WCTU placed considerable emphasis on the "Americanization" of immigrant groups through the inculcation of "American" values, not the least of which was temperance. Fluent in her native language, she reached German-speaking audiences in various parts of the country throughout the 1880s. For some of this time she edited *Der Bahnbrecher* (The Pioneer), a German-language temperance publication. In addition, she wrote a number of books on aspects of German life. Skelton won high praise from WCTU leadership for her efforts, which moved from lecturing and editing to organizing in the later 1880s. Working in Idaho in 1886 and 1887, she was the central figure in the establishment of the WCTU in that state. She remained in the field through the next decade, during which time she returned to California for organizational duties there. Skelton was at work when she died in 1900. Never a temperance leader of the first rank, Skelton's career still demonstrated the concern of the WCTU to reach out to immigrant groups, and that the effort bore at least some fruit.

**Bibliography:**

A. *The Christmas-Tree: A Story of German Domestic Life* (Cincinnati, OH, 1883).
B. SEAP 5, 2445; WW 1, 1131.

**SMITH, Addison Taylor**    (5 September 1862, Cambridge, OH—5 July 1956, Washington, DC). *Education*: studied at Cambridge (OH) Business Coll., 1883; LLB., Columbia (now George Washington) Univ., 1895; LLM., National Law Sch., Washington, DC, 1896. *Career*: committee clerk, U.S. Senate, Washington, DC, 1896; legal practice, ID, from 1905; U.S. Land Office register, ID, 1907–8; member, U.S. House of Representatives, 1913–32; associate member, Board of Veterans Appeals, 1934–42.

Aside from his being raised a Methodist, little is known about Smith's early inclination toward the temperance cause. Throughout his public career, however, the antiliquor forces found fewer more energetic allies. Although staunchly dry in his sympathies, Smith chose not to join the Prohibition Party but to work for the cause as a Republican—a course which offered greater political rewards. After clerking in the Senate for a decade, he passed the Washington, D.C., bar in 1899, only to move to Boise, Idaho, the following year. There he joined the Idaho bar in 1905, established a successful practice, and won election to the House of Representatives in 1913. Subsequently winning nine more terms, he devoted much of his time to the quest for National Prohibition. At the urging of the Anti-Saloon League and other dry organizations, Smith and Congressman Edwin Webb* of North Carolina submitted a Prohibition amendment in the House in 1915. Serving for most of his congressional career on the House Committee on the Alcoholic Liquor Traffic, Smith chaired that body for two sessions of Congress; and on different occasions he also pressed for the passage of prohibitory legislation in Washington, D.C., Idaho, and other states. At the same time, Smith was an influential voice in Idaho Republican circles, and after the end of his electoral service he remained active in state political and civic affairs. His House career seemingly justified the arguments of the Anti-Saloon League, which claimed that more could be done for the dry cause through the major parties than through the separate Prohibition Party.

**Bibliography:**

B. SEAP 6, 2449–50; WW 3, 793.

**SMITH, Gerrit**   (6 March 1797, Utica, NY—28 December 1874, New York, NY). *Education*: graduated from Hamilton Coll., NY, 1818. *Career*: major philanthropic interests, with income from family fortune, beginning 1820s; active in various reform societies, beginning 1820s; member, U.S. House of Representatives, 1853–54.

Born the son of a wealthy trading associate of John Jacob Astor, Gerrit Smith was a good example of the paradox of the fanatic who applies the fruits gained from questionable economic practices to causes aimed at rectifying the vices of others. Smith inherited many of his father's eccentricities, especially his gloomy religious obsessions and profound sense of social guilt, which, as one writer has suggested, verged "on the psychotic." His second wife (his first had died after bearing six children, only four of whom survived infancy) was a Southerner, and reflecting on being the son-in-law of a slaveholder led Smith to espouse the abolitionist cause. Over his long life, he supported a host of causes from vegetarianism and prison reform to temperance and women's rights; but before the Civil War, Smith emerged as one of the most prominent, if unpredictable, antislavery voices in the nation. Indeed, the intensity of his feelings about slavery brought him into a nearly disastrous involvement with John Brown, whom Gerrit considered "the man in all the world I think most truly Christian." He assisted in the Underground Railroad; he donated, in an experiment that on the whole failed, 4,000 fifty-acre parcels of poor agricultural land in upstate New York for blacks (and some indigent white females) to settle and cultivate; he gave 21,000 acres of Virginia wilderness to Oberlin College for the same purpose; and, most perilously, he offered direct support to Brown himself. When Brown was executed after government forces retook the Harper's Ferry arsenal in 1859, Smith was named an accessory in the proslavery press. He retreated into madness and had to be institutionalized for seven months. Despite all the evidence to the contrary (including the fact that Brown was buried on the Adirondack farm, near Lake Placid, that Smith had given him a decade earlier), Smith, as did his family after his demise, denied any knowledge of Brown and any complicity in his plans for insurrection. The denials, however, had a hollow ring, and for a time, Smith, who had been a lively force on the New York State political scene (in 1852 he had even won a seat in Congress, although he did not serve his full term), became more circumspect about his activities.

Alcohol was second only to slavery as an object of Smith's revulsion, and he had joined the crusade against it in the late 1820s. An early gesture was his following the example of his friend and fellow reformer, Edward Delavan,* in the construction of a "temperance hotel" to compete with the purveyors of liquor. At enormous expense, Smith built an impressive establishment in the family seat of Peterboro, which did not lie on a main travel route. Within two years, the venture proved an economic disaster, and he was forced to board it up as a failure. In 1833, however, the still-zealous dry helped to organize a county temperance society, and he began to speak at national temperance gatherings on the applications of total abstinence principles. Temperance played a part in his successful race for Congress in 1852 and an unsuccessful gubernatorial campaign six years later. Smith also took an active interest in the Maine Law, supporting similar legislation in his home state. Not least among his accomplishments was his inspiring of his cousin, Elizabeth Cady Stanton, to become a zealous worker on behalf of temperance as well as abolition. A charter subscriber to the New York "Anti-Dram-Shop" Party in 1869, he was a "conspicuous presence" among the founders of the national Prohibition Party the same year. Indeed, he delivered the keynote address at the new party's organizing convention in Chicago; and in 1872, the party honored him by placing his name in nomination for the presidency, along with such other reform luminaries as General Benjamin Butler,* Chief Justice Salmon Chase, Neal Dow,* and Wendell Phillips.* It was Smith who drafted the party's first official manifesto, "An address to the people of the United States," in which he crystallized the sentiments of a generation of temperance reformers. "Slavery is gone, but drunkenness stays," went its oft-quoted preamble. Smith's historic document went on to assert that "there is no security from drunkenness but total abstinence from all intoxicating drinks" and to call for outright government prohibition of the dramshop, "the great manufactory, not of paupers only, but also of incendiaries, madmen, and murderers." It was forceful stuff, but typical of Smith's flare for the dramatic and of the style that made him, for all of his eccentricities, one of the most fascinating speakers of his day.

**Bibliography:**

A. *Letter from Gerrit Smith to Edward C. Delavan . . . on the Reformation of the Intemperate* (n.p., 1833); *Government Board to Protect from the Dramshop . . .* (Washington, DC, 1854); *Sermons and Speeches of Gerrit Smith* (1861; New York, 1969); *Temperance: Gerrit Smith to John Stuart Mill . . .* (n.p., 1869); *Letter on Temperance: To the Thoughtful and Candid of the County of Madison . . .* (n.p., 1871).

B. DAB 17, 270–71; SEAP 6, 2454–55; WW H, 560; Octavius Brooks, *Gerrit Smith: A Biography* (New York, 1879); Ralph Volney Harlow, *Gerrit Smith: Philanthropist and Reformer* (New York, 1939); Microfilming Corporation of America, *Guide to the Microfilm Edition of the Peter Smith Papers, 1763–1850, and the Gerrit Smith Papers, 1775–1924* (Glen Rock, NJ, 1975).

**SMITH, Green Clay**    (4 July 1826, Madison, KY—29 June 1895, Washington, DC). *Education*: studied at Center Coll., 1840s; graduated from Transylvania Coll., 1849. *Career*: cavalry officer, Mexican War, 1846–48; admitted to bar, 1852; legal practice, Covington, KY, beginning 1852; school commissioner, KY, 1853–57; member, Kentucky House of Representatives, 1861–63; officer (enlisted as private), Union army, 1861–63; member, U.S. House of Representatives, 1863–66; governor of Montana Territory, 1866–69; Baptist minister, Louisville, KY, 1870–90, minister, Metropolitan Baptist Church, Washington, DC, 1890–95.

Soldier, lawyer, politician, and evangelist, Green Clay Smith was an early champion of the Temperance Movement. Before establishing a thriving legal office in Covington, Kentucky, Smith served as an officer in his native state's volunteers in the Mexican War. Back home, he followed the law into politics, where his early interests centered on the public school systems, of which he held the post of commissioner for four years. Reform activities, however, were also a major part of his antebellum years. Smith was a steadfast total abstainer, perhaps from religious conviction (he was a Baptist). A member of the Sons of Temperance and the Independent Order of Good Templars, he eventually headed both of the fraternal groups in Kentucky. Despite his dry beliefs, though, Smith had little chance to become involved in prohibitionist politics. As a crucial Border State, Kentucky was swept up in the sectional controversy as the Civil War loomed; and against the threat of the approaching conflict, local temperance activities held little place in the popular eye. Indeed, Smith became almost completely absorbed in the war. While a Democrat, he chose to stand by the Union and opposed secession as a member of the state legislature. He later served in the Union army (he was brevetted to major general in 1865) before going to Congress in 1863 and serving two terms. He was a serious contender for the vice presidential nomination at the 1864 Republican convention, losing to Andrew Johnson (and thus missing the presidency itself upon Lincoln's assassination) by the extraordinary margin of half a vote. In 1866, Johnson, by then president, appointed his former rival governor of Montana Territory.

At some point, however, Smith felt a religious calling and decided to leave politics for the ministry. Departing Montana at the end of his term in 1869, he sought ordination as a Baptist minister and took a pastorate in Louisville, Kentucky. The former political leader emerged as a forceful evangelical preacher, and he rose quickly in the church hierarchy. For nine years, Smith was the leader of state's General Association of the Baptist Church, and he became a prominent spokesman for the denomination on the social issues of the day. Notably, he spoke on the liquor question. Smith had never abandoned his old temperance sympathies, and his rise in the ministry allowed him to make his views influence public policy. He denounced the drink trade with vigor, and when the established political parties refused to attack it directly, the ardent parson joined the Prohibition Party. In 1876, in the second presidential election in which the Prohibitionists took part, Smith received the party's nomination for chief executive. He campaigned actively, but the party was not well organized in most states and the Kentucky reformer tallied under ten thousand votes, less than the Prohibition candidate in 1872. Yet Smith retained the esteem of the party, which again offered him the nomination in 1888. He declined, however, and allowed the honor to fall to General Clinton Fisk.* Smith continued to preach on behalf of the antiliquor cause and spent his last years as pastor of a large Baptist congregation in the national capital.

**Bibliography:**

B. SEAP 6, 2455–56; WW H, 560.

**SMITH, Hannah Whitall**    (7 February 1832, Philadelphia, PA—1 May 1911, Iffley, England). *Career*: interdenominational preaching with husband, Robert Pearsall Smith, United States and Great Britain, 1860s to 1875; writing on religious and reform subjects, beginning 1869; active on behalf of reform causes, United States and Great Britain, 1870s to 1899.

The evangelical spirit accounted for a good deal of nineteenth-century American temperance activity, and few reformers better demonstrated the spiritual roots of the antiliquor crusade than Hannah Whitall Smith. Raised a strict Quaker, upon her marriage to Robert Pearsall Smith (1851) she became acquainted with the Wesleyan doctrines of Methodism. Robert subsequently established himself as a noted evangelist and religious editor, while Hannah soon began to preach herself and to build a reputation as an author on religious topics. Together, the Smiths conducted a widely-heralded interdenominational revival tour in Great Britain from 1873 to 1875, which ended in scandal when Robert was accused of too much familiarity with female worshippers. While the incident later turned Robert away from religion, Mrs. Smith grew to fame as an internationally-recognized interpreter of religious themes. Her work in the 1870s focused on combining certain Quaker and Methodist beliefs; and her writings displayed a faith and subtlety of reason that won the admiration of the likes of Henry and William James, George Bernard Shaw, Bertrand Russell, Bernard Berenson, and George Santayana. Indeed, two of her daughters eventually married Russell and Berenson. Her relatively elevated literary style, however, was not without popular appeal. Her speeches and Bible readings were regarded as special attractions on the temperance and religious lecture circuit, and one of her books, *The Christian's Secret of a Happy Life* (1875) was a best seller. Smith garnered applause as well for her championing of a wide variety of reform causes and for successfully combining the roles of a public individual and homemaker.

In the later part of her career, Smith emphasized work on behalf of secular reform movements rather than religion (although she by no means lost any of her ardent faith). She had joined the Woman's Christian Temperance Union soon after its founding in the 1870s, and for a quarter of a century she was an intimate friend of WCTU president Frances E. Willard.* Her preaching and religious studies made her the logical choice for the post of superintendent when the union founded its Evangelical Department in 1883. Smith gave up the position, however, when she moved permanently to England in 1886. But she did not give up temperance. She quickly joined the British Women's Temperance Association, holding various executive roles from 1888 to 1906. From 1903 until her death she was honorary vice president. Her lecturing and organizing work made her a central figure in the transatlantic movement against liquor, as she kept up with the progress of the crusade back in America. Indeed, in 1891 she briefly returned to her native land to attend the founding meeting of the World's WCTU. With Robert Smith's death in 1899, Hannah withdrew from most of her public activities and concentrated on raising her two grandchildren. After 1904 she was severely crippled by arthritis, although until her death she retained the broad interests, literary grace, and tolerant outlook that marked her long and productive life.

### Bibliography:

A. *Frank; the Record of a Happy Life; Being Memorials of Franklin Whitall Smith...* (London, 1873); *The Christian's Secret of a Happy Life* (1875; Westwood, NJ, 1952); *Faith* (New York, circa 1900); *The Open Secret, or; the Bible Explaining Itself* (Chicago, 1902); *The Unselfishness of God and How I Discovered It: A Spiritual Autobiography* (New York, 1903); *Living in the Sunshine*, 2nd ed. (New York, 1906).

B. DAB 17, 274–75; NAW 3, 313–16; SEAP 6, 2456; Ray Strackey, *A Quaker Grandmother: Hannah Whitall Smith* (London, 1914); Frances E. Willard, *Glimpses of Fifty Years* (Chicago, 1889); Frances E. Willard, *Woman and Temperance* (Hartford, CT, 1883).

**SMITH, Ida Belle Speakman Wise**    (3 July 1871, Philadelphia, PA—16 February 1952, Des Moines, IA). *Education*: studied at Univ. of Nebraska, 1894; graduated from Kindergarten Teaching Normal Sch., IA, 1890s; LLD. (honorary), John Fletcher Coll., IA, 1927. *Career*: schoolteacher, IA, 1887–1901; public lecturer on reform subjects, 1900s–1940s; president, WCTU of Iowa, 1913–33, 1944–52; ordained, Disciples of Christ, 1923; president, National WCTU, 1933–44; honorary president, National WCTU, 1944–52.

Ida Speakman was born in 1871, just two years before the outbreak of the so-called Woman's War that led to the founding of the Woman's Christian Temperance Union. She grew up dry, became involved with temperance activities as a young woman, and ultimately made her mark in the world with the WCTU. In effect, they grew together as she served the organization over the years in offices of increasing responsibility. Beginning her public career as a schoolteacher, she married James A. Wise in 1889, and after moving with him to Lincoln, Nebraska, she became active in youth work for the local union. Settling later in Iowa again, she became a WCTU district president, and after her husband's death (1902) she was state corresponding secretary for more than a decade. Finally, from 1913 to 1933, she led the Iowa Union as president, as well as holding the position of National WCTU director of Christian citizenship. In all of these posts, Ida Wise acquired a reputation as a hard worker who got results. In 1926 she further ascended in the union hierarchy by winning election as national vice president at large. Although she remarried in 1912 (attorney Malcolm Smith), the affairs of the WCTU occupied most of her time. Mrs. Smith also had a considerable reputation as a reform lecturer. She travelled frequently to speak on temperance and suffrage, and she became one of the best-known officers in the WCTU among the general public and the organization's rank and file. A skilled administrator, she built the membership and effectiveness of the Iowa Union and on two occasions (1925 and 1928) was cited by the governor as one of the most distinguished women in the state. Reflecting her prominence in the union, in 1925 she was also named superintendent of the Citizenship Department of the World's WCTU. Clearly, she was one of the most accomplished temperance leaders the WCTU had, and when national president Ella Boole* completed her tenure in 1933, Smith was a logical successor.

The Iowa reformer was pleased with her new role, but 1933 was a hard time to assume the WCTU presidency. National Prohibition had been routed, and although dry die-hards, including Smith, urged a counterattack to restore the Eighteenth Amendment, it remained to be seen whether such a bold step could succeed. As it turned out, the public failed to rally to the antiliquor standard despite the best efforts of the WCTU and other temperance groups. Smith and her colleagues were disappointed but never gave up hope that a way could be found to roll back the wet tide. During the 1930s, Smith also found that the strength of the WCTU was falling precipitously. Memberships declined in the state chapters, which cost the organization most of its former political and social influence. Only briefly did the WCTU president see any reason to take heart: During World War II, temperance leaders generally hoped that the citizenry would consider a return to some sort of prohibition as a war-related measure, much as it had during World War I. Most Americans, though, were uninterested in the dry appeal, and Smith was never able to find an opening against effective wet lobbying to stall the antiliquor attempt. Frustrated by the low state of dry fortunes, Smith voluntarily stepped aside in 1944 and was succeeded by Mrs. D. Leigh Colvin* as head of the WCTU. Smith resumed the presidency of the Iowa Union (and was named honorary president of the National WCTU), in which post she served until her death. She had given the union her best, but for all of her considerable reform experience, the cause she had served so well was beyond help by the time she ever assumed the reins of national leadership.

### Bibliography:

A. *A Door Opened: Annual Address...* (San Francisco, 1938); *Building a Wall for the Home Front: A Discussion of the Liquor Problem During War and Reconstruction* (Evanston, IL, 1944); *Will Our Children Forgive Us? An Appraisal of the Liquor Problem in Wartime America* (Evanston, IL, 1944).

B. SEAP 5, 2457; WW 3, 796; Mrs. D. Leigh Colvin, "Mrs. Ida B. Wise Smith," *Union Signal* 78, No. 9 (1952):133; F.D.L. Squires, "Mrs. Ida B. Wise Smith," *Union Signal* 78, No. 9 (1952):133–35.

**SMITH, Robert Holbrook ("Dr. Bob")** (8 August 1879, St. Johnsbury, VT—16 November 1950, Akron, OH). *Education*: graduated from Dartmouth Coll., 1901; premedical study, Univ. of Michigan, 1905–7; M.D., Rush Medical Coll., 1910. *Career*: medical practice, Akron, OH, 1912–48; co-founder, Alcoholics Anonymous, 1935; treated alcoholics, St. Thomas Hosp., Akron, OH, beginning 1939.

One of the two men who founded Alcoholics Anonymous, Robert Smith grew up in rural Vermont in the late nineteenth century. Provided with a good elementary and secondary education, Smith took his baccalaureate at Dartmouth College. And it was at Dartmouth that drinking assumed a growing part in his life. Apparently having little sympathy with the rising prohibitionist sentiments of the day, he was a hard-drinking student, a habit he maintained through medical school and after establishing a medical practice in Akron, Ohio. By the time he had settled in Akron, however, Smith was probably an alcoholic. Despite his drinking, he was still able to function socially and professionally: He married Anne Ripley in 1915, began to raise a family, and continued to practice surgery. But as his drinking went out of control, so did Smith. He became increasingly erratic both as a doctor and a family man, all to the alarm of his wife and friends. In 1933, Mrs. Smith finally persuaded her husband to seek help at meetings of the Oxford Group, which had received considerable acclaim for helping a number of alcoholics through its program of "spiritual regeneration." Smith found some comfort with the Oxford members, whom he admired for "their seeming poise, health, and happiness." Yet it was not enough, and by 1935 Smith was seeking medical treatment. Fortuitously, though, as he was reaching "bottom," a local minister introduced the struggling doctor to stockbroker William Wilson,* another alcoholic looking for help. The two ailing men spent long hours discussing their mutual condition and slowly worked toward a means of supporting one another in their struggle with the bottle. A month after meeting Wilson, Smith took his last drink, and Alcoholics Anonymous had begun.

For the next fifteen years, Smith played a central role in the growth of the AA fellowship. While still in contact with the Oxford Group, Smith (now known as "Dr. Bob" in keeping with AA anonymity) was largely responsible for establishing the nation's first AA group in Akron in June 1935. Thereafter, he lent crucial help to other alcoholics as they formed AA meetings in other Midwestern cities and, by 1939, led the Akron AAs to total independence from the Oxford Group. There were some difficult times, especially when Smith and Wilson were accused of making excessive profits from AA publications, but the growth of the fellowship continued steadily. In addition to his work with AA, in 1939 Smith also began to treat alcoholics at St. Thomas Hospital in Akron, a practice he maintained until cancer forced his retirement in 1948. Anonymity was the sine qua non of the fellowship (the preferred term, as there was no formal AA organizational structure), and true to their principle, the founders long avoided divulging their identities. Only the death of Smith's wife in 1949 persuaded him to emerge into public view, and then only to give her a deserved share of the credit for the success of AA. Smith himself ultimately was to be the less visible of AA's founders: While Wilson took charge of the group's national growth and remained active until his death in 1971, the Akron doctor confined his work to the Midwest and did not live long enough to witness the dramatic growth of AA membership in the 1950s and 1960s. Yet his contributions were significant, and among those familiar with the origins of AA, Smith is justly remembered as a central figure in the rise of the single most successful approach to alcoholism treatment in history.

**Bibliography:**

A. Dr. Bob and Bill W., "Your Third Legacy," *AA Grapevine* 7, No. 7 (1950):6–9.

B. NYT, Nov. 17, 1950; *Time* 57 (Nov. 27, 1950), 97; Anonymous, *Dr. Bob and the Good Oldtimers: A Biography with Recollections of Early A.A. in the Midwest* (New York, 1980); Ernest Kurtz, *Not God: A History of Alcoholics Anonymous* (Center City, MN, 1979); Robert Thompson, *Bill W.* (New York, 1975); Bill W. [William Wilson], *Alcoholics Anonymous: A Brief History of A.A.* (New York, 1967); Bill W. [William Wilson], *Alcoholics Anonymous: The Story of How More than One Hundred Men Have Recovered from Alcoholism* (New York, 1939).


**SMITHERS, Robert Brinkley**   (30 July 1907, Glen Cove, NY— ). *Education*: studied at Johns Hopkins Univ., 1927–29; attended the Yale Summer Sch. of Alcohol Studies, 1956; LLD. (honorary), Rutgers Univ., 1964. *Career*: business management, Brown Brothers & Co., International Business Machines, Aircraft Marine Specialty Company, 1931–32, 1932–37, 1938–41; partner in investment banking firm, F. S. Smithers & Co., beginning 1950; founder, Christopher D. Smithers Foundation, 1952; officer, National Council on Alcoholism, 1955–65; member, Governor's Advisory Committee on Alcoholism, NY, 1962–72.

Philanthropy has always played an important role in the history of American reform. In the nineteenth and early twentieth centuries, the Temperance Movement received crucial financial support from private benefactors, and the modern effort to deal with drinking-related difficulties has found similar help. One of the most notable philanthropic efforts has been that of Robert Brinkley Smithers, who left a successful business career in the early 1950s to devote most of his subsequent attention to the alleviation of alcohol problems. A recovered alcoholic, he had stopped drinking about 1953 and had begun to work on an individual basis counseling other alcoholics. When a friend pointed out that he would be able to reach very few alcoholics with such an approach, Smithers joined the board of the National Council of Alcoholism in 1955, hoping to help popularize the disease conception of alcoholism nationally and to marshall popular support for alcoholism treatment. He had particular interests in encouraging the medical community to address alcohol problems: the creation of rehabilitation programs in industry, and the removal of the social stigma attached to alcoholism. Serving as treasurer of NCA from 1955 to 1958, he was elected president in 1958, holding the post until 1962, when he became chairman of the board (he also served another year as president in 1964). During these years, he not only helped with NCA fund-raising and organizational activities but also emerged as a national spokesman on alcohol-related issues and a member of a number of other groups (private and political) concerned with drinking problems. At the same time, Smithers was steadily expanding his role as one of the chief philanthropists in the alcoholism field.

The vehicle for most of his charitable work was the Christopher D. Smithers Foundation, established in 1952 and named after his father. Originally created to fund treatment and research efforts in cancer and alcoholism, a charter amendment in 1956 placed the entire focus on alcoholism. With money from the Smithers family, the foundation, with Robert Brinkley Smithers at its head, began underwriting certain NCA operations as early as 1955 and then took on an increasing number of projects in the field. Among the most important was a study of alcohol problems by E. M. Jellinek* (whom Smithers had first met at the Yale Summer School of Alcohol Studies in 1956) resulting in the 1960 publication of *The Disease Concept of Alcoholism*, a classic in the alcohol studies literature. The foundation also supported the publication of thousands of educational pamphlets which saw an international distribution. By the 1960s, the foundation had become a major and steady contributor to fourteen different alcohol-related charities. The largest foundation effort, however, came in 1962. When the Yale Center of Alcohol Studies moved to Rutgers University, the Smithers Foundation, Smithers personally, and the National Institute of Mental Health jointly contributed a total of $700,000 toward the construction of a new building, establishing the center in its new home. In response to this and his other work, Rutgers conferred on Smithers an honorary doctor of laws degree. After the completion of the Rutgers Center, Smithers devoted much of his time to assisting efforts to increase governmental aid to alcoholism programs. He encouraged politicians at all levels in this regard and worked closely with Senator Harold Hughes* of Iowa in the legislative process that finally created the Comprehensive Alcohol Abuse and Alcoholism Prevention, Treatment and Rehabilitation Act of 1970. Over the 1970s and 1980s, Smithers and the foundation remained active, placing special emphasis on the operations of the Smithers Alcoholism Treatment and Training Center at Roosevelt Hospital in New York City.

**Bibliography:**

B. *Who's Who in America*, 38th ed., vol. 2 (Chicago, 1974); Christopher D. Smithers Foundation, *Pioneers We Have Known in the Field of Alcoholism* (Mill Neck, NY, 1979).

**STEARNS, John Newton**   (24 May 1829, New Ipswich, NH—21 April 1895, Brooklyn, NY). *Career*: schoolteacher, New Ipswich, NH, 1840s to 1850; magazine salesman, New York City, 1850–53; publisher, *Merry's Museum*, beginning 1853; publishing agent, National Temperance Society and Publication House, 1865–95; editor, *National Temperance Advocate* and *Youth's Temperance Banner*, 1865–95.

John Stearns grew up with the Temperance Movement. It provided a social life, a political focus, and, importantly, a full and prosperous career. Stearns joined his first antiliquor organization, the "Cold Water Army," at the age of seven; dressed in its uniform, he and his small friends in reform marched the streets singing temperance songs. From that point on he was never without some formal group affiliation in the movement. Over the years, he was also a member of the Cadets of Temperance (1839), the Band of Hope (1842, a group inspired by the Washingtonian temperance revival), and the fraternal Sons of Temperance (1848) and Independent Order of Good Templars (1866). Not a mere joiner, Stearns played active roles in these groups whenever he could. In both the Sons and the Templars he achieved high office, and for a time was worthy patriarch of the National Division of the Sons of Temperance, the chief post in the order. His rise as a temperance leader, however, paralleled his rise in the publishing business. A schoolteacher until 1850, he had moved to New York City, where he sold magazines before purchasing *Merry's Museum*, a juvenile publication (he also wrote for the publication under the name "Robert Merry"). He handled the marketing of this journal personally and built it into a successful venture. His goal, though, was to combine his talents as a publisher with his enthusiasm for the temperance reform; and in 1865 he got his chance. That year, Stearns was the moving force behind a call for a temperance convention which met at Saratoga Springs, New York, and founded the National Temperance Society and Publication House. The group quickly named him publication agent and editor of its publications, the *National Temperance Advocate* and *Youth's Temperance Banner*. It was a new beginning for both Stearns and the movement.

The dry editor held his posts with the National Society for thirty years until his death in 1895. During that time, he made the group the single most prolific source of antiliquor publishing, while at the same time building an effective distribution network for the organization's books, hymnals, pamphlets, and various tracts. It was a dry effort unsurpassed until the rise of the Anti-Saloon League in the next generation. It was also a prodigious personal labor: Stearns not only ran the business operation, which probably spent some $1.5 million over the years, but wrote and edited many of the society's titles. While the Temperance Movement had long appreciated the value of the press and public education, its members soon came to prize the work of Stearns, for under his direction dry literature blanketed the land. The wet opposition had no comparable publication venture. His editing tasks, however, did not take Stearns away from other temperance activities. He continued in other organizations as well and even added new ones to his impressive list of memberships. In the mid-1870s he was president of the New York State Temperance Society and for eight years headed the state Constitutional Amendment Association. He also lent a hand in organizing efforts, speaking to the delegates who founded the Dominion Prohibitory Council in Canada and making the arrangements that resulted in the massive World's Temperance Congress in Chicago in 1893. To the end of his days, Stearns remained one of the most active leaders of the antiliquor cause and was accorded a respect and admiration enjoyed by relatively few others.

**Bibliography:**

A. *Temperance Hymn-book* (New York, 1869); ed., *Water Sports* (New York, 1879); *Prohibition Does Prohibit, or; Prohibition not a Failure* (New York,

1882); ed., *The Temperance Speaker*. . . (New York, 1884); comp., *The Prohibition Songster*. . . (New York, 1886); comp., *The Constitutional Prohibitionist, or; Prohibition by the People* (New York, 1891).

B. DAB 17, 546; NYT, April 23, 1895; SEAP 6, 2525; WW H, 574; W. H. Daniels, *The Temperance Reform and Its Great Reformers* (Cincinnati, OH, 1878); John A. Krout, *The Origins of Prohibition* (New York, 1925); *A Noble Life*. . .*a Memorial Pamphlet* (New York, n.d.).

**STELZLE, Charles**    (4 June 1869, New York, NY—27 February 1941, New York, NY). *Education*: training as machinist, R. Hoe & Co., NY, 1885–90; private study of theology, 1890–93; attended Moody Bible Inst., 1894–95; LLD. (honorary), Cumberland Univ., TN, 1933. *Career*: machinist, NY, 1885–93; layworker, Hope Chapel, Minneapolis, MN, 1895–97; layworker, Hope Chapel, New York, 1897–99; pastor, Marlsham Memorial Church, St. Louis, MO, 1899–1903; ordained, Presbyterian Church, 1900; superintendent, Department of Church and Labor, Presbyterian Home Board, 1903–13; author on religious, reform, and philanthropic subjects, 1900s to 1941.

The role of "apostle to labor" came naturally to Charles Stelzle. His father had owned a brewery in New York City, but his death left his family in desperate straits. To make ends meet, eight-year-old Charles worked stripping tobacco leaves in a sweatshop and at eleven dropped out of school to work as a cutter in an artificial flower shop. But the youth was determined to make something of himself, and he managed to gain instruction as machinist and to make a living in that role by his late teens. All of this was experience he never forgot, and upon entering the ministry he singled out the working population as the chief object of his compassion. As a proponent of the Progressive "social gospel," Stelzle consistently urged the church to address itself not only to the souls of working Americans but also to their social and economic needs. While often facing the disapproval of more conservative clergy, Stelzle fought consistently for church involvement with urban labor as he organized special self-help classes for working families, mediated labor disputes, wrote widely on social issues, evangelized the laboring population, and distributed enormous amounts of religious literature. His theology was generally conservative, but his efforts led the church to reach out to those it had often ignored. In 1903, the Presbyterian hierarchy named Stelzle the first superintendent of the Department of Church and Labor, which placed him in charge of relations with working families. In this capacity, he did good work in improving communications between the church and organized labor and in assuring that most working people did not come to see the church as mindful only of the views of the middle classes and the wealthy.

Stelzle accepted prohibition as part of the social gospel, convinced that alcohol lay at the root of much social misery. He wrote extensively on the liquor question, not only denouncing drink but taking pains to explain why working men in particular had a stake in drying out the nation. Nor did he write without firsthand knowledge: Shortly before World War I, Baltimore philanthropist William F.

Cochran supported Stelzle in an investigation of the impact of drinking problems in Europe and the United States. Stelzle reported the results in *Why Prohibition!* (1918), a study he later supplemented with similar research in some two hundred American cities and another tour of Europe in 1924 (to Great Britain and Germany). All of these studies received considerable publicity, and their conclusion that working families would see an improved standard of living and safer jobs under prohibition helped gain the Temperance Movement important labor support. Indeed, because of his credence with labor leaders, Stelzle could find a sympathetic hearing for the dry cause among working men where other antiliquor crusaders could not. On its part, the dry camp responded to the opportunities Stelzle's efforts created. The Anti-Saloon League named him director of a special Bureau of Labor, which targeted working Americans for temperance evangelizing, and named him editor of the league's *Worker* in 1915. The hard-working minister also contributed pieces to the *National Daily*, also a league publication, and lectured extensively in support of National Prohibition in many cities. Over the years, Stelzle did as much as any reformer to give temperance an urban face.

**Bibliography:**

A. *The Workingman and Social Problems* (New York, 1903); *Leaflets on the Liquor Problem* (Westerville, OH, 1914); *Liquor and Labor...* (Newark, NJ, 1917); *Why Prohibition!* (New York, 1918); *The Right to Drink: A Discussion of Personal Liberty* (New York, 1920); *A Son of the Bowery* (New York, 1926); *What Shall We Substitute for the Saloon?* (Westerville, OH, n.d.).

B. DAB Supp. 3, 733–35; DARB, 428–30; NCAB C, 160; NYT, Feb. 28, 1941; SEAP 6, 2528.

**STEVENS, Adie Allen**    (20 August 1845, Blair Co., PA—1 January 1917, Tyrone, PA). *Education*: private study of law, 1870–72. *Career*: photographer, 1859–64; enlisted man, Union army, 1864–65; admitted to bar, PA, 1872; legal practice, Tyrone, PA, 1872–1917; business interests in utilities, banking, lime, and stone, 1870–1917.

Adie Allen Stevens typifies the connection between the Temperance Movement and the development of American business and industry, a connection which rested on a mutual opposition to the economically and socially subversive influence of excessive drinking. Stevens was the classic self-made man: He quit school at fourteen years old to become a photographer, served in the Union army, read law privately, and upon passing the bar opened a flourishing legal office. He made a second fortune as an entrepreneur and corporate officer in gas, banking, and lime production. In such a man as Stevens, whose ambition and dedication to the work ethic were of the most rigorous and energetic kind (his photograph shows him determined, even grim), an interest in temperance demanded nothing less than total prohibition. In addition, he was a devout and active Methodist, and the dry posture of his church complemented the hostility toward alcohol he had gained from other quarters. The assistance the Temperance

Movement derived from such local business leaders can hardly be overestimated. They lent not only their influence (which was often considerable in their localities) but, as in the case of Adie Stevens, their time and organizing skills. Stevens was a leader in both the Pennsylvania Sons of Temperance lodge and the local Independent Order of Good Templars. Working with these groups and other antiliquor proponents, he took a central part in the successful drive to enact local-option laws in the state. Stevens also was instrumental in fostering the growth of the Prohibition Party. With James Black* (the party's presidential candidate in 1872), he organized the convention that founded the Pennsylvania branch of the party; and at various times over the 1880s and 1890s he held committee and convention posts on both the state and national levels for the Prohibitionists. Indeed, beyond these assignments, between 1888 and 1912 he was a member of the party's National Executive Committee. Dedicated and committed, Stevens represented the kind of support the antiliquor crusade depended upon to secure its fortunes in the business community. That so much business support was forthcoming in Pennsylvania was, in part, testimony to his labors.

**Bibliography:**

B. SEAP 6, 2529–30; WW 3, 819.

**STEVENS, Lillian Marion Norton Ames**    (1 March 1844, Dover, ME—6 April 1914, Portland, ME). *Education*: studied at Foxcroft Acad. and Westbrook Sem., ME, 1850s to 1862?; A.M. (honorary), Bates Coll., 1911. *Career*: schoolteacher, South Portland, ME, circa 1862–65; president, Maine WCTU, 1878–1914; various National WCTU offices, 1880–93; president, National WCTU, 1898–1914.

Born to a reform-oriented family, Lillian Ames married Michael T. Stevens, a well-to-do grain and salt merchant, in 1865. He was a firm temperance man, and when his wife showed an interest in the reviving Temperance Movement in the 1870s he encouraged her participation. She joined the cause as part of the Woman's Crusade of 1873 and 1874, and when the crusade coalesced into the more formally structured Woman's Christian Temperance Union, she helped found the Maine chapter in 1875. Stevens served until 1878 as the group's first treasurer, and then moved into the presidency. And she was no mere figurehead: Setting to work with enthusiasm, she spoke across Maine building WCTU membership, denouncing drink, and praising efforts to enact state-wide constitutional prohibition. In this latter cause, the WCTU officer became a fast friend of Neal Dow,* champion of the antebellum Maine Law and in the later nineteenth century a fighter once more for the legal abolition of the liquor traffic. With the final victory of Maine prohibition in 1884, Stevens shared a great deal of the credit with Dow. Throughout her campaigns, Michael Stevens remained a firm proponent of Lillian's work. And as her antiliquor responsibilities grew, he hired a governess to watch their daughter in order that Mrs. Stevens could keep the field. But temperance was hardly her only interest. She took special interest in the problems of delinquent women and children, sometimes giving them refuge in her own home. She also sought the improvement of prison conditions for women, while at the same time emerging as a zealous proponent of women's suffrage. Without question, Stevens was one of the premier reformers in the state.

Despite her other pursuits, however, temperance remained Stevens's chief interest, and it was there that she did her best work. While maintaining the presidency of the Maine Union, she became an officer (recording secretary) in the National WCTU in 1880 and became a confidant of union president Frances E. Willard.* Indeed, she became Willard's strong right arm, and in 1894 the union leader engineered Mrs. Stevens's election as vice president at large. Willard had in fact created the post for her, and the union membership widely assumed that the Maine reformer would succeed Mrs. Willard as president. She did. When Willard died in 1898, Stevens moved into the top office without appreciable opposition. She proved an able leader, although she never won the emotional devotion her predecessor had enjoyed. Still, Stevens presided over a campaign to expand the WCTU, and she watched with satisfaction as membership rose from 168,000 in 1900 to 248,000 by 1910. Stevens also maintained Willard's "Do Everything" reform policy, and the organization publicly backed Progressive measures across the board, from pure food and drug legislation to women's suffrage. Her chief objective, however, was a national prohibition amendment. In 1913, she spearheaded a major union drive to impress Congress with the depth of public sentiment on the question, which culminated in the presentation of massive dry petitions to the legislators. Stevens herself spent most of her time lobbying in Washington, D.C., although she kept up with her other duties. In addition to her post with the National WCTU, she was also vice president at large of the World's WCTU and editor-in-chief of the *Union Signal*. Yet Stevens was not to see the final dry victory. In failing health for some time, she succumbed to chronic nephritis in April 1914. When the Eighteenth Amendment was finally ratified in 1919, however, it could safely be said that Lillian Stevens had been a powerful force in its success.

**Bibliography:**

A. *What Lillian M.N. Stevens Said*, Anna A. Gordon, comp. (Evanston, IL, 1914).

B. NAW 3, 370–72; SEAP 6, 2530–31; WW 1, 1182; Gertrude Stevens Leavitt and Margaret L. Sargent, *Lillian M. N. Stevens: A Life Sketch* (Evanston, IL, 1921).

**STEVENSON, Katharine Adelia Lent**    (8 May 1853, Copake, NY—27 March 1919, Des Moines, IA). *Education*: graduated from Amenia (NY) Sem., 1873; graduated from Boston Univ. Sch. of Theology, 1881. *Career*: various offices, Massachusetts and National WCTU, 1870s–1900s; Methodist lay preacher, beginning 1890; editor for books and leaflets, Woman's Temperance Publishing Association, beginning 1894; associate editor, *Union Signal*, beginning 1894.

Long a dedicated total abstainer, Katharine Lent joined the Woman's Christian Temperance Union soon after its inception in 1874. She spent most of the rest of her life in its service. Her interest in the dry crusade probably stemmed from her devout Methodist faith; she pursued theological studies at Boston University and later served as a lay preacher in the denomination, and we can assume that much of her speaking focused on the liquor question. Over the years, the ardent reformer assumed increasingly more responsible positions in the WCTU hierarchy. After some fifteen years of service, Mrs. Stevenson (she married James Stevenson of Boston in 1883) became superintendent of the Franchise Department of the Massachusetts WCTU and used the post to proselytize for women's suffrage. She then went on to become state corresponding secretary in 1891 and to national duties in 1894 as associate editor of the *Union Signal*, the official organ of the WCTU. At the same time, she was made an editor with the Woman's Temperance Publishing Association, a venture strongly backed by the union. She served as national corresponding secretary in 1894. In each of her positions, Stevenson proved a tireless and capable worker with sound organizational and leadership skills. Thus it was no surprise when, in 1898, the Massachusetts Union elected her president, an honor she enjoyed for the following twenty years. Quite clearly, the WCTU was a career: It offered Stevenson not only an opportunity for service against liquor—a cause to which she was sincerely committed—but also a means to upward mobility in her chosen field, something American society too often denied women of her generation. And just as clearly, she made the most of her chances. The Massachusetts reformer received not only local applause for her work but also international recognition. In Boston in 1891 she took part in the founding of the World's WCTU and, while maintaining her post as head of the Bay State union, travelled a good deal of the world as superintendent of temperance and missions for the new organization. Between 1908 and 1910, Stevenson spoke to youth groups on the evils of drink in such diverse locations as China, Ceylon, Burma, India, Egypt, Greece, and Italy. While it would be difficult to assess the impact of such tours, her trips clearly demonstrated the confidence and ambitions of the cause in which she served. In addition, Stevenson found the time to write extensively on reform subjects, including a *Brief History of the Woman's Christian Temperance Union* (1906).

**Bibliography:**

A. *A Brief History of the Woman's Christian Temperance Union: An Outline Course of Study for Local Unions* (Evanston, IL, 1906); *Woman Suffrage . . .* (Chicago, 1913).

B. SEAP 6, 2531; WW 1, 1183.

**STEVENSON, Sarah Hackett**  (2 February 1843, Buffalo Grove, IL—14 August 1909, Chicago, IL). *Education*: graduated from State Normal Univ., IL,

1863; studied at Woman's Hosp. Medical Coll., Chicago, circa 1869–71; studied at South Kensington Science Sch., circa 1871–72; M.D., Woman's Hosp. Medical Coll., 1874. *Career*: school principal and teacher, IL, 1863 to circa 1869; medical practice, Chicago, 1875–1903; staff, Cook County Hosp., beginning 1881; member, Illinois State Board of Health, beginning 1893; professor of physiology, histology, and obstetrics, Woman's Hosp. Medical Coll., Chicago, 1875–94; writing on medical subjects, beginning 1870s.

After teaching in Illinois public schools for some six years, Sarah Stevenson left the classroom to pursue her interest in science. Thinking first to be a writer on the subject, she instead pursued a medical education in Chicago and abroad. For a time, she studied in London under renowned biologist Thomas Huxley, who considered her one of his best students. Launching her own practice in 1875, Stevenson went on to become one of the most prominent physicians of her region. As one of the relatively few women doctors in the nation, she compiled an impressive list of "firsts": the first female member of the American Medical Association (1876); the first woman to join the staff of the Cook County Hospital in Chicago (1881); the first woman appointed to the state Board of Health (1893). She also pioneered medical education for women, teaching for years at her alma mater, the Woman's Hospital Medical College in Chicago and helping to found the Illinois Training School for Nurses in 1880. A dedicated Methodist, many of her social views reflected the reforming sympathies of the denomination. At various times, she contributed to or spoke on behalf of foreign missionary work, temperance, women's rights (although she was never zealous in this area), and black civil rights. Active in many civic organizations as well, Stevenson moved comfortably among the Illinois social elite until a stroke compelled her retirement in 1903.

While Stevenson's first concern as a reformer was women's medical education, she placed an almost equal emphasis on the Temperance Movement. She viewed the liquor question not only as a moral and humanitarian concern but also as a health problem. Joining the Woman's Christian Temperance Union in 1881, she became the first superintendent of the organization's Department of Hygiene, responsible for the dissemination of information on the impact of drinking on health. She served in the post for two years, resigning in 1882 but retaining a keen interest in the dry reform. Four years later, when the Chicago chapter of the WCTU founded the National Temperance Hospital, Stevenson accepted an invitation to head the staff as president. The institution (later renamed the Frances Willard Hospital, after the National WCTU president), was a general service facility but strictly forbade the use of any medicines containing alcohol. The anti-alcohol policy stemmed from the longstanding debate within the medical community over the efficacy of alcohol in medicine and its place in the pharmacopoeia. The WCTU members were so adamant on the question that they were willing to establish the National Hospital to demonstrate that physicians could do nicely without the use of the drug they considered such an evil. In casting her lot with the temperance view on the matter, Stevenson in fact sided publicly with a position favored by many of the nation's better-trained practitioners anyway.

**Bibliography:**

A. *The Physiology of Woman*... (Chicago, 1880); *Boys and Girls in Biology*... (New York, 1975).

B. *Chicago Tribune*, Aug. 15, 1909; NAW 3, 374–76; WW 1, 1183; Chicago Medical Society, *History of Medicine and Surgery, and Physicians and Surgeons of Chicago* (Chicago, 1922); F. M. Sperry, comp., *A Group of Distinguished Physicians and Surgeons of Chicago* (Chicago, 1922).

**STEWART, Eliza Daniel**    ("Mother Stewart")(25 April 1816, Piketon, OH— 8 August 1908, Hicksville, OH). *Career*: assistant postmaster, Piketon, OH, 1833 to 1840s; schoolteacher, OH, 1840 to 1850s; relief work with Union troops, 1862–65; active reform work, chiefly temperance, 1860s–1900s.

One of the more radical founders of the Woman's Christian Temperance Union, Eliza Stewart's uncompromising views and impressive oratory won her a reputation as the dry crusade's "Wendell Phillips in Petticoats." Born Eliza Daniel, she was twice married, first to one Joseph Coover (who soon died) and then to a prominent local farmer, Hiram Stewart, in 1848. Stewart began her professional career as a teacher in the Ohio public schools, becoming one of the most highly regarded instructors in the state. Teaching gave her an appreciation of public affairs and social responsibility, an outlook further strengthened by a Methodist faith stressing moral reform and personal salvation. After settling with her husband in the town of Athens, Mrs. Stewart became involved with the reform activities that characterized the rest of her life. About 1858, she helped to organize a lodge of the Independent Order of Good Templars, a fraternal temperance group, and then gave her first temperance lecture to a Band of Hope gathering (a youth temperance organization) in nearby Pomeroy, Ohio. Stewart's interest in the dry crusade was intense, but she gave it up during the Civil War to help with relief work for Union wounded. The grateful troops began calling her Mother Stewart, and she carried the name as a public honor for the rest of her years. After the war, she reentered the reform lists, emerging as a champion of woman's suffrage (she was the first president of the suffrage organization in Springfield, Ohio) and of prison reform. Temperance, however, remained her chief interest, and she seldom missed an opportunity to attack the liquor traffic. Indeed, as the Temperance Movement began to rebuild its strength in the 1870s, Mother Stewart became one of its driving forces—first locally in the Midwest, and then in a role with national implications.

With slavery defeated in the Civil War, Stewart, like other reformers of similar bent, asserted that the next task Americans faced was a struggle against enslavement to drink. Public policy, she believed, needed changing in this regard, for the laws of the land fostered "a foe...even worse than the one the soldiers had just conquered by force of arms." In January 1872, she fired the opening salvoes of what she called "temperance warfare" in a speech in Springfield, Ohio. Stewart not only urged women to total abstinence but called on them to use the law in their favor. Specifically, she wanted the wives and mothers of problem drinkers to sue liquor dealers under Ohio's Adair Act, which made the traffic liable for damages coming in the wake of beverage sales to family members. Mrs. Stewart appeared in court herself to help in several of these suits, a number of which brought victories. Out of her inspirational example came mass meetings and antiliquor petitions and, on December 2, 1873, a Woman's Temperance League with Stewart as president. The league quickly became part of the "Woman's War" or "Woman's Crusade," which saw Ohio women praying in saloons and demanding an end to illegal liquor sales (the Woman's War also spread nationally). In 1874, the crusade gave birth to the Woman's Christian Temperance Union, with Mother Stewart chairing the organizational convention. Her election, however, was a touchy subject: To more moderate delegates, she represented the "extreme radical portion of the temperance women." But when Frances Willard* spoke on her behalf, emphasizing her contributions to the crusade, the convention acquiesced. Later, Stewart headed the National WCTU's committee on Southern work, helping to found both black and white local chapters of the organization. She also remained active with the Good Templars, lecturing for the group and attending national and international conventions. On one such sojourn in 1876 she was instrumental in the founding of the British Women's Temperance Association as well as the Scottish Christian Union. Throughout the later nineteenth century, the Ohio reformer proved one of the more effective speakers for the dry cause and she kept the field well into her eighties. Her account of the Woman's War, *Memories of the Crusade* (1888), was recognized as one of the classics of temperance history.

**Bibliography:**

A. *Memories of the Crusade: A Thrilling Account of the Uprising of the Women of Ohio in 1873, Against the Liquor Crime* (1888; New York, 1972); *The Crusader in Great Britain: Or, the History of the Origin and Organization of the British Women's Temperance Association* (Springfield, OH, 1893); with others, *The White Angel of the World, that Fortells the Freedom of the Nations from the Evils of Strong Drink* (Lynn, MA, 1893).

B. NAW 3, 376–77; SEAP 6, 2531–32; WW 1, 1184; Helen E. Tyler, *Where Prayer and Purpose Meet: The W.C.T.U. Story, 1874–1949* (Evanston, IL, 1949); Frances E. Willard, *Woman and Temperance* (Hartford, CT, 1883); Frances E. Willard and Mary A. Livermore, eds., *A Woman of the Century* (New York, 1893).

**STEWART, Gideon Tabor**    (7 August 1824, Johnstown, NY—9 June 1909, Pasadena, CA). *Education*: studied at Oberlin Coll., early 1840s? *Career*: admitted to bar, OH, 1846; legal practice, Norwalk, OH, 1846–1901.

Born in New York, Gideon Stewart spent most of his life in Ohio, where he established a reputation as one of the most ardent prohibitionists in the Midwest. Not much is known of his formative years, except that he was able to obtain a sound education which in 1846 enabled him to launch a prosperous legal practice in Norwalk, Ohio. He maintained his practice for some fifty-five years while at times dabbling in journalism. Over the years, he helped edit the *Norwalk Reflector* and the *Dubuque* (Iowa) *Daily Times* and was part owner and publisher of the *Toledo Blade* and *Toledo Commercial*. Yet despite his professional career, Stewart spent most of his free time in temperance activities. We know little of the origins of his long association with the dry crusade, save for the fact that he became involved soon after opening his legal office. In 1847, Stewart was a founder of the Norwalk division of the fraternal Sons of Temperance. The group rose nationally in the wake of the Washingtonian temperance revival, attracting many local community notables and professionals. While there was a sincere temperance motive for joining, there was evidently a social appeal as well for some members. At any rate, Stewart became one of the organization's most active participants, and he later served as its grand worthy patriarch. He was also connected with the Independent Order of Good Templars, another dry fraternal lodge, and he was three times grand worthy chief templar of Ohio. Like many others in the antiliquor movement, however, politics became Stewart's primary reform focus, and in 1853 he began agitation for a separate prohibition party. Four years later he organized a state-wide convention with the purpose of establishing such a group, although the effort came to nothing. Yet he kept the faith, insisting that the other parties would never fully commit themselves to political prohibition. Accordingly, he played an active role in the successful attempt to revive dry sentiments after the Civil War and to found the Prohibition Party in 1869. Thereafter, he was an almost perennial candidate for office: three times for governor of Ohio; eight times for judge of the State Supreme Court; and once, in 1876, for vice president. Such was Prohibitionist regard for the Ohioan that on three occasions, in 1876, 1880, and 1884, elements of the party wanted him to run for the presidency; but he would never permit his name to be placed in nomination. Finally, after more than half a century in Norwalk, Ohio, he retired and moved to Pasadena, California, where he spent his remaining three years working on behalf of his new state's Prohibition Party and the Anti-Saloon League.

**Bibliography:**

A. *How Shall We Best Secure State Prohibition?* (n.p., 1870); *The Constitutionality and Expediency of the Home Protection Bill* (Columbus, OH, 1881); *The Ballot Test of Temperance* (New York, 1882); *Christianity Against the Liquor Crime: Address* (New York, 1884); *Liberty and Union, and the Conflict of Liberty* (New York, 1885); *Early and Late Poems* (n.p., 1906).

B. SEAP 6, 2532; WW 1, 1185.

**STEWART, Oliver Wayne**   (22 May 1867, Mercer Co., IL—15 February 1937, Chicago, IL). *Education*: A.B., Eureka Coll., IL, 1890; LLD. (honorary),

Eureka Coll., 1916. *Career*: ordained, Church of Christ, 1887; evangelical preaching, 1890–93; officer, Illinois Christian Endeavor Union, 1893–97; chair, National Committee, Prohibition Party, 1899–1905; member, Illinois House of Representatives, 1903; vice president, Flying Squadron of America, 1915–20 (also president, 1920); active in various prohibitionist organizations, 1900 to 1930s.

Oliver Stewart was one of the Midwest's most ardent prohibitionists. A firm dry since his youth, he was seldom without a formal affiliation with a temperance group for the greater part of his life. As a young man, he was active with the Independent Order of Good Templars and for a number of years served as an officer in his local chapter in Illinois. A frequent speaker on the liquor question, his ordination in 1887 allowed him ample opportunity to use temperance themes in the pulpit over his next several years as an evangelist. From the beginning, however, Stewart's notions of reform were as much political as religious. Joining the Prohibition Party early, he became one of its more active members and a frequent party official and candidate. In 1890, he ran for Congress, sat on the state party committee from 1804 to 1908, chaired its annual convention for three years, and, in December 1900, was elected chair of the Prohibition Party National Committee. He served until 1905. In a brief exception to the usually dismal party record at the polls, Stewart also won an election: Running as a Prohibitionist in 1902, he captured a seat in the state legislature, which he filled in 1903. This victory alone was enough to bring him national attention in temperance circles, although his other work on behalf of the party was more than enough to guarantee his reputation as an antiliquor champion.

Most of Stewart's national recognition, however, was not dependent on his labors as a Prohibition Party standardbearer, for his other reform efforts were considerable. Indeed, he boasted a list of positions in other dry organizations that few of his colleagues could rival. Among these may be cited the post of chair of the National Prohibitionist Extension Committee (1907–11) and of field secretary of the National Temperance Society of New York (1910–12) and his participation in many law enforcement campaigns from 1921 to 1933 in defense of the Volstead Act. Perhaps his most noteworthy effort in this regard was his work as a member of the Flying Squadron. Between 1915 and 1920 this group of dedicated dry crusaders visited some 225 cities and towns in the United States speaking on behalf of the abolition of the liquor traffic. Stewart was vice president of the Squadron, and, on the death of J. Franklin Hanly,* succeeded him as the group's president in 1920. Enforcement of the Eighteenth Amendment to the Constitution was another of Stewart's pet projects, and he was associated with a large number of organizations that attempted to make the national dry laws effective. Among these were the United Committee for Prohibition Enforcement, the National Conference of Prohibition Organizations Supporting the 18th Amendment (of which he was the founder), the Cooperative Committee for Prohibition Enforcement, and the Allied Forces for Prohibition. Stewart also used his position as editor of the *National Enquirer* to rally popular opinion behind National Prohibition. Stewart, however unsuccessful he was in preserving the prohibition amendment, was certainly indefatigable: In the course of joining, organizing, and leading these various groups, he once held 2,312 meetings with temperance gatherings in as many days. In any event, the work apparently agreed with him, for he lived to be seventy and was still campaigning as late as 1935.

**Bibliography:**

A. with others, *The Battle of 1900...* (Chicago, 1900); with others, eds., *Speeches of the Flying Squadron* (Indianapolis, IN, 1915).

B. SEAP 6, 2533; WW 1, 1186.

**STODDARD, Cora Frances**    (17 September 1872, Irvington, NB—13 May 1936, Oxford, CT). *Education*: A.B., Wellesley Coll., 1896. *Career*: school-teacher, CT, 1897; business, Boston, 1897–98; secretary to Mary H. Hunt, Department of Scientific Temperance Instruction, National WCTU, 1899–1904; school administrator, NY, 1905–6; co-founder and executive secretary, Scientific Temperance Federation, 1906–36; editor, *Scientific Temperance Journal*, 1906–33; headed Scientific Temperance Instruction operations in National and World's WCTU, 1918–36; associate editor, *Standard Encyclopedia of the Alcohol Problem*, 1918–30.

Modern alcohol education has its roots in the "scientific temperance instruction" efforts of the Temperance Movement. During the late nineteenth and early twentieth centuries, most states required the public schools to teach dry-sponsored lessons on the nature and evils of alcohol and drink. The campaign to secure these laws was largely the work of the Woman's Christian Temperance Union and, even more particularly, of Mary H. Hunt.* But while Hunt orchestrated the WCTU educational drive, she had the assistance of dedicated lieutenants, not the least of whom was Cora Frances Stoddard. After a year of teaching and two of an unsuccessful business venture, Stoddard joined Hunt as her secretary; as such, she became familiar not only with the operations of Hunt's WCTU Department of Scientific Temperance Instruction but also with the Scientific Temperance Association. Hunt had founded the latter group to study and endorse temperance education texts—in return for which Hunt received royalties from text publishers. Stoddard worked closely with Hunt in both groups, although other WCTU leaders looked askance at the association because of its financial connections with publishers. Indeed, after Hunt's death in 1906 the union refused to incorporate the organization. Instead, after two years away from the dry crusade because of poor health, Stoddard helped to reconstitute the association as the Scientific Temperance Federation and then served as its executive secretary for the rest of her life. Over the years she became as adept as her mentor ever was at lobbying on behalf of antiliquor education and writing on the personal and social impact of drinking and intemperance.

Stoddard ran the Temperance Federation independent of the WCTU for over a decade, the rift following the death of Hunt not healing quickly. In the interim, she published an impressive number of titles on various aspects of the liquor question, including a number of detailed statistical studies. In addition, she began editing (1906) the *Scientific Temperance Journal*, a publication intended to provide a forum for research reports on the deleterious effects of alcohol on humans. In 1913, the Anti-Saloon League became the *Journal*'s publisher and Stoddard enthusiastically began an active association with that powerful and growing organization. Perhaps her most valuable contribution came between 1918 and 1930, when she served as an associate editor of the six-volume *Standard Encyclopedia of the Alcohol Problem* (1924–30), the league's attempt to compile an authoritative reference on all aspects of drinking-related questions. Stoddard's work with the Anti-Saloon League also brought about a reapproachment with the WCTU; for as her career progressed, it became impossible to deny her contributions to and importance in the alcohol education field. She continued to write extensively, attended a number of international meetings on alcohol problems as an official American delegate, and became the leading source people consulted on how to teach about drinking. The WCTU simply could not compete with Stoddard, so in 1918 it appointed her head of the Bureau of Scientific Temperance Investigation. Four years later she became director of the Department of Scientific Temperance Instruction, and still later she took charge of a similar division of the World's WCTU. With the passage of the Eighteenth Amendment, the tireless reformer produced a number of studies purporting to show that the dry laws had brought major social benefits to the nation, and she defended National Prohibition to the end. In her final years, however, Stoddard suffered severely from arthritis, and by 1933 she had withdrawn from all activity except her work with the Scientific Temperance Federation.

**Bibliography:**

A. *Alcohol's Ledger in Industry* (Westerville, OH, 1914); *Massachusetts' Experience with Exempting Beer from Prohibition* (Westerville, OH, 1919); *The Teacher's Place in the Anti-Alcohol Movement...* (Boston, 1927); *The World's New Day and Alcohol...* (Westerville, OH, 1929); *Science and Human Life in the Alcohol Problem* (Westerville, OH, 1930); *Alcohol in Experience and Experiment* (Evanston, IL, 1934).

B. NAW 3, 380–81; SEAP 6, 2535–36; WW 1, 1190; Norton Mezvinsky, "The White-Ribbon Reform, 1874–1920" (Ph.D. diss., Univ. of Wisconsin, 1959).

**STUART, George Rutledge**    (14 December 1857, Talbotts Station, TN—11 May 1926, Birmingham, AL). *Education*: A.B., Emory and Henry Coll., VA, 1882; A.M., Emory and Henry Coll., 1884; D.D. (honorary), Emory and Henry Coll., ?; LLD. (honorary), Birmingham-Southern Coll., AL, 1923. *Career*: ordained, Methodist Episcopal Church, South, 1883; minister, Cleveland, TN, 1883–84; professor of English and natural science, Centenary Coll., TN, 1885–90; minister, Chattanooga, TN, 1890–91; Methodist evangelist, 1892–1907;

lecturer on reform and religious subjects, 1907–12; minister, Birmingham, AL, 1916–26.

The career of George Rutledge Stuart offers another view of the power of the pulpit and the public podium in the spread of the temperance gospel during the late nineteenth and early twentieth centuries. He probably came to his temperance sympathies via the Methodist Church in which he had grown up and in which he was ordained in 1883. At any rate, Stuart's antiliquor ideals surfaced early. When he was nineteen, he did organizational work for the Independent Order of Good Templars and then for the Woman's Christian Temperance Union. Later, he lent a hand when Dr. J. K. Osgood* launched his Blue Ribbon Movement and began founding a chain of Reformed Men's Clubs across the nation. Thus by the time he had entered the active ministry, Stuart had already made substantial contributions to the war against the liquor traffic. After serving a number of Tennessee pulpits and teaching for some six years, the reform-minded minister went into full-time evangelical work. He proved an effective speaker on behalf of his church, and his humorous and anecdotal style made him a favorite of audiences throughout the South. After 1907, he worked for five years as an independent lecturer and proved just as successful. He dealt with many issues, although temperance remained his staple topic. At various times, he worked in tandem with the great revivalist Sam Jones* (he later compiled a volume of Jones's sermons). With the rise of the Anti-Saloon League in the 1890s and early 1900s, Stuart found another outlet for his oratorical talents. He spoke repeatedly at league gatherings, where he received uniformly good reviews. He was also a member of the Prohibition Party and generally took to the stump on its behalf during campaigns. As a temperance lecturer, then, Stuart held a long-standing and significant reputation. He was never of the stature of a Sam Jones or a John Gough;* yet he helped fill a vital contemporary demand for public speakers, which often combined elements of serious debate and discussion with entertainment. The fact that he could make his living from lecture fees for a good number of years was testimony to the drawing power of the public platform of the era, as well as to the Temperance Movement's ability to use that fact to its advantage. Stuart, however, finished his career back in the pulpit, taking a Birmingham church in 1916.

### Bibliography:

A. *Sermons, Stories, and Parables* (New York, 1907); *The Saloon Under the Searchlight*, 5th ed. (New York, 1908); comp., *Sam Jones' Famous Sayings* (New York, 1908); *What Every Methodist Should Know* (n.p., 1923).

B. SEAP 6, 2543–44; WW 1, 1201.

**STUART, Moses** (26 March 1780, Wilton, CT—4 January 1852, Andover, MA). *Education*: B.A., Yale Coll., 1799; legal study, Newtown, CT, 1801–2; *Career*: schoolteacher, North Fairfield, CT, 1799–1800; admitted to the bar,

CT, 1802; tutor, Yale Coll., 1802–4; licensed to preach, 1803; ordained, Congregational Church, 1806; minister, First Congregational Church, New Haven, CT, 1806–10; professor of sacred literature, Andover Theological Sem., 1810–48; retired, 1848.

After graduating at the head of his class at Yale, Stuart studied law and was admitted to the bar in 1802. Yet he found he had no love for the law and never practiced. Indeed, he returned to his alma mater as a tutor, and there, under the evangelical guidance of Yale president Timothy Dwight, he decided on a career in the pulpit. Ordained in 1806, he took a pastorate in New Haven and emerged as a bulwark of Calvinistic conservatism. His reputation in this regard was such that in 1810 Andover Theological Seminary offered him a professorship in sacred literature, despite the fact that he had few linguistic skills. Yet Stuart was as determined as he was pious, and he quickly set about mastering Hebrew and German. Indeed, he was the first American theologian to teach Hebrew, and in 1821 he authored a Hebrew grammar that became a standard text. At the height of his career he had few equals as a philologist, and he worked studiously over the years to apply his enormous store of knowledge to Biblical research. His goal was to rediscover the original meanings of scriptural passages and thus to reveal the divine inspirations behind them. His long tenure at Andover allowed him to impart his views on the divine nature of the Bible, and the search for meaning in its pages, to some fifteen thousand theological students, many of whom went on to distinguished careers in academia and the ministry. To the end, Stuart saw the way to religious vibrancy as the way of study, and his legacy of scholarship was testimony as much to his faith as to his learning.

Yet scholarly pursuits were only part of the man, for he was hardly unaware of the rising impact of social issues on the church. Stuart was well into his career at Andover when the Temperance Movement reached serious proportions, but he became one its most earnest champions. His participation in the struggle against drink, however, reflected his studious nature, and some of his most noteworthy contributions derived from his Biblical scholarship. Specifically, Stuart was one of the early participants in the so-called Bible wine controversy, in which drys claimed that the wines mentioned in scripture were either grape juice or otherwise nonalcoholic. Using his philological skills, the Andover professor came down on the temperance side of the issue, insisting in *The Scriptural View of the Wine Question* (1848) that the original Biblical texts did not indicate that Christ drank alcohol. The dispute raged for years, but Stuart's reputation as a religious scholar provided the drys with some of their most effective ammunition in the struggle. The Bible wine argument, however, was not his only foray against liquor. Stuart also was an early member of the American Temperance Union, a committed personal total abstainer, and an enthusiastic supporter of the Maine Laws of the 1850s. Never a zealot in his views, he could nevertheless be uncompromising on some matters: He once won a prize for an essay arguing that true Christians should never be drinkers or engage in the drink trade and that churches should exclude from membership any who did. So far as is known, he never changed his mind. Persuasive in argument, erudite in his writings, unswervingly devout, he was mourned by reformers as well as scholars.

**Bibliography:**

A. *A Hebrew Grammar* (Andover, MA, 1821); *Essay on the Prize Question, Whether the Use of Distilled Liquors, or Traffic in Them, is Compatible...with...Christianity* (Glasgow, Scotland, 1831); *An Essay Upon the Wines and Strong Drinks of the Ancient Hebrews...* (London, 1831); *A Critical History and Defense of the Old Testament Canon* (Andover, MA, 1845); *A Commentary on the Book of Daniel* (Boston, 1850); with Lucius M. Sargent, *The Maine Law...* (New York, 1851).

B. DAB 18, 174–75; DARB, 442–43; NCAB 6, 244–45; SEAP 6, 2545; WW H, 586; E. A. Park, *A Discourse Delivered at the Funeral of Professor Moses Stuart* (Boston, 1852).

**SULLIVAN, John Lawrence**    (15 October 1858, Boston, MA—2 February 1918, West Abington, MA). *Career*: assistant to plumber and tinsmith, Boston, 1874–77; semiprofessional baseball, Roxbury, MA, circa 1875–77; prize fighter, 1877–92 (heavyweight champion, 1882–92); vaudeville performer, late 1890s; saloon owner, New York City, 1900s to 1905; temperance lecturer, 1905–12; retired to farm, West Abington, MA, 1912.

John L. Sullivan, or "The Great John L.," as he became known in boxing legend, hardly seemed a candidate for temperance acclaim. His mother, who weighed in at some 180 pounds herself, had hoped her strapping son would take priestly orders, but he never showed an inclination in that direction. Instead, he preferred sports, and several years after finishing grammar school be began to play semiprofessional baseball. His rise to glory, however, began in 1877, when a local heavyweight challenged any man in the Dudley Street Opera House in Boston to last only three rounds in the ring. The stakes were ten dollars, and Sullivan knocked him out with one punch. After that, "The Boston Strong Boy" toured for a year, offering twenty-five dollars to anyone who lasted a single round with him—and he never lost. He then sought more serious fights, winning increasing respect as he won them easily. Finally, in 1882, he hammered Paddy Ryan to the turf to claim the national bare knuckle heavyweight championship. The victory made him a popular hero, and for the next decade he reigned supreme in the national and international ring. At five feet ten and a half inches tall and 180 pounds, he consistently smashed opponents senseless. The champion earned a fortune but spent it just as quickly, becoming a denizen of saloons and a lover of booze and the fast life. Even drunk, however, he was too much for other fighters: One stunned opponent literally thanked the Almighty that Sullivan had fought while in his cups—"Sober, he'd a killed me," was the reported comment. Yet the hard drinking (and eating) finally began to slow Sullivan down. He had to train desperately for his final championship victory in 1889, and he won only through a decision. Three years later, fighting under the new Marquis of Queensberry rules (not with bare knuckles), he went down under a barrage of punches from "Gentleman Jim" Corbett. "I fought once too often," the former champion admitted.

Sullivan did not leave the public eye, however. For several years he toured the country in vaudeville, in which he made a modest living. He performed as well in Canada and Australia. He then bought a saloon in New York City (which, at one point, Carry Nation* considered assaulting) as well as an interest in another in Boston. Although never again a rich man, Sullivan was generally prosperous and still popular enough for some local politicians to consider (briefly) as a congressional candidate. In 1905, due to what influence is unknown, the former champion suddenly announced that he had taken his last drink. Selling out his saloon, he became a temperance lecturer, roundly denouncing the liquor that had been so much a part of his life for years. Sullivan's notoriety as a fighter made him a celebrity as a dry speaker, although he never achieved lasting prominence in the field. His second wife, however, Kate Harkins, whom he married in 1908, was pleased with his new occupation. She had been his childhood sweetheart and had never approved of his drinking or boxing. The Sullivans retired to a small Massachusetts farm in 1912, where after his wife's death in 1917 the former heavyweight spent his final year with an old friend from fighting days.

**Bibliography:**

B. DAB 18, 193–94; NYT, Feb. 3, 1918; R. F. Dibble, *John L. Sullivan* (Boston, 1925); Ted Harris, "The Great John L., Himself," *NABCA Newsletter* (Dec. 1981).

**SUNDAY, William Ashley** ("Billy Sunday") (19 November 1862, Ames, IA—6 November 1935, Chicago, IL). *Education*: D.D. (honorary), Westminister Coll., 1896. *Career*: odd jobs, janitor, undertaker's assistant, salesman in furniture store, 1870s to 1883; professional baseball player, 1883–91; assistant secretary, Chicago YMCA, 1891–93; agent and assistant preacher for J. Wilbur Chapman, 1893–95; travelling evangelist, 1896–1935; ordained, Presbyterian Church, 1903.

"The liquor interests," an Anti-Saloon League writer noted in an *American Issue* of 1913, "hate Billy Sunday as they hate no other man." It was in some respects true, for William Ashley ("Billy") Sunday made drink a frequent target of his wrath during his many years as a fire-breathing revivalist. Yet Sunday hardly started life as a preacher, much less a temperance man. Orphaned as an infant, he never found a steady role in life in his early years, and he never fully escaped marginal circumstances until he began playing professional baseball in 1883. He spent most of his years with the Chicago White Sox, although he was never more than a journeyman outfielder with a lifetime batting average of .248. But he was fast, stealing 236 bases. It was the only stealing, however, that

Sunday condoned; for during his years on the diamond he had a conversion experience, and he was commonly known among the baseball fraternity as the Evangelist even before he rose to fame. Leaving sports in 1891, and after time with the YMCA and evangelist J. Wilbur Chapman, Sunday launched his own evangelical career and quickly brought a new dimension to American revivalism. Avoiding complex theology, he used his flare for the vernacular to spellbind audiences; his preaching had the support of massed singers, musicians, and acrobatics by Sunday. And it all worked. By the end of his career he was an international celebrity who probably had converted some 300,000 people and whose total audience may have reached 80 million. Part of his appeal lay in his preaching on popular topics, and temperance was one of his favorites. In sermons typically warning of divine wrath, he repeatedly flayed the liquor traffic and urged his listeners away from the sin of drinking. His standard jeremiad, "Get on the Water Wagon," became something of a classic dry stricture and aroused uncounted Americans against liquor as Sunday proclaimed, "Booze is the parent of crime and the mother of sin." While his precise impact is hard to judge, many contemporaries were convinced that the popular evangelist was of crucial importance in establishing public support for the passing of the Eighteenth Amendment.

Sunday's temperance work, however, was of a peculiar variety. Unlike the many prohibitionists who saw temperance as a way to ameliorate the ills of an urban, complex, and industrial society (advocates of the social gospel, Progressive reformers, business leaders, and others), there was little if anything subtle about Billy Sunday. Indeed, it is doubtful that he spent any thought on trying to reconcile traditional cultural or religious values with changing economic or social conditions. Instead, he simply labeled what he found disturbing to his simple—albeit sincere—values "evil" and railed against it. Thus he attacked not only alcohol but immigrants, blacks, Catholics, and liberalism generally, while accepting the support of such extreme nativist groups as the Ku Klux Klan. During World War I Sunday's overblown sermons did much to fan the flames of ethnic hatreds and to whip up public fears of the "reds." If he inspired the loyalties of many, then, he also provoked revulsion in others. Thus with his impassioned oratory, his unsophisticated religion, his warnings of divine wrath, and his crude bigotry and extremism, both Sunday's theology and his temperance views were easily caricatured in the worst of terms: Here was the classic confrontation between the reactionary rural fanatic and the liberal urban population that some historians saw as defining the nature of the struggle over National Prohibition. It did not. Yet Sunday in some respects did represent exaggerated variants of some widely held temperance concerns on such topics as immigration and plural cultural values; and it did the movement little credit when more moderate drys accepted Sunday's support for Prohibition without challenging his more outrageous statements and positions.

### Bibliography:

A. *The Second Coming* (Sturgis, MI, 1913); *Get on the Water Wagon* (Sturgis, MI, 1915); *Great Love Stories of the Bible* (New York, 1917); *Face to Face with Satan* (Knoxville, TN, 1923); *Billy Sunday Speaks: One Thousand Epigrams of the World Famous Evangelist* (Grand Rapids, MI, 1937).

B. DAB 21, 679; DARB, 443–44; NCAB A, 123; NYT, Nov. 7, 1935; SEAP 6, 2552–53; Elijah P. Brown, *The Real Billy Sunday* (New York, 1914); William T. Ellis, *Billy Sunday: The Man and His Message* (Philadelphia, 1914); William G. McLoughlin, *Billy Sunday Was His Real Name* (Chicago, 1955).

**SWALLOW, Silas Comfort**    (5 March 1839, near Wilkes-Barre, PA—13 August 1930, Harrisburg, PA). *Education*: studied at Susquehanna Sem., 1860s; D.D. (honorary), Taylor Univ., IN, 1889. *Career*: schoolteacher, PA, 1850s to 1862; minister, Methodist circuit, western PA, 1866–76; presiding elder, Altoona District, PA, 1876–86; financial agent, Dickinson Coll., 1886–92; superintendent, Methodist Book Rooms, Harrisburg, PA, beginning 1892; editor, *Pennsylvania Methodist*, 1892–1905.

Silas Comfort Swallow, the "Fighting Parson," was born and raised in the rural countryside near Wilkes-Barre, Pennsylvania. His early years were hard, but from the start he manifested the tenacity and self-confidence he was later to display in his conflicts with those whom he believed promoted evil in any form. When Silas was fourteen his father died, leaving him the management of the family farm. He worked it to such effect that he was able to save enough money to attend Wyoming Seminary in Kingston, Pennsylvania. He taught school for five years after graduating, then studied law briefly. But his real calling was to the ministry, and after attending Susquehanna Seminary in Binghamton, New York, he was ordained in the Methodist Episcopal Church in 1862. During the Civil War he served brief stints with the Pennsylvania Emergency Volunteers and in between preached on a circuit in western Pennsylvania. From the beginning of his long tenure in the pulpit, however, Swallow emerged as a man of strict moral standards and a zealous intolerance of those less strident than himself. That alone was disturbing enough to many Pennsylvanians, and when he coupled his abrasiveness with the advocacy of such causes as abolitionism and temperance, he more than once antagonized even his fellow Methodists. On one occasion, after he delivered a fiery attack on slavery, his disgruntled congregation responded by padlocking him out of the church. Further examples of his inflexible views abound. For instance: He attended only one theatrical performance in his life and walked out before it was over when an actor in Oliver Goldsmith's *She Stoops to Conquer* uttered a mild expletive. Not surprisingly, Swallow also saw only moral and social ruin in dancing, roller-skating, card playing, and other forms of diversion and hoped to see them banned. Naturally enough, he made plenty of enemies, and his blasts sometimes provoked heated volleys in kind. His charges of dubious conduct against a number of Republican politicians in Pennsylvania brought him repeatedly into court to defend himself against charges of libel. Even the Methodist hierarchy bristled at times, and his fellow churchmen suspended him in 1901 and charged him with "lying and insubordination." The charges were not proven, but he was found "guilty of highly imprudent and unministerial conduct.'' To put it mildly, the ''Fighting Parson'' fully earned his prickly reputation.

Swallow was at his acerbic best in his efforts against the liquor traffic. The man was nothing if not a magnificent hater, and he was uncompromising in his denunciation of booze and its kin. When he swore off tobacco in 1864, for example, he pledged with characteristic theatrics never to smoke again unless his life depended upon it (!), and only then if two physicians testified to its necessity. The struggle against drink he saw as not less important than the Civil War: ''With the close of the Civil War I quit fighting for the emancipation of the Afro-American slaves,'' he wrote, ''and began the battle anew for the emancipation of the liquor-license slaves.'' The zealous reverend also had the political courage of his convictions, and he took part actively in the affairs of the Prohibition Party. He won the party's nomination for state treasurer in 1897 and for governor the following year. He waged a vigorous campaign, and when the results came in, Swallow had tallied some 132,000 votes. It was a credible showing and was enough to convince the national Prohibitionist convention in 1904, after a tough debate, to nominate Swallow for the presidency. He never stood a chance in the general election against Theodore Roosevelt, but he attracted a respectable 258,847 voters. It was his final electoral contest, though, and he devoted the rest of his ninety-one years to lecturing and writing (notably his long and interesting memoirs). The Temperance Movement produced its share of zealous proponents over its long history; of them all, however, only a rare few could match the combativeness of the strident Pennsylvanian.

**Bibliography:**

A. *Camp Meetings: Their Origin, History, and Unity* (New York, 1879); ''The Prohibition Party's Appeal,'' *Independent* (New York), Oct. 13, 1904; *III Score & X: Or, Selections, Collections, Recollections of Seventy Busy Years* (Harrisburg, PA, 1909); *''Toasts'' and ''Roasts'' of Silas C. Swallow's III Score and 10''...* (n.p., 1911?); *Then and Now: Or, Some Reminiscences of an Octagenarian* (Harrisburg, PA, 1920); *Four Score, and More...* (Harrisburg, PA, 1922).

B. DAB 18, 233–34; NYT, Aug. 14, 1930; SEAP 6, 2558–59; WW 1, 1208; Jack S. Blocker, Jr., *Retreat from Reform: The Prohibition Movement in the United States, 1890–1913* (Westport, CT, 1976).

**SWENGEL, Uriah Frantz**    (28 October 1876, Middlebury, PA—8 March 1921, Harrisburg, PA). *Education*: graduated from Union Sem. (later Central Pennsylvania Coll., now Albright Coll.), 1864?; A.M., Central Pennsylvania Coll., 1898; D.D. (honorary), Richmond Coll., IN, 1899. *Career*: enlisted man, Union army, 1864–65; minister, Evangelical Association, PA, 1867–79; ordained in the United Evangelical Church, 1869; presiding elder, Juniata District, PA, 1880–84; editor, Sunday school publications, United Evangelical Church, 1884–87; minister and presiding elder, various pastorates and districts, PA, MD,

1887–10; bishop, United Evangelical Church, 1910–21; president, Board of Bishops, 1910–18.

Shortly after graduating from Union Seminary in New Berlin, Pennsylvania, Uriah Swengel enlisted in the Union army. Serving with a volunteer infantry regiment, he saw some tough action at the Battle of Hatcher's Run and during the campaign that finally brought Robert E. Lee's Army of Northern Virginia to bay at Appomattox Court House. Upon his discharge from the service in 1865, Swengel was free to pursue his ministerial calling, and in 1867 he began preaching in the United Evangelical Church. Ordained in 1869, he filled a number of pulpits in western Pennsylvania until 1879, when he became presiding elder of the Juniata District. He gave up active preaching in 1883 to edit his denomination's Sunday school literature but four years later returned to a succession of congregations in Maryland and Pennsylvania. In all of his posts, Swengel discharged his duties with ability, and he emerged over the years as one of the most visible spokesmen of his church. He strove as well to align the Evangelical Church with the temperance reform, and he used his pulpits to proclaim the dry gospel. While a minister in Baltimore, Maryland, Swengel was a leader in establishing the Maryland State Temperance Alliance and in founding the Anti-Saloon League of America. When serving a pastorate in Lewistown, Pennsylvania, he moved openly into politics, and the reform-minded minister was a key voice in a successful campaign to adopt a local-option law. Such activity increased his reputation as a clergyman and played a part in the church decision to elect him a bishop in 1910. It was a good choice, for Swengel brought energy and executive ability to the job. He was active in overseeing denominational missionary and educational work, encouraged the study of Evangelical history, sat on the Federal Council of Churches of Christ in America, and headed the Board of Bishops between 1910 and 1918. Bishop Swengel also kept up with temperance affairs. He represented his native state on the National Board of Trustees of the Anti-Saloon League until 1920 and spoke out forcefully in favor of National Prohibition. He died before popular opinion swung against the "noble experiment," satisfied that he had done his best to place his church on record against the "demon rum."

**Bibliography:**

A. *A Manual of the United Evangelical Church* (Reading, PA, 1896).
B. SEAP 6, 2577; WW 1, 1210.

**TAYLOR, Edward Thompson**   (25 December 1793, Richmond, VA—5 April 1871, Boston, MA). *Career*: cabin boy and sailor, 1800–14; peddler, odd jobs, farm hand, MA, 1815–19; itinerant preacher, MA, 1815–19; ordained, Methodist Church, 1819; minister, various Methodist pastorates, MA, 1819–29; minister, Seamen's Bethel, 1830–71.

The "drunken sailor" is one of the enduring stereotypes in social history, although it was not because the Temperance Movement failed to carry the dry gospel to American seamen. Indeed, Edward Taylor, a Methodist reverend renowned as the "seaman's chaplain" as well as a firm temperance man in the early and mid-nineteenth century, did yeoman service in the battle against liquor. Taylor's road to prominence as a preacher and reformer, however, was anything but easy. He had run away to sea as a cabin boy at age seven, and after ten years before the mast he was converted during a port call in Boston by the Reverend Elijah Hedding. Captured at sea by the British in the War of 1812, he served as chaplain to his fellow prisoners until their release. For Taylor, it was a new departure in life: He never stopped preaching. He became an itinerant exhorter after the war, supporting himself with marginal jobs until he received a Methodist ordination in 1819. He served pastorates along the Massachusetts coast for ten years, and thereafter he settled in Boston to work among the sailors of the port city. For some forty years he preached in the Seamen's Bethel, a Methodist church established especially to meet the needs of the mariners, and became famous for his forceful and blunt manner of speaking. Admired by many literary figures of the age, he was probably the model for Herman Melville's Father Mapple in *Moby Dick*. Yet as his reputation spread, Taylor never turned from his mission of service to the seafarers of Boston (in which he was ably assisted by his wife, Deborah). In fact, he never lost his own fascination with the sea, making a number of voyages to Europe over his years in the ministry, including chaplain service on a ship carrying supplies to Ireland during the Great Famine. His devoted labors earned him the sobriquet "Father Taylor" among the Boston sailors.

Part of Taylor's work involved protecting his nautical congregants from the perils of liquor. A personal dry, and fully reflecting the total abstinence sentiments of the Methodist Church, Taylor labored tirelessly to combat what many observers considered unacceptable levels of alcohol use in Boston. And during these efforts he became one of the region's leading temperance figures. When the Washingtonian Movement spread to Boston in 1841, Father Taylor readily embraced it and opened the doors of the Seamen's Bethel for a massive temperance rally. The result was the formation of the long-lived Boston Washingtonian Society shortly thereafter. In 1849, he took part in yet another major antiliquor event, this time the tumultuous public welcome for Father Theobald Mathew,* the Irish "Apostle of Temperance." Taylor remained a consistent foe of drink over the years, charging the liquor dealers with originating all manner of misery. Even Satan, he once proclaimed to a Methodist gathering, would have no truck with a member of the traffic. In return, the Temperance Movement proudly called attention to the fact that as prestigious a clergyman as Taylor had elected to champion the dry crusade. In fact, Taylor ultimately owed much of his national reputation as a reformer to temperance praise in his honor. For his own part, the Seaman's Chaplain considered his work against drink an integral part of his efforts to better the lot of the sailors with whom he had shared so much over his own lifetime.

**Bibliography:**

B. DAB 18, 321–22; SEAP 6, 2612; WW H, 592; Charles Jewett, *Forty Years' Fight with the Drink Demon* (New York, 1876).

**TENSKWATAWA (original name, Lalawethika, also called Elskwatawa and "The Prophet")** (17 March 1768, near present Old Chillicoth, OH— 1834?). *Career*: Shawnee leader; founder and leader of Indian spiritual revitalization movement, 1805–11.

One of the most notorious of Shawnee drunkards, Lalawethika experienced a deathlike trance in 1805 which changed his life. The Indian Master of Life spoke to Lalawethika in this trance, instructing him that the Indians should renounce white ways and return to more primitive and communal Indian traditions. After adopting the name "Tenskwatawa," "the Prophet" (as he was commonly called by whites) merged his religious revival with the political revival being undertaken by his twin brother Tecumseh. Adding significantly to their following through the correct prediction of an eclipse of the sun in 1806, the two leaders spread their message of revitalization to the Shawnee, Wyandot, Creek, Choctaw, Sauk, Fox, Winnebago, Arikara, Sioux, Mandan, and Blackfoot tribes. Their ultimate goal was to unite the tribes in the face of white encroachments and to regain a measure of Indian autonomy. William Henry Harrison, governor of Ohio Territory, concerned over the growing power of the Prophet, managed to maneuver him into the Battle of Tippecanoe in 1811. After his defeat, Tenskwatawa was banished from the tribe by Tecumseh. Abandoned by his family, tribe, and followers, Tenskwatawa spent the remainder of his life in obscurity among an Indian tribe to the west.

While he was in power, however, Tenskwatawa's reforms especially emphasized total abstinence from liquor, which he felt was a tool of the white man used to degrade the Indian. As a reformed drunkard himself, he recognized not only the vulnerability to the white man that alcohol occasioned but also the personal difficulties and community strife which resulted from drunkenness. The fiery eternal damnation he described as punishment for those who touched alcohol alarmed his followers to such a great degree that drunkenness among those Indians was, for a time, virtually unknown. In addition to the personal benefits of temperance, Tenskwatawa and Tecumseh also stressed the cultural virtues of abstinence. The elimination of the liquor trade, with all of its attendant evils, would allow the Indians to avoid victimization at the hands of whites. The force of the Prophet's teachings in regard to the entire alcohol question was such that temperance remained a Shawnee concern long after Tenskwatawa's personal disgrace and exile.

**Bibliography:**

B. DAB 18, 375–76; SEAP 1, 14; WW H 595; Angie Debo, *A History of the Indians of the United States* (Norman, OK, 1970); Alvin M. Josephy, *The Patriot Chiefs* (New York, 1961).

**THOMAS, John Lloyd**    (22 April 1857, Witton Park, Durham, England—6 February 1925, New York, NY). *Career*: assisted father in ironworks, MD, 1880s; writer and editor, New York City, 1888–96; manager, Mills Hotels and Model Dwellings, 1897–1918; manager, Business Men's Relief Committee of New York City, 1903–5.

Born in Great Britain, Thomas immigrated to the United States at age ten with his family. After spending his early years in Utica, New York, he took his first job in the 1880s in a Maryland ironworks supervised by his father. Maryland was also where Thomas first emerged as a reformer, although little is known of his precise motives. For whatever reasons, however, he became a firm temperance stalwart. The young ironworker joined the Independent Order of Good Templars in 1886 and took a post as one of its most effective field organizers. In one six-month period, he founded some one hundred new lodges and enlisted three thousand new members. He also advocated a strong political effort against booze and elected to work on behalf of the Prohibition Party rather than urge either of the major parties to a dry course. Travelling the South for the Prohibitionists, he helped establish branches of the party in several states. Thus by the later 1880s Thomas had become a recognized antiliquor champion, and his effectiveness in the South, where dry sentiments had previously lagged, won special applause from his fellow reformers. The South, though, did not hold him; for Thomas elected to pursue what he saw as a more satisfying employment opportunity in the North. In 1888, he took up residence in New York City, working as a writer and editor. The city would be his home for the rest of his life.

Leaving the South, however, did not mean leaving reform. On the contrary,

Thomas became even more deeply involved with humanitarian causes. He quickly reestablished his antiliquor ties, becoming secretary of the National Prohibition Bureau and managing much of its publicity effort until 1892. In addition, he served as secretary of the dry National Constitutional League and from 1890 to 1896 edited its newspaper, the *Constitution*. The paper sought to demonstrate the unconstitutional nature of liquor license laws. In both of these positions, Thomas wrote widely and prepared syndicated material on the liquor question for over a hundred newspapers throughout the world. His temperance work, though, led him to explore other social issues as well, and he eventually took a particular interest in the welfare of industrial working families. In 1897, he left the *Constitution* to become manager of a model housing complex for working people, the Mills Hotels and Model Dwellings. He held the position for more than twenty years, during which time he became an expert on the sociology of the American urban scene. He wrote and spoke widely on the subject, travelled to Europe to study urban life there, and took part in philanthropic efforts to aid New York's poor. All the while, however, Thomas saw temperance as a reform central to progress in the rest of society, and he remained a firm believer in the dry cause to the end.

**Bibliography:**

B. SEAP 6, 2641; WW 1, 1229–30.

**THOMPSON, Eliza Jane Trimble**    ("Mother Thompson") (24 August 1816, Hillsboro, OH—3 November 1905, Hillsboro, OH). *Education*: secondary education at private schools in Cincinnati and Chillicothe, OH.

Eliza Thompson's strong religious background—her mother was a Quaker while her father was a staunch Methodist—instilled in her a strong will and a certain idealism. Both of these traits stood her in good stead in her subsequent involvement with the antiliquor crusade. She was familiar with temperance issues since childhood. The Trimbles did not drink, and her father, Allen*—acting governor of Ohio in 1822 and governor from 1826 to 1830—was the first president of the Ohio Temperance Society. In 1836 she accompanied him to the National Temperance Convention in Saratoga, New York, and had the distinction of being the only woman in attendance. With such an early exposure to the dry movement it is rather surprising that she did not remain actively involved with temperance organizations while a young woman. She did not, however; and this may be attributed in part to her marriage to Kentucky lawyer James Thompson in 1837—which took her briefly out of the state—and her subsequent rearing of eight children. But her interest was rekindled in 1873 when Dr. Dioclesian Lewis,* a Massachusetts reformer and lecturer, spoke at a Hillsboro gathering. He recalled how his mother, years before, had successfully used prayer to convince an owner to close a tavern frequented by his father. Inspired, a number of local women called on Mrs. Thompson, who had not heard Lewis's talk, and asked for her help in a similar venture in Hillsboro. Despite her husband's distinct lack of enthusiasm, she agreed.

Mrs. Thompson's support for this undertaking may have been critical. As the daughter of an ex-governor and wife of a prominent attorney, she was one of Hillsboro's most influential women. Led by Eliza, some fifty women formed a "praying band" on December 24, 1873, and visited liquor-selling drugstores. Singing, praying, and using temperance arguments, they appealed to the owners to stop their liquor sales. Soon after this they invaded local saloons employing the same tactics and continued the practice almost daily for several months. From Hillsboro, the movement spread to other parts of the nation, becoming known as the Woman's Crusade or Woman's War. It was easily the most enthusiastic and spontaneous outpouring of antiliquor sentiment to that point in the post–Civil War period; and in order to preserve the gains of the crusade and to institutionalize it for future work, a number of the most active women met in Cleveland in late 1874 to found the Woman's Christian Temperance Union. Thompson—now known as "Mother Thompson," in honor of her role in the original Hillsboro uprising—was a delegate to the Cleveland meeting; but thereafter she played at best a minimal role in the ongoing temperance reform. The rest of the dry movement, however, and particularly the WCTU, always regarded her fondly as one of the founders of the postwar antiliquor reform.

**Bibliography:**

A. with Mary McArthur Tuttle, Marie Rives and Frances Elizabeth Willard, *Hillsboro's Crusade Sketches and Family Records* (Cincinnati, OH, 1896).

B. NAW 3, 451–52; SEAP 6, 2643; Eliza Stewart, *Memories of the Crusade* (Columbus, OH, 1889); Frances E. Willard, *Woman and Temperance* (Hartford, CT, 1883); Frances E. Willard and Mary Livermore, eds., *A Woman of the Century* (New York, 1893); Annie T. Wittenmeyer, *History of the Woman's Temperance Crusade* (Philadelphia, 1878).

**THOMPSON, Henry Adams**    (23 March 1837, Stormstown, PA—3 July 1920, Dayton, OH). *Education*: A.B., Jefferson Coll., PA, 1858; studied at Western Theological Sem., PA, 1858–59?; D.D. (honorary), Jefferson Coll., 1873; LLD. (honorary), Westfield Coll., IL, 1886. *Career*: schoolteacher, IN, circa 1859–61; professor of mathematics, Western Coll., IA, 1862–87; professor of mathematics, Otterbein Coll., OH, 1862–67; superintendent of schools, Troy, OH, 1867–71; professor of mathematics, Westfield Coll., IL, 1871–72; president, Otterbein Coll., 1872–86; editor, United Brethren Sunday school literature, 1893–1901; editor, *United Brethren Quarterly Review*, 1901–9.

A deeply religious member of the United Brethren Church, with some theological training, Henry Thompson evidently considered a career in the ministry before deciding that his true calling was education. Over the 1860s and 1880s he compiled an outstanding record as a teacher and academic administrator, finally serving as president of Otterbein College (where he had previously been a professor of mathematics) between 1872 and 1886. It was during these years at Otterbein that he surfaced as a temperance reformer, gradually emerging as one of the more active prohibitionists of the Midwest. We know little of the direct roots of his dry sentiments, although his activities probably reflected the antiliquor stance of most of the United Brethren denomination, and perhaps something of his experience as an educator. In the post–Civil War period, many teachers came out against drink as an enemy of the nation's youth and therefore as an impediment to successful education. At any rate, Thompson was a zealous foe of the traffic, becoming an activist in the Prohibition Party. His first venture in politics came in 1874, when he ran unsuccessfully for Congress on the Prohibition ticket. The defeat, however, seemed only to whet his enthusiasm for the political side of temperance work, and thereafter he ran for office several more times and sought additional dry organizational responsibilities. In both 1875 and 1877, the reform-minded college president stood as a candidate for lieutenant governor of Ohio; and when the National Prohibition Alliance was founded in New York in the latter year, Thompson was elected its first president. This position increased his national visibility in temperance circles, and three years later he received the Prohibition Party's nomination for vice president. He was the running mate of prohibition champion Neal Dow,* of Maine Law fame, and the two men waged a spirited (if losing) campaign. While directing his labors against the "demon rum," Thompson always placed a great emphasis on service to his church as well; and during his later years the United Brethren claimed an increasing amount of his attention. Attending religious conferences and serving in various lay administrative capacities, by the 1890s he had entered the work of the denomination full time. He first took charge of the editing of Sunday school literature and then directed the publication of the church's official organ, the *United Brethren Quarterly Review*, until 1909. His interest in denomination affairs also led to his authoring a number of books and articles on various aspects of church history, doctrine, and Bible study.

**Bibliography:**

A. *Demand for an Educated Ministry! An Address...* (Dayton, OH, 1865); *The Power of the Invisible, and Other Lectures and Addresses, Chiefly Educational and Baccalaureate* (Dayton, OH, 1882); *Biography of Jonathan Weaver, D.D....* (Dayton, OH, 1901); *Our Bishops: A Sketch of the Origin and Growth of the Church of the United Brethren in Christ*, rev. ed. (Dayton, OH, 1906); *Women of the Bible...* (Dayton, OH, 1914).

B. SEAP 6, 2644–45; WW 1, 1233.

**THOMPSON, Ralph Seymour** (19 December 1847, Albion, IL—6 February 1925, Columbus, OH). *Career*: drugstore owner, Albion, IL, 1865–73; publisher, *Albion Pioneer*, 1869–73; printing business, Cincinnati, OH, 1873–76; published agricultural journal, Springfield, OH, 1876 to 1880s; lecturer, Ohio State Grange, 1878–82; publisher, *New Era*, 1885 to 1900s; manager, New Era

Publishing Co., 1886 to 1890s; general manager, Ideal Heating Co., Columbus, OH, beginning 1909.

Thompson joined the ranks of the temperance reform at the age of sixteen, an affiliation he maintained for the rest of his life. He belonged first to the Cadets of Temperance and then went on to the fraternal Sons of Temperance and the Independent Order of Good Templars. He took the dry gospel seriously, even when it went against his own best economic interest. At eighteen years old, after an education received largely at home, he opened a drugstore in his home town of Albion. But the business ultimately clashed with his temperance principles: Among his merchandise were various patent medicines with high alcohol content, and his conscience finally compelled him to pour his wares into the street. Thompson then founded the *Albion Pioneer*, in which he put his reform views into print. While the Illinois crusader may have eased his feelings by attacking alcohol, he enraged local wets, who evidently boycotted both his newspaper and his drug business. By 1873, Thompson had had enough. He sold out and moved to Ohio, where, after several years as a printer, he brought out an agricultural journal and became a lecturer for the Grange. He remained a loyal temperance man, but the antiliquor cause claimed less of his time as he gave his efforts to the interests of the Grange and Midwestern farmers. Yet Thompson kept abreast of dry developments, especially as the movement increased its pace over the late 1870s and early 1880s, and he apparently was simply waiting for an opportune moment to take out after the "demon rum" again.

In 1881, Thompson returned to the temperance wars, this time on a political basis. Forsaking any hope that the major political parties would launch a determined assault on the liquor traffic, he joined the Prohibition Party and quickly plunged into the electoral arena. In 1884 he ran unsuccessfully for mayor of Springfield, and thereafter he made a number of unsuccessful bids for Congress as well. Elected chairman of the Illinois party in 1885, Thompson also put his editorial skills to work again, bringing out the *New Era* as the Prohibitionists' official organ. Later, he merged it with the *Delaware Signal*, another dry paper he founded. In addition, he established and managed the New Era Publishing Company, which handled the literature needs of the party. Thompson was an active participant in the affairs of the national Prohibition Party, attending its conventions, seeking to influence its directions, and, over the years, attempting to broaden its political base. A believer in the necessity of other political and social reforms, such as women's suffrage, the Illinois crusader insisted that Prohibitionists also include these causes in their national platforms, although he met with limited success. The issue came to a head at the party convention of 1896, when the majority of the party rejected a Thompson-inspired movement to endorse measures other than prohibition. Thompson and the others in the "broad-gauge" faction then walked out, and two years later he organized a rival Union Reform Party. This effort, however, went nowhere. Yet he remained loyal to temperance, continuing to speak and write widely on the evils of drink until his death.

**Bibliography:**

A. *Science in Farming*... (Springfield, OH, 1882); *Profit or Plunder, Which?* (Springfield, OH, 1890); *A Pure Democracy*... *(Springfield, OH, 1898); The Party or the People?* (Springfield, OH, 1899).

B. SEAP 6, 2645; WW 4, 939.


**THORNBURGH, George**   (25 January 1847, Havana, IL—9 March 1923, Little Rock, AR). *Education*: studied law at Cumberland Univ., TN, 1860s. *Career*: private, Confederate army, 1865; admitted to bar, AR, 1868; legal practice, AR, beginning 1868; publisher, *Walnut Ridge* (TN) *Telephone*, 1868 to circa 1887; member, Arkansas House of Representatives, 1871, 1873, 1881, 1885; publisher, *Masonic Travel*, 1887–1919; manager, *Arkansas Methodist*, 1889–1903; director, Arkansas Building and Loan Association, beginning 1890s?

George Thornburgh spent most of his life as a firm adherent of the Temperance Movement. Born in Illinois, his family moved to Smithville, Arkansas, before the Civil War, and young Thornburgh began his antiliquor work there in the late 1850s. Most probably, he became involved in the prohibitionist agitation that disturbed state politics as Maine Law sentiments spread from the East, although the controversy died as the sectional war approached. Too young to fight when the guns opened, Thornburgh nevertheless enlisted in the Confederate army upon turning eighteen in 1865. After the Southern defeat, he started a legal practice in Arkansas, ultimately settling in Little Rock. Over the years, he also prospered in publishing and banking and acquired a reputation as one of the state's most dedicated men in civic affairs: He was an active and devout Methodist; he retained his interest in temperance, becoming one of the most influential drys of the region; he took a prominent role in founding schools for the blind, an orphanage, and a state-wide Sunday school association; he was an officer in the Arkansas militia; and he was a leader in the state's Masonic order. Thornburgh also used his considerable social prestige politically, serving four terms in the state legislature, one of them (1881) as speaker of the state House of Representatives. Yet his many interests and responsibilities never prevented him from devoting the time he considered necessary to the cause he held most important—the battle against drink. Indeed, his standing in the public eye made Thornburgh an especially effective spokesman for the reform position.

In his various professional and civic capacities, Thornburgh had always flayed the liquor traffic. As an editor and publisher, for example, he saw to it that the *Arkansas Methodist* (which he managed for years) spread the antiliquor gospel, while he proved an articulate advocate of political prohibition in the state legislature. His most important work, however, came with the rise of the Anti-Saloon League, the Arkansas chapter of which he helped to found in 1899. Thornburgh easily won election as league president, and soon after he became state superintendent as well (the superintendent was the actual operating officer). He held both posts until his death. He also edited the *Searchlight*, the official journal of the Arkansas League, in 1906 and 1908. At the head of the league, Thornburgh conducted an ongoing campaign against the liquor traffic, speaking widely on the subject, writing on prohibitionist subjects, and marshalling support for the enforcement of the state's dry laws. In 1916, when local wets mounted a determined counterattack against state-wide prohibition in the legislature, Thornburgh skillfully managed the effort that turned them back; he then went on to write an even more stringent enforcement measure. The Arkansas reformer also used his position within the state Masonic order—he was one of its most prominent members—to rally its lodges against the saloon, and he received credit for making the Freemasons a bulwark of temperance support. Although Thornburgh had little national reputation as a reformer, he still did good service in his area, and his career was indicative of the earnest and skillful support that made the Anti-Saloon League, and thus the Temperance Movement generally, a force to be reckoned with for so many years.

**Bibliography:**

A. *Freemasonry: When, Where, How? A History*. . . (Little Rock, AR, 1914).
B. SEAP 6, 1645–46; WW 1, 1236.

**TOPE, Homer**    (28 May 1859, Del Roy, OH—4 June 1936, Philadelphia, PA). *Education*: studied at Mt. Union Coll., Oberlin Coll., and Capital Univ., OH, all early 1880s; A.B., Harlem Springs Coll., OH, 1885; A.M., Harlem Springs Coll., 1888; graduated from Mt. Airy Theological Sem., PA, 1888; D.D. (honorary), Carthage Coll., IL, 1898; private study of law, 1905–7. *Career*: schoolteacher, OH, 1881–88; ordained, Lutheran Church, 1888; minister, Grace Lutheran Church, Youngstown, OH, 1888–97; minister, Grace Lutheran Church, Chicago, 1897–99; minister, Lutheran Church, Freeport, IL, 1900; various district and assistant state superintendencies, Anti-Saloon League, NY, MA, PA, 1900–19; state superintendent, Pennsylvania Anti-Saloon League, beginning 1919.

Active, dedicated, and productive in the temperance cause, there was something of the wanderer in most phases of Homer Tope's adult life. He was well educated but had difficulty settling in at college: Tope attended Mt. Union College, Oberlin, and Capital University in Columbus, Ohio, before finally obtaining a degree from Harlem Springs College in 1885. There was similar difficulty in settling on a career. Tope taught school, read for the law, and finally studied for the ministry. After ordination in 1888 as a Lutheran, he served three pulpits until 1900, when he left the ministry to work full time on behalf of the Temperance Movement. He accepted the post of superintendent of the Poughkeepsie District of the New York Anti-Saloon League. This began a peripatetic period of service with the Anti-Saloon League, and over the course of the next twenty years, Tope held positions in a number of cities and states. He did good work in Albany, New York, where he supervised prohibitionist legislative activities in the New York state legislature; and he was effective as well in the cities of Syracuse and Rochester, where he was league district superintendent and helped secure passage of township option laws and amendments to the Raines Law. Subsequently, he moved on to the Anti-Saloon League of Massachusetts, where he served as assistant superintendent. In the Bay State, Tope was instrumental in lining up support for the league among the various churches and in marshalling enough popular support to elect sympathetic representatives to the state legislature. Next, Tope went to Pennsylvania and performed similar work in Pittsburgh and Philadelphia. He was district superintendent in Philadelphia from 1907 to 1919, when he was elected superintendent of the Pennsylvania League. He led Pennsylvania drys in efforts to enforce National Prohibition and garnered national attention as a popular writer and speaker on dry themes. He frequently addressed audiences on such topics as "America's Greatest Shame," "Patriotism and Prohibition," "King Alcohol Dethroned," and the like. In general, Tope was a steady if unspectacular temperance leader. Never in the first rank of antiliquor reformers, he was typical of the dry organizational stalwarts who provided the operational backbone of the league in its heyday of national power.

**Bibliography:**

A. *The Overthrow of the Saloon* (Philadelphia, 1916); *The Why, What and How*, Pamphlets on Prohibition in the U.S., No. 95 (n.p., 1921); *Lecture on Gustavus Adolphus* (Lebanon, PA, 1922).

B. SEAP 6, 2657–58; WW 1, 1246.

**TRIMBLE, Allen**    (24 November 1783, Augusta Co., VA—3 February 1870, Hillsboro, OH). *Career*: farmer, Highland Co., OH, beginning 1804; county recorder and common pleas court clerk, Highland Co., OH, circa 1809–16; officer, volunteer troops, War of 1812, 1812–15; member, Ohio House of Representatives, 1816–17; member, Ohio Senate, 1817–25; acting governor of Ohio, 1821–22; state canal fund commissioner, 1824–25; governor of Ohio, 1826–30; president, Ohio Board of Agriculture, 1846–48.

A distinguished frontier soldier and Ohio politician, Allen Trimble's interest in the temperance reform was one of the early indications that the dry movement would find hospitable ground in the Midwest. The Trimble family had moved west with the frontier in the first years of the nineteenth century: Allen was born in Virginia, spent his early days in Kentucky, and reached maturity in Ohio. There he prospered, playing an active role in local politics and civil affairs. During the War of 1812, Trimble led an expedition against the Indians in relief of besieged Fort Wayne and briefly commanded a battalion under General (and later President) William Henry Harrison. After the war, he served some nine years in the Ohio legislature and in 1821 and 1822 sat as acting governor. In office, he emerged as a champion of governmental involvement in civic and economic matters. As acting governor, Trimble appointed the state committee on common schools, which laid the basis for Ohio's public school system; and in 1824 and 1825 he served as one of the canal fund commissioners who negotiated the financing for the state canal system. On a personal basis, he was also an innovator: Far in advance of public opinion, which condoned hard drinking, he became a total abstainer and publicly urged others to the same course. His political allies feared that his abstinence would hurt his political fortunes, but Trimble still proved an effective campaigner. He was elected governor twice, in 1826 and 1828, and when his political career ran aground, his temperance sentiments were not the cause. Rather, he was caught up in the internecine strife that gripped the old Jeffersonian Republican Party in the early 1820s. Trimble sided with the John Quincy Adams–Henry Clay faction of the party against Andrew Jackson, and when Jackson's partisans carried the state in the presidential election of 1828, Trimble retired from politics in 1830 (although he became an active member of the new Whig Party over the 1830s and 1840s).

When Trimble first declared his temperance sympathies there was no organized Temperance Movement in the United States, much less on the early frontier. It was certainly rather novel for a prominent regional politician to declare himself against liquor. Trimble's outlook on the nascent drinking question, however, perhaps mirrored his general social and political outlook: He believed firmly in a nation bound together politically, economically (thus his approval of internal improvements such as canals with government aid), culturally, and morally. Temperance reinforced this theme of shared common values, calling as it did for nationally-recognized norms of behavior. In addition, Trimble also pointed to the adverse economic impact of drinking: Claiming that providing agricultural help with traditional beverage rations led to decreased productivity, he was one of the first landowners in the region to discontinue the practice. Later, as organized temperance gathered momentum, the Ohio politician became one of its most articulate proponents; indeed, he had helped lay the foundations upon which the movement built. In 1836, he attended the National Temperance Convention in Saratoga Springs, New York, accompanied by his daughter, Eliza.* Miss Trimble fully absorbed her father's antiliquor sentiments; in a later day she went on to national fame as a dry leader herself in the so-called Woman's War that after the Civil War reignited the temperance flame her father had kindled a generation earlier.

**Bibliography:**

B. DAB 18, 641; SEAP 6, 2671; WW H, 609.

**TURNER, Joseph E.**     (1832, Bath, ME—1889, Wilton, CT?). *Career*: physician and proselytizer for inebriate asylums, to 1864; superintendent, New York State Inebriate Asylum, Binghamton, NY, 1864–67; proprietory asylum promoter, mostly in CT, to 1889.

Ever since the work of Benjamin Rush* and Thomas Trotter in the late eighteenth and early nineteenth centuries, a growing number of physicians and laymen had viewed chronic drunkenness as a disease. Indeed, the idea had become fairly well diffused in the medical community in the decades before the Civil War, even though the concept lacked an empirical foundation or a serious theory on the causes of addiction. The disease and addiction models, however, came into sharper focus shortly after the war, with a good deal of the impetus for the increased interest growing from the labors of Dr. Joseph E. Turner. We know relatively little of Turner's background, except that he spent his childhood in Maine and for a time practiced medicine in Trenton, New Jersey. The origins of his fascination with alcohol problems are equally sketchy, although he apparently chose the subject as his life's work quite early in his career. He rather uncritically accepted the prevalent notions on the disease conception as established facts and did little to clarify or refine them. His theoretical contributions to the understanding of alcoholism were therefore minimal. On the practical side, however, Turner launched a crusade for the medical treatment of alcoholics and urged the construction of special "inebriate asylums" for that purpose. Only in these institutions, he claimed, could alcoholics get the professional care that would allow them to escape the chains of their addiction. And with genuine foresight, he also stressed an equally important justification for the asylums: He believed that studies of patient populations would lead to new knowledge in the medical battle against alcoholism. Thus, in Turner's view, research and new insights could come later—the asylums had to come first.

Turner carried this message to all who would hear it. He actually went from door to door in the medical and philanthropic communities of the 1850s, pleading for stock subscriptions to finance the construction of an asylum. His missionary approach won the support (and the money) of many prominent politicians, doctors, and reformers, including surgeons Valentine Mott* and Willard Parker.* After years of proselytizing, Turner's dream became a reality in 1864 with the opening of the New York State Inebriate Asylum in Binghamton. The doctor himself was superintendent of the venture, which was housed in a single handsome and well-appointed building. Yet his tenure proved an exercise in frustration. He proved a better crusader than a manager and showed little aptitude for administration and finance (a situation not helped by a serious fire soon after the asylum opened). To make matters worse, Turner also differed seriously with much of his staff over treatment practices: The superintendent favored a strict regimen, with patients accorded little freedom to come and go as they pleased; others wanted a more relaxed approach with patients able to visit out of the building. Turner claimed that such privileges would only invite patients to relapse. All of these issues finally came to a head in 1867, when the institution's board of trustees, led by Parker, voted to dismiss Turner. The founding superintendent fought the action in court but lost, and the trustees ultimately conferred title of the asylum to the state, which later turned it into a mental facility.

The failure of the New York Asylum, however, was not the end of the treatment idea in alcoholism. Turner remained a promoter for asylums, concentrating in particular on a project for an institution for women alcoholics in Wilton, Connecticut. Unfavorable publicity from the Binghamton experiment, however, finally frustrated his plans in the late 1870s. Yet he had left a profound influence on other doctors interested in alcohol problems, some of whom had worked with him at Binghamton, and they carried on with the asylum idea and the disease conception. By 1900, some eleven years after Turner's death, over fifty public or private facilities had opened around the nation to deal with alcoholism and addictions; and as early as 1870, a number of doctors already had founded the American Association for the Study and Cure of Inebriety, dedicated to the study of the disease conception and to asylum construction. (Turner never joined, as he was never reconciled with Parker, who was a founder of the association.) While his own ventures had been business failures, then, many who followed Turner, at least in retrospect, considered him no less "a discoverer of a new realm of scientific medicine."

## Bibliography:

A. *The History of the First Inebriate Asylum in the World. . .* (New York, 1888).

B. T. D. Crothers, ed., *The Diseases of Inebriety* (New York, 1893); E. M. Jellinek, *The Disease Concept of Alcoholism* (Highland Park, NJ, 1960); Mark Edward Lender, "Jellinek's Typology of Alcoholism," *Journal of Studies on Alcohol* 40(1979):361–75; Senta Rypins, "Joseph Turner and the First Inebriate Asylum," *Quarterly Journal of Studies on Alcohol* 10(1949):127–34; A. E. Wilkerson, "A History of the Concept of Alcoholism as a Disease" (DSW. diss., University of Pennsylvania, 1967).

# U

**UPSHAW, William David**   (15 October 1866, Newman, GA—21 November 1952, Glendale, CA). *Education*: studied at Mercer Univ., 1895–96. *Career*: author, lecturer, evangelist, mid-1880s to 1952; publisher, *Golden Age*, 1906–18; member, U.S. House of Representatives, 1918–26; president, National Christian Citizenship Foundation, 1933–52; vice president, Linda Vista Baptist Coll. and Sem., San Diego, CA, 1949–52.

Known as "the driest of the drys," Upshaw in his career displayed a combination of Baptist piety, militant social reform activity, and virulent political and racial hatreds. While slowly recovering from a crippling injury in his youth, Upshaw gained his first public attention under the pen name "Earnest Willie," writing and giving public readings of articles and poems on religious themes. After two years at Mercer University, he began publishing the Atlanta-based *Golden Age* in 1906—a magazine, as the young Upshaw put it, of "militant Christian citizenship." Using the *Golden Age* and the public podium, he became a champion of fundamentalist Christianity, prohibition (he had helped found the Anti-Saloon League of Georgia in 1905), woman's suffrage, labor reform, and white supremacy. As vice president of the state Anti-Saloon League, he was instrumental in directing the enactment of prohibition in Georgia in 1907, and he gained a national reputation as a dry spokesman while lecturing under the auspices of the league and of the WCTU. This reputation carried him to the House of Representatives in 1918 as a Democrat, where he subsequently served four terms. In Congress, he was renowned for his zealous support of the Eighteenth Amendment and the Volstead Act (he frequently asked other congressmen to sign temperance pledges), his ardent racism and vocal sympathies for the Ku Klux Klan, and his work on behalf of labor, education (he wanted a cabinet-rank Department of Education), agriculture, and suffrage reforms. Later he added anticommunism to his repertoire—which further marked him for blending an extraordinary diversity of enthusiasms.

Upshaw's fortunes declined in the 1920s. His close affiliation with the KKK hurt him as the secret organization gradually came under political fire; and his substantial antiliquor lecture fees led to charges that his attachments to Prohibition were largely monetary. Losing his bid for reelection in 1926, he then broke with the Democrats in 1928 when he supported the presidential race of Republican

Herbert Hoover instead of the wet and Catholic Democrat, Al Smith. Still active in temperance affairs, Upshaw subsequently became so disenchanted with the liquor policies of both parties that he joined the Prohibition Party; he received 81,000 votes as its presidential standardbearer in 1932. After Repeal he continued to lecture for nineteen years—travelling the nation to inveigh against the "twin devils" of liquor and communism. He remained an active Baptist, was ordained in that denomination in 1938, and for a time was vice president of the Southern Baptist Convention. After an unsuccessful political comeback as a Democrat in 1942, he moved to California, where from 1949 until his death he served as vice president of Linda Vista Baptist College and Seminary.

### Bibliography:

A. *Earnest Willie, or Echoes from a Recluse* (Atlanta, GA, 1893); *Clarion Calls from Capital Hill* (New York, 1923); *Bombshells for Wets and Reds: The Twin Devils of America* (Cincinnati, OH, 1936).

B. DAB Supp. 5, 701–2; SEAP 6, 2729; "The 'Georgia Cyclone' for President," *Literary Digest*, July 23, 1932; Charleston Moseley, "Invisible Empire: A History of the Ku Klux Klan in Georgia, 1915–1965" (Ph.D. diss., Univ. of Georgia, 1968); Peter H. Odegard, *Pressure Politics: The Story of the Anti-Saloon League* (New York, 1928).

# V

VAN RENSSELEAR, Stephen (1 November 1764, New York, NY—26 January 1839, Albany, NY). *Education*: studied at Coll. of New Jersey (now Princeton Univ.); graduated from Harvard Coll., 1782. *Career*: member, New York Assembly, 1789–90, 1798, 1818; member, New York Senate, 1791–96; lieutenant governor of New York, 1795–1801; major general, New York militia, 1812; member, Erie Canal Commission, 1816–39; member, Board of Regents, Univ. of New York, 1819–39; president, New York Board of Agriculture, 1820; member, U.S. House of Representatives, 1822–29.

Remembered as the "last of the patroons," the great landowning families of New York State, Stephen Van Rennselear was the scion of two of the most distinguished families of the region. Related to the notable Livingstons of New York on his mother's side, he married into the equally prestigious Schuylers (indeed, his wife was the daughter of Revolutionary General Philip Schuyler). As befitted one who could boast such a lineage, he was educated at Princeton (then the College of New Jersey) and Harvard before following the traditional family duties of managing the Van Rensselear estates and entering politics. He did well in both areas. Noted as a generous and astute landlord, he substantially increased the already considerable family fortune; and from 1789 to 1801, he served variously in the state legislature and as lieutenant governor. In the War of 1812, he led the New York militia on the ill-conceived assault on Queenston Heights, Canada. Repulsed with heavy loss, Van Rensselear called off the attack and soon after resigned. Later, he returned to politics, serving in Congress from 1822 to 1829. Over the years, he did a great deal to foster various civic, reform, and philanthropic causes in his region; and in most cases, the activities he chose to support prospered through his efforts. He was an articulate and creditable spokesman for the early Temperance Movement, a driving force behind the construction of the Erie Canal, a regent of the University of New York, president of the Albany Lyceum of Natural History, founder of the school that ultimately became Rensselear Polytechnic Institute, and a generous contributor to charities. Quite clearly, he saw his role in society as a cultural as well as a political and economic leader.

This perspective may help explain much of Van Rensselear's original interest in the Temperance Movement. In his early years he showed no interest in the question, which was not surprising, for there was little organized temperance sentiment in the early nineteenth century. Yet with the rise of the Temperance Movement the prominent New Yorker became what one dry account termed ''an ardent advocate.'' He donated funds to distribute antiliquor tracts, while in 1833 he was a delegate to the first national temperance convention in Philadelphia. Concerned that the message of that gathering reach the widest possible audience, he personally financed the printing and distribution of 100,000 copies of its proceedings. It was a gesture that only a true believer would have made, although we can only speculate about his motives. On one level, he was genuinely concerned about the health and social problems associated with intemperance, matters amply discussed in the temperance convention proceedings he so prized. But there was also the matter of politics: Van Rensselear had been a firm and committed Federalist, a member of a party that in some important respects had spoken for the cultural and moral views of the established American social elite. With the Federalist Party shattered and groups from outside of the power structure formerly dominated by men like Van Rensselear reaching for national power, a number of historians have suggested that some of the old elite may have seen moral reform (and especially temperance) as a way of trying to retain cultural preeminence in the republic. If so, then perhaps Van Rensselear's interest in temperance (at least in part) was of a piece with other old Federalists seeking ways to reassert social norms they could no longer enforce through political means. One suspects, however, that the New Yorker's aristocratic sense of noblesse oblige was also at work, and that he supported temperance out of the same concern for the public good that prompted his efforts on behalf of state agriculture, the state university, the Albany Lyceum, and other philanthropic causes. At any rate, he was remembered fondly by a movement that benefitted greatly from his contributions, no matter what their origins.

**Bibliography:**

B. DAB 19, 211–12; SEAP 6, 2742; WW H, 620; Daniel Dewey Barnard, *A Discourse on the Life, Services, and Character of Stephen Van Rensselear...* (Albany, NY, 1839); Mark Edward Lender and James Kirby Martin, *Drinking in America: A History* (New York, 1982); William Buel Sprague, *Religion and Rank: A Sermon...Succeeding the Funeral of the Hon. Stephen Van Rensselear* (Albany, NY, 1839).

**VAYHINGER, Culla Johnson** (25 September 1867, Bennington, VT—15 August 1924, Upland, IN). *Education*: M.A. (honorary), Moores Hill Coll., IN, 1914. *Career*: temperance organizer and WCTU officer, 1800s–1924.

The wife of a Methodist minister (who was also president of Taylor University in Indiana), Vayhinger devoted most of her adult life to the crusade against drink. While little is known of her early years, she apparently became involved with temperance work at about seventeen years of age, joining the Woman's Christian Temperance Union in her adopted state of Indiana. Over the 1880s and 1890s she served in a succession of local, county, and state positions with the union, gaining in effectiveness and confidence as a leader and public speaker. In 1903, Vayhinger won election as president of the state organization, holding the post until 1920. Her long tenure gave continuity to the WCTU's leadership during the crucial years that saw the successful drive for the framing and ratification of National Prohibition—an event in which the Indiana president played an active role. She became a familiar figure on the public platform during this period, proclaiming the merits of prohibition and belaboring the evils of the liquor traffic before state and national audiences. Much of her speaking came under the aegis of the Flying Squadron, a group of dry orators who stumped the country for the antiliquor cause in 1914 and who captured considerable popular attention. Vayhinger also worked to influence temperance legislation in Indiana, where she proved an effective lobbyist with state lawmakers. Her work earned the minister's wife a reputation as one of the most capable dry leaders in the region, and when she stepped down as leader of the Indiana WCTU, she did so only to move on to increased responsibility.

The reform interests of the WCTU had always been greater than the struggle for prohibition alone. Even after the death of Frances Willard,* when the wide-ranging "Do Everything" policy began to narrow, the union still maintained departments to address concerns other than drinking and the saloon. In 1920, Vayhinger took charge of the National WCTU's "Americanization" program, which dealt only indirectly with the national prohibition question but which nevertheless was an important issue for many temperance workers. Americanization was the WCTU attempt to assist in the assimilation of immigrant populations, to wean them from their European (or other) cultural backgrounds, and to train them in "American" values and traditions. Union members taught classes in English and civics and offered other social work services at times. Much of this activity was based on a humanitarian premise but was often coupled with a desire to reduce "foreign" influences in the United States and to safeguard traditional cultural norms (as the WCTU interpreted them). Thus, in its way, Americanization was as much an attempt to protect national order and perfect society as the drive to outlaw the saloon. Vayhinger wrote unfortunately little on the subject, so her personal views on the matter remain obscure. But she devoted the rest of her career to the Americanization effort, holding her post until her death in 1924.

**Bibliography:**

B. SEAP 6, 2744; Mark Edward Lender and James Kirby Martin, *Drinking in America: A History* (New York, 1982).

# W

WALLACE, Zarelda Gray Sanders (6 August 1817, Millersburg, KY—March 1901, Cataract, IN). *Career*: president, Indiana WCTU, 1874–77, 1879–83; superintendent, Franchise Department, National WCTU, 1883–88; active lecturing on behalf of temperance and suffrage, 1874 to 1880s.

One of the most prominent temperance and suffrage reformers of the Midwest during the last quarter of the nineteenth century, Zarelda Wallace had shown little interest in activities outside of her home and her church in her earlier years. She was the daughter of a successful Indianapolis physician, John Sanders, and later wife of lieutenant governor and congressman David Wallace. Consequently, she wanted for little and concentrated on raising her six children (only three of whom lived beyond childhood) and three stepchildren (including Lew Wallace, later author of *Ben Hur* and a Civil War general). Extremely devout, Wallace also devoted much of her energy to the Indianapolis Christian Church. In 1859, however, her husband died, and although the value of her real estate holdings eventually left her financially secure, there was a brief period of uncertainty when the lack of David Wallace's income and a cash shortage forced her to take in boarders to make ends meet. The experience made her touchy about the status of her home and family and about the position of women in American society generally. Thus when the Woman's Crusade of 1873 identified the saloon as a threat to hearth and home, Wallace enlisted with a fervent dedication. By the time the crusade had gathered enough strength to take on permanent form as the Woman's Christian Temperance Union in 1874, she was one of the best-known antiliquor campaigners in the region. She helped organize the founding convention of the WCTU and shortly thereafter was the central figure in establishing its Indiana chapter. Wallace proved an effective leader, serving as president of the Indiana Union for some seven years (although with a break in 1878), molding it as an effective lobby against drink in her home state, as well as using her position to speak out on national temperance concerns.

Her work in temperance led directly to her involvement with the suffrage movement as well. In 1875, Wallace presented a temperance petition signed by ten thousand women to the Indiana legislature, only to see it virtually ignored. Outraged, she reached the unsurprising conclusion that prohibition could succeed only after women secured the vote. Accordingly, she persuaded the WCTU to call for women's suffrage, at least when it came to temperance issues, and to create a special Franchise Department. Wallace became the first national superintendent of the new unit and established herself as an effective advocate for the woman's ballot. Soon after assuming this post, however, she also helped organize the Indianapolis Equal Suffrage Society (and served as its first president in 1878) as well as the Indiana Woman Suffrage Association. For Mrs. Wallace, the vote was not an end in itself but only "the most potent means for all moral and social reforms." She was an effective and popular speaker, often talking extemporaneously for as much as two hours at a time. She boasted of making no notes before her talks, depending instead, as she put it, "on circumstances to afford me a suggestion for my beginning." Her stepson, General Lew Wallace, claimed that she was the model for the mother of the title character in his highly popular novel, *Ben Hur* (1880). Her work on behalf of temperance and women's suffrage ended when she collapsed while speaking in the late 1880s, and though she lived until 1901, she seldom appeared on the public platform again. In her later years she lived with a daughter in Cataract, Indiana, where she died at the age of eighty-four.

**Bibliography:**

B. NAW 3, 535–36; SEAP 6, 2796; "Fourteenth Annual Convention of the National W.C.T.U.," *Union Signal* 13 (Dec. 1, 1887):22; Frances E. Willard, *Woman and Temperance* (Hartford, CT, 1883); Frances E. Willard and Mary A. Livermore, eds., *A Woman of the Century* (New York, 1893).

**WALWORTH, Reuben Hyde**     (26 October 1786, Bozrah, CT—27 November 1867, Saratoga, NY). *Education*: studied law, Troy, NY, circa 1808–9; LLD. (honorary), Princeton Univ., 1835. *Career*: admitted to bar, NY, 1809; legal practice, Plattsburgh, NY, beginning 1909; justice of the peace, master in chancery, 1811–21; adjutant general to General Benjamin Mooers, 1812–15; member, U.S. House of Representatives, 1821–23; circuit judge, New York Supreme Court, 1823–28; chancellor of New York, 1828–48.

Reuben Hyde Walworth grew up in Hoosick, New York, working on a farm to which his family had moved from Connecticut not long after he was born. At the age of seventeen, after having acquired the elements of an education at home, he read for the law in Troy, New York, and opened his own practice in Plattsburgh in 1809. Thereafter, his professional star rose quickly, as Walworth emerged as a legal, political, and cultural leader in his state. In 1811, he was appointed master in chancery while also serving as a county justice of the peace. During the War of 1812, Walworth joined the New York militia as adjutant general and played a notable part in the Battle of Plattsburgh. After a term in Congress as a Democrat (1821–23), he took a seat on the bench as a circuit court judge, a post he held until elevated to the post of chancellor of New York in 1828. He was chancellor for twenty years, and by most accounts he was a capable if somewhat irascible one. Considered an expert in equity law, he was held in high esteem by such legal lights as James Kent and Joseph Story; on the other hand, his sarcastic manner on the bench enraged many attorneys. Walworth, however, had interests beyond the courtroom. He used his position to speak out on matters of moral reform, especially temperance. The antiliquor crusade was in its infancy in the 1820s, but the chancellor saw it as a vehicle to uplift the populace and to assure social order. Accordingly, he was the first president of the New York State Temperance Society, founded in Albany in 1829, and served as a vice president of the American Temperance Union in 1836 and subsequently as president. Busy with his legal career, he did not devote a great deal of personal attention to the direction of the daily affairs of these groups; but his prestige brought the rising dry movement badly needed visibility and public credence. At the time, contemporary reformers recognized Walworth's contributions, and later generations of temperance workers rightly considered him an influential pioneer. This popularity with reformers, though, did not translate into political success generally. With the elimination of the court of chancery in 1848, Walworth ran for governor but lost badly. His last public service came in the month just before the Civil War, when he tried to aid conciliation efforts between North and South. He then spent his remaining years researching and writing a voluminous family genealogy.

**Bibliography:**

A. *Circular of the New York State Temperance Society to the Citizens of the State* (Albany, NY?, 1829?); *Hyde Genealogy*... (Albany, NY, 1864).
B. DAB 19, 406–7; SEAP 6, 2797; WW H, 632.

**WARREN, John Collins**   (1 August 1778, Boston, MA—4 May 1856, Boston, MA). *Education*: graduated from Harvard Univ., 1797; studied medicine, London, Edinburgh, Paris, 1799–1802; M.D. (honorary), Harvard Univ., 1819. *Career*: medical practice, Boston, beginning 1802; assistant professor, professor, professor emeritus, Harvard Medical Sch., 1806–15, 1815–47, 1847–56; founder and editor, *Boston Medical and Surgical Journal*.

A member of a long and distinguished line of Boston surgeons, John Collins Warren was also one of the temperance pioneers of his native state of Massachusetts. The prestige he brought to the struggling young Temperance Movement when he joined its ranks in the 1820s was considerable: By any measure, he was one of the outstanding physicians of his generation. Warren was the first American to operate successfully for strangulated hernia and aneurism, and one of the earliest to use ether as an anesthetic during surgery. He authored a number of highly respected titles on medical subjects, conducted agricultural experiments on his family estate, and as a talented amateur even made some interesting contributions to paleontology. Despite these many other pursuits, however, Warren managed to devote a great deal of time to the fight against intemperance, and he emerged as one of the most visible early leaders of the reform crusade in New England. In 1827, he became president of the Massachusetts Society for the Suppression of Intemperance, and over the years he was instrumental in building it into an effective organization. In addition, Warren convinced the Massachusetts Medical Society (of which he was an influential member) to sponsor an annual essay contest on the deleterious effects of alcohol beverages, and he served on the prize committee. In 1837, he visited Europe, doing research and speaking on temperance-related issues, including compiling historical information on alcohol-related questions. Temperance, in Warren's view, was a reform vital to the good of society, and he clearly dealt with it accordingly.

Warren's temperance activities reflected much of the changing nature of the antebellum dry reform movement. When he first announced himself as a foe of intemperance, the Boston doctor was not a total abstainer. Rather, he drank wine in moderation, believing that ardent spirits posed the chief danger to human health. Arguing that position, he discouraged the medical use of distilled liquors and saw no contradiction between his temperance work and his own drinking (or, for that matter, the drinking of anyone else who used alcohol as he did). It was a position many reformers adopted; it put a premium on civil order, the leadership and example of community notables (who generally headed such groups as the Massachusetts Society for the Supervision of Intemperance), while doing little to disturb the imbibing of the temperate elements of society. Yet as total abstinence sentiments gained ground in the movement over the 1830s and 1840s, Warren reconsidered his position and in about 1841 became a teetotaler. It was hardly a unique transition. Many other reformers also abandoned moderate drinking, and by the end of the 1840s temperance had become largely synonymous with total abstinence. The fact that Warren became a spokesman for abstinence helped give the more extreme position credence. Indeed, he believed in it so strongly that he donated considerable sums to the Massachusetts Society to aid in its work. In 1853, he gave ten thousand dollars, and he bequeathed another two thousand dollars in his will. Such generosity was in character for Warren, as he also contributed to other civic causes and philanthropic ventures, including the construction of the Bunker Hill Monument. At his death in 1856 the old campaigner was still president of the temperance society he had led for so long.

### Bibliography:

A. *Physical Education and the Preservation of Health* (Boston, 1845); *Etherization, with Surgical Remarks* (Boston, 1848); *The Mastodon Giganteus of North America* (Boston, 1852); *The Preservation of Health* (Boston, 1854).

B. DAB 19, 480–81; SEAP 6, 2798–99; W. L. Burrage, *A History of the Massachusetts Medical Society* (Boston, 1923); Edward Warren, *The Life of John Collins Warren* (Boston, 1860).

**WATKINS, Aaron Sherman**   (29 November 1863, Rushsylvania, OH—10 February 1941, Rushsylvania, OH). *Education*: B.S., Ohio Northern Univ.,

1886; legal study in private law office, OH, 1886–89; M.S., Ohio Northern Univ., 1907; LLD. (honorary), Taylor Univ., 1902; LHD. (honorary), Ohio Northern Univ., 1923; D.D. (honorary), Asbury Coll., 1930. *Career*: schoolteacher, OH, 1880–83, 1890–93; admitted to bar, OH, 1889; minister, various Methodist pastorates, OH, 1893–1905, 1915–35; ordained, Methodist Episcopal Church, 1845; professor of literature and philosophy, Ohio Northern Univ., 1905–9; vice president, Ohio Northern Univ., 1907–9; president, Asbury Coll., KY, 1909–10; public lecturer, 1910–15; professor, Miami Military Institute, OH, 1918–20.

A stalwart of the Prohibition Party, the Reverend Aaron Watkins fully reflected the antiliquor zeal of his Methodist denomination. Trained originally as a lawyer, Watkins entered the bar only to find he had no taste for it, deciding instead on a career in the pulpit. Over the years, he served a number of Ohio pastorates as well as devoting five years to college teaching and administration. At the same time, he was an enthusiastic participant in organized temperance activities. Watkins decided early that the only practical approach to the liquor question was politics, but he eschewed the Republicans and Democrats, considering them hopelessly entangled with the beverage industry. He therefore joined the small but, as he saw things, morally correct Prohibition Party. The reformer-minister held a number of party offices, initially at the local level, where he got his first experience as a dry organizer and campaigner. He also took his politics before the public: His pulpits rang with denunciations of drink; and between 1910 and 1915, when Watkins supported himself as a speaker on the Chautauqua circuit, prohibition was his favorite theme. By the turn of the century he was a familiar figure in Midwestern reform circles, known for his uncompromising positions on temperance matters. Not surprisingly, the Prohibition Party turned to him to head its state ticket, and in 1908 and 1912 he ran for governor. The Prohibitionists did not capture the entire dry vote, much of which went to candidates of other parties endorsed by the nonpartisan Anti-Saloon League. But Watkins himself won applause from local drys for his campaign, and he kept his party a visible part of the Ohio political scene.

In addition to his work with Ohio prohibition advocates, Watkins also contributed to national temperance affairs. But his work on the national scene still was bound closely to the Prohibition Party. Indeed, he became one of its most visible figures. In the elections of 1908 and 1912, the Ohio minister ran for vice president as the running mate of Eugene W. Chafin.* He expected to win in neither case, only to demonstrate the continued vitality of the party and to publicly air its views. An effective campaigner, he impressed Prohibitionist rank and file with his efforts (even if the general electorate had little idea of who he was), and in 1920 he received the party's nomination for the presidency. Watkins took to the stump in a spirited bid. He spoke before dry audiences across the nation while his vice presidential candidate, David Leigh Colvin,* traveled the country as well. When the ballots were counted, Republican Warren G. Harding had won in a landslide, but Watkins had polled some 188,678 votes. It was hardly the best showing for a Prohibition Party candidate, but it was at least a respectable tally for a party that relied more on enthusiasm than financial backing in its campaigns. Watkins made one more electoral bid, mounting a final effort for the Ohio governorship in 1932. By then, however, the public had turned against the "noble experiment," and the campaign never reached the intensity of his earlier challenges. In his final years, Watkins remained active in the affairs of his denomination, and he never relented in his hatred for the traffic. But his long years as a dry campaigner ended with the fall of National Prohibition.

**Bibliography:**

A. *Why Am I a Prohibitionist?* (Chicago, 1920).
B. SEAP 6, 2808–9; WW 1, 1306.

**WAY, Amanda**    (10 July 1828, Winchester, IN—24 February 1914, Whittier, CA). *Career*: schoolteacher, dressmaker, tailor, 1840s to 1851; antislavery, suffrage, and temperance organizing and lecturing, 1850s to 1861, 1869–1914; editor, *Woman's Tribune*, 1859; nurse, Union army, 1861–65; travelling preacher, Methodist Church, IN, KS, 1871–80; minister, Quaker meetings, KS, ID, CA, 1880–1914.

Pious, tireless, unassuming, Amanda Way devoted over sixty years to work on behalf of social reform causes. As a young woman, she worked as a school-teacher, milliner, dressmaker, and tailor shop operator in order to support her family after her father's death. But she had a lively interest in public affairs and, following the example of relatives, became involved in the antislavery movement. Over the 1860s, she worked with the Underground Railroad to assist escaping slaves. At an antislavery convention in 1851, Way took still another step: She called for the founding of an Indiana suffrage association and then headed it for the rest of the decade. Way soon established a reputation as one of the chief advocates of women's rights in the Midwest, while at the same time becoming deeply involved in the Temperance Movement. Way saw the various reform causes as interrelated, arguing that as women were the chief victims of the saloon—which threatened their families—women ought to take a direct role in the war against booze. Accordingly, she joined the Independent Order of Good Templars in 1854, holding a series of high offices in the lodge and lecturing throughout the nation on behalf of the antiliquor position. Perhaps more impor-tant, Way launched a "Woman's Temperance Army" in 1854 to attack the saloons in her native Winchester, Indiana. Using tactics later employed on a broader basis during the Woman's War of 1873 and 1874, she led women into the saloons to call attention to their complaints against the traffic. Her early crusading ended, however, when she volunteered as a nurse with the Union during the Civil War.

Way returned to reform activities at the close of the sectional conflict, playing an important part in reestablishing the momentum of the Temperance Movement. In 1869, the Indiana reformer participated in the founding convention of the

Prohibition Party, and she remained a vital force in the Good Templars. Indeed, after moving to Kansas in 1872, Way joined two more fraternal temperance groups, the Sons of Temperance and the Rechabites. The battle against drink, however, did not limit her other interests. She continued as a suffrage leader and also obtained a license to preach as a Methodist. But in 1880, when the Methodists sought to discontinue licensing women, Way returned to her original Quaker faith. Meanwhile, the same year she campaigned hard for prohibition in Kansas and received some modest public acclaim when the measure became part of the state constitution. Way proved an effective dry organizer as well, founding the Kansas branch of the Woman's Christian Temperance Union and serving as its president. Increasingly, though, her life centered on church affairs. She ministered to a number of Quaker meetings over her later years, finally leaving Kansas to continue her preaching in Southern California (although she lived briefly in Idaho first). She was still active in the pulpit when she died, recognized as a pioneer of women's rights and of women's participation in the social causes for which she had fought so long.

### Bibliography:

B. NAW 3, 552–53; SEAP 6, 2811; James Black, *Brief History of Prohibition and of the Prohibition Reform Party* (New York, 1880).

**WAYLAND, Francis**    (11 March 1796, New York, NY—30 September 1865, Providence, RI). *Education*: B.A., Union Coll., NY, 1813; medical studies, Troy, NY, and New York City, 1814–16; student at Andover Sem., 1816–17; D.D. (honorary), Union Coll., 1828, Harvard Univ., 1829; LLD. (honorary), Harvard Univ., 1852. *Career*: tutor, Union Coll., 1817–21; ordained, Baptist Church, 1821; pastor, First Baptist Church, Boston, 1821–26; professor of mathematics and moral philosophy, Union Coll., 1826–27; president and professor, Brown Univ., 1827–55; pastor, First Baptist Church, Providence, RI, 1855–57; retirement, 1857–65.

Although remembered most for his contributions to higher education and American religious thought, Francis Wayland also devoted considerable energy to questions of moral reform, including the Temperance Movement. Indeed, later generations of antiliquor workers considered the Baptist minister "a true temperance pioneer" to whom the growth of the dry crusade owed much. As a young minister he was not noted as an especially good speaker, but his sermons won considerable applause for their literary grace and forceful reasoning. He dealt frequently with ethical concerns, stressing the importance of right living and the utility of Christianity as a guide to everyday life. In 1827, he gave up his ministerial duties to assume the presidency of Brown University, then in a state of fiscal disarray. Wayland set to work raising money and elevating educational standards, ultimately building the institution into one of the finest universities in the nation. Throughout his years at Brown, however, he continued to preach and to write, maintaining his focus on ethical standards and Christian morality as a basis of personal and civil conduct. As part of this commitment, Wayland lent his support to the struggle against intemperance, seeing in drunkenness one of those evils he frequently denounced as incompatible with Christianity and social virtue. He was an original member of the American Temperance Society (founded in 1826), and he spoke before the group on a number of occasions. Typically, he called attention to the moral aspects of the Temperance Movement, urging its mission upon fellow reformers and the citizenry generally.

Given his choice, Wayland's reform temperament would have led him away from a prohibitionist position. He placed considerable value on spreading reform ideas throughout the republic, and he wrote and spoke widely on many of them besides temperance: Slavery, labor unions, prisons, public libraries, and other subjects all received his attention. But in all of these cases, his hope was to achieve results through reason and persuasion and through reaching the hearts of Americans. Compelling change through the force of legislation, in his view, was only a second-best remedy. The liquor question, however, presented particular problems. Wayland believed that the legal restraint of the beverage traffic would produce "the most happy results" and that, at least in the case of distilled spirits, prohibitory legislation was in order. The Rhode Island reformer took this rather advanced position quite early, in 1833. It was a sentiment well beyond most popular opinion or even temperance thinking at the time and marked Wayland as one of the first responsible reform advocates to lend credence to such a drastic step. Aside from offering this view of the temperance question, though, he took no other direct or organizational part in the rising assault on drink. Rather, he devoted his energies to the leadership of Brown, a task which earned him an honored position in the annals of American education. His stance on prohibition, however, was enough to secure the gratitude of temperance reformers as well.

### Bibliography:

A. *An Address Delivered Before the Providence Association for the Promotion of Temperance*... (Cincinnati, OH, 1832); *The Elements of Moral Science* (Boston, 1835, and subsequent editions); *The Elements of Political Economy* (Boston, 1837, and subsequent editions); *Thoughts on the Present Collegiate System in the United States* (1842; New York, 1969); *A Memoir of the Life and Labors of the Rev. Adoniram Judson*, 2 vols. (Boston, 1853); *Letters on the Ministry of the Gospel* (New York, 1863).

B. DAB 19, 558–60; DARB, 494–95; NCAB 8, 22–24; NYT, Oct. 2, 1865; SEAP 6, 2811–12; James O. Murray, *Francis Wayland* (New York, 1891); Francis Wayland and H. L. Wayland, *A Memoir of the Life and Labors of Francis Wayland, D.D., LL.D.*, 2 vols. (New York, 1867).

**WEAKLEY, Samuel David**  (16 July 1860, Somerville, AL—14 February 1921, Birmingham, AL). *Education*: graduated from State Normal Sch., AL, 1879; legal studies in private law office, Florence, AL, 1879–80. *Career*: admitted to bar, 1880; legal practice, Memphis, TN, 1880–87; assistant attorney general, Shelby Co., TN, circa 1882–87; legal practice, Birmingham, AL, beginning 1887; city attorney, Birmingham, 1889–90; chief justice, Supreme Court of Alabama, 1906; special counsel, state of Alabama, beginning 1907.

One of the most distinguished Southern jurists of his generation, Samuel Weakley was also one of the South's most ardent prohibitionists. His dry sympathies formed early, although from motives which remain obscure. At any rate, Weakley was chief templar of the Junior Templars' Lodge (a youth branch of the Independent Order of Good Templars) while in college at the Alabama State Normal School in Florence. At the same time, he also took part in the antiliquor activities sparked by the spread of the so-called Murphy Movement into Alabama. Francis Murphy,* a former alcoholic and a powerful temperance orator, made a dramatic impact in reform circles nationally, and young Weakley apparently admired him deeply. The war against liquor, then, formed an essential part of Weakley's background as he prepared for his professional future, and it continued to inform his perspectives on contemporary issues thereafter. He completed his legal education in 1880 and for seven years maintained law offices in Memphis, Tennessee (where he also served as a county prosecutor), before settling permanently in Birmingham, Alabama. In practice with his brother, Weakley was an influential and successful man, emerging as a specialist in railroad law. As special counsel for the state, he tried cases in this field in both the state and federal courts, including the Supreme Court. His reputation was such that in 1906 the legislature appointed him chief justice of the State Supreme Court, filling the unexpired term of his deceased predecessor. At the end of the term, however, he refused reappointment, preferring to return to his practice.

Throughout these years of rising legal stature, Weakley remained a firm temperance adherent and, beginning in the early 1900s, a stalwart partisan of the Anti-Saloon League. Ultimately, his association with the league brought him fame as an expert on legal aspects of the liquor question as well. Weakley, in fact, became the legal mastermind of the Anti-Saloon League's efforts to dry out Alabama and a number of neighboring Southern states. A crucial part of the prohibitionist campaign was the attempt to pass dry legislation, both prohibitory laws and enforcement measures, all of which required the acumen to write statutes that would not only pass but stand up under wet challenges of their constitutionality. And it was in precisely this area that Weakley offered the league invaluable help. He drafted the 1907 bill that finally emerged as Alabama's state prohibition law and then led the defense in the courts that ultimately sustained it against all attacks. In addition, Weakley worked closely with the league in monitoring its effectiveness and in drafting necessary changes. Indeed, from 1907 until his death in 1921, the liquor-hating attorney authored every piece of temperance legislation to go on the Alabama statute books. Few other temperance advocates could match his record in the legal arena, and dry leaders in the region looked to him for advice on matters of legislation whenever possible. As a consequence, he also wrote prohibition laws for Georgia (1915) and Mississippi

(1919). Temperance success, though, made Weakley some bitter enemies, and he lost a hard-fought bid for the Democratic nomination for senator in 1920. Still, his legal activities and his reform career had brought him major public recognition, and at his death he was clearly one of the most influential drys in the South.

**Bibliography:**

B. SEAP 6, 2812; WW 1, 1311.

**WEBB, Edwin Yates**    (23 May 1872, Shelby, NC—7 February 1955, Shelby, NC). *Education*: A.B., Wake Forrest Coll., 1893; studied law, Univ. of North Carolina, 1893–94; studied law, Univ. of Virginia, 1896; LLD. (honorary), Wake Forrest Coll., Davidson Coll., 1918. *Career*: legal practice, NC, 1894–1903; member, North Carolina Senate, 1900–1902; member, U.S. House of Representatives, 1903–19; federal district court judge, NC, 1919–48; retirement, 1948.

The ability of the Temperance Movement to win the cooperation and loyalty of influential political leaders was a source of constant frustration to opponents of National Prohibition. Such was the case with Edwin Webb, a man who rose to prominence relatively quickly and spent a great deal of his time in Congress giving wets ample cause for alarm. Active in Democratic Party affairs in North Carolina, he served two years in the State Senate before moving on in 1903 to Congress, where he remained until 1919. He had long been a convinced dry himself, and the fact that his constituents shared his sentiments on the liquor question allowed him considerable freedom to flay the beverage traffic on the floor of the House without fear of political retaliation at the polls. He worked on behalf of a number of dry measures, relentlessly keeping the pressure on the wets. His first major contribution came with his successful sponsorship of legislation to bar the shipment of liquor from wet into dry states, a statute wets fought doggedly. The Webb Law—later called the Webb-Kenyon Act, to note the efforts of its sponsor in the Senate—passed Congress in 1913 only to meet a veto from President William Howard Taft. But the veto did not stand as both houses of Congress quickly voted to override it. The Supreme Court later sustained the constitutionality of the Webb-Kenyon Act in a test case in 1917. After this victory, which drys correctly interpreted as a major step on the path toward the Eighteenth Amendment, Webb maintained the offensive. He co-authored the dry amendment and served as one of the House leaders in the legislative fight to have it passed. Indeed, he opened the first debate on its behalf. The North Carolinian also took a leading role in framing the statutes that dried out Washington, D.C., and in establishing War Prohibition when the United States entered World War I. In 1919, however, Webb left the House for a place on the federal bench in his native state. He remained a judge until his retirement in 1948, no longer a combatant in the legislative wars over liquor. Yet Webb's chief claim on public attention remained his efforts to drive beverage alcohol from the American scene.

**Bibliography:**

B. SEAP 6, 2812–13; WW 3, 897.

**WHEELER, Wayne Bidwell**   (10 November 1869, Brookfield, OH—5 September 1927, Battle Creek, MI). *Education*: A.B., Oberlin Coll., 1893; A.M., Oberlin Coll., 1894; LLB., Western Reserve Univ., 1898; LLD. (honorary), Muskingum Coll., 1917, Oberlin Coll., 1919. *Career*: officer, Ohio Anti-Saloon League (state superintendent after 1903), 1894–1916; general counsel, Anti-Saloon League of America, 1916–27, legislative superintendent, Anti-Saloon League of America, 1919–27.

When the Reverend Howard Hyde Russell* organized the Anti-Saloon League, he asked the reform-minded faculty of Oberlin College in Ohio for a likely assistant. Reportedly, their answers were unanimous—Wayne Bidwell Wheeler. They were right: Starting as the Ohio League's field secretary in May 1894, Wheeler remained with the antiliquor group for the rest of his life; indeed, he rapidly became the driving force behind the league's rise to national influence. Working tirelessly in Ohio, he pioneered the nonpartisan organizing techniques and local-option campaigns that later dried out much of the nation. By the turn of the century, he was producing dramatic results. The league could bring out entire church congregations (its basic organizational blocs) and other local drys for friendly candidates, Republican or Democrat. Large parts of Ohio went dry, and wets were clearly on the defensive. In 1905, Wheeler won the league's greatest victory to that point, marshalling the votes to upset Republican Governor Myron Herrick when he refused to follow a staunchly prohibitionist path. Called to Washington, D.C., as general counsel of the Anti-Saloon League of America in 1916 (and as legislative superintendent in 1919), he directed dry lobbying efforts with extraordinary skill. He took a direct role in frustrating wet attempts to stop the antiliquor drive and in framing temperance legislation, including the Eighteenth Amendment and the Volstead Act. Over the years, he also personally led the assault on drink in the courts. From the local courts of Ohio to the U.S. Supreme Court, he took part in over two thousand cases, both prosecuting liquor law violations as well as defending dry measures. In the nation's capital he was known for his insistence on vigorous steps against the liquor traffic, especially in defense of the Volstead Act. At one point, for example, he reportedly promised to make wets "believe in punishment after death," and he no doubt meant it. By any standard, then, Wheeler was one of the most committed and capable reformers the dry crusade ever produced.

For at least the final years of his activity on the national scene, Wheeler, more than anyone else, came to embody the zealous drive and political acumen of the Temperance Movement. As legislative superintendent, he presided over a well-oiled and tested lobbying organization that kept league headquarters in the nation's capital easily in touch with state groups and individual church congregations. The existence of this network allowed Wheeler to develop enormous influence on Capitol Hill: With minimal effort, he could barrage a wavering or hostile legislator with telegrams from irate constituents, a tactic only the most secure wets could ignore. Assured of such support, Wheeler rarely lost his temper in debate; rather, he had a reputation for urbanity that, at times, wets found unnerving when coupled with his willingness to resort to pressure tactics. Alarmed at his power to marshall the strength of the league, opponents of Prohibition referred to his often strong-armed methods as Wheelerism, a term which stuck. Indeed, drys began to use it too; and in that it produced results they were just as happy with it. "Wheelerism," wrote league founder Howard Hyde Russell, was "the embodiment in life and service of the Highest Possible Patriotism." Even his enemies admitted his consummate political skill and mastery of the legislative process as well as his singular dedication to the Anti-Saloon League and its cause. For good or ill, however, Wheeler clearly pioneered the high-powered lobbying techniques so prevalent in modern American politics.

Wheeler, having led the temperance cause to the heights of its legislative influence, never lived to see Prohibition's fall from grace. His health was failing by 1926, and his insistence on maintaining his usual schedule in Washington, D.C., provided little opportunity for needed rest. During that year, he defended the league in a grueling session of hearings dominated by the hostile "grilling" of Senator Reed of Missouri, after which he finally (1927) agreed to take some time off. Wheeler retired to Michigan, where tragedy struck: His wife died as the result of a stove explosion in their home, and his elderly father-in-law succumbed soon after the incident. Wheeler tried to carry on, addressing an Anti-Saloon League gathering in the wake of the family deaths, but he died of kidney trouble less than three weeks after his wife's funeral. The leadership of the league was never the same, as Wheeler's successors lacked his command of the dry lobby. Final estimates of his career generally differed according to views on the Prohibition question. Many drys were convinced that Repeal never would have occurred had Wheeler lived to direct the defense of the Eighteenth Amendment. On the other hand, wets claimed that the bitterness engendered by "Wheelerism" hastened the collapse of the "noble experiment." Both views are wide of the mark: Wayne Wheeler could not have stopped Repeal, but he was too good at what he did to have damaged his cause mortally. In an exaggerated comment on his passing, the *Washington Post* at least captured something of his influence on the affairs of his day: "No other private citizen of the United States," the editorial noted, "has left such an impress upon national history."

## Bibliography:

A. *The Federal and State Laws Relating to Intoxicating Liquor* (Westerville, OH, 1916).

B. DAB 20, 54–55; NCAB 20, 13–14; NYT, Sept. 6, 1927; SEAP 6, 2832–35; WW 1, 1329; Peter Odegard, *Pressure Politics: The Story of the Anti-Saloon*

*League* (New York, 1928); Justin Stewart, *Wayne Wheeler: Dry Boss* (New York, 1928).

**WHITMAN, Charles Seymour**    (28 August 1868, Hanover, CT—29 March 1947, New York, NY). *Education*: A.B., Amherst Coll., 1890; LLB., New York Univ., 1894; M.A. (honorary), Williams Coll., 1904; LLD. (honorary), New York Univ., Amherst Coll., 1913, Williams Coll., 1914, Hamilton Coll., 1918. *Career*: assistant corporation counsel, New York City, 1901–3; member, Board of City Magistrates, 1904–7; district attorney, New York Co., 1910–14; governor of New York, 1915–18; legal practice, New York City, from 1919.

One temperance worker called Whitman "the first Prohibition governor New York ever had." His attachments to Prohibition, however, were more the results of political expediency than belief (Whitman was in fact an extremely heavy drinker). He made his initial reputation in New York City politics, at the age of forty, as chief of the city's Board of Magistrates in 1907. In that position he launched a crusade against police corruption—a standard ploy of the era to build a "reform" image while ignoring more serious aspects of city problems. Whitman was nothing if not an ambitious and practical politician. On the other hand, during this period he did initiate an effective program to enforce liquor and gambling laws, a practice he continued after he was elected New York County district attorney in 1910 as a reform candidate. He made national headlines in prosecuting the sensational Herman Rosenthal murder case. In a highly controversial trial, five men, including a police lieutenant, were ultimately sent to the electric chair for the killing of gambler Rosenthal. Largely on the basis of the publicity he received during this case (or at least this was the argument of the man who arranged for most of it: journalist, and future editor of the *New York World*, Herbert Swope), Whitman won the governorship in 1914, and many observers considered him a potential Republican presidential candidate for the 1916 election.

During his term as governor Whitman vigorously and consistently supported the work of the Anti-Saloon League and the drive for National Prohibition. In turn, the league winked at the fact that the governor had no prior record of commitment to prohibition, much less the fact that his drinking had become something of a public scandal. But Whitman justified the league's argument that the best way for the dry movement to get results was to back anyone willing to cooperate in return for the league's help at the polls. He fought attempts to weaken local-option laws in favor of the liquor traffic, and he prevented a popular referendum on the National Prohibition question, which the league opposed. If many drys were happy with Whitman, however, other New Yorkers were not. He made no real impact on state politics and proved uninterested in reform— perhaps because he devoted most of his time to his presidential aspirations. Whatever the reason, the victory of wet Democrat Al Smith in the race for the governorship in 1918 ended Whitman's political career forever. As if to emphasize his bogus position as a "Prohibition governor," he showed no further interest in the cause after leaving office.

**Bibliography:**

B. DAB Supp. 4, 884–86; NYT, March 30, 1947; SEAP 6, 2840–41; WW 2, 574; E. J. Kahn, Jr., *The World of Swope* (New York, 1965); Andy Logan, *Against the Evidence: The Becker-Rosenthal Affair* (New York, 1970).

**WILCOX, Ella Wheeler**    (5 November 1850, Johnstown Center, WI—30 October 1919, Short Beach, CT). *Education*: attended Univ. of Wisconsin, 1867–68. *Career*: author and poet, 1860s to 1919.

While she has never received recognition as a particularly good or original writer, Ella Wilcox was one of the most prolific and popular authors of the late nineteenth century. Interested in literature since childhood, her short stories, essays, and poems began earning her a respectable income by the time she was eighteen. Her primary interest was poetry, and her verses attained a modest popularity in the 1870s. Wilcox's first major success, however, was fortuitous: A Chicago publisher refused a volume of her poems entitled *Poems of Passion* on the grounds of alleged immorality. This had the effect of guaranteeing an extensive sale of the book once another publisher released it in 1883. Popular recognition of her work soared thereafter; and although literary critics seldom took her seriously (a fact which nagged at her throughout her career), she was established as one of the best-known writers of her era. After 1884 she lectured widely in the United States and Europe, took on free-lance writing assignments, and at one point was producing a poem a day for a newspaper syndicate.

Wilcox's writing, however, did not prevent her from pursuing a variety of reform and religious interests, and temperance was one of the chief of these. Her family had been Good Templars, and Ella participated in that group's activities. Her dry sentiments were evident in a number of her poems, and in fact her first book was a collection of temperance verses entitled *Drops of Water* (1872). Typical of the era's temperance literature, *Drops of Water* carried the total abstinence message to a children's audience and enjoyed a wide reading. Subsequent works, such as *Shells* (1873), dealt in similar fashion with moral subjects; and there is no doubt that she was genuinely concerned with the morality and well-being of the younger generation. Wilcox was also an ardent spiritualist and regularly attended seances; in her declining years she announced that she had established communication with her dead husband through the medium of a ouija board. She kept writing to the end, and temperance workers considered her one of the most important literary contributors to the dry cause.

**Bibliography:**

A. *Drops of Water* (Chicago, 1872); *Poems of Passion* (Chicago, 1883); "Literary Confessions of a Western Poetess," *Lippincott's Monthly Magazine*

(May 1886); *The Heart of the New Thought* (Chicago, 1911); *The Worlds and I* (Chicago, 1918).

B. DAB 20, 203–4; NAW 3, 607–8; NYT, Oct. 31, 1919; SEAP 6, 2846–47; Jenny Ballou, *Period Piece: Ella Wheeler Wilcox and Her Times* (Boston, 1940).

**WILEY, Harvey Washington**    (18 October 1844, Kent, IN—30 June 1930, Washington, DC). *Education*: A.B., Hanover Coll., IN, 1867; A.M., Hanover Coll., 1870; M.D., Indiana Medical Coll., 1871; B.S., Harvard Univ., 1873; Ph.D. (honorary), Hanover Coll., 1876; LLD. (honorary), Hanover Coll., 1898, Univ. of Vermont, 1911; D.Sc. (honorary), Lafayette Coll., 1912; A.M. (honorary), Hahnemann Medical Coll., 1912. *Career*: professor of chemistry, Purdue Univ., and state chemist of Indiana, 1874–83; chief chemist, U.S. Department of Agriculture, 1888–1912; professor of agricultural chemistry, George Washington Univ., 1899–1914; active writing and lecturing, 1900s to 1930; contributing editor, *Good Housekeeping*, 1912–30.

One of the most prominent figures of the Progressive era, Dr. Harvey Wiley's career offered a clear demonstration of the links between the Temperance Movement and the broader reform impulse of the period. Trained in chemistry and medicine, he became chief chemist in the federal Department of Agriculture in 1883, and over his almost thirty years in the post he transformed an office of six individuals into one of the most effective agencies in the government, with over five hundred employees. Wiley used them to pursue research and investigations in a wide variety of areas, from dairy products and soils to public health and sanitation. Perhaps his most significant contribution, however, was his exposure of industrial food adulteration practices. Wiley's articulate and tireless campaign to correct these evils finally led to the passage of the 1906 Pure Food and Drugs Act. Yet even after this victory, the chief chemist maintained a careful scrutiny of the food processing business, as well as a vocal criticism of the dietary and medical uses of what he claimed were dangerous substances—not the least of which was alcohol. While he had no early interest in prohibition, Wiley did take the lead in campaigning against the presence of whiskey in the national pharmacopoeia, and he ultimately concluded "that alcohol in its various forms is an unmitigated evil." Given his pronounced views on food safety, it came as no surprise to Wiley's associates when, once he became convinced of the dangers of alcohol, he became a dedicated antiliquor reformer as well. It was not in his nature to level criticisms without taking action.

Wiley's temperance activities quickly joined the mainstream of organized antiliquor politics. In 1912, the same year he stepped down as chief chemist, he announced his support for national prohibition—and later stated that he considered the drink problem so serious that "world-wide prohibition" was an even better solution. Wiley admitted that he was not a teetotaler himself (old habits were evidently hard to break) but that the general good demanded governmental action against liquor. And apparently he finally gave up his own alcohol, probably by the time the nation ratified the Eighteenth Amendment. A gifted speaker and writer, he lectured frequently on temperance issues and lent his testimony as a scientist against alcohol on a number of official occasions. In 1925, Wiley joined the Anti-Saloon League, sitting for a number of years as a vice president of its District of Columbia chapter. He took the duty to heart, standing with the league to defend the Volstead Act and Prohibition as popular sentiments shifted against the "noble experiment" in the later 1920s. To the end, he described himself as "an ardent prohibitionist," holding that the Eighteenth Amendment had done more good for the public welfare than any other part of the Constitution. Wets, the reformer claimed, were engaged in nothing less than a "second 'Whiskey Rebellion' " in opposing the measure.

**Bibliography:**

A. *Foods and Their Adulteration*... (Philadelphia, 1907, and later editions); *Wiley's Health Series* (Chicago, 1917); *Beverages and Their Adulteration* (Philadelphia, 1919).

B. DAB 20, 215–16; NYT, July 1, 1930; SEAP 6, 2847–48; Oscar Edward Anderson, *The Health of a Nation: Harvey W. Wiley and the Fight for Pure Food* (Chicago, 1958).

**WILLARD, Frances Elizabeth Caroline**   (28 September 1839, Churchville, NY—17 February 1898, New York, NY). *Education*: studied at Milwaukee Female Coll., 1857; L.S., North Western Female Coll., 1859; studied at the Collège de France and the Sorbonne, 1869–70. *Career*: teacher, various women's academies in IL, PA, and NY, 1860–67; president, Evanston Coll. for Ladies, Evanston, IL, 1871–73; dean, Woman's Coll. of Northwestern Univ., Evanston, IL, 1873–74; president, WCTU of Chicago, 1874; corresponding secretary, National WCTU, 1875–79; president, National WCTU, 1879–98; founder and acting president, then president, World's WCTU, 1883–98.

Of all the leaders of the Temperance Movement, Willard was one of the most respected and influential. Although raised in a strictly Protestant and dry family, she expressed no special interest in temperance as a young woman, pursuing instead a distinguished career in education. She ultimately became dean of the Woman's College of Northwestern University but resigned after a prolonged clash with the university president and faculty. Willard was then caught up in the excitement of the Woman's Crusade of 1873–74 and resolved to make temperance her life's work. She helped found the Woman's Christian Temperance Union of Chicago, after which she quickly assumed leadership roles in the Illinois and National Unions. From 1879 to her death, Willard served as president of the National WCTU; and from 1883 she also led the World's WCTU. She had considerable talents as a speaker, author, and organizer, and during her tenure she worked devotedly to build unions and antiliquor sentiment throughout the United States, Canada, and Western Europe. Under her guidance, the WCTU combined two general approaches to alcohol-related problems: In a reflection of her own religious faith in individual salvation and the redemption of sinners, the union waged a long "gospel temperance" campaign to win drinkers away from the bottle, supported institutional medical care for alcoholics, and fostered a variety of other measures aimed at the "rescue" of problem drinkers. However, Willard also held that preventive social measures—such as alcohol education and prohibition—were critical, arguing that it was more logical to stop drunkenness before it started than to deal afterward with its consequences. She finally emphasized this later view, and her efforts to influence legislation on behalf of these ends made her a nationally recognized political figure.

The key to Willard's temperance commitment was her "home protection" credo. She became convinced that national stability, morality, and social justice all rested on the preservation of the family unit, which therefore had to be defended against all threats. In this regard, Willard saw the liquor traffic not only as a threat in itself—one too often embodied in drunken fathers and sons—but also as a breeding ground for prostitution, the oppression of labor, political corruption, poor schools, disease, poverty, and a host of other social evils. Thus for Willard, temperance work, and particularly the destruction of "the traffic," was intended to cure an entire range of national ills, which would consequently assure the safety of the family. This broadly-conceived outlook on the meaning of temperance was reflected in her attempts to join forces with the Populists and labor reformers, the launching of the prohibitionist "Home Protection Party" in the 1880s, and her advocacy of the WCTU's "Do Everything" policy, which obligated the union to enter as many fields of reform work as possible. She felt that women in particular, the guardians of the sanctity of the home in her view, should spearhead the reform; and this belief explained much of her staunch support for women's suffrage. In the face of initial opposition, she persuaded the WCTU to endorse suffrage as a home protection measure in 1883.

Willard's zeal for reform never flagged. In her final years, probably due to her exposure to European politics while on an extended visit with Lady Henry Somerset in Britain, she developed a strong interest in socialism. She even suggested, in a reversal of temperance dogma, that alcoholism was as much an effect as a cause of poverty and that education would prove more helpful than prohibition in fighting intemperance. Despite some internal challenges, sparked largely by these controversial views, the WCTU remained loyal to its president and to her multifaceted reform posture. Upon her death, however, while venerating her memory, the organization gradually abandoned broad reform goals in favor of a narrower concentration on prohibition.

### Bibliography:

A. *Home Protection Manual* (New York, 1879); *Woman and Temperance* (Hartford, CT, 1883); *How to Win* (New York, 1886); *Glimpses of Fifty Years* (Chicago, 1889); *The Modern Temperance Movement* (London, 1893); *Do Everything* (Chicago, 1895).

B. DAB 20, 233–34; NAW 3, 613–19; NCAB 1, 376–77; SEAP 6, 2848–

51; Mary Earhart, *Frances Willard: From Prayers to Politics* (Chicago, 1944); Anna A. Gordon, *The Beautiful Life of Frances E. Willard* (Chicago, 1898); Lydia A. Trowbridge, *Frances Willard of Evanston* (New York, 1938).

**WILLIAMS, Wayne Cullen**    (20 September 1878, near Indianola, IL—15 August 1953, Denver, CO). *Education*: studied at Univ. of Denver, 1898–1900; LLB., Univ. of Denver, 1906. *Career*: reporter, *Rocky Mountain News*, Denver, 1906; admitted to bar, CO, 1906; legal practice, Denver, beginning 1906; county judge, Denver, 1912; assistant district attorney, Denver, 1913–15; member, Colorado Industrial Commission, 1915–17; state attorney general, CO, 1917–25; special assistant to U.S. attorney general, 1926–33.

Completing his legal education in 1906, Williams began a distinguished legal and civil career in his adopted state of Colorado. In addition to a successful private practice, he also served successively as a county judge, a Denver prosecutor, attorney general of Colorado, and finally as a special assistant to the federal attorney general. Intertwined with his activities in the law, however, was a fervent commitment to the Temperance Movement. The same year he passed the bar, Williams became affiliated with the Colorado Anti-Saloon League, serving as a member of its Board of Trustees. He quickly became immersed in the state-wide battle against the traffic, and when the campaign for actual prohibition started in 1910, he volunteered to chair the Denver Dry Committee. This initial assault, though, proved premature: Coloradans were willing to put limits on the drink trade but not to abolish it. Yet the effort brought the reforming attorney considerable popular exposure, and when he became an assistant district attorney in Denver, he surprised no one when he used his position to crack down on illegal alcohol sales. He captured national attention in his legal crusade against saloons trying to find loopholes in the state dry statutes (some establishments tried to masquerade as "cafes"). And when Colorado did go dry in 1914, Williams (who had joined still another group, the Dry Colorado Federation Committee, during the effort) received much of the credit.

As he fought for prohibition, Williams remained active in public service; and after several years on the state Industrial Commission, he took office in 1917 as Colorado attorney general, a post he retained until 1925. His tenure in the state administration saw him cling firmly to his dry loyalties, presiding over Colorado's efforts to sustain not only its own antiliquor statutes but the Volstead Act as well during National Prohibition. Williams also devoted considerable time to the Methodist Church, serving for a number of years on the Board of Trustees of its Board of Temperance, Prohibition and Public Morals. His efforts on behalf of the dry crusade, in aggregate, established him as one of the premier reform workers in his region, and there is little question that he did much to advance public support for prohibition in the West. As sympathies for the Eighteenth Amendment waned, however, Williams no longer served the state, and he took little active role in the political efforts to stem the advancing wet tide. Serving as an assistant to the federal attorney general after 1926, he was largely removed from day-to-day legislative battles against drink. And after Repeal, he spent most of his time on civic and religious activity or in writing.

**Bibliography:**

A. *Workmen's Compensation in Colorado* (Denver, 1916?); *William Jennings Bryan* (New York, 1936); *American Tomorrows* (New York, 1939); *Sweet of Colorado* (New York, 1943); *A Rail Splitter for President* (Denver, 1951).
B. SEAP 6, 2854; WW 3, 923.

**WILLING, Jennie Fowler**    (22 January 1834, Buford, Canada—6 October 1916, New York, NY). *Education*: A.M. (honorary), Evanston Coll. for Ladies, IL, 1872. *Career*: schoolteacher, Newark, IL, circa 1849–53; extensive work with foreign and home missionary groups, Methodist Church, 1869–89; organizer and officer, WCTU, IL, NY, 1874–1916; professor of English, Illinois Wesleyan Univ., 1874–89?; founder and principal, New York Evangelistic Training Sch., 1895–1916.

The daughter of one of the founders of Methodism in Canada, Jennie Fowler moved from her native country to the United States after her parents lost their home in the aftermath of the Canadian rebellion of 1837. Staying briefly in New York State, the Fowlers settled in Newark, Illinois, in 1842, where Jennie spent her childhood. With little formal education, she nevertheless was an intelligent young woman, and by age fifteen she was teaching in a local school. Married at nineteen years old to the Reverend William C. Willing, she followed him from pastorate to pastorate in New York State and, eventually, back to Illinois. Along the way, Reverend Willing encouraged her to pursue her own interests, and over the years she emerged as a prolific writer on religious and reform subjects. She also became an able preacher herself, and her husband arranged for licensing in 1874. At the same time, Willing devoted considerable attention to Methodist missionary efforts. She was an officer of the Woman's Foreign Missionary Society for years (1869 to 1880s), and of the Woman's Home Missionary Society from 1880 to 1889. Her other major interest was the Temperance Movement, a reform she hoped would rid America of an evil she considered as monstrous as human slavery. She took part in the Woman's Crusade that spread out of Ohio in 1874 when she helped organize a crackdown on illegal liquor sales in her home town of Bloomington. Later in the year, Willing also played a central role in organizing the Cleveland convention that founded the National Woman's Christian Temperance Union. She was a member of the WCTU for the rest of her life.

Willing's career as an antiliquor reformer never lessened her interests in other activities, but she made some notable contributions. Immediately after presiding over the National WCTU's organizing convention, the press of her other responsibilities compelled her to refuse any office with the new group. For the same reason, she turned down a dry attempt to nominate her for the post of Illinois superintendent of public instruction. Yet she did agree to serve as president of the Illinois chapter of the union, a step which shortly thereafter (also in late 1874) led her to accept the editorship of the WCTU's official publication. At first, the journal was known as *Our Union*, but it subsequently merged with another dry paper, the *Signal*, to form the *Union Signal* (the name it still maintains). Willing held the post only for a year, but her literary and administrative skills put the organ on a solid footing. After her move to New York City in 1889 (where she founded and operated a training school for immigrant girls), she continued with the WCTU. She attended the World's WCTU convention in 1895 and then ran a union department on evangelical training. At her death, she was president of the Frances Willard* chapter of the WCTU in New York and active in the affairs of the state organization. Her leadership of the Willard chapter—named after the union president who died in 1898—continued an old relationship: Willing had been a trustee of Evanston College for Ladies in the 1870s when Willard had headed the school, and when Willing's brother, C. H. Fowler,* had been engaged briefly to Willard. When the engagement soured, however, Willing evidently did not try to dissuade her brother, the president of Northwestern University, from pushing Willard out of her position. Willing left half of her estate to the union and half to her girls' school.

### Bibliography:

A. *Through the Dark to the Day: A Story of Discipline* (Cincinnati, OH, 1868); *The Only Way Out* (Boston, 1881); *A Bunch of Flowers for Girls* (Boston, 1888); *How to Win Souls* (Chicago, 1919); *From Fifteen to Twenty-five: A Book for Young Men* (Chicago, 1920).

B. NAW 3, 623–25; NYT, Oct. 7, 27, 1916; SEAP 6, 2855–56; Frances E. Willard, *Woman and Temperance* (Hartford, CT, 1883).

**WILSON, Alonzo Edes**  (5 February 1868, Madison, WI—17 June 1949, Evanston, IL). *Career*: assistant editor, *St. Paul* (MN) *Times*, 1886–90; editorial staff, Chicago *Lever*, 1890–95; assistant editor, *Chicago Record*, 1896; freelance journalist, late 1890s; secretary and manager, United Prohibition Press, 1903–5; member, Illinois House of Representatives, 1904; president, Lincoln Temperance Press, and manager, Lincoln Temperance Chautauqua System, 1910–18; field director, Near East Relief Organization, 1919–29; national director, American Business Men's Prohibition Foundation, beginning 1930.

Wilson, a Wisconsin-born journalist and propagandist on behalf of prohibition, was not educated beyond the secondary level and spent most of his life in the Midwest. Yet over the course of a long reform career he was able to garner a modest national reputation as a temperance crusader, largely as a writer and organizer for various antiliquor groups. His interest in the liquor question began at the age of sixteen, when he attended the 1884 national convention of the Prohibition Party. He became a party activist, chairing the Prohibitionist Chicago Central Committee by 1889 and holding a succession of increasingly important party posts (state committeeman, treasurer and secretary, national committeeman) between then and 1916. Wilson even ran for office himself, providing a rare Prohibition Party victory in 1904 when he won a seat in the Illinois legislature. His campaign for the national Senate in 1916, however, was unsuccessful. Between 1904 and 1911, he was treasurer of the Temperance Society of the Methodist Episcopal Church, which later became the politically influential Methodist Board of Temperance, Prohibition and Public Morals, and from 1910 to 1918 he was an organizer of the Lincoln Temperance Chautauqua System and its publications program. Wilson served with ability in all of these positions, offering a further example of the steady mid-level leadership that made the national drive for prohibition so effective in most parts of the country.

The coming of National Prohibition found Wilson's role little changed. He remained busy in various organizational capacities, although he devoted a great deal of time to the leadership of relief efforts in the Near East. For a number of years, he served as a vice president of the World's Prohibition Confederation, but the group made only minimal headway in spreading the dry gospel to any effect. More substantial were his labors with the American Business Men's Prohibition Foundation. Wilson helped to establish the group along with an old associate from his Chautauqua management days. He took the position of national director in 1930, with the responsibility of leading the foundation's efforts to collect and disseminate information on the impact of the country's antiliquor statutes on the nation's commercial and business communities. At various times he argued vigorously that Prohibition had proven a major help in stimulating business productivity, safety, and efficiency; and he bitterly attacked the drive for the repeal of the Eighteenth Amendment as dangerous as to the nation's economic health. In defense of the dry laws, Wilson was also an active member of the Joint Committee for the Enforcement of the Eighteenth Amendment. The collapse of the "noble experiment" found the Business Men's Foundation leaders disappointed, although the organization continued to press its case with the public long after popular support for the antiliquor cause had evaporated.

**Bibliography:**

A. *Prohibition Handbook and Voters' Manual* (Chicago, 1900); *American Prohibition Year Book...* (Chicago, 1901–10).

B. SEAP 6, 2857–58; WW 2, 588.

**WILSON, Clarence True**     (24 April 1872, Milton, DE—16 February 1939, Gresham, OR). *Education*: studied at St. John's Coll., MD, 1890s; A.B., Univ. of Southern California, 1894; B.D., McClay Coll. of Theology, CA, 1895; Ph.D. (honorary), San Joaquin Valley Coll., CA, 1897; D.D. (honorary), St. John's Coll., 1900; LLD. (honorary), Washington Coll., MD, 1925. *Career*: minister, various pastorates in DE, NY, CA, NJ, OR, 1890–1910; president, Oregon Anti-Saloon League, 1908–10; general secretary, Temperance Society of the Methodist Episcopal Church (later the Board of Temperance, Prohibition, and Public Morals), 1910–39.

Born the son of Methodist clergyman John A. B. Wilson, a founding member of the Prohibition Party in the state of Delaware, Clarence True Wilson followed in his father's footsteps: He became both a man of the cloth and a devoted champion of the Temperance Movement. His initial involvement with the antiliquor crusade came early. At only sixteen years old, Wilson joined the Independent Order of Good Templars and became one of the group's regular lecturers; and two years later, still too young to vote, he was elected secretary of the state committee of the Delaware Prohibition Party (1890). The same year, Wilson was ordained a deacon in the Methodist Episcopal Church (and two years later an elder) and took his first pastorate in Seaford, Delaware; he served a total of seven congregations in five states before leaving the pulpit in 1910. At each of his churches, Wilson made a practice of reserving the first Sunday evening of each month to discussions of temperance and other aspects of moral reform. Like his father before him, he considered total abstinence as nothing less than an article of faith, and he tirelessly urged his congregations and society in general to that course. On the other hand, his militancy left little room for compromise with or tolerance for wet arguments, and he carried the battle to the enemy on whatever front he could. Thus while a minister in Pasadena, California (1894–97), he waged a spirited (if unsuccessful) campaign for Congress on the Prohibition Party ticket. And when leading a church in Portland, Oregon (1902–10), he simultaneously served as president of the state Anti-Saloon League. By the early 1900s, then, Wilson had emerged as one of America's most implacable foes of the traffic.

In 1910, Wilson's reputation as a prohibition worker brought him to a crossroads in his career: He accepted a full-time appointment as general secretary of the Methodist Church Temperance Society (renamed in 1916 the Board of Temperance, Prohibition, and Public Morals), and over the years he built the organization into one of the most effective dry lobbies in the nation. The board kept Methodists in constant communication on the liquor question, served as a clearinghouse for information and propaganda, and spoke with the authority of the denomination on temperance matters. Among other projects, the crusading minister successfully led a building fund to construct a national headquarters— the Methodist Building—for the board in Washington, D.C. In addition, Wilson emerged as a prolific dry author. Until 1910, he had published only one temperance-related work; as the head of the board, however, he wrote a number of popular and influential titles on various aspects of the liquor question. Wilson presided over the board as the nation ratified the Eighteenth Amendment and then led an active defense of the measure against wet assaults. In 1928, Wilson became vice president of the National Conference of Organizations Supporting the Eighteenth Amendment and held a similar office with the International Reform Federation. As the popular tide rose against Prohibition, though, Wilson characteristically refused to give an inch. At one point, the angry crusader advocated calling out the Marines to assure compliance with the Volstead Act, and he summed up his resolve on prohibition enforcement in one pithy sentence: "The putting of the fear of God in the minds of those who fear neither God nor man is the chief function of good government.''

**Bibliography:**

A. *The Next Step Toward National Prohibition* (Chicago, 1911); *Dry or Die: The Anglo-Saxon Dilemma*, 2nd ed. (Topeka, KS, 1913); with Deets Pickett and Ernest Dailey Smith, eds., *The Cyclopedia of Temperance, Prohibition and Public Morals* (New York, 1917); *What Has Prohibition Done...* (Westerville, OH, 1927); with Deets Pickett, *The Case for Prohibition: Its Past, Present Accomplishments, and Future in America*, 2nd ed. (New York, 1930).
B. SEAP 6, 2858; WW 1, 1359; John Kobler, *Ardent Spirits: The Rise and Fall of Prohibition* (New York, 1973).

**WILSON, Henry**    (16 February 1812, Farmingham, NH—22 November 1875, Washington, DC). *Career*: indentured to farmer, NH, 1822–33; indentured to shoemaker, MA, 1833; shoemaker, Natick, MA, 1833–35; owner of shoe factory, 1830s–1840s; member, Massachusetts House of Representatives, 1841–42; member, Massachusetts Senate, 1844–53; editor, *Boston Republican*, 1848–51; member, U.S. Senate, 1855–73; vice president of the United States, 1873–75.

Born Jeremiah Colbath to a rural New Hampshire family in circumstances of abject poverty, the abolitionist Henry Wilson, as he was legally known after 1832, rose in veritable Horatio Alger fashion to occupy the vice presidency in the administration of Ulysses S. Grant. So extreme was his family's poverty that young Colbath served some eleven years as an indentured servant. But he was a quick study and possessed of enormous drive: Except for some courses at New Hampshire academies in the 1830s, he largely educated himself and ultimately prospered as a shoe manufacturer in Natick, Massachusetts. By this time having changed his name to Wilson, he also entered politics as a Whig, winning election to the state legislature in 1840. With only brief interruptions, he won reelection repeatedly, sitting until 1853. Over his years in the Massachusetts Senate, Wilson emerged as a firm proponent of reform. He advocated measures in support of Northern manufacturing, public education, the Temperance Movement, and other causes. Most of all, though, Wilson was a staunch abolitionist, a loyalty he retained as he passed through affiliations with the Whig, American (Know-Nothing), Free Soil, and, finally, Republican parties. In the national Senate, he was first a prominent foe of slavery and then an advocate of vigorous military measures against the Confederacy. After the war, the Bay State senator bitterly fought President Andrew Johnson's Reconstruction policies as well as championing the rights of the freedmen. He also flourished as a contemporary historian, authoring a number of volumes on the Civil War years and on the history of American slavery, some of which remain notable works. As a vice presidential candidate in 1872, he was more conciliatory toward the

South, although with his death from a stroke in 1875 he was able to make little mark on Grant's policies.

Wilson's temperance work was never of a caliber equal to his contributions on behalf of abolitionism. But the nature of his commitment to the struggle against drink was indicative of the force behind much of the nation's postwar temperance drive. He had long been a firm total abstinence man, and he had favored the passage of the Massachusetts state prohibition law. Indeed, when the statute came under fire in 1867, he defended it passionately, reputedly stating that he would rather see the repeal of the Thirteenth Amendment (which had abolished slavery). He had nothing but contempt for proponents of an attempt to replace state prohibition with license laws. "I look upon the liquor trade," he announced, "as grossly immoral, causing more evil than anything else in this country." Those who would buy or sell licenses to take part in the traffic were lacking, he believed, in all public spirit. Wilson was not active with mass temperance organizations, but he did take a hand in reactivating the moribund Congressional Temperance Society in 1867, and then served a term as its president. A highly moral man with a perfectionist outlook on humanity, Wilson saw the war on liquor in much the same terms as the war against slavery: an effort to purge mankind of a sin and an impediment to human betterment.

### Bibliography:

A. *Speech of Hon. Henry Wilson, at the First New England Convention...* (Boston, 1866); *Senator Wilson's Speech on Prohibition...* (Boston, 1867); *The Relation of Churches and Ministers to the Temperance Cause* (Boston, 1870); *Father Mathew, The Temperance Apostle: An Address...* (New York, 1873); *History of the Rise and Fall of the Slave Power in America*, 3 vols. (Boston, 1872–77).

B. DAB 20, 322–25; SEAP 6, 2860; Richard H. Allot, *Cobbler in Congress: The Life of Henry Wilson, 1812–1875* (Lexington, KY, 1972); Ernest McKay, *Henry Wilson: Practical Radical: A Portrait of a Politician* (Washington, NY, 1971); *Memorial Addresses on the Life and Character of Henry Wilson...Delivered in the Senate and House of Representatives...* (Washington, DC, 1876); Elias Nason and Thomas Nason, *The Life and Public Services of Henry Wilson...* (Boston, 1876).

**WILSON, Luther Barton**    (14 November 1856, Baltimore, MD—4 June 1918, Baltimore, MD). *Education*: A.B., Dickinson Coll., 1875; M.D., Univ. of Maryland, 1877; A.M., Dickinson Coll., 1878; D.D. (honorary), Dickinson Coll., 1892; LLD. (honorary), Dickinson Coll., 1904; LHD. (honorary), Syracuse Univ., 1912; LLD. (honorary), Wesleyan Univ., 1913. *Career*: minister, Methodist Episcopal Church, MD, DC, 1878–94; presiding elder, Washington District, 1894–1900; presiding elder, West Baltimore District, 1903–4; elected bishop, 1904; resident bishop, Chattanooga, TN (1904–8), Philadelphia (1908–12), New York (1912–28); president, Board of Foreign Missions, 1912–28.

Methodist bishop and president of the Anti-Saloon League of America, Luther Barton Wilson originally set his sights on a medical career. The son of a physician, he completed his medical degree at the University of Maryland in 1897 and joined his father's practice. Within a year, however, he had a change of heart and obtained a license to preach as a Methodist. Taking charge of pastorates in western Maryland and the District of Columbia, Wilson compiled a successful record in the pulpit and his denomination rewarded him with election as a bishop in 1904. As bishop, he presided over Methodist affairs in the districts of Chattanooga, Philadelphia, and New York as well as serving as head of the church's Board of Foreign Missions after 1912. Over the years, Wilson proved an activist on social issues of concern to Methodism, not the least of which was the liquor question. And in this regard, he acquired a considerable reputation as a reformer even before his election as bishop. While a minister, his pulpits fully reflected his denomination's hatred of the beverage traffic and support for prohibition. Indeed, he became one of the most prominent and tireless workers in the founding of the Anti-Saloon League in the nation's capital, and he played a leading role in 1895 in the establishment of the Anti-Saloon League of America. In fact, the impetus for calling a national organizing convention came from discussions between himself, the Reverend A. J. Kynett,* Catholic Archbishop John Ireland,* and several others who sought to unite local groups opposed to the traffic with the league already in the field under Howard Hyde Russell.*

Wilson was named a vice president of the new and enlarged organization, a post he held until 1901, when he succeeded to the presidency. The league president was in some respects less powerful than the various league superintendents, who were the group's actual operating officers. Yet the post carried enormous prestige among temperance faithful as well as major public visibility— especially since Wilson held the job for twenty years, through the successful struggle for National Prohibition. With Prohibition a reality, though, the reform-minded bishop finally stepped down, considering that the battle had been won and pointing to the demands of church responsibilities. He devoted his final years to the service of his denomination and to the leadership of the many additional organizations he had become affiliated with over his tenure as bishop (he was on the boards, for example, of some five colleges and universities). His temperance colleagues recalled him as a man of sound judgement and vision, one who "brought. . .the prestige of his ecclesiastical position" to the league he had served with such dedication.

## Bibliography:

A. *Doctrines and Discipline of the Methodist Episcopal Church. . .* (Cincinnati, OH, 1912); *The Trend of the Anti-Saloon League Movement. . .* , Pamphlets on Prohibition in the United States, No. 99 (Westerville, OH, 1913); with others, *Marshalling the Forces of Patriotism. . .* (New York, 1918).

B. SEAP 6, 2861; WW 1, 1363; Ernest Cherrington, *History of the Anti-*

*Saloon League* (Westerville, OH, 1913); Peter Odegard, *Pressure Politics: The Story of the Anti-Saloon League* (New York, 1928).

**WILSON, William Griffith ("Bill W.")**    (26 November 1895, East Dorset, VT—24 January 1971, Miami Beach, FL). *Education*: studied engineering, Norwich Univ., 1914–17; *Career*: artillery officer, U.S. army, 1917–18; stock analyst and broker, New York City, 1920s–1930s; co-founder, Alcoholics Anonymous, 1935; active in fostering growth and managing central affairs of AA, 1935–62; semiretirement, with AA and securities business activity, beginning 1962.

William Wilson, the famous "Bill W." who co-founded Alcoholics Anonymous, grew up in turn-of-the-century Vermont. In his youth, he was physically frail and painfully aware of his inadequacy, he drove himself to excel. He became the captain of his high school baseball team, an accomplished violinist, and conductor of the school orchestra. But that sense of inferiority never left him, and when as an artillery officer in World War I he took his first drink, he found he could bolster his self-confidence with alcohol. Thereafter, like his alcoholic father, he took willingly to the bottle. For the most part, he kept his early drinking under control, but it was already an important part of his life when he entered Wall Street as a securities analyst after the war. Wilson was good at what he did, his acumen earning handsome profits for his employers and for himself during the boom years of the 1920s. But while he could advise clients on their conduct, his own was increasingly mortgaged to alcohol. When his wife, Lois, became alarmed, he excused his drinking with the claim that geniuses did their best work "when drunk." When the Great Crash hit Wall Street in 1929, however, Wilson crashed with it. In his own words, he "became a falling down drunk." From the heights he had plummeted to become "just another guy named Bill who couldn't handle booze."

It was while he was in this condition that Wilson had an experience that changed not only his life but countless thousands of others as well. Recovering from a three-day drunk in the Towns Hospital in New York in 1934, he had recourse to the only solution he believed remained to him—he prayed: "If there is a God let Him show Himself. I am ready to do anything, anything." By his own account, "the room lit up with a great white light. I was caught up into an ecstasy which there are no words to describe." Then came a second fortuitous stroke: a chance meeting with Dr. Robert Holbrook Smith,* an Akron, Ohio, surgeon, who had been seeking a medical cure for alcoholism. The answer, they concluded, was not science but self-help, not medicine but fellowship. Thus was born Alcoholics Anonymous, an organization of alcoholics whose only qualification for membership was and is "a sincere desire to stop drinking." At first, Wilson and Smith believed they needed substantial outside monetary assistance. They approached John D. Rockefeller, Jr., for a major contribution. Mr. Rockefeller, whose father had built something of a reputation for distributing dimes to the needy, turned them down. "I think money will spoil this," he remarked.

(Rockefeller, however, did make a modest contribution which enabled Wilson to maintain his organizational work.) After swallowing his initial disappointment, Wilson concluded that Rockefeller had been right. There would be very little outside money. And there would be total anonymity for everyone, including the founders. In this manner no one would be able to capitalize monetarily on his AA experience. Wilson assumed the cognomen of "Bill W.," and Smith of "Dr. Bob." Wilson took no salary: His only income came from royalties of the books he wrote and some small support from the Rockefeller money. The organization flourished until, at the time of his death, it had 475,000 members in 15,000 chapters in over 100 countries. It was only at the time of his death, on January 24, 1971, that his true identity, known only to intimate acquaintances, was revealed to the public.

Throughout his long years of service to AA, "Bill W." was more than a proselytizer. He was the key figure in the shaping of AA practices and ideas. More than any other single individual, Wilson, drawing on the work of the Oxford Group (to which he acknowledged his intellectual debt), William James, and other sources of inspiration, was responsible for codifying the Twelve Steps and the Twelve Traditions of AA. He also administered the establishment of a central General Service Office for the group in New York City, which assumed the duties of an AA information clearinghouse and publisher of AA literature. It was not all easy: There were serious funding problems from time to time, and at one point critics charged that Wilson and Smith were collecting exorbitant royalties from AA books. Yet on the whole, Wilson kept ahead of the problems and the criticisms and gave the AA fellowship the substance it needed to endure over the long term. Upon his retirement, he could look back on a career that did as much as anyone in American history to bring help to the alcoholic. We should note as well that he did not work alone: Over the years, Lois Wilson, who had stood by him during his drinking, was his strong right arm in nurturing AA and was largely responsible for the establishment of Al-Anon for the families of alcoholics.

### Bibliography:

A. *Alcoholics Anonymous: The Story of How More than One Hundred Men Have Recovered from Alcoholism* (New York, 1939, and many subsequent editions); *Twelve Steps and Twelve Traditions* (New York, 1953); *Twelve Concepts for World Service...* (New York, 1962); *The A.A. Way of Life: Selected Writings of A.A.'s Co-founder: A Reader* (New York, 1967); *Alcoholics Anonymous Comes of Age: A Brief History of A.A.* (New York, 1967).

B. *Newsweek* 77 (Feb. 8, 1971):102; NYT, Jan. 26, 1971; *Time* 97 (Feb. 8, 1971):52; Mark Keller, " 'Bill W.' 1895–1971," *Quarterly Journal of Studies on Alcohol* 32(1971):186–87; Ernest Kurtz, *Not God: A History of Alcoholics Anonymous* (Center City, MN, 1979); Christopher D. Smithers Foundation, *Pioneers We Have Known in the Field of Alcoholism* (Mill Neck, NY, 1979); Robert Thompson, *Bill W.* (New York, 1975).

**WITTENMYER, Annie Turner**    (26 August 1827, Sandy Springs, OH—2 February 1900, Sanatoga, PA). *Education*: secondary education at private sem., 1840s. *Career*: relief agent, various soldiers' aid groups, 1861–65; religious and social charity work, 1865–1900; editor, *Christian Woman*, 1871–82; temperance reformer, 1873–98.

A deeply religious Methodist with an acute sense of social responsibility for the poor and disadvantaged, Annie Wittenmyer made active reform and charitable work an integral part of her life. During the 1850s she devoted most of her time to the affairs of her local (Keokuk, Iowa) Methodist church, which she helped found, and to the support of a school for poor children. But her talents as a reformer came into full flower with the coming of the Civil War. Working with a number of relief agencies, she organized the collection and distribution of medical and other supplies among Union troops throughout the war years. Wittenmyer also served as a front-line nurse and came under enemy fire more than once. Following the war she took the lead in convincing Iowa to assist the orphans of state war dead and used her influence within the Methodist Church to generate denominational action on behalf of the poor. Mrs. Wittenmyer, however, was best known for her labors in the Temperance Movement. Soon after the upsurge of dry sentiment in the "Women's Crusade" of 1873–74, she committed herself to the new cause; and when veterans of the crusade met in Cleveland in late 1874 to found the Woman's Christian Temperance Union, her reputation as an established reformer led to her election as the group's first president. Assisted primarily by WCTU corresponding secretary Frances E. Willard,* Wittenmyer toured the nation lecturing and organizing local unions and rallying support for a federal investigation of the liquor traffic. Characteristically, she interpreted the use of the WCTU in religious terms, believing God had brought it into the field to save the nation from the drink trade.

Mrs. Wittenmyer's presidency ended with some acrimony in 1879, when the union elected Miss Willard in her place. The conflict between the two women had been building for some time, and the younger Willard had, despite her past cooperation with Wittenmyer, already mounted strong challenges for the WCTU presidency in 1877 and 1878. Wittenmyer had always maintained that the union's proper function was a nonpartisan concentration on temperance closely directed by a strong National WCTU, without alliances with any single political party and without becoming involved with other reforms—particularly women's suffrage, which she adamantly opposed. On the other hand, Willard was a champion of suffrage, which she considered an integral and indispensable part of the Temperance Movement, a proponent of cooperation with the Prohibition Party, and an advocate of involving the union with other reform causes. She also favored deemphasizing the authority of the National Union and allowing local chapters considerable freedom of action. Willard's victory was a milestone in the history of the WCTU, and although Mrs. Wittenmyer remained active in the group's affairs, she continued, unsuccessfully, to oppose many of Willard's policies. In 1890, however, along with a number of other dissidents, she formally broke with the group she had once led and helped organize the Non-Partisan Woman's Christian Temperance Union. This new "counter union" was more conservative on social issues than the parent WCTU and opposed women's suffrage; Mrs. Wittenmyer, more comfortable with this than with Willard's group, served as president from 1896 to 1898. At the same time, she remained active in veteran's relief efforts, especially on behalf of former Civil War nurses. At her death she was mourned as one of the premier reformers of her day.

### Bibliography:

A. *Women's Work for Jesus* (Philadelphia?, 1871); *History of the Women's Temperance Crusade* (Philadelphia, 1878); *Women of the Reformation* (Philadelphia, 1884); *Under the Guns* (Philadelphia, 1895).

B. NAW 3, 636–38; SEAP 6, 2888–89; Mary Earhart, *Frances Willard: From Prayers to Politics* (Chicago, 1944); Helen E. Tyler, *Where Prayer and Purpose Meet* (Evanston, IL, 1949); Frances E. Willard, *Woman and Temperance* (Hartford, CT, 1883); Frances E. Willard and Mary A. Livermore, eds., *A Woman of the Century* (New York, 1893).

**WOLFENBARGER, Andrew Givens**   (24 March 1856, Greenbank, VA— 1923, Lincoln, NB). *Education*: LLB., Univ. of Nebraska, circa 1890. *Career*: schoolteacher, IA, NB, 1875–80; editor and co-publisher, *David City* (NB) *Republican*, 1880–85; managing editor, *New Republic*, 1885–90; admitted to bar, NB, 1890.

Born in Virginia, young Andrew Wolfenbarger grew up in Iowa, where his parents moved in 1859. In marginal economic circumstances, the family farm offered Andrew no prospects, and he was forced to shift for himself as an agricultural laborer at age sixteen. By 1875, he had drifted into teaching in both Iowa and Nebraska, a profession he followed until 1880, when he settled in David City, Nebraska, and became editor and part owner of the *David City Republican*. He specialized in political reporting, earning a reputation as a partisan of the Republican Party. Yet over his five years in David City his interest in temperance also grew, and in time he grew disillusioned with the GOP's reluctance to fully embrace the temperance cause. He had joined the Independent Order of Good Templars in 1880, becoming an active and dedicated member. Three years later, his antiliquor sentiments were strong enough to carry him out of the Republican Party and to the small but zealous Prohibition Party. In 1885, he combined his journalistic skills with his temperance dedication, helping to launch and manage a dry publication in the state capital at Lincoln. The journal was titled the *New Republic*, and it soon became one of the more widely-read temperance papers. Of equal importance, in founding the *New Republic* Wolfenbarger brought to public attention one William "Pussyfoot" Johnson,* his co-editor and future giant of the Temperance Movement. Wolfenbarger stayed with the paper until 1890, when he was admitted to the bar.

Though the Prohibition Party was a decade old when Wolfenbarger joined its ranks, he made his presence felt relatively quickly. The Nebraska reformer became an activist whose efforts were visible on both the state and national levels. For example, he led the party and other drys in the battle for state-wide prohibition, and when the drive succeeded, Wolfenbarger received much of the credit. The victory brought him considerable recognition in reform circles across the country. He was also secretary and field manager of the Prohibition State Committee of Nebraska and in 1887 became his state's representative on the Prohibition Party's National Committee. By any standard he was a party war-horse, serving for some fifteen years with genuine dedication in a variety of leading party positions. Among Wolfenbarger's other achievements was his purported ''discovery'' of ''Pussyfoot'' Johnson, a Nebraska Good Templar, Anti-Saloon League worker, and also founding editor of the *New Republic*. Johnson subsequently rose to national fame as a special government officer for the enforcement of the ban on liquor sales in Indian Territory (later Oklahoma). Much later, Johnson recalled that much of his original interest in full-time temperance work had been stimulated by Wolfenbarger. The Nebraska editor also attained eminence as a Templar, acquiring a succession of those grandiose titles (''deputy right worthy grand templar for the Western Hemisphere,'' and others) to which that organization was addicted. He made lecture tours through thirty-one states on behalf of Good Templary and National Prohibition, and twice visited Canada on similar missions.

**Bibliography:**

A. ed., *Nebraska Legislative Yearbook for 1897...* (Lincoln, NB, 1897).
B. SEAP 6, 2890.

**WOOLLEY, John Granville**   (15 February 1850, Collinsville, OH—13 August 1922, Spain). *Education*: A.B., Ohio Wesleyan Univ., 1871; A.M., Ohio Wesleyan Univ., 1874; LLD., Ohio Wesleyan Univ., 1906; B.L., Univ. of Michigan, 1873. *Career*: legal practice in IL, MN, NY, 1873–86; temperance lecturer, editor, politician, and author, 1888–1922.

John Granville Woolley was one of the great travelling orators in the Prohibition movement. Himself a victim of alcoholism, Woolley in 1888 ''became,'' in his own words, ''a Christian and a party Prohibitionist at the same instant.'' He left what had been, apparently a successful career as an attorney (in Paris, Illinois, Minneapolis, and New York City), and followed a calling that would lead him to a strenuous life of speaking engagements and publication efforts throughout the United States and the world. He became the Prohibitionist candidate for the presidency in 1900 (he had refused the nomination in 1896), campaigned energetically on a ''Prohibition Special'' train, and obtained a vote of over 209,000, the biggest ever for a candidate of that party. While active in Prohibition Party politics, Woolley attempted to heal the rift between the party and the nonpartisan Anti-Saloon League—which preferred working with Republican and Democratic candidates. He argued that while the Prohibitionists could not win elections, temperance workers should affiliate with the party out of moral conviction, while as a practical measure voting for the league-endorsed candidates of the major parties. Woolley's position, articulated in 1903, was a sign of recognition in temperance ranks that third-party politics was ineffective as a means of bringing about national prohibition.

Besides his formidable oratorical talent, the key to Woolley's special appeal was his fusion of prohibitionism with the Gospel of Christianity. In particular he regarded the saloon as an antithesis to the church, and prohibitionism as an agent for renewal of the church's influence. (He himself had joined the Church of the Strangers in New York upon his conversion.) From 1899 to 1906 Woolley brought this point of view to the editorship of the *New Voice*, which developed under his hand into the preeminent periodical of the Prohibitionist cause. In 1892–93, under the auspices of Lady Somerset, he had evangelized with spectacular success in England, and after the election of 1900 he returned to England with identical results. In 1901 and 1905 he toured the world. The enthusiastic response of huge audiences in New Zealand, especially, is reported to have powerfully catalyzed the Prohibition movement in that country. His seemingly indefatigable zeal for lecturing was nearly matched by his literary output, most of which consisted, however, simply of reprints of his speeches and editorials. Though his books have been described as "ephemeral and superficial," they were popular types of the prohibitionist genre and embodied the tone of Christian warmth and humanity that was a critical element in his speaking style as well. Aside from such works, he also produced (with W. E. Johnson*) the more substantial *Temperance Progress in the Nineteenth Century* (1903) and conceived the *Standard Encyclopedia of the Alcohol Problem*, which was completed after his death. Failing health brought Woolley to retirement in 1921; but when his wife died a short while later he sought consolation in studying the alcohol problem in Europe for the World League Against Alcoholism. He died at this task in 1922 while in Spain, and is said to have wished for just such an end, "in active service for the cause of sobriety."

### Bibliography:

A. *The Christian Citizen* (Chicago, 1900); *Seed* (New York, 1903); with William E. Johnson, *Temperance Progress in the Nineteenth Century* (Philadelphia, 1903); with Mary V. Woolley, *South Sea Letters* (Chicago, 1906).

B. DAB 20, 515–16; NYT, Aug. 14, 1922; SEAP 6, 2909–10; WW 1, 1381; W.D.P. Bliss, ed., *New Encyclopedia of Social Reform* (New York, 1908); Jack S. Blocker, Jr., *Retreat from Reform: The Prohibition Movement in the United States, 1890–1913* (Westport, CT, 1976).

# X Y Z

**YEAMES, James** (7 January 1843, Dover, England—?). *Education*: private study of theology, 1860s. *Career*: schoolteacher, 1860s; ordained, Church of England, 1863; publisher, *The Templar*, 1871–83; minister, Boston, 1883–97; minister, St. John's Episcopal Church, Arlington, MA, 1897–1912; retirement, 1912.

The career of James Yeames illustrates something of the international character of the Temperance Movement. Born in Dover, England, after several years of teaching and study for the ministry he was ordained in the Church of England (1863). But his immediate concern was not the pulpit; rather, Yeames became deeply involved with British temperance activities. He had developed a keen interest in the liquor question by age thirteen, and he remained active in the dry cause for more than sixty years thereafter. In 1871, along with a fellow member of the fraternal Independent Order of Good Templars, he founded and edited Britain's first illustrated weekly temperance journal, *The Templar*. As the official publication of the Grand Lodge of the Templars, it enjoyed a circulation of thirty thousand. Yeames also tried to appeal to young readers with the *Juvenile Templar* and *Sunrise*, magazines he also originated. Indeed, the young had a special appeal for Yeames, a fact further reflected in his appointment as grand superintendent of juvenile templars, a post he held between 1871 and 1878. He took the job seriously indeed, and personally wrote the group's constitution and developed its ritual. Tireless in the reform effort, by the 1880s he was one of the best-known drys in his native country. In 1885, however, perhaps answering a call to a parish, Yeames immigrated to the United States. He took up residence first in Boston, later moving to Arlington, Massachusetts, where he became rector of St. John's Episcopal Church (he remained there until his retirement in 1912). Yeames remained active in antiliquor matters in his new home, soon joining the Good Templars in America. He was a bulwark of the lodge and even organized a highly novel charity: Under his direction, the local Templars financed the outfitting of a "Good Templar lifeboat" on the Massachusetts coast. On at least one occasion the boat rescued the crew of a German ship wrecked in the locale. The incident brought the fraternal order and Yeames considerable publicity, although upon his retirement the British-born reformer and minister dropped out of the public eye.

**Bibliography:**

A. *The Book of Temperance Songs* (n.p., 1869).
B. SEAP 6, 2929.

# APPENDICES

# APPENDIX I
# Listing by Birthplace

This appendix offers an alphabetical listing of temperance leaders by their states or countries of birth. The first section lists all individuals born in the United States; the second holds those from other countries. All former colonies, territories, and other political units are listed under their current names. Missing or questionable information is designated with a question mark.

While the information presented here can support certain inferences about the geographical origins and spread of the Temperance Movement and related activity, it is well to keep in mind the limits of the data. The following entries do *not* constitute a random sample of temperance leadership. In the first place, as I noted in the Preface, *leadership* is a subjective term: My list includes some individuals whom many drys would not have considered leaders. It excludes others with valid claims. I did not include everyone; I did not try. Rather, my concern was to show the variety in temperance thought and action, as well as to demonstrate the diversity of persons who in some manner contributed to the cause. Also, temperance careers often developed in areas far removed from an individual's birthplace. New York, for example, was the original home of many drys who never expressed any interest in the antiliquor reform until long after settling elsewhere. Still, the following tabulation provides one of the largest available sources of demographic information on the men and women who lent their efforts against alcohol-related problems in the United States.

## UNITED STATES

| *Name* | *Birthdate* | *Birthplace* |
| --- | --- | --- |
| ALABAMA | | |
| Horace Mellard Du Bose | 7 November 1858 | Mobile |
| Richmond Pearson Hobson | 17 August 1870 | Greensboro |
| Samuel Porter Jones | 16 October 1847 | Chambers County |
| Samuel David Weakley | 16 July 1860 | Somerville |
| ARKANSAS | | |
| Arthur James Barton | 2 February 1867 | near Jamesboro |
| CALIFORNIA | | |
| Arthur Hislop Briggs | ? 1858 | San Francisco |
| Alexander Patrick Doyle | 28 February 1857 | San Francisco |

| Name | Birthdate | Birthplace |
|------|-----------|------------|

**CONNECTICUT**

| Name | Birthdate | Birthplace |
|------|-----------|------------|
| Phineas Taylor Barnum | 5 July 1810 | Bethel |
| Lyman Beecher | 12 October 1775 | New Haven |
| Sarah Knowles Bolton | 15 September 1841 | Farmington |
| William Alfred Buckingham | 28 May 1804 | Norwich |
| William Henry Burleigh | 2 February 1812 | Woodstock |
| William Earl Dodge | 4 September 1805 | Hartford |
| Andrew Hull Foote | 12 September 1806 | New Haven |
| Nathaniel Hewit | 28 August 1788 | New London |
| Heman Humphrey | 26 March 1779 | West Simsbury |
| Mary Hannah Hanchett Hunt | 4 June 1830 | Canaan |
| Charles Jewett | 5 September 1807 | Lisbon |
| John Marsh | 12 April 1788 | Wethersfield |
| Emily Clark Huntington Miller | 22 October 1833 | Brooklyn |
| Eliphalet Nott | 25 June 1773 | Ashford |
| John Pierpont | 6 April 1785 | Litchfield |
| Gifford Pinchot | 11 August 1865 | Simsbury |
| Moses Stuart | 26 March 1780 | Wilton |
| Reuben Hyde Walworth | 26 October 1786 | Bozrah |
| Charles Seymour Whitman | 28 August 1868 | Hanover |

**DELAWARE**

| Name | Birthdate | Birthplace |
|------|-----------|------------|
| Clarence True Wilson | 24 April 1872 | Milton |

**GEORGIA**

| Name | Birthdate | Birthplace |
|------|-----------|------------|
| Mary Harris Armor | 9 March 1863 | Penfield |
| Alfred Holt Colquitt | 20 April 1824 | Waltor County |
| Rebecca Latimer Felton | 10 June 1835 | DeKalb County |
| Henry Woodfin Grady | 1 December 1832 | Athens |
| Lamartine Griffin Hardman | 14 April 1856 | Commerce |
| Joseph Henry Lumpkin | 23 December 1799 | Oglethorpe |
| William Jonathan Northen | 9 July 1835 | Jones County |
| Colemen Roberson Pringle | 1830s | Monroe County? |
| William David Upshaw | 15 October 1866 | Newman |

**ILLINOIS**

| Name | Birthdate | Birthplace |
|------|-----------|------------|
| William Hamilton Anderson | 8 August 1874 | Carlinville |
| William Wirt Bennett | 10 October 1869 | Oregon |
| William Jennings Bryan | 19 March 1860 | Salem |
| Anna Marden De Yo | 18 October 1868 | Glasgow |
| Jasper L. Douthit | 10 October 1834 | Shelby County |
| Jervice Gaylord Evans | 19 December 1833 | Wenona |
| James Franklin Hanly | 4 April 1863 | St. Joseph |
| Wesley Livsey Jones | 9 October 1863 | Bethany |
| George McGinnis | 28 July 1858 | Mendota |

| Name | Birthdate | Birthplace |
|------|-----------|------------|
| Eugenia Florenci St. John Mann | ? 1847 | Kane County |
| Marty Mann | 15 October 1904 | Chicago |
| George Washington Morrow | 27 May 1863 | Champaign County |
| Margaret Cairns Munns | 10 August 1870 | Fairbury |
| Robert Howard Patton | 18 January 1860 | Auburn |
| Frank Stewart Regan | 3 October 1862 | Rockford |
| Sarah Hackett Stevenson | 2 February 1843 | Buffalo Grove |
| Oliver Wayne Stewart | 22 May 1867 | Mercer County |
| Ralph Seymour Thompson | 19 December 1847 | Albion |
| George Thornburgh | 25 January 1847 | Havana |
| Wayne Cullen Williams | 20 September 1878 | near Indianola |

## INDIANA

| | | |
|------|-----------|------------|
| Elizabeth Preston Anderson | 27 April 1861 | Decatur |
| Howard Wilcox Haggard | 18 July 1891 | LaPorte |
| Mary Garrett Hay | 29 August 1857 | Charlestown |
| Ferdinand Cowle Inglehart | 8 December 1845 | Warrick County |
| Little Turtle | 1752? | near Fort Wayne |
| Samuel Edgar Nicholson | 29 June 1862 | Azalia |
| John Pierce St. John | 25 February 1833 | Brookville |
| Newell Sanders | 12 July 1850 | Owen County |
| Amanda Way | 10 July 1828 | Winchester |
| Harvey Washington Wiley | 18 October 1834 | Kent |

## IOWA

| | | |
|------|-----------|------------|
| Virgil Goodman Hinshaw | 15 January 1876 | Woolson |
| Harold Everett Hughes | 10 February 1922 | Ida Grove |
| William Ashley Sunday | 19 November 1862 | Ames |

## KANSAS

| | | |
|------|-----------|------------|
| Karl Murdock Bowman | 4 November 1888 | Topeka |
| Arthur Capper | 14 July 1865 | Garnett |

## KENTUCKY

| | | |
|------|-----------|------------|
| George Washington Bain | 24 September 1840 | Lexington |
| Alben William Barkley | 24 November 1877 | Grover County |
| Yandell Henderson | 23 April 1873 | Louisville |
| Thomas Francis Marshall | 7 June 1801 | Frankfort |
| Carry Amelia Moore Nation | 25 November 1846 | Garrard County |
| Green Clay Smith | 4 July 1826 | Madison |
| Zarelda Gray Sanders Wallace | 6 August 1817 | Millersburg |

## LOUISIANA

| | | |
|------|-----------|------------|
| Caroline Elizabeth Thomas Merrick | 24 November 1825 | East Feliciana Parish |

| *Name* | *Birthdate* | *Birthplace* |
|--------|-------------|--------------|

**MAINE**

| | | |
|--------|-------------|--------------|
| George Barrell Cheever | 6 February 1814 | Hallowell |
| Wilbur Fisk Crafts | 12 January 1850 | Fryeburg |
| Albert Day | ? October 1812 | Wells |
| Nelson Dingley | 15 February 1832 | Durham |
| Neal Dow | 20 March 1804 | Portland |
| William Thomas Haines | 7 August 1854 | Levant |
| Oliver Otis Howard | 8 November 1830 | Leeds |
| Charles Edgar Littlefield | 21 June 1851 | Lebanon |
| John Davis Long | 27 October 1838 | Buckfield |
| Joshua Knox Osgood | 11 November 1816 | Gardiner |
| Sidney Perham | 27 March 1819 | Woodstock |
| Henry Augustus Reynolds | 9 November 1839 | Bangor |
| Lillian Marion Norton Ames Stevens | 1 March 1844 | Dover |
| Joseph E. Turner | ? 1832 | Bath |

**MARYLAND**

| | | |
|--------|-------------|--------------|
| Martha McClellan Brown | 18 April 1838 | Baltimore |
| Charles Force Deems | 4 December 1820 | Baltimore |
| Ninian Edwards | 17 March 1775 | Montgomery County |
| Frances Ellen Watkins Harper | 24 September 1825 | Baltimore |
| John Henry Willis Hawkins | 23 October 1799 | Baltimore |
| Joshua Levering | 12 September 1845 | Baltimore |
| Mervin Louis Maus | 8 May 1851 | Burnt Mills |
| Luther Barton Wilson | 14 November 1856 | Baltimore |

**MASSACHUSETTS**

| | | |
|--------|-------------|--------------|
| Susan Brownell Anthony | 15 February 1820 | Adams |
| James Appleton | 14 February 1785 | Ipswich |
| Melbourne Parker Boynton | 6 November 1867 | Lynn |
| George Nixon Briggs | 12 April 1796 | Adams |
| Caroline Brown Buell | 24 October 1843 | Marlboro |
| Morris Edward Chafetz | 20 April 1924 | Worcester |
| James Mathew Cleary | 8 September 1849 | Dedham |
| Russell Herman Conwell | 15 Feburary 1843 | Worthington |
| David Daggett | 31 December 1764 | Attleboro |
| Samuel Dexter | 14 May 1761 | Boston |
| Daniel Dorchester | 11 March 1827 | Duxbury |
| Justin Edwards | 25 April 1787 | Westhampton |
| Judith Ellen Horton Foster | 3 November 1840 | Lowell |
| Lydia Folger Fowler | 5 May 1822 | Nantucket |
| William Lloyd Garrison | 10 December 1805 | Newburyport |
| Anna Adams Gordon | 21 July 1853 | Boston |
| Edward Everett Hale | 3 April 1822 | Boston |
| Samuel Dexter Hastings | 24 July 1816 | Leicester |

| *Name* | *Birthdate* | *Birthplace* |
|---|---|---|
| Mark Hopkins | 4 February 1802 | Stockbridge |
| Nathan Whitman Littlefield | 21 May 1846 | Bridgewater |
| Mary Ashton Livermore | 19 December 1821 | Boston |
| Raymond Gerald McCarthy | 30 April 1901 | Brockton |
| Horace Mann | 4 May 1796 | Franklin |
| Increase Mather | 21 June 1639 | Dorchester |
| Frederick Merrick | 29 January 1810 | Wilbraham |
| Dwight Lyman Moody | 5 February 1837 | Northfield |
| Lucretia Coffin Mott | 3 January 1793 | Nantucket |
| Peter Joseph O'Callaghan | 6 August 1866 | Mulford |
| Charles Henry Payne | 24 October 1830 | Taunton |
| Samuel Freeman Pearson | 16 July 1841 | Roxbury |
| Wendell Phillips | 29 November 1811 | Boston |
| Lucius Manlius Sargent | 25 June 1786 | Boston |
| John Lawrence Sullivan | 15 October 1858 | Boston |
| John Collins Warren | 1 August 1778 | Boston |

## MICHIGAN

| | | |
|---|---|---|
| Leonard Bacon | 19 February 1802 | Detroit |
| Helen Mar Jackson Gougar | 18 July 1843 | Litchfield |
| John Harvey Kellogg | 26 February 1852 | Tyrone |

## MINNESOTA

| | | |
|---|---|---|
| Bertha Rachel Palmer | 31 August 1880 | Graham Lakes |
| Howard Hyde Russell | 21 October 1855 | Stillwater |

## MISSISSIPPI

| | | |
|---|---|---|
| Belle Kearney | 6 March 1863 | Vernon |

## MISSOURI

| | | |
|---|---|---|
| James Cannon, Jr. | 13 November 1864 | Salisbury |
| Charles Martin Hay | 10 November 1879 | Wayne County |
| Eliza Buckley Ingalls | 24 August 1848 | St. Louis |
| William Jefferson Pollard | 1 May 1860 | Kingston |

## NEBRASKA

| | | |
|---|---|---|
| Charles Hiram Randall | 23 July 1865 | Auburn |
| Cora Frances Stoddard | 17 September 1872 | Irvington |

## NEVADA

| | | |
|---|---|---|
| Johnson Sides | ? | ? |

| *Name* | *Birthdate* | *Birthplace* |
|---|---|---|

**NEW HAMPSHIRE**

| | | |
|---|---|---|
| Henry William Blair | 6 December 1834 | Campton |
| Benjamin Franklin Butler | 5 November 1818 | Deerfield |
| Lewis Cass | 9 October 1782 | Exeter |
| Lorenzo Sweet Coffin | 9 April 1823 | Alton |
| Noah Davis | 10 September 1818 | Haverhill |
| Adoniram Judson Gordon | 19 April 1836 | New Hampton |
| Horace Greeley | 3 February 1811 | Amherst |
| Edward Kent | 8 January 1802 | Concord |
| Mary Greenleaf Clement Leavitt | 22 September 1830 | Hopkinton |
| Alonzo Ames Miner | 17 August 1814 | Lempster |
| Reuben Dimond Mussey | 23 June 1780 | Pelham |
| Willard Parker | 2 September 1800 | Lyndeborough |
| John Newton Stearns | 24 May 1829 | New Ipswich |
| Henry Wilson | 12 February 1812 | Farmington |

**NEW JERSEY**

| | | |
|---|---|---|
| Daniel Agnew | 5 January 1809 | Trenton |
| Theodore Frelinghuysen | 28 March 1787 | Franklin Township |
| Matthew Newkirk | 31 May 1794 | Pittsgrove |

**NEW YORK**

| | | |
|---|---|---|
| Timothy Shay Arthur | 6 June 1809 | Newburgh |
| Henry Warren Austin | 1 August 1828 | Skaneateles |
| James Emory Norton Backus | 13 September 1835 | Minden |
| Seldon Daskam Bacon | 10 December 1909 | Pleasantville |
| Hannah Johnston Bailey | 5 July 1839 | Cornwall-on-the-Hudson |
| Helen Morton Barker | 7 or 8 December 1834 | Rickville |
| Albert Barnes | 1 December 1789 | Rome |
| Frances Julia Allis Barnes | 14 April 1846 | Skaneateles |
| John Bascom | 1 May 1827 | Genoa |
| Josephine Abiah Penfield Cushman Bateham | 1 November 1829 | Alden |
| Charles Eugene Bentley | 30 April 1841 | Warner's |
| John Bidwell | 5 August 1819 | Ripley Hills |
| Amelia Jenks Bloomer | 27 May 1818 | Homer |
| Helen Louise Bullock | 29 April 1836 | Norwich |
| Myron Holley Clark | 23 October 1806 | Naples |
| Julia Colman | 16 February 1828 | Troy |
| Howard Crosby | 21 February 1826 | New York |
| Thomas Davidson Crothers | 21 September 1842 | Charlton |
| Theodore Ledyard Cuyler | 10 January 1822 | Aurora |
| Nathan Smith Davis | 9 January 1817 | Greene |
| Edward Cornelius Delavan | 6 January 1793 | Westchester County |
| Elmer Ephraim Ellsworth | 11 April 1837 | Malta |

| Name | Birthdate | Birthplace |
| --- | --- | --- |
| William Porter Frisbee Ferguson | 13 December 1861 | Delhi |
| Irving Fisher | 27 February 1867 | Saugerties |
| Clinton Bowen Fisk | 8 December 1828 | Clapp's Corners |
| William Goodell | 25 October 1792 | Coventry |
| Elizabeth Ward Greenwood | 6 February 1850 | Brooklyn |
| Emil Louis George Hohenthal | 15 October 1864 | New York |
| Alphonso Alva Hopkins | 27 March 1843 | Burlington Flats |
| Elvin Morton Jellinek | 15 August 1890 | New York |
| William Eugene Johnson | 25 March 1862 | Coventry |
| Edward Norris Kirk | 14 August 1802 | New York |
| Albert Gallatin Lawson | 5 June 1842 | Poughkeepsie |
| Dioclesian Lewis | 3 March 1823 | Auburn |
| David Ross Locke | 20 September 1833 | Vestal |
| Harriet Calista Clark McCabe | 19 January 1827 | Sidney Plains |
| Catherine Gouger Waugh McCulloch | 4 June 1862 | Ransomville |
| Lewis Duncan Mason | 20 June 1843 | Brooklyn |
| James Burtis Merwin | 22 May 1822 | Cairo |
| Edward Jay Moore | 6 September 1861 | Norwich |
| Valentine Mott | 20 August 1785 | Glen Cove |
| Charles Andrew Pollack | 21 September 1853 | Elizabethtown |
| Alonzo Potter | 6 July 1800 | Beekman |
| Nathaniel Scudder Prime | 21 April 1785 | Huntington |
| Seth Reed | 2 June 1823 | Hartwick |
| Tapping Reeve | ? October 1744 | Brookhaven |
| Louise S. Jones Rounds | 6 July 1839 | Heuvelton |
| John Russell | 20 September 1822 | Livingston County |
| Charles Henry St. John | 18 September 1843 | near Auburn |
| John Savage | 22 February 1779 | New York |
| Charles Moore Sheldon | 26 February 1857 | Wellsville |
| Frank J. Sibley | 11 August 1847 | Royalton |
| William Duncan Silkworth | 22 July 1877 | Brooklyn |
| Gerrit Smith | 6 March 1797 | Utica |
| Robert Brinkley Smithers | 30 July 1907 | Glen Cove |
| Charles Stelzle | 4 June 1869 | New York |
| Katharine Adelia Lent Stevenson | 8 May 1853 | Copake |
| Gideon Tabor Stewart | 7 August 1824 | Johnston |
| Stephen Van Rensselear | 1 November 1764 | New York |
| Francis Wayland | 11 March 1796 | New York |
| Frances Elizabeth Caroline Willard | 28 September 1839 | Churchville |

NORTH CAROLINA

| Name | Birthdate | Birthplace |
| --- | --- | --- |
| Josephus Daniels | 18 May 1862 | Washington |
| Robert Brodnax Glenn | 11 August 1854 | Rockingham County |
| Timothy Nicholson | 9 November 1828 | Belvidere |
| Edwin Yates Webb | 23 May 1872 | Shelby |

| *Name* | *Birthdate* | *Birthplace* |
|--------|-------------|--------------|
| **OHIO** | | |
| Purley Albert Baker | 10 April 1858 | Jackson County |
| Lou Jenks Beauchamp | 14 January 1851 | Cincinnati |
| Ella Alexander Boole | 26 July 1858 | Van Wert |
| Justin Dewitt Bowersock | 19 September 1842 | New Alexander |
| Marie Caroline Brehm | 30 June 1859 | Sandusky |
| Samuel Fenton Cary | 18 February 1814 | Cincinnati |
| Ernest Hurst Cherrington | 24 November 1877 | Hamden |
| David Leigh Colvin | 28 January 1880 | South Charleston |
| Mamie White Colvin | 12 June 1883 | Westview |
| Edwin Courtland Dinwiddie | 29 September 1867 | Springfield |
| Edwin Othello Excell | 13 December 1851 | Uniontown |
| Herman Preston Faris | 25 December 1858 | Bellefontaine |
| Isaac Kaufman Funk | 10 September 1839 | Clifton |
| Frances Dana Barker Gage | 12 October 1808 | Marietta |
| David Harvey Goodell | 6 May 1834 | Hillsboro |
| Lucy Ware Webb Hayes | 28 August 1831 | Chillicothe |
| Grant Martin Hudson | 23 July 1868 | Eaton Township |
| Lewis Henry Keller | 24 February 1858 | Upper Sandusky |
| William Squire Kenyon | 10 June 1869 | Elyria |
| Adna Wright Leonard | 2 November 1874 | Cincinnati |
| Francis Scott McBride | 29 July 1872 | Carroll County |
| George Martin Mathews | 22 August 1848 | Hamilton County |
| Duncan Chambers Milner | 10 March 1841 | Mt. Pleasant |
| Henrietta Greer Moore | 2 September 1844 | Newark |
| Norman Austin Palmer | 3 February 1853 | Pataskal |
| Preston Bierce Plumb | 12 October 1837 | Delaware County |
| Esther Pugh | 31 August 1834 | Cincinnati |
| Edward Seitz Shumaker | 30 July 1867 | Greenville |
| Addison Taylor Smith | 5 September 1862 | Cambridge |
| Eliza Daniel Stewart | 25 April 1816 | Piketon |
| Tenkswatawa | 17 March 1768 | near Old Chillicothe |
| Eliza Jane Trimble Thompson | 24 August 1816 | Hillsboro |
| Homer Tope | 28 May 1859 | Del Roy |
| Aaron Sherman Watkins | 29 November 1863 | Rushsylvania |
| Wayne Bidwell Wheeler | 10 November 1869 | Brookfield |
| Annie Turner Wittenmyer | 26 August 1827 | Sandy Springs |
| John Granville Woolley | 15 February 1850 | Collinsville |
| **OREGON** | | |
| Louis Albert Banks | 12 November 1855 | Corvallis |
| Daniel Alfred Poling | 30 November 1884 | Portland |
| **PENNSYLVANIA** | | |
| Ernest Francis Acheson | 19 September 1855 | Washington |
| Robert Baird | 6 October 1798 | near Pittsburgh |

| Name | Birthdate | Birthplace |
|------|-----------|------------|
| James Addams Beaver | 21 October 1837 | Millerstown |
| Ada Matilda Cole Bittenbender | 3 August 1848 | Macedonia |
| James Black | 23 September 1823 | Lewisburg |
| David James Burrell | 1 August 1844 | Mt. Pleasant |
| Harry Malcolm Chalfant | 26 June 1869 | Coal Center |
| Joshua Reed Giddings | 6 October 1795 | Athens |
| Solomon Washington Gladden | 11 February 1836 | Pottsgrove |
| Sarepta M. Henry | 4 November 1839 | Albion |
| Jacob Hostetter Hoofstitler | 9 January 1846 | Salunga |
| Clinton Norman Howard | 28 July 1868 | Pottsville |
| Charles Reading Jones | 9 November 1862 | near Philadelphia |
| Sabastian Spering Kresge | 31 July 1867 | Bald Mount |
| Alpha Jefferson Kynett | 12 August 1829 | Adams County |
| John Alexander Martin | 10 March 1839 | Brownsville |
| Joseph Parrish | 11 November 1818 | Philadelphia |
| Hiram Price | 10 January 1814 | Washington County |
| Benjamin Rush | 24 December 1746 | Philadelphia |
| Hannah Whitall Smith | 7 February 1832 | Philadelphia |
| Ida Belle Speakman Wise Smith | 3 July 1871 | Philadelphia |
| Adie Allen Stevens | 20 August 1845 | Blair County |
| Silas Comfort Swallow | 5 March 1839 | near Wilkes Barre |
| Uriah Frantz Swengel | 28 October 1876 | Middlebury |
| Henry Adams Thompson | 23 March 1837 | Stormstown |

RHODE ISLAND

| William Ellery Channing | 7 April 1780 | Newport |

SOUTH CAROLINA

| Sarah Flournoy Moore Chapin | 14 March 1830? | Charleston |
| John Belton O'Neall | 10 April 1793 | Bush River |

TENNESSEE

| Edgar Estes Folk | 6 September 1856 | Haywood County |
| Joseph Wingate Folk | 28 October 1869 | Brownsville |
| Elijah Embree Hoss | 14 April 1849 | Washington County |
| David Campbell Kelley | 25 December 1833 | Wilson County |
| George Rutledge Stuart | 14 December 1857 | Talbotts Station |

TEXAS

| James Britton Cranfill | 12 September 1858 | Parker County |
| Ira Landrith | 23 March 1865 | Milford |
| William Henry Murray | 21 November 1869 | Collinsville |
| Morris Sheppard | 28 May 1875 | Wheatville |

VERMONT

| Jeremiah Evarts | 3 February 1781 | Sunderland |

| Name | Birthdate | Birthplace |
|------|-----------|------------|
| Wilbur Fisk | 31 August 1792 | Brattleboro |
| James Willis Gleed | 8 March 1859 | Morrisville |
| Angelina French Thurston Kilgore Newman | 4 December 1837 | Montpelier |
| Robert Holbrook Smith | 8 August 1879 | St. Johnsbury |
| Culla Johnson Vayhinger | 25 September 1867 | Bennington |
| William Griffith Wilson | 26 November 1895 | East Dorset |

VIRGINIA

| | | |
|------|-----------|------------|
| Jacob Smith Boreman | 4 August 1831 | Middlebourne |
| William Gannaway Brownlow | 29 August 1805 | Wythe County |
| Thomas Rosabaum Carskadon | 17 May 1837 | Sheetz's Mill |
| John Hartwell Cocke | 19 September 1780 | Surry County |
| Josiah Flournoy | 17 March 1789 | Dinwiddie County |
| Felix Grundy | 11 September 1777 | Berkeley County |
| Matthew Simpson Hughes | 2 February 1863 | Doddridge County |
| Robert Latham Owen | 2 February 1856 | Lynchburg |
| Frederick Dunglison Power | 23 January 1851 | Yorktown |
| Emma Frances Sanford Shelton | ? | Montrose |
| Edward Thompson Taylor | 25 December 1793 | Richmond |
| Allen Trimble | 24 November 1783 | Augusta County |
| Andrew Givens Wolfenbarger | 24 March 1856 | Greenback |

WEST VIRGINIA

| | | |
|------|-----------|------------|
| Norman Hayhurst Jolliffe | 18 August 1901 | Knob Fork |
| Charles Scanlon | 5 October 1869 | Three Churches |

WISCONSIN

| | | |
|------|-----------|------------|
| Eugene Wilder Chafin | 1 November 1852 | East Troy |
| Edith Smith Davis | 20 January 1859 | Milton |
| John Faville | 7 July 1847 | Milford |
| George Hartshorn Hodges | 6 February 1866 | Orion |
| Stella Blanchard Irvine | 21 July 1859 | Beaver Dam |
| John Brown Lennon | 12 October 1850 | Lafayette County |
| Ella Wheeler Wilcox | 5 November 1850 | Johnston Center |
| Alonzo Edes Wilson | 5 February 1868 | Madison |

## OTHER COUNTRIES

AUSTRIA

| | | |
|------|-----------|------------|
| Mark Keller | 21 February 1907 | ? |

CANADA

| | | |
|------|-----------|------------|
| Joseph Flintoft Berry | 13 May 1856 | Aylmer |
| Samuel Dickie | 6 June 1851 | Oxford |
| Charles Henry Fowler | 11 August 1837 | Burford |

| Name | Birthdate | Birthplace |
|------|-----------|------------|
| Jacob H. Gallinger | 28 March 1837 | Cornwall |
| John Henry Hector | 17 March 1847 | Windsor |
| Donald Campbell MacCleod | 13 November 1869 | Nova Scotia |
| Thomas Nicholson | 27 January 1862 | Woodburn |
| Richard Hugh Scott | 23 July 1869 | Renfrew |
| Jennie Fowler Willing | 22 January 1834 | Buford |

ENGLAND

| | | |
|------|-----------|------------|
| Francis Asbury | 20 August 1745 | Handsworth |
| Evangeline Cory Booth | 25 December 1865 | London |
| Elizabeth Leslie Rous Comstock | 30 October 1815 | Maidenhead |
| George Fletcher Cotterill | 18 November 1865 | Oxford |
| Samuel Fallows | 13 December 1835 | Pendleton |
| John Bartholomew Gough | 22 August 1817 | Sandgate |
| Joseph Malins | 21 October 1844 | Worcester |
| Alfred Noon | 8 December 1845 | Elstead |
| William Ross | 25 December 1812 | London |
| Anna Howard Shaw | 14 February 1847 | Newcastle-upon-Tyne |
| John Lloyd Thomas | 22 April 1857 | Wilton Park |
| James Yeames | 7 January 1843 | Dover |

FRANCE

| | | |
|------|-----------|------------|
| Anthony Benezet | 31 January 1713 | St. Quentin |

GERMANY

| | | |
|------|-----------|------------|
| Simon Bamberger | 27 February 1847 | Darmstadt |
| Henrietta Skelton | 5 November 1842 | Giessen |

IRELAND

| | | |
|------|-----------|------------|
| Matilda Bradley Carse | 19 November 1835 | Saintfield |
| John Chambers | 19 December 1797 | Stewartstown |
| John Francis Cunneen | 21 May 1868 | Limrick |
| John Ireland | ? 1838 | Burnchurch |
| Leslie Enraught Keeley | ? 1832 | Kings County |
| Jeremiah McAuley | 1839? | ? |
| Theobald Mathew | 10 October 1790 | Thomastown House |
| Francis Murphy | 24 April 1836 | Wexford |

NETHERLANDS

| | | |
|------|-----------|------------|
| Edward William Bok | 9 October 1863 | Helder |

SCOTLAND

| | | |
|------|-----------|------------|
| Robert McIntyre | 20 November 1851 | Selkirk |
| Robert Valentine Muir | 23 October 1826 | ? |

SWEDEN

| | | |
|------|-----------|------------|
| David Ostlund | 19 May 1870 | Orebro |

# APPENDIX II
# Listing by Religious Affiliation

Religion was often an important element in the shaping of temperance sympathies, and most of the individuals included in this volume (although by no means all of them) maintained a denominational affiliation. They are listed below by denomination, subject to the same statistical cautions noted in Appendix I. Again, doubtful or missing information is noted with a question mark. All individuals are classed in the denomination in which they maintained their longest affiliation or made their most substantial expression of faith. A denomination in parentheses represents a former affiliation from which the person converted. People not listed in any category were not necessarily unchurched; most were evidently Protestants, although there was insufficient information to place them in a specific denominational group.

AFRICAN METHODIST

John Henry Hector

BAPTIST

Arthur James Barton
Charles Eugene Bentley
Melbourne Parker Boynton
George Nixon Briggs
Lorenzo Sweet Coffin
Russell Herman Conwell
James Britton Cranfill
Josiah Flournoy?
Adoniram Judson Gordon
Lamartine Griffin Hardman
Richmond Pearson Hobson
Clinton Norman Howard
Grant Martin Hudson
Albert Gallatin Lawson

Mary Greenleaf Clement Leavitt
Joshua Levering
George McGinnis
Margaret Cairns Munns
William Jonathan Northen
John Belton O'Neall
David Ostlund (Seventh Day Adventist)
Coleman Roberson Pringle?
Newell Sanders
Green Clay Smith
Lillian Marion Norton Ames Stevens
William David Upshaw
Francis Wayland
Samuel David Weakley?

CONGREGATIONALIST

James Appleton
Leonard Bacon
John Bascom

Lyman Beecher
William Wirt Bennett
Sarah Knowles Bolton

Justine Dewitt Bowersock
William Alfred Buckingham
Matilda Bradley Carse
George Barrell Cheever
Myron Holley Clark?
Thomas Davidson Crothers?
David Daggett
Edward Cornelius Delavan?
Samuel Dexter
Justin Edwards
Jeremiah Evarts
Irving Fisher
Lydia Folger Fowler
Solomon Washington Gladden
Edward Everett Hale
Samuel Dexter Hastings
Nathaniel Hewit

Emil Louis George Hohenthal
Mark Hopkins
Oliver Otis Howard
Heman Humphrey
Charles Jewett
Lewis Henry Keller
Edward Kent?
Nathan Whitman Littlefield
John Davis Long?
Catherine Gouger Waugh McCulloch
John Marsh
Increase Mather
Reuben Dimond Mussey?
Howard Hyde Russell
Charles Moore Sheldon
Cora Frances Stoddard
Moses Stuart

## DISCIPLES OF CHRIST

George Hartshorn Hodges
Carry Amelia Moore Nation
Frederick Dunglison Power
Emma Frances Sanford Shelton

Ida Belle Speakman Wise Smith
Oliver Wayne Stewart
Zarelda Gray Sanders Wallace

## DUTCH REFORMED

Edward William Bok
Theodore Frelinghuysen

Daniel Alfred Poling
Stephen Van Rensselear?

## EPISCOPAL

Selden Daskam Bacon
John Hartwell Cocke
George Fletcher Cotterill?
Andrew Hull Foote
Joseph Malins

Robert Latham Owen
Alonzo Potter
William Ross?
James Yeames

## JEWISH

Simon Bamberger

Mark Keller

## LUTHERAN

Edwin Courtland Dinwiddie
Isaac Kaufman Funk

Henrietta Skelton
Homer Tope

## METHODIST

Ernest Francis Acheson
Elizabeth Preston Anderson
William Hamilton Anderson

Mary Harris Armor?
Francis Asbury
George Washington Bain

Purley Albert Baker
Louis Albert Banks
Helen Morton Barker
Josephine Abiah Penfield Cushman Bateham
Joseph Flintoft Berry
James Black
Ella Alexander Boole
Jacob Smith Boreman
Arthur Hislop Briggs
William Gannaway Brownlow
James Cannon, Jr.
Thomas Rosabaum Carskadon
Eugene Wilder Chafin
Harry Malcolm Chalfant
Sarah Flournoy Moore Chapin
Ernest Hurst Cherrington
Julia Colman
Alfred Holt Colquitt
David Leigh Colvin
Mamie White Colvin
Wilbur Fisk Crafts
Josephus Daniels
Edith Smith Davis
Noah Davis
Anna Marden DeYo
Samuel Dickie
Daniel Dorchester
Horace Mellard Du Bose
Jervice Gaylord Evans
Edwin Othello Excell
Samuel Fallows
John Faville
Rebecca Latimer Felton
William Porter Frisbee Ferguson
Clinton Bowen Fisk
Wilbur Fisk
Joseph Wingate Folk
Judith Ellen Horton Foster
Charles Henry Fowler
Anna Adams Gordon (Congregational)
Henry Woodfin Grady
James Franklin Hanly?
Charles Martin Hay
Lucy Ware Webb Hayes
Sarepta M. Henry
Virgil Goodman Hinshaw (Quaker)
Jacob Hostetter Hoofstitler?
Alphonso Alva Hopkins?

Elijah Embree Hoss
Harold Everett Hughes
Matthew Simpson Hughes
Mary Hannah Hanchett Hunt?
Ferdinand Cowle Iglehart
Eliza Buckley Ingalls
Stella Blanchard Irvine
Charles Reading Jones?
Belle Kearney
David Campbell Kelley
Sabastian Spering Kresge
Alpha Jefferson Kynett
Adna Wright Leonard
Harriet Calista Clark McCabe
Robert McIntyre
Eugenia Florenci St. John Mann
Caroline Elizabeth Thomas Merrick
Frederick Merrick
Emily Clark Huntington Miller
Edward Jay Moore
Angelina French Thurston Kilgore Newman
Thomas Nicholson
Alfred Noon
Norman Austin Palmer
Robert Howard Patton
Charles Henry Payne
Charles Andrew Pollack
Hiram Price
Charles Hiram Randall
Seth Reed
John Russell
Charles Henry St. John
John Pierce St. John
Richard Hugh Scott
Anna Howard Shaw
Edward Seitz Shumaker
Addison Taylor Smith
Adie Allen Stevens
Katharine Adelia Lent Stevenson
Sarah Hackett Stevenson
Eliza Daniel Stewart
Gideon Tabor Stewart
George Rutledge Stuart
Silas Comfort Swallow
Edward Thompson Taylor
Eliza Jane Trimble Thompson
Ralph Seyour Thompson?
George Thornburgh

Allen Trimble
Culla Johnson Vayhinger
Aaron Sherman Watkins
Wayne Cullen Williams
Jennie Fowler Willing

Alonzo Edes Wilson
Clarence True Wilson
Luther Barton Wilson
Annie Turner Wittenmyer

## NONDENOMINATIONAL PROTESTANTS AND INDEPENDENT EVANGELISTS

Caroline Brown Buell (Congregational)
Helen Louise Bullock
Arthur Capper (Quaker)
Charles Force Deems (Methodist)
Ninian Edwards
Frances Dana Barker Gage (Universalist)
William Goodell
John Bartholomew Gough
Elizabeth Ward Greenwood
Samuel Porter Jones (Methodist)
Edward Norris Kirk
Jeremiah McAuley

Dwight Lyman Moody
George Washington Morrow
Francis Murphy
Joshua Cox Osgood
Samuel Freeman Pearson
Henry Augustus Reynolds
Louise S. Jones Rounds
Hannah Whitall Smith (Quaker)
William Ashley Sunday
Uriah Frantz Swengel
William Griffith Wilson (Congregational)
John Granville Woolley

## PRESBYTERIAN

Robert Baird
Albert Barnes
Lou Jenks Beauchamp
James Addams Beaver
Ada Matilda Cole Bittenbender
Henry William Blair
Marie Caroline Brehm
Martha McClellan Brown
William Jennings Bryan
David James Burrell
Samuel Fenton Cary
John Chambers
Howard Crosby
Theodore Ledyard Cuyler
Herman Preston Faris
Robert Brodnax Glenn
Helen Mar Jackson Gougar
Felix Grundy
Mary Garrett Hay
William Eugene Johnson
Ira Landrith

John Brown Lennon
Joseph Henry Lumpkin?
Francis Scott McBride
Donald Campbell MacCleod
Lewis Duncan Mason?
Duncan Chambers Milner
Robert Valentine Muir?
Matthew Newkirk
Eliphalet Nott
Bertha Rachel Palmer
Willard Parker?
Gifford Pinchot
Nathaniel Scudder Prime
Tapping Reeve
Benjamin Rush
Charles Scanlon
Charles Stelzle
Reuben Hyde Walworth
John Collins Warren?
Charles Seymour Whitman

QUAKER

Susan Brownell Anthony
Hannah Johnston Bailey
Francis Julia Allis Barnes
Anthony Benezet
Amelia Jenks Bloomer
Elizabeth Leslie Rous Comstock

Lucretia Coffin Mott
Valentine Mott?
Samuel Edgar Nicholson
Timothy Nicholson
Joseph Parrish
Amanda Way

ROMAN CATHOLIC

James Mathew Cleary
John Francis Cunneen
Alexander Patrick Doyle
John Ireland
Leslie Enraught Keeley

Raymond Gerald McCarthy
Theobald Mathew
Peter Joseph O'Callaghan
John Lawrence Sullivan

SALVATION ARMY

Evangeline Cory Booth

SEVENTH DAY ADVENTIST

John Harvey Kellogg

SPIRITUALIST

Ella Wheeler Wilcox

SWEDENBORGIAN

Timothy Shay Arthur

UNITARIAN-UNIVERSALIST

William Henry Burleigh
William Ellery Channing
Jasper L. Douthit
William Thomas Haines
Frances Ellen Watkins Harper

Mary Ashton Livermore
Alonzo Ames Miner
Henrietta Greer Moore
John Pierpont

UNITED BRETHREN

George Martin Mathews

Henry Adams Thompson

# Index

Note: The location of main entries in the dictionary is indicated in the index by italic page numbers.

## About the Author

MARK EDWARD LENDER is Director of Grants, Kean College of New Jersey, and Visiting Professor at the Rutgers University Center of Alcohol Studies. He is the author of many articles and reviews and co-author of *A Respectable Army: The Military Origins of America, 1763-1783, Citizen-Soldier: The Revolutionary War Journal of Joseph Bloomfield*, and *Drinking in America: A History*. He is also the editor of *New Jersey History*.